Pancreatitis

Pancreatitis
Medical and surgical management

EDITED BY

David B. Adams
Medical University of South Carolina, US

Peter B. Cotton
Medical University of South Carolina, Charleston, South Carolina, US

Nicholas J. Zyromski
Indiana University School of Medicine, US

John Windsor
The University of Auckland, NZ

WILEY Blackwell

Contents

List of contributors

Ulrich Adam
Department of Surgery
Vivantes Hospital Humboldt, Berlin, Germany

Kiran Altaf
NIHR Liverpool Pancreas Biomedical Research Unit
Institute of Translational Medicine
Royal Liverpool University Hospital, Liverpool, UK
Institute of Translational Medicine
University of Liverpool, Liverpool, UK

Dana K. Andersen
Division of Digestive Diseases and Nutrition
National Institute of Diabetes and Digestive and Kidney
Diseases
National Institutes of Health, Bethesda, MD, USA

Minoti V. Apte
Pancreatic Research Group, South Western Sydney Clinical
School, Faculty of Medicine
University of New South Wales, Sydney, NSW, Australia
Ingham Institute for Applied Medical Research
Liverpool Hospital, Liverpool, NSW, Australia

Appakalai N. Balamurugan
Clinical Islet Cell Laboratory
Cardiovascular Innovation Institute
Department of Surgery, University of Louisville
Louisville, KY, USA
Islet Transplantation Program
University of Louisville, Louisville, KY, USA

Chad G. Ball
Departments of Surgery and Oncology
Foothills Medical Centre and the University of Calgary
Calgary, AB, Canada

Peter A. Banks
Department of Medicine, Harvard Medical School
Boston MA, USA
Center for Pancreatic Disease, Brigham and Women's Hospital
Boston, MA, USA

Greg Beilman
Department of Surgery & Medicine, University of Minnesota
Minneapolis, MN, USA

Melena D. Bellin
Schulze Diabetes Institute
University of Minnesota, Minneapolis, MN, USA

Marc G.H. Besselink
Department of Surgery, Academic Medical Center, Amsterdam
the Netherlands

Deepak Bhasin
Department of Gastroenterology
PGIMER, Chandigarh, India

Thomas L. Bollen
Department of Radiology, St. Antonius Hospital, Nieuwegein
the Netherlands

Philippus C. Bornman
Department of Surgery
University of Cape Town, Cape Town, South Africa
Groote Schuur Hospital, Cape Town, South Africa

Stefan A.W. Bouwense
Department of Surgery, Radboudumc, Nijmegen
the Netherlands

Alexsander K. Bressan
Department of Surgery
Foothills Medical Centre and the University of Calgary
Calgary, AB, Canada

Suresh T. Chari
Division of Gastroenterology and Hepatology
Mayo Clinic College of Medicine, Rochester, MN, USA

Gregory A. Coté
Division of Gastroenterology, Hepatology, and Nutrition
Department of Medicine
Medical University of South Carolina, Charleston, SC, USA

Kristopher P. Croome
Division of Transplant Surgery
Mayo Clinic Florida, Jacksonville, FL, USA

Ferenc Czeyda-Pommersheim
Department of Medical Imaging
University of Arizona, College of Medicine, Tucson, AZ, USA

Ashley Dennison
Department of Hepato-Pancreato-Biliary Surgery
Leicester General Hospital
University Hospitals of Leicester NHS Trust, Leicester, UK

Dana A. Dominguez
Department of Surgery
University of California, San Francisco, San Francisco, CA, USA

Alistair B.J. Escott
Department of Surgery
University of Auckland, Auckland, New Zealand

Michael B. Farnell
Department of Surgery
Mayo Clinic Rochester, Rochester, MN, USA

Paul Fockens
Department of Gastroenterology and Hepatology
Academic Medical Center, Amsterdam, the Netherlands

Chris E. Forsmark
Division of Gastroenterology, Hepatology, and Nutrition
University of Florida, Gainesville, FL, USA

Martin Freeman
Department of Surgery & Medicine
University of Minnesota, Minneapolis, MN, USA

Charles F. Frey
Department of General Surgery
University of California Sacramento, Sacramento, CA, USA

Giuseppe Garcea
Department of Hepato-Pancreato-Biliary Surgery
Leicester General Hospital
University Hospitals of Leicester NHS Trust, Leicester, UK

Timothy B. Gardner
Department of Medicine
Geisel School of Medicine at Dartmouth, Hanover, NH, USA

Pramod Kumar Garg
Department of Gastroenterology
All India Institute of Medical Sciences, New Delhi, India

Dirk J. Gouma
Academic Medical Center, Amsterdam, the Netherlands

Julia Greer
Division of Gastroenterology & Hepatology
Department of Medicine
University of Pittsburgh Medical Center, Pittsburgh, PA, USA

Rajesh Gupta
Division of Surgical Gastroenterology
Department of General Surgery, PGIMER, Chandigarh, India

Brenda Hoffman
Division of Hepatology and Gastroenterology
Medical University of South Carolina, Charleston, SC, USA

Muhammad A. Javed
NIHR Liverpool Pancreas Biomedical Research Unit
Institute of Translational Medicine
Royal Liverpool University Hospital, Liverpool, UK
Institute of Translational Medicine
University of Liverpool, Liverpool, UK

Bobby Kalb
Department of Medical Imaging
University of Arizona, College of Medicine, Tucson, AZ, USA

Matthew Kappus
Division of Gastroenterology
Department of Medicine, Duke University, Durham, NC, USA

Tobias Keck
Department of Surgery
University Medical Center Schleswig Holstein, Lübeck, Germany

Kimberly S. Kirkwood
Department of Surgery
University of California, San Francisco, San Francisco, CA, USA

Andree H. Koop
Department of Medicine
Geisel School of Medicine at Dartmouth, Hanover, NH, USA

Efstratios Koutroumpakis
Division of Gastroenterology, Hepatology and Nutrition
University of Pittsburgh Medical Center, Pittsburgh, PA, USA

Jake E. J. Krige
Department of Surgery
University of Cape Town, Cape Town, South Africa
Groote Schuur Hospital, Cape Town, South Africa

William Lancaster
Department of Surgery
Medical University of South Carolina, Charleston, SC, USA

Diego Martin
Department of Medical Imaging
University of Arizona, College of Medicine, Tucson, AZ, USA

Robert Martindale
Department of Surgery
Oregon Health and Sciences University, Portland, OR, USA

Lucas McDuffie
Department of Surgery
Indiana University School of Medicine, Indianapolis, IN, USA

Thiruvengadam Muniraj
Section of Digestive Diseases
Yale University School of Medicine, New Haven, CT, USA

Sydne Muratore
Department of Surgery & Medicine
University of Minnesota, Minneapolis, MN, USA

Ritambhra Nada
Department of Histopathology, PGIMER, Chandigarh, India

Duvvur Nageshwar Reddy
Department of Gastroenterology
Asian Institute of Gastroenterology, Hyderabad, India

Stephen J. Pandol
Basic and Translational Pancreas Research Program
Cedars-Sinai Medical Center, Los Angeles, CA, USA

Georgios I. Papachristou
Division of Gastroenterology, Hepatology and Nutrition
University of Pittsburgh Medical Center, Pittsburgh, PA, USA

Maxim S. Petrov
Department of Surgery
University of Auckland, Auckland, New Zealand

Anthony J. Phillips
Applied Surgery and Metabolism Laboratory
School of Biological Sciences and Department of Surgery
University of Auckland, Auckland, New Zealand

Ron C. Pirola
Pancreatic Research Group
South Western Sydney Clinical School, Faculty of Medicine
University of New South Wales, Sydney, NSW, Australia
Ingham Institute for Applied Medical Research
Liverpool Hospital, Liverpool, NSW, Australia

Ravi K. Prakash
Division of Gastroenterology, Hepatology, and Nutrition
University of Florida, Gainesville, FL, USA

Surinder S. Rana
Department of Gastroenterology, PGIMER, Chandigarh, India

Nathaniel Ranney
Division of Hepatology and Gastroenterology
Medical University of South Carolina, Charleston, SC, USA

Wiriyaporn Ridtitid
Division of Gastroenterology and Hepatology, Indiana
University School of Medicine, Indianapolis, IN, USA

Raghuwansh P. Sah
Division of Gastroenterology and Hepatology
Mayo Clinic College of Medicine, Rochester, MN, USA

Michael G. Sarr
Department of Surgery, Mayo Clinic, Rochester, MN, USA

Alexander Schlachterman
Division of Gastroenterology, Hepatology, and Nutrition
University of Florida, Gainesville, FL, USA

Thomas Schnelldorfer
Department of Surgery
Lahey Clinic, Burlington, MA, USA

Sunil D. Shenvi
Department of Surgery
Division of Transplant Surgery, MUSC, Charleston, SC, USA

Stuart Sherman
Division of Gastroenterology and Hepatology, Chulalongkorn
University
King Chulalongkorn Memorial Hospital, Thai Red Cross
Society, Bangkok, Thailand

Marsela Sina
University Clinic of Gastrohepatology
University Hospital Center Mother Theresa, Tirana, Albania

Vikesh K. Singh
Division of Gastroenterology
Johns Hopkins University School of Medicine, Baltimore, MD
USA

Ajith K. Siriwardena
Department of Hepatobiliary Surgery
University of Manchester, Manchester, UK
Regional Hepato-Pancreato-Biliary Surgery Unit
Manchester Royal Infirmary, Manchester, UK

Robert Sutton
NIHR Liverpool Pancreas Biomedical Research Unit
Institute of Translational Medicine
Royal Liverpool University Hospital, Liverpool, UK
Institute of Translational Medicine
University of Liverpool, Liverpool, UK

Peter Szatmary
NIHR Liverpool Pancreas Biomedical Research Unit
Institute of Translational Medicine
Royal Liverpool University Hospital, Liverpool, UK
Institute of Translational Medicine
University of Liverpool, Liverpool, UK

Rupjyoti Talukdar
Department of Gastroenterology
Asian Institute of Gastroenterology, Hyderabad, India
Wellcome DBT India Alliance Laboratory
Asian Healthcare Foundation, Hyderabad, India

Sandie R. Thomson
Groote Schuur Hospital, Cape Town, South Africa
Division of Gastroenterology
Department of Medicine, University of Cape Town, Cape
Town, South Africa

Ulrich Wellner
Department of Surgery
University Medical Center Schleswig Holstein, Lübeck,
Germany

Li Wen
NIHR Liverpool Pancreas Biomedical Research Unit
Institute of Translational Medicine
Royal Liverpool University Hospital, Liverpool, UK
Institute of Translational Medicine
University of Liverpool, Liverpool, UK

David C. Whitcomb
Division of Gastroenterology, Hepatology and Nutrition
Departments of Medicine, Cell Biology & Physiology, and
Human Genetics
University of Pittsburgh/UPMC, Pittsburgh, PA, USA

Jeremy S. Wilson
Pancreatic Research Group
South Western Sydney Clinical School
Faculty of Medicine
University of New South Wales, Sydney, NSW, Australia
Ingham Institute for Applied Medical Research
Liverpool Hospital, Liverpool, NSW, Australia

John A. Windsor
Department of Surgery
University of Auckland, Auckland, New Zealand
Applied Surgery and Metabolism Laboratory
School of Biological Sciences and Department of Surgery
University of Auckland, Auckland, New Zealand

Zhihong Xu
Pancreatic Research Group
South Western Sydney Clinical School
Faculty of Medicine
University of New South Wales, Sydney, NSW, Australia
Ingham Institute for Applied Medical Research
Liverpool Hospital, Liverpool, NSW, Australia

Dhiraj Yadav
Division of Gastroenterology & Hepatology
Department of Medicine
University of Pittsburgh Medical Center, Pittsburgh, PA, USA

Nicholas J. Zyromski
Department of Surgery
Indiana University School of Medicine, Indianapolis, IN, USA

CHAPTER 1

Epidemiology and genetics of pancreatitis

David C. Whitcomb

Division of Gastroenterology, Hepatology and Nutrition, Departments of Medicine, Cell Biology & Physiology, and Human Genetics, University of Pittsburgh/UPMC, Pittsburgh, PA, USA

Definition

Chronic pancreatitis (CP) can be defined as "a continuing inflammatory disease of the pancreas, characterized by irreversible morphological change, and typically causing pain and/or permanent loss of function" [1]. This definition is intentionally pragmatic, as developed by the members of the Pancreatic Society of Great Britain and Ireland in March 1983 in Cambridge, England as a pretext to the morphology-based Cambridge classification of CP severity [1]. The definition is vague but has stood the test of time and has been followed in consensus statements by nearly all societies and expert groups for the subsequent two decades.

The pragmatic nature of the Cambridge definition speaks to the challenges in defining a syndrome with multiple etiologies, variable features, unpredictable clinical course, and inadequate treatment [2]. As a morphology-based definition, it also ignores key histologic, clinical, and functional features that dominate the definitions from the Marseilles meetings [3, 4] and ignores the possibility of "minimal change" CP [5a], functional changes such as pancreatitis-associated chronic pain syndrome and/or pancreatic insufficiency, or autoimmune pancreatitis. Furthermore, the definition is independent of etiology, it cannot differentiate progressive disease from old scars from a bout of acute pancreatitis (AP), and it has little prognostic value. A new, two-part mechanistic definition of CP has been proposed that focuses on disruption of the normal injury → inflammation → resolution → regeneration sequence. The definition includes the *essence* of CP,

"Chronic pancreatitis is a pathologic fibro-inflammatory syndrome of the pancreas in individuals with genetic, environmental and/or other risk factors who develop persistent pathologic responses to parenchymal injury or stress," and the characteristics of CP, "Common features of established and advanced CP include pancreatic atrophy, fibrosis, pain syndromes, duct distortion and strictures, calcifications, pancreatic exocrine dysfunction, pancreatic endocrine dysfunction, and dysplasia." This new definition opens the door to new diagnostic criteria that distinguishes CP from other disorders with CP-like features, provides a method for diagnosing "early CP," and may improve methods of mechanism-based therapies – which is the goal of personalized medicine [5b].

Burden of disease

Epidemiologists struggle to determine the incidence and prevalence of CP – in part because of the vague definitions and different detection approaches [6, 7]. Administrative data, such as ICD-9 codes used in the United States, have limited value because the same code, 577.1, is used for recurrent acute pancreatitis (RAP) as well as CP. Indeed, authoritative studies of the burden of digestive diseases in the United States found it impossible to distinguish AP from CP using public records and grouped the two entities into one big problem [8].

Autopsy studies using histologic criteria such as duct ectasia, periductal fibrosis, ductular proliferation, acinar ductular metaplasia, and interstitial inflammation or fibrosis suggest that the incidence of CP is as high as 12–14% [9, 10], with abnormal fibrosis in up to 39% [10]. Histologic changes suggestive of CP are even more prevalent in patients with very common chronic disorders such as renal disease (up to 56%) [9] and diabetes mellitus (DM) (~7% by clinical evaluation but much higher in diabetes autopsy databases such as nPOD [11] – noting the problem of reverse causality [12]). However, it is well recognized that interstitial inflammation and fibrosis alone are not sufficient to make a diagnosis of CP [13].

The emergence and widespread use of sensitive abdominal imaging techniques has helped standardize epidemiological approaches when morphologic criteria are used. While morphology is not the only criteria used in epidemiology studies, it does serve as an equalizing factor. Thus, the burden of CP in terms of disease prevalence from more recent surveys is more useful.

In the United States the best estimate comes from Minnesota, where the age-adjusted prevalence of CP was estimated at 41.8 cases per 100,000 population [7]. In contrast to earlier studies, the prevalence between males and females was similar, as reported in the North American Pancreatitis Study 2 (NAPS2) reports [14, 15]. In Japan the prevalence of CP was similar to the United States, with 36.9 cases per 100,000 population [16]. In France the prevalence of CP was 26.4 cases per 100,000 population [17], with a strong male predominance. The lowest prevalence was in China, which was only 3 cases of CP per 100,000 population in 1996 but had risen rapidly to 13.5 per 100,000 population by 2003 [18]. The highest rates were in Southern India, where the prevalence of CP is 114–200 per 100,000 population [19]. In addition to difference in prevalence, there are marked differences in rates of the etiologic diagnoses, with alcoholic and idiopathic being the most common causes in all studies. Alcohol etiology is consistently more common in men than in women.

Clinical features

The clinical features of CP include recurrent and chronic inflammation, fibrosis, duct distortion, pseudocysts, atrophy, pancreatic exocrine insufficiency, DM, multiple pain patterns, stones, and risk of pancreatic cancer. These features vary with etiology and environmental factors, and none of them are present in all

patients – except for when duct distortion is used as the diagnostic criteria as in the Cambridge definition [1].

Diagnosis

Using the Cambridge definition of CP, a "clinical" diagnosis of CP can usually be made without ambiguity when significant morphologic features are documented. The problem with the Cambridge definition is the requirement of "irreversible morphological change" in the pancreas, how it is defined, and when it occurs. Indeed, patients may have symptoms of CP for 5–10 years before irreversible morphologic changes are documented, resulting in presumably unnecessary pain, anxiety, uncertainty, suffering, and numerous diagnostic tests. The result of the process is a "diagnosis," with continued symptomatic treatment. Furthermore, the consequence of classifying CP based on morphologic criteria is that, while all investigators and clinicians agree on what end-stage CP looks like, they continue to sharply disagree on the border between "normal" and "abnormal" and on the minimal required features.

Many experts also deviate from the Cambridge definition, recognizing the limitations of morphology alone and the possibility of minimal change CP with prominent functional features such as pancreatic juice with low bicarbonate concentrations or pancreatitis-like pain syndromes. This view is supported by the clinical improvement in some patients diagnosed with minimal change pancreatitis and pain who find relief with total pancreatectomy and islet autotransplantation (TPIAT) [20–23]. These differences in perspectives on traditional views of CP make a consensus definition of early CP nearly impossible, with a ripple effect of making the criteria for early diagnosis somewhat arbitrary.

Animal models of early CP

The use of model organisms to understand human diseases remains a critical component of biomedical research. A good model should be a simplified version of something that reflects its primary components and is useful to study its characteristics under a variety of conditions. In the case of CP, animal models demonstrated that multiple injuries and inflammation resulted in parenchymal pathology, including scaring, but did not provide insight into human disease, which appeared stochastic in onset and highly variable in progression, clinical features, and outcomes. Thus, animal models provided insight into downstream pathology but failed to provide insight into etiologies, susceptibility, and variable progression.

Genetic risk factors for CP

In 1996 we discovered that hereditary pancreatitis (HP), a rare, autosomal dominant, highly penetrant, and early-onset syndrome of RAP and CP, was caused by a *gain-of-function* mutation in the cationic trypsinogen gene (*PRSS1*) [24–26]. The discovery immediately implicated prematurely activated trypsin as a key factor in the pathogenesis of AP and CP in humans, indicated that RAP can lead to typical CP, and introduced the possibility that other genetic factors associated with trypsin regulation may increase the risk of RAP and/or CP. Further, study of HP families indicated that even with inheritance of the most virulent of pathogenic variants, the age of onset, the progression to CP, DM, pain syndromes, and PDAC were highly variable – even among identical twins [27]. Finally, the high sensitivity of HP patients to alcohol and the strong effect of smoking on the risk of PDAC provided new insights into the role of environmental modifying factors [28].

Since 1996, many additional genetic factors linked to trypsin regulation proved to be strongly associated with susceptibility to and severity of RAP and CP. These include *SPINK1* [29, 30], cystic fibrosis transmembrane conductance regulator (*CFTR*) [31, 32], and *CTRC* [33–36]. In our US population pathogenic mutations in these four genes are found in 26% of RAP patients and 21% of CP patients [37], not counting the common *CTRC* G60G risk allele, which is in another 18% of CP patients [36]. Other CP risk genes were also discovered using other candidate gene approaches, including *CPA1* [38], and linkage studies including *CEL* [39] or other approaches such as *GGT1* [40].

In 2012 we published the first pancreatitis genome-wide association study (GWAS) [41]. This study identified two major loci, a common *PRSS1–PRSS2* haplotype with reduced PRSS1 expression that is *protective* for multiple etiologies and a common *CLDN2* haplotype on the X chromosome, associated with risk of CP, especially in alcoholics. These findings have recently

been replicated in a European cohort [42]. These data suggest multiple etiologies and susceptibility factors, with several strong modifying factors that determine the risk of progression and other clinical features of CP. This concept is extended with a recent paper demonstrating that the risk of the common *CTRC* G60G haplotype is for CP, but not RAP, and is strongly associated with *smoking* [36].

Mendelian genetic syndromes

An understanding of genetic should begin with simple Mendelian disorders. These disorders are caused by strong pathogenic variants in a single gene that cause well-defined syndromes. In the case of CP, the two most important Mendelian disorders are HP and cystic fibrosis (CF).

Hereditary pancreatitis

HP is defined either by two or more individuals with pancreatitis in two or more generations of the family (i.e., an autosomal dominant pattern of inheritance) or pancreatitis associated with a known disease-causing germ line mutation in the cationic trypsinogen gene *PRSS1*. The term *familial pancreatitis* is used when more than one person in the family has RAP or CP – regardless of etiology – since the incidence is above the expected rate in the population by chance alone.

HP has been conclusively linked with gain-of-function mutations in *PRSS1* [43–46]. Gain-of-function mutations increase autocatalytic conversion of trypsinogen to active trypsin causing premature, intrapancreatic trypsinogen activation. Trypsin, as the master enzyme regulating activation of the other pancreatic zymogens, is thought to cause widespread enzyme activation, autodigestion of the pancreatic parenchyma, and release of danger-associated molecular pattern (DAMP) molecules that activate the immune system causing AP. Trypsin, chymotrypsin, and other digestive enzymes may also cross-activate the immune system by activating the thrombin pathway or protease-activated receptors [47–51].

Many rare genetic variants in *PRSS1* have been reported (see www.pancreasgenetics.org), but the majorities of families either have the *PRSS1* N34S or R122H gain-of-function mutation or less commonly, copy number variants (CNV). The other variants may be loss-of-function variants that cause pancreatic stress and injury signaling through an unfolded protein response [52, 53].

The clinical features of HP have been defined in several large studies [54, 55]. In the European Registry of Hereditary Pancreatitis and Pancreatic Cancer [54], the cumulative risk at 50 years of age for patient with HP for exocrine failure was 37.2%, for endocrine failure 47.6%, and pancreatic resection for pain 17.5%. The cumulative risk of pancreatic cancer was 44.0% at 70 years. In a French study patients with HP reported pancreatic pain (83%), AP (69%), pseudo-cysts (23%), cholestasis (3%), pancreatic calcifications (61%), exocrine pancreatic insufficiency (34%), DM (26%), and pancreatic adenocarcinoma (5%). In both studies the median age of onset of symptoms was about age 10, with about half the patients developing CP by age 20 years, followed over the next 10 years by pancreatic exocrine insufficiency and DM in up to 40% of patients. The risk of cancer in the fifth to sixth decade of life replicated the studies by Lowenfels [28, 56]. Of note, the incidence of pancreatic cancer is cut in half and delayed by a decade in patients who do not smoke [56].

The diagnosis of HP is made on clinical grounds and genetic testing (see www.pancreas.org). Genetic testing is warranted when there is unexplained documented episode of AP in childhood; recurrent acute attacks of pancreatitis of unknown cause; CP of unknown cause, particularly with onset before age 25 years; and a family history of RAP, CP, or childhood pancreatitis of unknown cause in first-, second-, or third-degree relatives or relatives known to have a mutation in a gene associated with HP [46, 57, 58].

The utility of genetic testing is in making an early diagnosis of a high-risk condition that may explain early functional symptoms and signal the likelihood that the person may develop some or all of the complications of CP. A positive result, in the context of pancreatitis-like symptoms, has a very high likelihood of the symptoms coming from the pancreas. No further diagnostic testing for the etiology of CP-like symptoms is needed. A negative genetic testing result for HP suggests that the etiology is not pathogenic *PRSS1* variants, although many other pathogenic genetic variants in other loci are also possible (see Chapter 12). Genetic testing, in the future, may also provide guidance on likelihood of specific syndromes, such as constant pain or diabetes,

although these ideas currently remain at a research stage.

Cystic fibrosis

CF refers to an autosomal recessive disorder affecting secretory epithelial cells of glands, respiratory mucosa, and the digestive system. The term "cystic fibrosis" refers to the CP (with pseudocysts and fibrosis) that occurs in all affected individuals, beginning *in utero*.

The disease is caused by mutations in the *CFTR* gene [59–61]. The CFTR protein forms a regulated anion channel that facilitates transport of chloride and bicarbonate across the apical membrane of epithelial cells during active secretion and/or absorption. CFTR is the most important molecule for the function of the pancreatic duct cell – there are no significant alternate molecules for physiologic anion secretion. Loss of CFTR results in failed flushing of digestive zymogens out of the pancreas and into the intestine. Thus, dysfunction of CFTR results in retention of zymogens in the duct where they can become active and begin digesting the surrounding pancreas, leading to AP. Since the pancreas is so strongly dependent on CFTR function, the severity of pathogenic *CFTR* variants can be estimated from the effects on the pancreas. Furthermore, pancreatic injury can typically be detected at birth, justifying CF screening using serum trypsinogen measurements, and end-stage CP with pancreatic exocrine insufficiency often occurs during the first year of life. Thus, the disease was characterized by failure to thrive and salty sweat with death in infancy until pancreatic enzyme replacement therapy was developed. Only after surviving pancreatic exocrine insufficiency will a child begin developing respiratory failure.

The organs that are most strongly affected by *CFTR* mutations include the pancreas, sweat glands, sinuses, respiratory system, gastrointestinal track, male reproductive system, and liver. The features of *CFTR*-associated diseases depend on the functional consequences of specific mutations on the two *CFTR* alleles [62, 63], as well as mutations in modifier genes and effects of environmental factors. CF is caused by two severe mutations ($CFTR^{sev}/CFTR^{sev}$). Residual CFTR function can occur with some milder mutations, and the severity of CF is linked to the *least* severe mutation. The milder forms of CF can be referred to as atypical CF (aCF) and are caused by mild-variable mutations with two possible genotypes: ($CFTR^{m-v}/CFTR^{sev}$) or

($CFTR^{m-v}/CFTR^{m-v}$). In these cases there is residual function of the various organs that use CFTR for fluid secretion, and disease occurs later in life, with organ specificity determined by modifying genetic and environmental factors [61, 64].

In 1989 two groups reported that patients with idiopathic CP had a greater-than-expected prevalence of pathogenic *CFTR* variants [31, 32]. In many CP cases it appeared that heterozygous pathogenic *CFTR* variants were found in individuals who also harbored *SPINK1* variants as ($CFTR^{sev}/CFTR^{wt}$; $SPINK1^{N34S}/SPINK1^{wt}$) genotypes [65–67], a phenomenon called epistasis. Thus, these cases of idiopathic CP were clearly examples of complex trait genetics.

In 2011 we reported that a common *CFTR* variant, R75Q, affected bicarbonate conductance while maintaining chloride conductance and had major effects on the pancreas but minimal effects on the lungs, presumably because the pancreas uses CFTR as a bicarbonate channel [67]. Since the functional effect of *CFTR* genotypes is determined by the least severe mutation, either two bicarbonate defective (BD) variants ($CFTR^{BD}/CFTR^{BD}$) or one BD and one severe variant ($CFTR^{BD}/CFTR^{sev}$) can result in a monogenic pancreatitis-predominant disorder. We then made a screening panel of 81 previously reported CFTR single-nucleotide polymorphisms (SNPs) and screened nearly a thousand patients with pancreatitis from the North American Pancreatitis Study 2 (NAPS2) cohort [68]. We identified nine *CFTR* SNPs that were classified as benign by pulmonologists but were associated with pancreatitis: R74Q, R75Q, R117H, R170H, L967S, L997F, D1152H, S1235R, and D1270N. When these variants were cloned into wild-type CFTR genes and expressed in experimental cells, they had normal chloride conductance but failed to transform into bicarbonate-conducting channels when CFTR was activated with WNK1/SPAK [68]. Molecular modeling demonstrated that four different mechanisms were involved in this transformation and/or regulation of bicarbonate conductance.

The pancreas is susceptible to variants that impair CFTR-mediated bicarbonate conductance because of the way it makes bicarbonate-rich pancreatic juice [68, 69]. Since other organs also use CFTR to secrete bicarbonate, we evaluated the risk of rhinosinusitis and male infertility in patients with CP, with or without the $CFTR^{BD}/CFTR^{other}$ genotypes. We found that $CFTR^{BD}$

significantly increased the risk of rhinosinusitis (OR 2.3, $P < 0.005$) and male infertility (OR 395, $P \ll 0.0001$). Thus, a variant subtype of CF has been defined that is characterized by CP and dysfunction of other organs that utilize CFTR for bicarbonate secretion, but without lung disease.

A new paradigm of personalized medicine

To advance our understanding of CP, we require a paradigm shift. It is recognized that CP is a *complex disorder*. It is useful to understand a complex disorder in contrast to a simple disorder [70]. A simple disorder is when a specific microorganism invades a host and causes a specific clinical syndrome. Modern Western medicine has been built on the germ theory of disease, which organizes the study of simple disorders using Koch's postulates to test a defined hypothesis. In simple diseases the pathologic agent is sufficient to cause the disease syndrome. In contrast, complex disorders typically include acquired conditions caused by complex gene–environment, gene–gene, or multiple gene–environmental interactions where the pathologic agents are neither necessary nor sufficient to cause the disorder. Further complexity occurs if a sequence of pathologic events is needed before enough qualifying features of the syndrome emerge to meet diagnostic criteria. In complex disorders the "scientific method" used in medical research to identify the etiology of disease by applying Koch's postulates fail, since none of the hypothesized pathogenic agents will meet the four criteria. The challenges of evaluating and managing a complex disorder include developing a new way of thinking about the diagnosis and management of these disorders, integration of complex genetic risk into the paradigm, and developing new tools to assist the practitioner. Specifically, personalized medicine demands going beyond a simple Boolean operator of the germ theory (is a pathologic agent present, yes or no?) to more sophisticated disease modeling and outcome simulation where the influence of multiple variables of different effects can be assessed under different conditions.

The terms personalized medicine and precision medicine are used interchangeably. We will use the term *personalized medicine* as a medical model that utilizes genetic information and biomarkers of disease activity to define the specific mechanism of disease within a subject from among multiple possibilities and target disease management at the specific mechanism. In contrast, we use the term *precision medicine* to define a medical model that optimizes the treatment of the patient within a disease mechanism. Thus, in our view, personalized medicine defines the underlying problem, whereas precision medicine defines the optimal treatment for the problem.

Driven by multiple genetic discoveries and environmental risk assessments on the one hand and a failure to effectively define and treat pancreatic diseases on the other, the CP disease model shifted from "germ theory" (a single agent causing a stereotypic disorder) to a "complex genetic disorder" with individual patients harboring different combinations of pathogenic factors that alone are neither necessary nor sufficient to cause pancreatic disease [70]. This approach may have profound implications for both early detection and disease management. The new and exciting opportunity is to define the *specific risk complex* in individual patients, to monitor disease activity and to target pathogenic pathways so that the pathologic endpoints are never reached (see Chapter 12b). This is personalized medicine [70, 71], and this must be the future direction for the pancreatic diseases management since the end stages are irreversible.

References

1 Sarner M, Cotton PB. Classification of pancreatitis. Gut. 1984;25(7):756–759. PMID: 6735257

2 Steer ML, Waxman I, Freedman S. Chronic pancreatitis. New England Journal of Medicine. 1995;332(22):1482–1490. PMID: 7739686

3 Sarles H. Proposal adopted unanimously by the participants of the Symposium, Marseilles 1963. Bibliotheca Gastroenterologica. 1965;7:7–8

4 Sarles H, Adler G, Dani R, Frey C, Gullo L, Harada H, et al. The pancreatitis classification of Marseilles, Rome 1988. Scandinavian Journal of Gastroenterology. 1989;24:641-642.

5 (a) Walsh TN, Rode J, Theis BA, Russell RCG. Minimal change chronic pancreatitis. Gut 1992;33:1566–1571; (b) Whitcomb DC, Frulloni L, Garg P, Greer JB, Schneider A, Yadav D, et al. Chronic pancreatitis: an international draft consensus proposal for a new mechanistic definition. Pancreatology. 2016;16:218–224. PMID: 26924663

6 Levy P, Dominguez-Munoz E, Imrie C, Lohr M, Maisonneuve P. Epidemiology of chronic pancreatitis: burden of the disease and consequences. United European gastroenterology journal. 2014;2(5):345–354. PMID: 25360312

7 Yadav D, Timmons L, Benson JT, Dierkhising RA, Chari ST. Incidence, prevalence, and survival of chronic pancreatitis: a population-based study. The American Journal of Gastroenterology. 2011;106(12):2192–2199. PMID: 21946280

8 Peery AF, Dellon ES, Lund J, Crockett SD, McGowan CE, Bulsiewicz WJ, et al. Burden of gastrointestinal disease in the United States: 2012 update. Gastroenterology. 2012;143(5):1179–1187 e1–3. PMID: 22885331

9 Avram MM. High prevalence of pancreatic disease in chronic renal failure. Nephron. 1977;18(1):68–71.

10 Pace A, de Weerth A, Berna M, Hillbricht K, Tsokos M, Blaker M, et al. Pancreas and liver injury are associated in individuals with increased alcohol consumption. Clinical Gastroenterology and Hepatology. 2009;7(11):1241–1246. PMID: 19560556

11 Butler AE, Campbell-Thompson M, Gurlo T, Dawson DW, Atkinson M, Butler PC. Marked expansion of exocrine and endocrine pancreas with incretin therapy in humans with increased exocrine pancreas dysplasia and the potential for glucagon-producing neuroendocrine tumors. Diabetes. 2013;62(7):2595–2604. PMID: 23524641

12 Andersen DK, Andren-Sandberg A, Duell EJ, Goggins M, Korc M, Petersen GM, et al. Pancreatitis-diabetes-pancreatic cancer: summary of an NIDDK-NCI workshop. Pancreas. 2013;42(8):1227–1237. PMID: 24152948

13 Homma T, Harada H, Koizumi M. Diagnostic criteria for chronic pancreatitis by the Japan Pancreas Society. Pancreas. 1997;15:14–15.

14 Whitcomb DC, Yadav D, Adam S, Hawes RH, Brand RE, Anderson MA, et al. Multicenter approach to recurrent acute and chronic pancreatitis in the United States: the North American Pancreatitis Study 2 (NAPS2). Pancreatology. 2008;8(4–5):520–531. PMID: 18765957

15 Yadav D, Hawes RH, Brand RE, Anderson MA, Money ME, Banks PA, et al. Alcohol consumption, cigarette smoking, and the risk of recurrent acute and chronic pancreatitis. Archives of Internal Medicine. 2009;169(11):1035–1045. PMID: 19506173

16 Hirota M, Shimosegawa T, Masamune A, Kikuta K, Kume K, Hamada S, et al. The sixth nationwide epidemiological survey of chronic pancreatitis in Japan. Pancreatology. 2012;12(2):79–84. PMID: 22487515

17 Levy P, Barthet M, Mollard BR, Amouretti M, Marion-Audibert AM, Dyard F. Estimation of the prevalence and incidence of chronic pancreatitis and its complications. Gastroentérologie Clinique et Biologique. 2006;30(6–7):838–844. PMID: 16885867

18 Wang LW, Li ZS, Li SD, Jin ZD, Zou DW, Chen F. Prevalence and clinical features of chronic pancreatitis in China: a retrospective multicenter analysis over 10 years. Pancreas. 2009;38(3):248–254. PMID: 19034057

19 Garg PK, Tandon RK. Survey on chronic pancreatitis in the Asia-Pacific region. Journal of Gastroenterology and Hepatology. 2004;19(9):998–1004. PMID: 15304116

20 Blondet JJ, Carlson AM, Kobayashi T, Jie T, Bellin M, Hering BJ, et al. The role of total pancreatectomy and islet autotransplantation for chronic pancreatitis. Surgical Clinics of North America. 2007;87(6):1477–1501. PMID: 18053843

21 Bellin MD, Freeman ML, Schwarzenberg SJ, Dunn TB, Beilman GJ, Vickers SM, et al. Quality of life improves for pediatric patients after total pancreatectomy and islet autotransplant for chronic pancreatitis. Clinical Gastroenterology and Hepatology: The Official Clinical Practice Journal of the American Gastroenterological Association. 2011;9(9):793–799. PMID: 21683160

22 Bellin MD, Freeman ML, Gelrud A, Slivka A, Clavel A, Humar A, et al. Total pancreatectomy and islet autotransplantation in chronic pancreatitis: Recommendations from PancreasFest. Pancreatology. 2014;14(1):27–35. PMID: 24555976

23 Chinnakotla S, Radosevich DM, Dunn TB, Bellin MD, Freeman ML, Schwarzenberg SJ, et al. Long-term outcomes of total pancreatectomy and islet auto transplantation for hereditary/genetic pancreatitis. Journal of the American College of Surgeons. 2014;218(4):530–543. PMID: 24655839

24 Whitcomb DC, Gorry MC, Preston RA, Furey W, Sossenheimer MJ, Ulrich CD, et al. Hereditary pancreatitis is caused by a mutation in the cationic trypsinogen gene. Nature Genetics. 1996;14(2):141–145. PMID: 8841182

25 Gorry MC, Gabbaizedeh D, Furey W, Gates LK, Jr., Preston RA, Aston CE, et al. Mutations in the cationic trypsinogen gene are associated with recurrent acute and chronic pancreatitis. Gastroenterology. 1997;113(4):1063–1068.

26 Sossenheimer MJ, Aston CE, Preston RA, Gates LK, Jr.,, Ulrich CD, Martin SP, et al. Clinical characteristics of hereditary pancreatitis in a large family, based on high-risk haplotype. The Midwest Multicenter Pancreatic Study Group (MMPSG). The American Journal of Gastroenterology. 1997;92(7):1113–1116. PMID: 9219780

27 Amann ST, Gates LK, Aston CE, Pandya A, Whitcomb DC. Expression and penetrance of the hereditary pancreatitis phenotype in monozygotic twins. Gut. 2001;48(4):542–547.

28 Lowenfels A, Maisonneuve P, DiMagno E, Elitsur Y, Gates L, Perrault J, et al. Hereditary pancreatitis and the risk of pancreatic cancer. Journal of the National Cancer Institute. 1997;89(6):442–446.

29 Witt H, Luck W, Hennies HC, Classen M, Kage A, Lass U, et al. Mutations in the gene encoding the serine protease inhibitor, Kazal type 1 are associated with chronic pancreatitis. Nature Genetics. 2000;25(2):213–216. PMID: 10835640

30 Pfutzer RH, Barmada MM, Brunskill AP, Finch R, Hart PS, Neoptolemos J, et al. SPINK1/PSTI polymorphisms act as disease modifiers in familial and idiopathic chronic pancreatitis. Gastroenterology. 2000;119(3):615–623. PMID: 10982753

31 Cohn JA, Friedman KJ, Noone PG, Knowles MR, Silverman LM, Jowell PS. Relation between mutations of the cystic fibrosis gene and idiopathic pancreatitis. The New England Journal of Medicine. 1998;339(10):653–658. PMID: 9725922

32 Sharer N, Schwarz M, Malone G, Howarth A, Painter J, Super M, et al. Mutations of the cystic fibrosis gene in patients with chronic pancreatitis. New England Journal of Medicine. 1998;339(10):645–652.

33 Rosendahl J, Witt H, Szmola R, Bhatia E, Ozsvari B, Landt O, et al. Chymotrypsin C (CTRC) variants that diminish activity or secretion are associated with chronic pancreatitis. Nature Genetics. 2008;40(1):78–82. PMID: 18059268

34 Masson E, Chen JM, Scotet V, Le Marechal C, Ferec C. Association of rare chymotrypsinogen C (CTRC) gene variations in patients with idiopathic chronic pancreatitis. Human Genetics. 2008;123(1):83–91. PMID: 18172691

35 Beer S, Zhou J, Szabo A, Keiles S, Chandak GR, Witt H, et al. Comprehensive functional analysis of chymotrypsin C (CTRC) variants reveals distinct loss-of-function mechanisms associated with pancreatitis risk. Gut. 2012;62(11):1616–1624. PMID: 22942235

36 LaRusch J, Lozano-Leon A, Stello K, Moore A, Muddana V, O'Connell M, et al. The common chymotrypsinogen C (CTRC) variant G60G (C.180T) increases risk of chronic pancreatitis but not recurrent acute pancreatitis in a North American population. Clinical and Translational Gastroenterology. 2015;6:e68. PMID: 25569187

37 LaRusch J, Stello K, Yadav D, Whitcomb DC. CFTR, PRSS1, SPINK1 and CTRC mutations in the final NAPS2 Cohort. Pancreatology. 2015;15(3):S79. EPC Abstract Book.

38 Witt H, Beer S, Rosendahl J, Chen JM, Chandak GR, Masamune A, et al. Variants in CPA1 are strongly associated with early onset chronic pancreatitis. Nature Genetics. 2013;45(10):1216–1220. PMID: 23955596

39 Fjeld K, Weiss FU, Lasher D, Rosendahl J, Chen JM, Johansson BB, et al. A recombined allele of the lipase gene CEL and its pseudogene CELP confers susceptibility to chronic pancreatitis. Nature Genetics. 2015;47:518–522. PMID: 25774637

40 Brand H, Diergaarde B, O'Connell MR, Whitcomb DC, Brand RE. Variation in the gamma-glutamyltransferase 1 gene and risk of chronic pancreatitis. Pancreas. 2013;42(5):836–840. PMID: 23462328

41 Whitcomb DC, LaRusch J, Krasinskas AM, Klei L, Smith JP, Brand RE, et al. Common genetic variants in the CLDN2 and PRSS1-PRSS2 loci alter risk for alcohol-related and sporadic pancreatitis. Nature genetics. 2012;44(12):1349–1354. PMID: 23143602

42 Derikx MH, Kovacs P, Scholz M, Masson E, Chen JM, Ruffert C, et al. Polymorphisms at PRSS1-PRSS2 and CLDN2-MORC4 loci associate with alcoholic and

non-alcoholic chronic pancreatitis in a European replication study. Gut. 2014; 64:1426–1433. PMID: 25253127

43 Teich N, Mossner J. Hereditary chronic pancreatitis. Best Practice & Research Clinical Gastroenterology. 2008;22(1):115–130. PMID: 18206817

44 Chen JM, Ferec C. Chronic pancreatitis: genetics and pathogenesis. Annual Review of Genomics and Human Genetics 2009;10:63–87. PMID: 19453252

45 LaRusch J, Whitcomb DC. Genetics of pancreatitis. Current Opinion in Gastroenterology. 2011;27(5):467–474. PMID: 21844754

46 Solomon S, Whitcomb DC, LaRusch J. PRSS1-related hereditary pancreatitis. In: Pagon RA, Bird TD, Dolan CR, Stephens K, editors. GeneReviews, University of Washington Seattle. Seattle, WA 2012.

47 Alvarez C, Regan JP, Merianos D, Bass BL. Protease-activated receptor-2 regulates bicarbonate secretion by pancreatic duct cells in vitro. Surgery. 2004;136(3):669–676. PMID: 15349117

48 Namkung W, Han W, Luo X, Muallem S, Cho KH, Kim KH, et al. Protease-activated receptor 2 exerts local protection and mediates some systemic complications in acute pancreatitis. Gastroenterology. 2004;126(7):1844–1859.

49 Masamune A, Kikuta K, Satoh M, Suzuki N, Shimosegawa T. Protease-activated receptor-2-mediated proliferation and collagen production of rat pancreatic stellate cells. Journal of Pharmacology and Experimental Therapeutics. 2005;312(2):651–658. PMID: 15367578

50 Sharma A, Tao X, Gopal A, Ligon B, Andrade-Gordon P, Steer ML, et al. Protection against acute pancreatitis by activation of protease-activated receptor-2. American Journal of Physiology: Gastrointestinal and Liver Physiology. 2005;288(2):G388-G395. PMID: 15458925

51 Pasricha PJ. Unraveling the mystery of pain in chronic pancreatitis. Nature Reviews Gastroenterology & Hepatology. 2012;9(3):140–151. PMID: 22269952

52 Nemeth BC, Sahin-Toth M. Human cationic trypsinogen (PRSS1) variants and chronic pancreatitis. American Journal of Physiology: Gastrointestinal and Liver Physiology. 2014;306(6):G466-G473. PMID: 24458023

53 Schnur A, Beer S, Witt H, Hegyi P, Sahin-Toth M. Functional effects of 13 rare PRSS1 variants presumed to cause chronic pancreatitis. Gut. 2014;63(2):337–343. PMID: 23455445

54 Howes N, Lerch MM, Greenhalf W, Stocken DD, Ellis I, Simon P, et al. Clinical and genetic characteristics of hereditary pancreatitis in Europe. Clinical Gastroenterology and Hepatology. 2004;2(3):252–261. PMID: 15017610

55 Rebours V, Boutron-Ruault MC, Schnee M, Ferec C, Le Marechal C, Hentic O, et al. The natural history of hereditary pancreatitis: a national series. Gut. 2009;58(1):97–103. PMID: 18755888

56 Lowenfels AB, Maisonneuve P, Whitcomb DC, Lerch MM, DiMagno EP. Cigarette smoking as a risk factor for pancreatic cancer in patients with hereditary pancreatitis. Journal of the American Medical Association. 2001;286(2):169–170.

57 Ellis I. Genetic counseling for hereditary pancreatitis--the role of molecular genetics testing for the cationic trypsinogen gene, cystic fibrosis and serine protease inhibitor Kazal type 1. Gastroenterology Clinics of North America. 2004;33(4):839–854. PMID: 15528021

58 LaRusch J, Solomon S, Whitcomb D. Pancreatitis Overview. In: Pagon RA, Adam MP, Bird TD, Dolan CR, Fong CT, Smith RJH, et al., editors. GeneReviews® [Internet]. Seattle, WA: University of Washington Seattle; 2014.

59 Riordan JR, Rommens JM, Kerem B, Alon N, Rozmahel R, Grzelczak Z, et al. Identification of the cystic fibrosis gene: cloning and characterization of complementary DNA. Science. 1989;245(4922):1066–1073.

60 Zielenski J, Rozmahel R, Bozon D, Kerem B, Grzelczak Z, Riordan JR, et al. Genomic DNA sequence of the cystic fibrosis transmembrane conductance regulator (CFTR) gene. Genomics. 1991;10(1):214–228.

61 Zielenski J, Tsui LC. Cystic fibrosis: genotypic and phenotypic variations. Annual Review of Genetics. 1995;29:777–807.

62 Moskowitz SM, Chmiel JF, Sternen DL, Cheng E, Cutting GR. CFTR-related disorders. In: Pagon RA, Adam MP, Ardinger HH, Bird TD, Dolan CR, Fong CT, et al., editors. GeneReviews®. Seattle, WA: University of Washington Seattle, 1993.

63 Bombieri C, Claustres M, De Boeck K, Derichs N, Dodge J, Girodon E, et al. Recommendations for the classification of diseases as CFTR-related disorders. Journal of Cystic Fibrosis: Official Journal of the European Cystic Fibrosis Society. 2011;10 Suppl 2:S86-S102. PMID: 21658649

64 Kerem E. Atypical CF and CF related diseases. Paediatric Respiratory Reviews 2006;7 Suppl 1:S144-S146. PMID: 16798544

65 Noone PG, Zhou Z, Silverman LM, Jowell PS, Knowles MR, Cohn JA. Cystic fibrosis gene mutations and pancreatitis risk: relation to epithelial ion transport and trypsin inhibitor gene mutations. Gastroenterology. 2001;121(6):1310–1319.

66 Cohn JA, Noone PG, Jowell PS. Idiopathic pancreatitis related to CFTR: complex inheritance and identification of a modifier gene. Journal of Investigative Medicine. 2002;50(5):247S-255S.

67 Schneider A, LaRusch J, Sun X, Aloe A, Lamb J, Hawes R, et al. Combined bicarbonate conductance-impairing variants in CFTR and SPINK1 variants are associated with chronic pancreatitis in patients without cystic fibrosis. Gastroenterology. 2011;140(1):162–171. PMID: 20977904

68 LaRusch J, Jung J, General IJ, Lewis MD, Park HW, Brand RE, et al. Mechanisms of CFTR functional variants that impair regulated bicarbonate permeation and increase risk for pancreatitis but not for cystic fibrosis. PLoS Genetics. 2014;10(7):e1004376. PMID: 25033378

69 Whitcomb DC, Ermentrout GB. A mathematical model of the pancreatic duct cell generating high bicarbonate concentrations in pancreatic juice. Pancreas. 2004;29(2):E30-E40. PMID: 15257112

70 Whitcomb DC. What is personalized medicine and what should it replace? Nature Reviews Gastroenterology & Hepatology. 2012;9(7):418–424. PMID: 22614753

71 Whitcomb DC. Genetic risk factors for pancreatic disorders. Gastroenterology. 2013;144(6):1292–1302. PMID: 23622139

CHAPTER 2

PART A: Pathobiology of the acinar cell in acute pancreatitis

Stephen J. Pandol

Basic and Translational Pancreas Research Program, Cedars-Sinai Medical Center, Los Angeles, CA, USA

Overview of the acinar cell morphology and function

The acinar cell of the exocrine pancreas is responsible for the synthesis, storage, and secretion of digestive enzymes. Acinar cells are organized into spherical and tubular clusters called acini with a central lumen. With neurohumoral stimulation as what occurs during a meal, the acinar cells secrete their digestive enzyme stores into the lumenal space which is connected to the pancreatic ductal system for transport of the digestive enzymes into the gastrointestinal tract.

The acinar cell's organization and function are customized to perform its major tasks of synthesis, storage, and secretion of large amounts of protein in the form of digestive enzymes (Figure 2A.1). The basal aspect of the acinar cell contains abundant rough endoplasmic reticulum (ER) for the synthesis of proteins, while the apical region of the cell contains electron-dense zymogen granules, the store of digestive enzymes. The apical surface of the acinar cell also possesses microvilli. Within the microvilli and in the cytoplasm underlying the apical plasma membrane is a filamentous actin meshwork that is involved in the exocytosis of the contents of the zymogen granules [1, 2]. Secretion is into the lumen of the acinus which is connected to the ductal system. The importance of the ductal system is that its cells (ductal cells) secrete large amounts of fluid rich in bicarbonate ion necessary to carry the digestive enzymes to the gastrointestinal lumen (Figure 2A.1). Of note, blockade of

secretion due to total obstruction of the ductal system as occurs in biliary pancreatitis, defect ductal secretion as occurs with cystic fibrosis, or destruction of the filamentous actin network all lead to injury of the acinar cell and pancreatitis [2–5].

Tight junctions between acinar cells and duct cells form bands around the apical aspects of the cells and act as a barrier to prevent passage of large molecules such as the digestive enzymes into the blood [6]. Injury to the tight junctions between the cells of the acinus as occurs in pancreatitis leads to "leakage" of the digestive enzymes into the blood resulting in the increased concentrations of digestive enzymes in the blood as a hallmark of pancreatitis.

The acinar cell is endowed with a highly developed ER to accomplish its function of protein synthesis. In addition, the ER is also the major store of intracellular calcium which the acinar cell uses to signal exocytosis and secretion of stored digestive enzymes [7–9]. Abnormalities in calcium signaling are also involved in causing pancreatitis as will be discussed later [9]. Each protein synthesized in the ER must undergo specific secondary modifications as well as folding in order for it to be properly transported to destination organelles such as Golgi, zymogen granule (storage for the digestive enzymes), and lysosome or membrane sites (Figure 2A.2). Furthermore, the acinar cell systems for protein synthesis and processing must be able to adapt because of variation in the demand for protein synthesis as a function of diet and because protein processing in

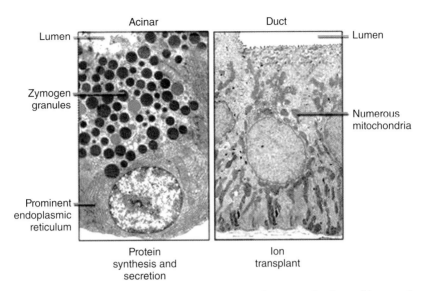

Figure 2A.1 Ultrastructure of acinar and duct cells of the exocrine pancreas. The pancreatic acinar cell has prominent basally located rough endoplasmic reticulum for the synthesis of digestive enzymes and apically located zymogen granules for the storage and secretion of the digestive enzymes. The zymogen granules undergo exocytosis with stimulation of secretion. The secretion is into the lumen of the acinar formed by the apical surfaces of the acinar cells with their projecting microvilli. Not visualized because of the relatively low magnification is the subapical actin network, the tight junctions, and the gap junctions. Pancreatic duct cells contain abundant mitochondria for energy generation needed for its ion transport functions. The ductal cells also project microvilli into the luminal space. Adapted from Gorelick F, Pandol, SJ, Topazian M. Pancreatic physiology, pathophysiology, acute and chronic pancreatitis. Gastrointestinal Teaching Project, American Gastroenterological Association. 2003.

the ER could be adversely affected by environmental factors such as alcohol, smoking, metabolic disorders, and xenobiotics. As discussed later, inability to adapt completely to these environmental factors can also lead to acinar cell injury and pancreatitis [10–14]. Secretion of the digestive enzymes occurs by exocytosis as a result of hormone- and neurotransmitter-generated intracellular signals [15].

Environmental and genetic stressors and the exocrine pancreatic unfolded protein response (UPR)

Because its chief function is to synthesize, store, and secrete large amounts of protein, the acinar cell has a highly developed ER system for protein translation and modification as well as a set of organelles such as the Golgi, lysosomes, and zymogen granules to further process the proteins using internal bonds for folding (i.e., disulfide bonds) and secondary modifications (i.e., glycosylation) for transport and targeting the proteins to the correct destination including zymogen secretory

granules for exocytosis. Factors such as mutations in digestive enzymes, alcohol abuse, smoking, diabetes, and medications can put stresses on the system by preventing proper folding and other necessary post-translational modifications because of a critically located mutation or an abnormal physiochemical environment altering catalytic reactions. In order to adapt to the ER stressors that the genetic and environmental factors pose, the ER of the pancreatic acinar cell has a highly responsive sensing and signaling system called the unfolded protein response (UPR) [13]. The sensors of the UPR are responsive to unfolded and misfolded proteins by initiating several processes that are needed to alleviate the ER stress. These include synthesis of chaperones and foldases to facilitate increased capacity as well as upregulation of the systems involved in the degradation of unfolded and misfolded proteins called ER-associated protein degradation (ERAD), which is required to rid the cell from accumulation of permanently misfolded and unfolded proteins that are toxic to the cell. If the ER stress exceeds the capacity of the UPR to correct the problem or if the mechanisms

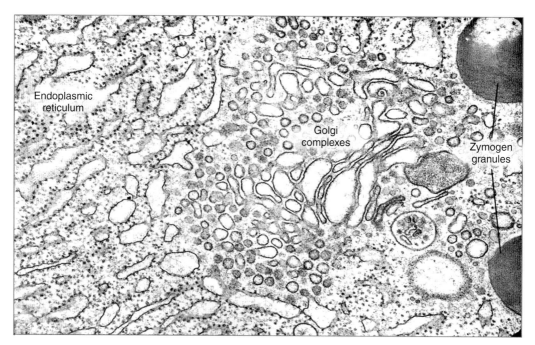

Figure 2A.2 Electron micrograph of the pancreatic acinar cell. This electron micrograph shows the key cellular structures involved in synthesis, processing, and storage of digestive enzymes. On the left is the rough endoplasmic reticulum, in the middle is the Golgi complex, and on the right are zymogen granules. Adapted from Gorelick F, Pandol, SJ, Topazian M. Pancreatic physiology, pathophysiology, acute and chronic pancreatitis. Gastrointestinal Teaching Project, American Gastroenterological Association. 2003.

for correction are blocked, the ER initiates a death response to rid the organ of dysfunctional cells. The death response can be associated with inflammation (pancreatitis).

Both ER-initiated adaptive responses to prevent the effect of toxic insults on cell death and inflammatory responses have been found in exocrine pancreas with stress insults [10, 12–14, 16–20]. An important and provocative observation in these studies is that alcohol abuse causes upregulation of an adaptive and protective UPR [12]. This may explain why alcohol abuse only uncommonly results in pancreatitis. Also, these studies suggest the possibility that treatments and strategies that promote the adaptive and protective UPR in the acinar cell can be used to prevent acute pancreatitis (AP) and recurrent acute pancreatitis.

Calcium signaling and pancreatitis

Intracellular changes in ionized calcium $[Ca^{2+}]_i$ represent the major signaling system mediating protein secretory responses [8]. Activation of G-protein coupled receptors for agonists cholecystokinin and acetylcholine receptors leads to a phospholipase C–mediated hydrolysis of phosphatidylinositol 4,5-bisphosphate to 1,2-diacylglycerol and inositol 1,4,5-triphosphate (IP_3) [7, 21]. IP_3, in turn, releases calcium from ER stores through IP_3 receptors on the ER [22, 23]. The calcium release into the cytosol causes a rapid rise in $[Ca^{2+}]_i$, which mediates the secretory response. With physiologic concentrations of agonists, the increase in $[Ca^{2+}]_i$ initiates in the apical area of acinar cell in the vicinity of the zymogen granules followed by a propagated "wave" toward the basolateral area of the cell [24–27]. Also, the increases in $[Ca^{2+}]_i$ are transient giving an oscillatory pattern. Each spike in $[Ca^{2+}]_i$ leads to a "burst" in zymogen granule exocytosis and secretion. Calcium release into the cytosol is also mediated by other intracellular mediators and receptors as well which are involved in propagating and regulating the "waves" and "oscillations" that are essential for physiologic $[Ca^{2+}]_i$ signaling [7].

In contrast to the "waves" and "oscillations" that comprise physiologic $[Ca^{2+}]_i$, pathologic stimuli can cause sustained increases in $[Ca^{2+}]_i$ that result in pancreatic acinar cell injury and necrosis. This pattern of $[Ca^{2+}]_i$ signaling is due to the influx of Ca^{2+} from the extracellular space through a channel called ORAI-1 that is regulated by the depletion of the amount of Ca^{2+} that is in the ER [9, 28–37]. Examples of pathologic stimuli that deplete ER Ca^{2+} stores resulting in ORAI-1 mediated Ca^{2+} entry and sustained $[Ca^{2+}]_i$ are high doses of the cholecystokinin, acetylcholine, and physiologic concentrations of bile acids [9, 36]. Of considerable importance are findings that pharmacologic agents specific for inhibition of ORAI-1 are able to inhibit ER store activation Ca^{2+} entry and prevent pancreatic necrosis in human acinar cells and pancreatitis in different models of experimental pancreatitis [36]. Inhibition of Ca^{2+} entry with pancreatitis causing stimuli acts in good part by preventing mitochondrial failure as discussed in the next section.

Mitochondrial function in pancreatitis

Mitochondria play a central role in generating energy for sustaining function in the pancreatic acinar cell. There is increased energy demand during secretion that is met by rises in $[Ca^{2+}]_i$ with physiologic neurohumoral stimulation which, in turn, leads to increased production of NADH through the effect of Ca^{2+} on Krebs cycle enzymes [38–40]. The increase in NADH generates a proton motive force resulting in ATP production needed for the energy of secretion. On the other hand, when the increase in $[Ca^{2+}]_i$ is sustained, the ability of the mitochondria to produce ATP stops because the Ca^{2+} overload causes dissipation of the proton motive force preventing ATP production [41–44]. This process leads to cellular failure and necrosis.

Recent evidence indicates that the effect of excess mitochondrial Ca^{2+} on mitochondrial function is due to the opening of a mitochondrial pore termed the mitochondrial permeability transition pore (MPTP) [45, 46]. The opening has been found to require the presence of a mitochondrial matrix protein cyclophilin D (CypD) [45, 46]. Both genetic deletion and pharmacologic inhibition of CypD prevent the pathologic responses in several models of experimental pancreatitis [45, 46].

Inflammatory signaling of pancreatitis

Inflammation is the hallmark of AP and the inflammatory response begins in the acinar cell [47–51]. In most cases the acute inflammatory response is limited to the pancreas, but in severe cases there can be progression to a systemic inflammatory response syndrome (SIRS) causing organ failure which can lead to mortality [52–54]. SIRS is mediated by pancreas-generated increased levels of circulating cytokines that affect several organs especially the lungs leading to pulmonary failure [55].

The studies that show that the acinar cell is the initial site of inflammatory signaling come from experiments that show that this cell produces a variety of inflammatory mediators with stressors that cause pancreatitis [47, 56, 57]. These mediators are then involved in the recruitment of neutrophils followed by macrophages, monocytes, and lymphocytes into the pancreas. Importantly, infiltrating inflammatory cells (both neutrophils and macrophages) mediate the pathologic, intra-acinar activation of trypsinogen which is involved in the promotion of the acinar cell injury and is a key feature of pancreatitis [58–61]. Furthermore, the inflammatory cell infiltrate exacerbates pancreatic necrosis. Although all the mechanisms for promotion of necrosis are not elucidated, another feature of inflammation is that it shifts apoptosis–necrosis balance of acinar cell death toward necrosis of the parenchymal tissue which is associated with a greater severity of disease [4, 62–69]. The severity of pancreatitis in experimental models improves with various strategies that inhibit inflammatory cell recruitment including neutralizing antibodies [58, 59, 70, 71], genetic deletion of specific integrins [59, 61], or inhibition of complement [72].

Although the exact mechanisms involved in initiating inflammatory signaling in the acinar cell are not completely understood, there are key transcription factors that are involved which are generally known to regulate inflammatory mediators. These include nuclear factor kappa-B (NF-κB), activator protein-1 (AP-1), and nuclear factor of activated T-cells (NFAT) [56, 73–82]. These transcription factors are, in turn, regulated by upstream intracellular signaling systems that include $[Ca^{2+}]_i$, calcineurin, novel isoforms of protein kinase C, and protein kinase D [48, 50, 51, 82–95]. For both the transcription factors and the signals that regulate

Summary of therapeutic targets for acute pancreatitis and acute recurrent pancreatitis

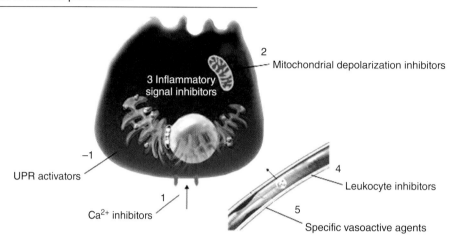

Figure 2A.3 Potential therapeutic targets. (−1) UPR activators to enhance the adaptive response to injurious agents; (1) inhibitors of Ca^{2+} influx to prevent the effect of increased $[Ca^{2+}]_i$ on mitochondrial function and inflammatory signaling; (2) mitochondrial depolarization inhibitors to prevent cellular ATP depletion; (3) inflammatory signal inhibitors to attenuate the inflammatory response and its effect on promoting further cellular injury; (4) leukocyte inhibitors to prevent infiltration and/or activation of leukocytes to prevent their injurious effects on the acinar cell; (5) specific vasoactive agents to both prevent inflammatory cell infiltration and promote the microcirculation which is compromised during pancreatitis.

them, the studies cited show that in animal models and *in vitro* studies using acinar cells, the inhibition of the pathways leads to attenuation of the severity of pancreatitis (and cellular injury) pointing to the central role played by the acinar cell and its inflammatory signaling in pancreatitis.

Summary and potential therapeutic targets

The elucidation of the roles of the acinar cell pathophysiology in AP allows for predicting classes of agents that should be considered for potential therapy. Figure 2A.3 provides a summary of these targets. Moreover, as indicated earlier, treatments for one class of targets can have beneficial effects on a broad set of pathologic responses as discussed with respect to the inflammatory response. In this context, recent reports show that supporting organellar function can lead to attenuation of several pathophysiologic responses. For example, prevention of mitochondrial failure by blocking the opening of the mitochondrial permeability pore with

pharmacologic and genetic inhibitors of CypD has effects on inflammation [45, 46].

References

1 Muallem S, Kwiatkowska K, Xu X, Yin HL. Actin filament disassembly is a sufficient final trigger for exocytosis in nonexcitable cells. Journal of Cell Biology 1995;128:589–598.

2 O'Konski MS, Pandol SJ. Effects of caerulein on the apical cytoskeleton of the pancreatic acinar cell. Journal of Clinical Investigation 1990;86:1649–1657.

3 Hegyi P, Pandol S, Venglovecz V, Rakonczay Z. The acinar-ductal tango in the pathogenesis of acute pancreatitis. Gut 2011;60:544–552.

4 Gukovskaya AS, Perkins P, Zaninovic V, Sandoval D, Rutherford R, Fitzsimmons T, Pandol SJ, Poucell-Hatton S. Mechanisms of cell death after pancreatic duct obstruction in the opossum and the rat. Gastroenterology 1996;110:875–884.

5 Lerch MM, Saluja AK, Rünzi M, Dawra R, Saluja M, Steer ML. Pancreatic duct obstruction triggers acute necrotizing pancreatitis in the opossum. Gastroenterology 1993;104:853–861.

6 Fallon MB, Gorelick FS, Anderson JM, Mennone A, Saluja A, Steer ML. Effect of cerulein hyperstimulation

on the paracellular barrier of rat exocrine pancreas. Gastroenterology 1995;108:1863–1872.

7 Petersen OH, Tepikin AV. Polarized calcium signaling in exocrine gland cells. Annual Review of Physiology 2008;70:273–299.

8 Pandol SJ, Schoeffield MS, Sachs G, Muallem S. Role of free cytosolic calcium in secretagogue-stimulated amylase release from dispersed acini from guinea pig pancreas. Journal of Biological Chemistry 1985;260:10081–10086.

9 Sutton R, Petersen OH, Pandol SJ. Pancreatitis and calcium signaling: report of an international workshop. Pancreas 2008;36:e1–e14.

10 Kubisch CH, Logsdon CD. Secretagogues differentially activate endoplasmic reticulum stress responses in pancreatic acinar cells. American Journal of Physiology: Gastrointestinal and Liver Physiology 2007;292:G1804–G1812.

11 Kubisch CH, Logsdon CD. Endoplasmic reticulum stress and the pancreatic acinar cell. Expert Review of Gastroenterology & Hepatology 2008;2:249–260.

12 Lugea A, Tischler D, Nguyen J, Gong J, Gukovsky I, French SW, Gorelick FS, Pandol SJ. Adaptive unfolded protein response attenuates alcohol-induced pancreatic damage. Gastroenterology 2011;140:987–997.

13 Pandol SJ, Gorelick FS, Lugea A. Environmental and genetic stressors and the unfolded protein response in exocrine pancreatic function – a hypothesis. Frontiers in Physiology 2011;2:8.

14 Seyhun E, Malo A, Schäfer C, Moskaluk CA, Hoffmann RT, Göke B, Kubisch CH. Tauroursodeoxycholic acid reduces endoplasmic reticulum stress, acinar cell damage, and systemic inflammation in acute pancreatitis. American Journal of Physiology: Gastrointestinal and Liver Physiology 2011;301:G773–G782.

15 Williams JA. Receptor-mediated signal transduction pathways and the regulation of pancreatic acinar cell function. Current Opinion in Gastroenterology 2008;24:573–579.

16 Kubisch CH, Sans MD, Arumugam T, Ernst SA, Williams JA, Logsdon CD. Early activation of endoplasmic reticulum stress is associated with arginine-induced acute pancreatitis. American Journal of Physiology: Gastrointestinal and Liver Physiology 2006;291:G238–G245.

17 Suyama K, Ohmuraya M, Hirota M, Ozaki N, Ida S, Endo M, Araki K, Gotoh T, Baba H, Yamamura K. C/EBP homologous protein is crucial for the acceleration of experimental pancreatitis. Biochemical and Biophysical Research Communications 2008;367:176–182.

18 Malo A, Krüger B, Seyhun E, Schäfer C, Hoffmann RT, Göke B, Kubisch CH. Tauroursodeoxycholic acid reduces endoplasmic reticulum stress, trypsin activation, and acinar cell apoptosis while increasing secretion in rat pancreatic acini. American Journal of Physiology: Gastrointestinal and Liver Physiology 2010;299:G877–G886.

19 Zeng Y, Wang X, Zhang W, Wu K, Ma J. Hypertriglyceridemia aggravates ER stress and pathogenesis of acute pancreatitis. Hepatogastroenterology 2012;59:2318–2326.

20 Mimori S, Ohtaka H, Koshikawa Y, Kawada K, Kaneko M, Okuma Y, Nomura Y, Murakami Y, Hamana H. 4-Phenylbutyric acid protects against neuronal cell death by primarily acting as a chemical chaperone rather than histone deacetylase inhibitor. Bioorganic & Medicinal Chemistry Letters 2013;23:6015–6018.

21 Williams JA. Intracellular signaling mechanisms activated by cholecystokinin-regulating synthesis and secretion of digestive enzymes in pancreatic acinar cells. Annual Review of Physiology 2001;63:77–97.

22 Muallem S, Schoeffield M, Pandol S, Sachs G. Inositol triphosphate modification of ion transport in rough endoplasmic reticulum. Proceedings of the National Academy of Sciences of the United States of America 1985; 82:4433–4437.

23 Streb H, Irvine RF, Berridge MJ, Schulz I. Release of Ca^{2+} from a nonmitochondrial intracellular store in pancreatic acinar cells by inositol-1,4,5-trisphosphate. Nature 1983;306:67–69.

24 Petersen OH, Petersen CC, Kasai H. Calcium and hormone action. Annual Review of Physiology 1994;56:297–319.

25 Kasai H, Petersen OH. Spatial dynamics of second messengers: IP3 and cAMP as long-range and associative messengers. Trends in Neurosciences 1994;17:95–101.

26 Kasai H, Li YX, Miyashita Y. Subcellular distribution of Ca^{2+} release channels underlying Ca^{2+} waves and oscillations in exocrine pancreas. Cell 1993;74:669–677.

27 Maruyama Y, Inooka G, Li YX, Miyashita Y, Kasai H. Agonist-induced localized Ca^{2+} spikes directly triggering exocytotic secretion in exocrine pancreas. EMBO Journal 1993;12:3017–3022.

28 Pandol SJ, Schoeffield MS, Fimmel CJ, Muallem S. The agonist-sensitive calcium pool in the pancreatic acinar cell. Activation of plasma membrane Ca^{2+} influx mechanism. Journal of Biological Chemistry 1987;262:16963–16968.

29 Muallem S, Schoeffield MS, Fimmel CJ, Pandol SJ. Agonist-sensitive calcium pool in the pancreatic acinar cell. I. Permeability properties. American Journal of Physiology 1988;255:G221–G228.

30 Muallem S, Schoeffield MS, Fimmel CJ, Pandol SJ. Agonist-sensitive calcium pool in the pancreatic acinar cell. II. Characterization of reloading. American Journal of Physiology 1988;255:G229–G235.

31 Pandol SJ, Gukovskaya A, Bahnson TD, Dionne VE. Cellular mechanisms mediating agonist-stimulated calcium influx in the pancreatic acinar cell. Annals of the New York Academy of Sciences 1994;713:41–48.

32 Prakriya M, Feske S, Gwack Y, Srikanth S, Rao A, Hogan PG. Orai1 is an essential pore subunit of the CRAC channel. Nature 2006;443:230–233.

33 Voronina SG, Barrow SL, Gerasimenko OV, Petersen OH, Tepikin AV. Effects of secretagogues and bile acids on mitochondrial membrane potential of pancreatic acinar cells: comparison of different modes of evaluating DeltaPsim. Journal of Biological Chemistry 2004;279:27327–27338.

34 Gerasimenko JV, Gryshchenko O, Ferdek PE, Stapleton E, Hébert TO, Bychkova S, Peng S, Begg M, Gerasimenko OV, Petersen OH. Ca^{2+} release-activated Ca^{2+} channel blockade as a potential tool in antipancreatitis therapy. Proceedings of the National Academy of Sciences of the United States of America 2013;110:13186–13191.

35 Gerasimenko JV, Gerasimenko OV, Petersen OH. The role of Ca^{2+} in the pathophysiology of pancreatitis. Journal of Physiology 2014;592:269–280.

36 Wen L, Voronina S, Javed MA, Awais M, Szatmary P, Latawiec D, Chvanov M, Collier D, Huang W, Barrett J, Begg M, Stauderman K, Roos J, Grigoryev S, Ramos S, Rogers E, Whitten J, Velicelebi G, Dunn M, Tepikin AV, Criddle DN, Sutton R. Inhibitors of ORAI1 prevent cytosolic calcium-associated injury of human pancreatic acinar cells and acute pancreatitis in 3 mouse models. Gastroenterology 2015;149:481–492. e487

37 Kim MS, Hong JH, Li Q, Shin DM, Abramowitz J, Birnbaumer L, Muallem S. Deletion of TRPC3 in mice reduces store-operated Ca^{2+} influx and the severity of acute pancreatitis. Gastroenterology 2009;137:1509–1517.

38 Murphy JA, Criddle DN, Sherwood M, Chvanov M, Mukherjee R, McLaughlin E, Booth D, Gerasimenko JV, Raraty MG, Ghaneh P, Neoptolemos JP, Gerasimenko OV, Tepikin AV, Green GM, Reeve JR, Jr., Petersen OH, Sutton R. Direct activation of cytosolic Ca^{2+} signaling and enzyme secretion by cholecystokinin in human pancreatic acinar cells. Gastroenterology 2008;135:632–641.

39 Criddle DN, Booth DM, Mukherjee R, McLaughlin E, Green GM, Sutton R, Petersen OH, Reeve JR, Jr., Cholecystokinin-58 and cholecystokinin-8 exhibit similar actions on calcium signaling, zymogen secretion, and cell fate in murine pancreatic acinar cells. American Journal of Physiology: Gastrointestinal and Liver Physiology 2009;297:G1085–G1092.

40 Voronina S, Sukhomlin T, Johnson PR, Erdemli G, Petersen OH, Tepikin A. Correlation of NADH and Ca^{2+} signals in mouse pancreatic acinar cells. Journal of Physiology 2002;539:41–52.

41 Criddle DN, Gerasimenko JV, Baumgartner HK, Jaffar M, Voronina S, Sutton R, Petersen OH, Gerasimenko OV. Calcium signalling and pancreatic cell death: apoptosis or necrosis? Cell Death & Differentiation 2007;14:1285–1294.

42 Mukherjee R, Criddle DN, Gukvoskaya A, Pandol S, Petersen OH, Sutton R. Mitochondrial injury in pancreatitis. Cell Calcium 2008; 44:14–23.

43 Gukovsky I, Pandol SJ, Gukovskaya AS. Organellar dysfunction in the pathogenesis of pancreatitis. Antioxidants & Redox Signaling 2011;15:2699–2710.

44 Criddle DN, Raraty MG, Neoptolemos JP, Tepikin AV, Petersen OH, Sutton R. Ethanol toxicity in pancreatic acinar cells: mediation by nonoxidative fatty acid metabolites. Proceedings of the National Academy of Sciences of the United States of America 2004;101:10738–10743.

45 Shalbueva N, Mareninova OA, Gerloff A, Yuan J, Waldron RT, Pandol SJ, Gukovskaya AS. Effects of oxidative alcohol metabolism on the mitochondrial permeability transition pore and necrosis in a mouse model of alcoholic pancreatitis. Gastroenterology 2013;144:437–446 e436.

46 Mukherjee R, Mareninova OA, Odinokova IV, Huang W, Murphy J, Chvanov M, Javed MA, Wen L, Booth DM, Cane MC, Awais M, Gavillet B, Pruss RM, Schaller S, Molkentin JD, Tepikin AV, Petersen OH, Pandol SJ, Gukovsky I, Criddle DN, Gukovskaya AS, Sutton R, and NPBRU. Mechanism of mitochondrial permeability transition pore induction and damage in the pancreas: inhibition prevents acute pancreatitis by protecting production of ATP. Gut 2015 doi: 10.1136/gutjnl-2014-308553.

47 Gukovskaya AS, Gukovsky I, Zaninovic V, Song M, Sandoval D, Gukovsky S, Pandol SJ. Pancreatic acinar cells produce, release, and respond to tumor necrosis factor-alpha. Role in regulating cell death and pancreatitis. Journal of Clinical Investigation 1997;100:1853–1862.

48 Blinman TA, Gukovsky I, Mouria M, Zaninovic V, Livingston E, Pandol SJ, Gukovskaya AS. Activation of pancreatic acinar cells on isolation from tissue: cytokine upregulation via p38 MAP kinase. American Journal of Physiology: Cell Physiology 2000;279:C1993–C2003.

49 Gukovskaya AS, Hosseini S, Satoh A, Cheng JH, Nam KJ, Gukovsky I, Pandol SJ. Ethanol differentially regulates NF-kappaB activation in pancreatic acinar cells through calcium and protein kinase C pathways. American Journal of Physiology: Gastrointestinal and Liver Physiology 2004;286:G204–G213.

50 Satoh A, Gukovskaya AS, Nieto JM, Cheng JH, Gukovsky I, Reeve JR, Shimosegawa T, Pandol SJ. PKC-delta and -epsilon regulate NF-kappaB activation induced by cholecystokinin and TNF-alpha in pancreatic acinar cells. American Journal of Physiology: Gastrointestinal and Liver Physiology 2004;287:G582–G591.

51 Satoh A, Gukovskaya AS, Edderkaoui M, Daghighian MS, Reeve JR, Shimosegawa T, Pandol SJ. Tumor necrosis factor-alpha mediates pancreatitis responses in acinar cells via protein kinase C and proline-rich tyrosine kinase 2. Gastroenterology 2005;129:639–651.

52 Pandol SJ, Saluja AK, Imrie CW, Banks PA. Acute pancreatitis: bench to the bedside. Gastroenterology 2007;132:1127–1151.

53 Mofidi R, Duff MD, Wigmore SJ, Madhavan KK, Garden OJ, Parks RW. Association between early systemic inflammatory response, severity of multiorgan dysfunction and death in acute pancreatitis. British Journal of Surgery 2006;93:738–744.

54 Singh VK, Wu BU, Bollen TL, Repas K, Maurer R, Mortele KJ, Banks PA. Early systemic inflammatory response syndrome is associated with severe acute pancreatitis. Clinical Gastroenterology and Hepatology 2009;7:1247–1251.

55 Norman J. The role of cytokines in the pathogenesis of acute pancreatitis. American Journal of Surgery 1998;175:76–83.

56 Gukovsky I, Gukovskaya AS, Blinman TA, Zaninovic V, Pandol SJ. Early NF-kappaB activation is associated with hormone-induced pancreatitis. American Journal of Physiology 1998;275:G1402–G1414.

57 Grady T, Liang P, Ernst SA, Logsdon CD. Chemokine gene expression in rat pancreatic acinar cells is an early event associated with acute pancreatitis. Gastroenterology 1997;113:1966–1975.

58 Gukovskaya AS, Vaquero E, Zaninovic V, Gorelick FS, Lusis AJ, Brennan ML, Holland S, Pandol SJ. Neutrophils and NADPH oxidase mediate intrapancreatic trypsin activation in murine experimental acute pancreatitis. Gastroenterology 2002;122:974–984.

59 Abdulla A, Awla D, Thorlacius H, Regnér S. Role of neutrophils in the activation of trypsinogen in severe acute pancreatitis. Journal of Leukocyte Biology 2011;90:975–982.

60 Awla D, Abdulla A, Syk I, Jeppsson B, Regnér S, Thorlacius H. Neutrophil-derived matrix metalloproteinase-9 is a potent activator of trypsinogen in acinar cells in acute pancreatitis. Journal of Leukocyte Biology 2012;91:711–719.

61 Sendler M, Dummer A, Weiss FU, Krüger B, Wartmann T, Scharffetter-Kochanek K, van Rooijen N, Malla SR, Aghdassi A, Halangk W, Lerch MM, Mayerle J. Tumour necrosis factor α secretion induces protease activation and acinar cell necrosis in acute experimental pancreatitis in mice. Gut 2013;62:430–439.

62 Sandoval D, Gukovskaya A, Reavey P, Gukovsky S, Sisk A, Braquet P, Pandol SJ, Poucell-Hatton S. The role of neutrophils and platelet-activating factor in mediating experimental pancreatitis. Gastroenterology 1996;111:1081–1091.

63 Mayerle J, Schnekenburger J, Krüger B, Kellermann J, Ruthenbürger M, Weiss FU, Nalli A, Domschke W, Lerch MM. Extracellular cleavage of E-cadherin by leukocyte elastase during acute experimental pancreatitis in rats. Gastroenterology 2005;129:1251–1267.

64 Mayerle J, Dummer A, Sendler M, Malla SR, van den Brandt C, Teller S, Aghdassi A, Nitsche C, Lerch MM. Differential roles of inflammatory cells in pancreatitis. Journal of Gastroenterology and Hepatology 2012;27 Suppl 2:47–51.

65 Demols A, Le Moine O, Desalle F, Quertinmont E, Van Laethem JL, Devière J. CD4(+)T cells play an important role in acute experimental pancreatitis in mice. Gastroenterology 2000;118:582–590.

66 Kaiser AM, Saluja AK, Sengupta A, Saluja M, Steer ML. Relationship between severity, necrosis, and apoptosis in five models of experimental acute pancreatitis. American Journal of Physiology 1995;269:C1295–C1304.

67 Hoque R, Sohail M, Malik A, Sarwar S, Luo Y, Shah A, Barrat F, Flavell R, Gorelick F, Husain S, Mehal W. TLR9 and the NLRP3 inflammasome link acinar cell death with inflammation in acute pancreatitis. Gastroenterology 2011;141:358–369.

68 Bhatia M. Apoptosis versus necrosis in acute pancreatitis. American Journal of Physiology: Gastrointestinal and Liver Physiology 2004;286:G189–G196.

69 Mareninova OA, Sung KF, Hong P, Lugea A, Pandol SJ, Gukovsky I, Gukovskaya AS. Cell death in pancreatitis: caspases protect from necrotizing pancreatitis. Journal of Biological Chemistry 2006;281:3370–3381.

70 Frossard JL, Saluja A, Bhagat L, Lee HS, Bhatia M, Hofbauer B, Steer ML. The role of intercellular adhesion molecule 1 and neutrophils in acute pancreatitis and pancreatitis-associated lung injury. Gastroenterology 1999;116:694–701.

71 Hartman H, Abdulla A, Awla D, Lindkvist B, Jeppsson B, Thorlacius H, Regnér S. P-selectin mediates neutrophil rolling and recruitment in acute pancreatitis. British Journal of Surgery 2012;99:246–255.

72 Hartwig W, Klafs M, Kirschfink M, Hackert T, Schneider L, Gebhard MM, Büchler MW, Werner J. Interaction of complement and leukocytes in severe acute pancreatitis: potential for therapeutic intervention. American Journal of Physiology: Gastrointestinal and Liver Physiology 2006;291:G844–G850.

73 Vaquero E, Gukovsky I, Zaninovic V, Gukovskaya AS, Pandol SJ. Localized pancreatic NF-kappaB activation and inflammatory response in taurocholate-induced pancreatitis. American Journal of Physiology: Gastrointestinal and Liver Physiology 2001;280:G1197–G1208.

74 Orlichenko LS, Behari J, Yeh TH, Liu S, Stolz DB, Saluja AK, Singh VP. Transcriptional regulation of CXC-ELR chemokines KC and MIP-2 in mouse pancreatic acini. American Journal of Physiology: Gastrointestinal and Liver Physiology 2010;299:G867–G876.

75 Steinle AU, Weidenbach H, Wagner M, Adler G, Schmid RM. NF-kappaB/Rel activation in cerulein pancreatitis. Gastroenterology 1999;116:420–430.

76 Chen X, Ji B, Han B, Ernst SA, Simeone D, Logsdon CD. NF-kappaB activation in pancreas induces pancreatic and systemic inflammatory response. Gastroenterology 2002;122:448–457.

77 Altavilla D, Famulari C, Passaniti M, Galeano M, Macrì A, Seminara P, Minutoli L, Marini H, Calò M, Venuti FS, Esposito M, Squadrito F. Attenuated cerulein-induced pancreatitis in nuclear factor-kappaB-deficient mice. Laboratory Investigation 2003;83:1723–1732.

78 Rakonczay Z, Hegyi P, Takács T, McCarroll J, Saluja AK. The role of NF-kappaB activation in the pathogenesis of acute pancreatitis. Gut 2008;57:259–267.

79 Neuhöfer P, Liang S, Einwächter H, Schwerdtfeger C, Wartmann T, Treiber M, Zhang H, Schulz HU, Dlubatz K, Lesina M, Diakopoulos KN, Wörmann S, Halangk W, Witt H, Schmid RM, Algül H. Deletion of IkBα activates RelA to reduce acute pancreatitis in mice through up-regulation of Spi2A. Gastroenterology 2013;144:192–201.

80 Gukovsky I, Gukovskaya A. Nuclear factor-kB in pancreatitis: Jack-of-all-trades, but which one is more important? Gastroenterology 2013;144:26–29.

81 Gukovsky I, Li N, Todoric J, Gukovskaya A, Karin M. Inflammation, autophagy, and obesity: common features in the pathogenesis of pancreatitis and pancreatic cancer. Gastroenterology 2013;144:1199–1209 e1194.

82 Awla D, Zetterqvist AV, Abdulla A, Camello C, Berglund LM, Spégel P, Pozo MJ, Camello PJ, Regnér S, Gomez MF, Thorlacius H. NFATc3 regulates trypsinogen activation, neutrophil recruitment, and tissue damage in acute pancreatitis in mice. Gastroenterology 2012;143:1352–1360. e1351–1357

83 Satoh A, Gukovskaya AS, Reeve JR, Shimosegawa T, Pandol SJ. Ethanol sensitizes NF-kappaB activation in pancreatic acinar cells through effects on protein kinase C-epsilon. American Journal of Physiology: Gastrointestinal and Liver Physiology 2006;291:G432–G438.

84 Gorelick F, Pandol S, Thrower E. Protein kinase C in the pancreatic acinar cell. Journal of Gastroenterology and Hepatology 2008;23 Suppl 1:S37–S41.

85 Thrower EC, Osgood S, Shugrue CA, Kolodecik TR, Chaudhuri AM, Reeve JR, Pandol SJ, Gorelick FS. The novel protein kinase C isoforms -delta and -epsilon modulate caerulein-induced zymogen activation in pancreatic acinar cells. American Journal of Physiology: Gastrointestinal and Liver Physiology 2008;294:G1344–G1353.

86 Yuan J, Lugea A, Zheng L, Gukovsky I, Edderkaoui M, Rozengurt E, Pandol SJ. Protein kinase D1 mediates NF-kappaB activation induced by cholecystokinin and cholinergic signaling in pancreatic acinar cells. American Journal of Physiology: Gastrointestinal and Liver Physiology 2008;295:G1190–G1201.

87 Thrower EC, Wang J, Cheriyan S, Lugea A, Kolodecik TR, Yuan J, Reeve JR, Gorelick FS, Pandol SJ. Protein kinase C delta-mediated processes in cholecystokinin-8-stimulated pancreatic acini. Pancreas 2009;38:930–935.

88 Thrower EC, Yuan J, Usmani A, Liu Y, Jones C, Minervini SN, Alexandre M, Pandol SJ, Guha S. A novel protein kinase D inhibitor attenuates early events of experimental pancreatitis in isolated rat acini. American Journal of Physiology: Gastrointestinal and Liver Physiology 2011;300:G120–G129.

89 Yuan J, Liu Y, Tan T, Guha S, Gukovsky I, Gukovskaya A, Pandol SJ. Protein kinase d regulates cell death pathways in experimental pancreatitis. Frontiers in Physiology 2012;3:60.

90 Han B, Logsdon CD. CCK stimulates mob-1 expression and NF-kappaB activation via protein kinase C and intracellular Ca(2+). American Journal of Physiology: Cell Physiology 2000;278:C344–C351.

91 Tando Y, Algül H, Wagner M, Weidenbach H, Adler G, Schmid RM. Caerulein-induced NF-kappaB/Rel activation requires both Ca^{2+} and protein kinase C as messengers. American Journal of Physiology 1999;277:G678–G686.

92 Thrower EC, Gorelick FS, Husain SZ. Molecular and cellular mechanisms of pancreatic injury. Current Opinion in Gastroenterology 2010;26:484–489.

93 Muili KA, Wang D, Orabi AI, Sarwar S, Luo Y, Javed TA, Eisses JF, Mahmood SM, Jin S, Singh VP, Ananthanaravanan M, Perides G, Williams JA, Molkentin JD, Husain SZ. Bile acids induce pancreatic acinar cell injury and pancreatitis by activating calcineurin. Journal of Biological Chemistry 2013;288:570–580.

94 Muili KA, Jin S, Orabi AI, Eisses JF, Javed TA, Le T, Bottino R, Jayaraman T, Husain SZ. Pancreatic acinar cell nuclear factor kB activation because of bile acid exposure is dependent on calcineurin. Journal of Biological Chemistry 2013;288:21065–21073.

95 Jin S, Orabi AI, Le T, Javed TA, Sah S, Eisses JF, Bottino R, Molkentin JD, Husain SZ. Exposure to radiocontrast agents induces pancreatic inflammation by activation of nuclear factor-kB, calcium signaling, and calcineurin. Gastroenterology 2015;149:753–764 e711.

PART B: Locoregional pathophysiology in acute pancreatitis: pancreas and intestine

Alistair B.J. Escott[1], Anthony J. Phillips[2] & John A. Windsor[1,2]

[1] Department of Surgery, University of Auckland, Auckland, New Zealand
[2] Applied Surgery and Metabolism Laboratory, School of Biological Sciences and Department of Surgery, University of Auckland, Auckland, New Zealand

Introduction

Acute pancreatitis (AP) is initiated in the acinar cell, but the prime determinants of severity occur at the tissue and organ levels [1]. The key intra-acinar events (see Chapter 2a) are important in understanding the common pathways by which the diverse etiologies initiate AP. The extra-acinar events are important in understanding the local and systemic complications of AP which determine the severity and outcome or more specifically the development of infected pancreatic necrosis and persistent organ failure [1]. This chapter focuses on the locoregional pathophysiology of AP with a specific emphasis on the key pancreatic and intestinal events and their interplay and contribution to the development of the local and systemic complications of AP (Figure 2B.1). Aspects of the pathophysiology that are of relevance to the management of AP will be highlighted.

Pancreatic pathophysiology

Morphology and local complications of acute pancreatitis

AP is a protean disease with a range of etiologies, severities, complications, and outcomes. The acute inflammatory process in the pancreas results in edema of the pancreatic interstitium and peripancreatic tissues. The development of edema is due to capillary leak, a cardinal feature of inflammation. Morphologically on computed tomography (CT), interstitial edematous pancreatitis (IEP) (Figure 2B.2a) is characterized by enlargement of the pancreas, homogenous enhancement, and peripancreatic fat stranding [4].

The presence or absence of necrosis on contrast-enhanced CT is important because it is an independent predictor of severity [4, 5] (Figure 2B.2b). Pancreatic necrosis is due to microcirculatory stasis [6] and/or failure [7, 8]. Three morphological forms of pancreatic necrosis have been described [9] based on their histological appearance. Type I, the most common (95%), is characterized by perilobular fatty tissue necrosis with subsequent necrosis of surrounding blood vessels, acinar cells, and ducts. Type II begins with ductal necrosis and is seen more often in patients with prolonged circulatory failure. Type III represents acinar cell necrosis without pancreatic autodigestion [9]. Peripancreatic necrosis can occur with or without pancreatic necrosis [4]. It has been suggested that peripancreatic necrosis is due to the liberation of activated lipase into peripancreatic fat [10].

The local complications of AP can be classified on the basis of chronicity, content, and infection (Table 2B.1) [11]. Acute peripancreatic fluid collections (APFCs) have no defined wall, have a homogenous appearance, rarely become infected, and usually resolve without intervention [4]. APFCs are thought to derive from aggregated loci of inflammatory edema and exudate. When an APFC is present in this state for more than 4 weeks, it is defined as a "pseudocyst." A pseudocyst only contains fluid and is not diagnosed in the presence of necrotizing pancreatitis. In the situation where there are also disrupted pancreatic ductules (in the absence of necrosis), the fluid collection is more likely to persist and becomes walled off. The underlying duct disruption involved in the etiology of this lesion also explains why

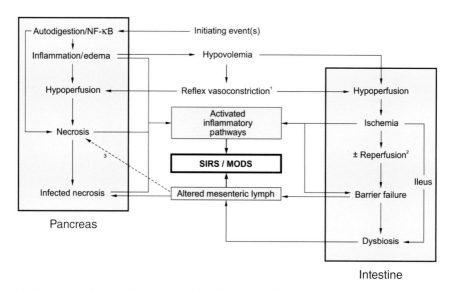

Figure 2B.1 Complex interactions between the pancreas and the intestine in the pathogenesis of severe acute pancreatitis. [1. Reflex vasoconstriction can be increased by nonselective inotropes; 2. fluid resuscitation can promote reperfusion injury; 3. experimental evidence suggests that altered mesenteric lymph can promote necrosis, but this requires confirmation.] Modified from [2].

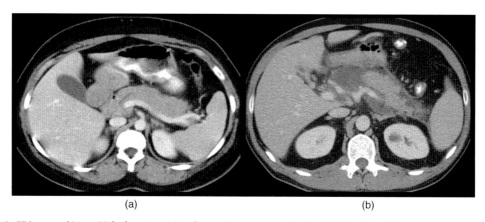

Figure 2B.2 CT images of interstitial edematous (a) and necrotizing pancreatitis (b). Modified from [3].

the pseudocyst fluid has an elevated pancreatic enzyme concentration.

The development of necrosis occurs in 5–10% of patients with AP [4]. The natural history of necrosis is variable, as it can liquefy or remain solid, be sterile or become infected, and persist or resolve. Morphologically this can result in an acute necrotic collection (ANC) or walled-off necrosis (WON), both of which can remain sterile or become infected (Table 2B.1). Disruption of the main pancreatic duct by necrosis results in a fluid

collection and potentially the "disconnected pancreatic duct syndrome" (Table 2B.1) [7] with almost certain persistence of what is now termed WON.

Pancreatic microcirculation

Before discussing the development of pancreatic necrosis in detail, it is important to review the control of normal pancreatic vascular perfusion. The pancreas is richly supplied by both the celiac and superior mesenteric arteries. The head of the pancreas has an anterior

Table 2B.1 Definitions of local complications of acute pancreatitis based on CT morphology.

Content	Acute (<4 weeks, no defined wall)		Chronic (<4 weeks, defined wall)	
	No infection	Infection	No infection	Infection
Fluid	Acute pancreatic fluid collection	Infected APFC	Pseudocyst	Infected pseudocyst
Solid ± fluid	Acute necrotic collection	Infected ANC	Walled-off necrosis	Infected WON

Modified from [11].

and posterior arcade derived from both of these arteries, while the pancreatic body and tail is supplied primarily from the splenic artery. Blood flow to the pancreas is regulated by neural, hormonal, and local (paracrine) factors [12]. Neural control is by dual sympathetic and parasympathetic innervation. Parasympathetic fibers release acetylcholine to cause vasodilation. Postganglionic sympathetic fibers release noradrenaline during hypovolemia resulting in vasoconstriction and a reduction in pancreatic blood flow. Autoregulation by local paracrine factors includes nitric oxide and endothelin modulation of the sympathetic response through reactive hyperemia and hypoxic vasodilation [13]. Animal models suggest that pancreatic tissue oxygen extraction is maintained via this mechanism until blood flow is reduced to 60% of the normal flow [12]. The pancreas has endocrine islets juxtaposed beside exocrine tissue, and the existence of an insuloacinar portal venous system suggests that the hormones from the pancreatic islet cells might influence the exocrine pancreas and blood flow [14]. Experimental studies of sepsis and hemorrhage [11, 12] have also demonstrated that pancreatic perfusion is affected to a greater extent than in other splanchnic organs (Figure 2B.3) and does not readily recover after intestinal ischemia–reperfusion [16]. The failure of autoregulation in the pancreas compared with the intestine (see Figure 2B.3) shows that there is no significant improvement in perfusion during the period of hypotension. There is also a significant regional variation in the blood flow in the pancreas during severe AP, with some areas of vasoconstriction/necrosis alongside other areas of normal perfusion. The extent to which the regulatory elements have a role in severe AP remains uncertain. And the failure of the microcirculation in regions of necrosis is also due, in part, to the proteolytic action of pancreatic enzymes.

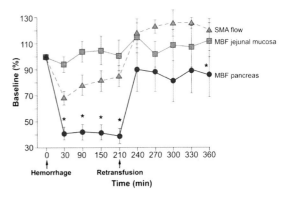

Figure 2B.3 Changes in the superior mesenteric artery (SMA) flow and in microcirculatory blood flow (MF) in the jejunal mucosa and in the pancreas after hemorrhage and after retransfusion of shed blood. (*$P < 0.05$ compared with baseline.) Redrawn from [15].

Pancreatic inflammation and interstitial edema

The release of activated pancreatic enzymes from the acinar cell into the interstitium promotes autodigestion of the pancreas and initiates an inflammatory response (see Chapter 2a). This response consists of recruitment and activation of inflammatory cells [17] and initiation of plasma-derived inflammatory pathways (including complement, coagulation, kallikrein–kinin, and fibrinolysis) [10]. Early in the inflammatory process, there is an increased vascular permeability ("capillary leak") due to a number of different factors. Neutrophils increase capillary permeability following adherence to postcapillary venules [6], while activated pancreatic enzymes attack the components of the endothelial wall. Both cellular and humoral mediators of inflammation have been implicated in the development of increased capillary permeability. Substance P, a neuropeptide released from nerve endings, increases the permeability of the vascular endothelium in AP [17]. The inflammatory mediator platelet-activating factor (PAF) released by a number of cells (e.g., endothelial, epithelial, mast, macrophages) also increases capillary permeability [17]. Bradykinin and thromboxane A2 are also associated with early increased capillary permeability in AP [6].

Pancreatic hypoperfusion

The arrangement of the pancreatic microcirculation makes it susceptible to ischemia [6], and the severity of AP was reported to be proportional to the severity of microvascular dysfunction [18]. The microcirculatory changes occur early with histological confirmation occurring within 30 minutes of the onset of AP in an animal model [19]. Local vasoconstriction in response to endothelins [8] results in progressive exclusion of capillaries from the pancreatic circulation. This creates discrete areas of physiological shunt within the pancreas leading to areas of pancreatic ischemia. The heterogeneous distribution of the shunting leads to other areas of vasodilation and hyperemia [6] contributing to edema formation.

Vascular luminal factors also impact blood flow through the pancreatic capillary bed by promoting microcirculatory stasis. Leukocytes also have a role in promoting plaque formation and obstruction of postcapillary venules [6]. The coagulation cascade activated early in AP [10] leads to multiple intravascular thrombi [6]. This hypercoagulable state appears to be mediated by both activated pancreatic proteases and fibrinolysis [20, 21]. The empiric evidence to support this hypothesis includes the fact that both fibrinogen and D-dimer (a marker of fibrinolysis) levels are raised in humans with AP [20]. The role of coagulation in pancreatic microcirculatory failure in AP is supported by the fact that heparin administration in experimental AP improves pancreatic blood flow [22]. Furthermore, platelet levels [21] are increased and activated in AP [23]. Hemoconcentration [24] from third-space fluid loss in AP also contributes to microcirculatory stasis.

Pancreatic necrosis

Persisting microcirculatory stasis contributes to pancreatic necrosis [18]. A recent observational study demonstrated that pancreatic necrosis was not detected within the first 4 days of hospital admission [25]. CT imaging of necrotizing pancreatitis reveals progressive changes from patchy attenuation in the early stages to areas of hypoperfusion before these become well demarcated and confluent [10, 26] (Figure 2B.2b). These observations suggest that this necrosis develops over several days. While some microcirculatory factors (e.g., reduced capillary flow, vasoconstriction, and shunting) are important early in AP [8, 19, 27], other factors must come into play during the development of necrosis. In promoting the inflammatory response and the development of severe pancreatitis [10], tumor necrosis factor α (TNF-α) can act directly on the pancreas to cause death by either apoptosis [28] or necrosis [25]. A porcine model of AP has demonstrated that apoptosis is associated with interstitial oedematous pancreatitis (IOP), while necrotic cell death is a feature of pancreatic necrosis [29]. The effect of fluid resuscitation on the development of pancreatic necrosis requires further study, as ischemia–reperfusion injury of the pancreas is likely to be an important factor in the development of pancreatic necrosis [13].

Infection of pancreatic necrosis

The infection of pancreatic necrosis usually heralds a worse clinical outcome and is an important determinant of AP severity [1, 5]. Although it may develop at any time during the disease course, infection most often occurs 2 weeks or more after the onset (Figure 2B.4) [30]; however up to a quarter of infected necrosis occurs before this time [31]. The bacteriology of the infected necrosis indicates that roughly half of the bacteria cultured are of enteric origin [32–34]. There has been a

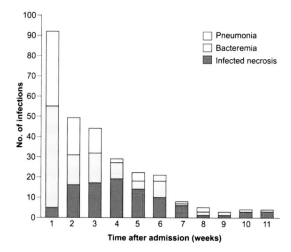

Figure 2B.4 Timing of diagnosis of infections (pneumonia, bacteremia, and infected necrosis) in 173 patients during a first episode of acute pancreatitis. Modified from [30].

shift toward gram-positive cocci and fungi in cultures from infected pancreatic necrosis, possibly due to the use of prophylactic antibiotics in some centers [32, 35]. A recent systematic review has highlighted the potential importance of extrapancreatic infections as a potential source of seeding bacteria and most notably bacteremia and pneumonia [36]. The extrapancreatic infections occur in a third of patients and at a mean interval of a week, which is well before the mean interval to infection of pancreatic necrosis (Figure 2B.4). It has been shown that bacteremia doubles the risk of infected necrosis and mortality [30]. The route by which bacteria infect the necrosis has been the subject of speculation, but the aforementioned evidence supports a hematogenous route, at least in some cases [37]. The paradox of this route is that antibiotics are currently delivered to the vascular compartment despite the fact that the target areas in the pancreas are necrotic and therefore lack a blood supply to deliver them. Other routes of infection seeding from the intestine are possible, including from duodeno-biliary–pancreatic reflux [38], bacterial translocation [39], transperitoneal [40], and lymphogenous [40]. Our group recently demonstrated in an experimental model that bacteria can rapidly pass by mesenteric lymph from the intestine into the pancreas through peripancreatic nodes [41]. It has been shown that mesenteric lymph can promote growth (or not) depending on the bacterial species and the inoculum size [42].

Intestinal pathophysiology

The intestine is no longer considered a passive bystander but an active contributor to the course and complications of AP [43]. As such the intestinal dysfunction associated with AP can be both a consequence and a cause of pathophysiology. Further, aspects of AP management can induce or exacerbate this intestinal dysfunction, including fluid resuscitation (ischemia–reperfusion injury), "nil per os" (failure of gut barrier), narcotic analgesia (ileus), nonselective inotropes (ischemia), and antibiotics (dysbiosis) (Figure 2B.1). The intestine, in its own right, should be considered one of the end organs that become dysfunctional and fail in AP, but current accepted organ failure scoring systems (e.g., SOFA, Marshall, and APACHE II) do not include the intestine.

Intestinal morphology and local complications in acute pancreatitis

The intestine undergoes characteristic changes in severe AP. While the intestine often appears normal on inspection during laparotomy, there can be significant underlying mucosal ischemia [44, 45]. The intestine may also become distended and adynamic [46], especially with heavy narcotic requirements, developing intestinal ileus. These patients might also develop enteral feeding intolerance [47]. Patients who remain hypovolemic, especially those on inotropes, may develop more obvious intestinal ischemia [48], often evidenced by *Pneumatosis intestinalis*. Rarely the intestine can become necrotic and perforate, leading to contamination and peritonitis [49].

Intestinal barrier

The intestine forms an anatomical, functional, and immunological barrier between the external environment (including intestinal lumen) and the internal milieu [50, 51]. The intestinal epithelium has several important roles including nutrient homeostasis, as a source of hormones, cytokines, and antimicrobial peptides as well as a physical barrier against pathogens [51]. The integrity of this epithelial layer is maintained by apical tight junctions and junctional adherens molecules regulated by myosin phosphorylation and the contraction of actomyosin complexes [52]. Disruption of these junctions increases intestinal permeability exposing the intestinal wall and the immune system to luminal content [52]. In addition to the epithelial layer and the junctional complexes, the intestinal barrier is maintained with the aid of other elements including the mucus layer, intestinal blood flow, lymphoid tissue, enteric nervous system, and the luminal microbiome [50–52]. A recent meta-analysis revealed that 60% of patients with AP have measurable intestinal barrier dysfunction [53]. An example of the significance of this dysfunction is the correlation between endotoxemia and outcome in AP [43, 53].

Intestinal mucus

The mucus layer, comprised of mucin glycoproteins, oligosaccharides, antimicrobial products, and secretory IgA, provides a hydrophobic barrier preventing microflora from adhering to the gut wall and digestive enzymes from disrupting the epithelial barrier [51]. Intestinal ischemia–reperfusion injury causes an acute loss in the mucus layer, which increases gut permeability [54]. Experimentally, pancreatic proteases in the intestinal lumen have been shown to compound mucus injury [55, 56]. In hemorrhagic shock ligation of the pancreatic duct reduced the effect of mucosal villous injury and mucus loss suggesting that luminal pancreatic proteases are involved in these events [57].

Intestinal blood flow

The arterial supply to the intestine is from the celiac trunk and superior and inferior mesenteric arteries [58]. Ultimately blood flow from these major vessels reaches the serosal, submucosal, and mucosal plexi of the intestine. It is the mucosal plexi that ultimately supply the intestinal mucosa, including the villi [59]. In the villous the artery and vein run parallel to form a rich capillary network at the tip. As blood flows in opposite directions, a countercurrent flow of oxygen results, lowering the pO_2 at the tip rendering it susceptible to ischemia [58].

Intestinal blood flow is regulated by intrinsic and extrinsic mechanisms. Intrinsic mechanisms include local metabolic and myogenic control, reflexes, and the paracrine influence of vasoactive substances. Extrinsic mechanisms are sympathetic innervation, humoral vasoactive substances, and hemodynamic changes. Both septic [60] and hemorrhagic [15] models of shock have demonstrated an ability to maintain microcirculatory flow to jejunal mucosa indicating the presence of an autoregulatory mechanism (Figure 2B.3). Potentially, blood flow from the muscularis layer is directed by neurohumoral factors to the mucosa probably by increased vascular tone in tissues with low oxygen demand to supply tissues with higher demand [15]. Prolonged hypoperfusion mediated by splanchnic vasoconstriction leads to regional ischemia (nonocclusive mesenteric ischemia or NOMI) [13] as the autoregulatory mechanisms that extract oxygen to perfuse tissues become saturated [2].

Intestinal ischemia–reperfusion injury

Important to the development of intestinal dysfunction/failure is the role of ischemia–reperfusion injury. Hypotension is a feature of severe AP and is largely due to third-space fluid loss secondary to increased capillary permeability and the development of edema [2, 6]. Reflex sympathetic vasoconstriction of splanchnic post-capillary veins and venules in response to hypotension is necessary to maintain perfusion of vital end organs

[61]. The consequence of this in the intestine is mucosal ischemia. Nasogastric tonometry has demonstrated that a low pHi (derived gastric intramucosal pH) correlates with severity and outcome in AP [44, 45]. This intestinal ischemia is an early event in AP with experimental studies documenting mitochondrial dysfunction in both the pancreas and jejunum within hours of the onset of AP [62]. With ischemia the epithelial cells separate at the tip and then down the sides of the villous [63]. Fluid resuscitation exposes tissue to a reoxygenation injury as the splanchnic bed is reperfused [64], but since it is the last organ to be reperfused, the intestine is subjected to an ongoing ischemic injury, compounding by the subsequent reperfusion injury. Reperfusion exacerbates microvascular dysfunction by impairing arteriolar dilation, leukocyte–endothelial adherence, enhancing fluid leak, and leukocyte plugging of capillaries [65]. There is also a surge in the production of oxygen radicals and a reduction in nitric oxide leading to increased inflammatory mediators (PAF, TNF-α). Together these events, which are characteristic of ischemia–reperfusion injury, lead to mucosal cell apoptosis [66] and disruption of the intestinal mucosal barrier [13]. Intestinal ischemia also impairs pancreatic microcirculation (velocity mm/s) on intravital microscopy (Figure 2B.5) and increases the severity of experimental AP through the effect of mesenteric lymph [15]. Periods of fasting (nil by mouth), including during parenteral nutrition, induce atrophy of the intestinal mucosa [68] and increase enterocyte apoptosis [69]. Histologically, villous atrophy has been documented in patients with AP [70]. And the histological changes seen following intestinal ischemia–reperfusion in experimental models are similar to that seen following AP [67, 71], including following pancreatic transplantation [72].

Intestinal microbiome

The human microbiome consists of more than 100 trillion microorganisms [73]. These organisms interact with their human host in a mutualistic relationship by producing vitamins and hormones and consuming nutrients necessary for pathogenic organisms as well as secreting substances to inhibit their growth [52]. Microbes indirectly affect epithelial permeability by acting on host immune cells via cytokines to increase (TFG-β IL-10) or decrease (TNF-α IFN-γ) permeability [74]. In acute and critical illness, including AP, the microbiome can sense host factors that lead to the

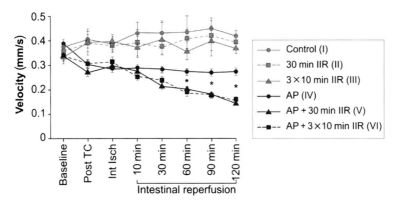

Figure 2B.5 Intravital microscopy sodium taurocholate model of acute pancreatitis effect on erythrocyte velocity (mm/s) with intestinal ischemia. (*$P < 0.05$ for difference between IV with both V and VI). Modified from [67].

development of increased virulence factors [51]. The predominance of enteric organisms cultured from infected pancreatic necrosis suggests that the intestinal microbiome is a major source of pathogens [75]. Lacto-bacilli are important in regulating the microbiome and are significantly reduced early in AP coinciding with a subsequent increase in enterobacterial overgrowth [76, 77]. Overgrowth is associated with translocation and ileus, where the interstitial cells of Cajal and myenteric neurons modulate slow wave propagation [78]. It is common in traditional Chinese medicine to administer an oral cathartic agent to cause diarrhea and decrease the bacterial load [79]. Prebiotics and probiotics have been promoted as possible treatment for restoring the dysbiosis in AP [51]. One study when *Lactobacillus* was administered early in AP documented a significant reduction in the subsequent rate of infected pancreatic necrosis [80]. Oral or enteral feeding is also important to prevent bacterial overgrowth, as well as maintain the enterocyte population, prevent mucosal and villous atrophy, and increased intestinal permeability [81]. By these means enteral nutrition in AP reduces infectious complications, pancreatic infections, and mortality [82]. But there is evidence from critically ill patients that standard enteral feeding (lacking in fiber) with proton-pump inhibitors is associated with dysbiosis [83].

Intestinal lymph

Intestinal barrier dysfunction is related to end-organ failure (see Chapter 2c). Throughout the 1980s the intestine was thought to contribute to multiorgan failure (MOF) through bacterial translocation [51], which has been documented in AP [53]. However,

this theory was challenged by Moore in 1994 [84] who proposed that neutrophils are primed by passing through the mesenteric circulation after it has been exposed to ischemia and reperfusion. It was proposed that activated neutrophils via the portal venous circulation mediate end-organ dysfunction/failure. A third model has been proposed by Deitch in which intestinal lymph containing toxic factors released from the ischemic intestine, transported by the thoracic duct, and bypassing the portal venous circulation and liver are responsible for driving organ dysfunction/failure [85, 86]. It is likely that both neutrophils primed in the ischemic intestine and toxic lymph derived from the intestine have important roles in the development of the systemic complications of AP.

Conclusion

The impact of AP on the pancreas and the intestine is profound. The pathophysiological events in these organs and the complex interplay between them are important in driving the disease course. These events include activation of the inflammatory pathways, microcirculatory failure, alterations in the microbiome, and breakdown of the intestinal barrier. Research priorities include understanding the mechanisms that determine why some patients develop pancreatic necrosis and why some subsequently develop infection. It is time that the intestine is considered an end organ in its own right, which necessitates an understanding of how the intestine fails and contributes to the severity of AP. The role of altered mesenteric lymph in the development of infected necrosis and end-organ dysfunction warrants further investigation, and this might offer new targets for treatment.

References

1 Petrov MS, Shanbhag S, Chakraborty M, Phillips ARJ, Windsor JA. Organ failure and infection of pancreatic necrosis as determinants of mortality in patients with acute pancreatitis. Gastroenterology. 2010;139(3):813–820.

2 Flint RS, Windsor JA. The role of the intestine in the pathophysiology and management of severe acute pancreatitis. Hepato Pancreato Biliary. 2003;5(2):69–85.

3 Bollen TL. Imaging of acute pancreatitis: update of the revised Atlanta classification. Radiologic Clinics of North America. 2012;50(3):429–445.

4 Banks PA, Bollen TL, Dervenis C, Gooszen HG, Johnson CD, Sarr MG, et al. Classification of acute pancreatitis-2012: revision of the Atlanta classification and definitions by international consensus. Gut. 2013;62(1):102–111.

5 Dellinger EP, Forsmark CE, Layer P, Levy P, Maravi-Poma E, Petrov MS, et al. Determinant-based classification of acute pancreatitis severity: an international multidisciplinary consultation. Ann Surg. 2012;256(6):875–880.

6 Cuthbertson CM, Christophi C. Disturbances of the microcirculation in acute pancreatitis. British Journal of Surgery. 2006;93(5):518–530.

7 Menger MD, Plusczyk T, Vollmar B. Microcirculatory derangements in acute pancreatitis. Journal of Hepato-Biliary-Pancreatic Surgery. 2001;8(3):187–194.

8 Plusczyk T, Witzel B, Menger MD, Schilling M. ETA and ETB receptor function in pancreatitis-associated microcirculatory failure, inflammation, and parenchymal injury. American Journal of Physiology: Gastrointestinal and Liver Physiology. 2003;285(1):G145-G153.

9 Kloppel G. Pathomorphology of acute pancreatitis. Annali Italiani di Chirurgia 1995;66(2):149–154.

10 Khokhar AS, Seidner DL. The pathophysiology of pancreatitis. Nutrition in Clinical Practice. 2004;19(1):5–15.

11 Windsor JA, Petrov MS. Acute pancreatitis reclassified. Gut. 2013;62(1):4–5.

12 Lewis MP, Reber HA, Ashley SW. Pancreatic blood flow and its role in the pathophysiology of pancreatitis. Journal of Surgical Research. 1998;75(1):81–89.

13 Oldenburg WA, Lau LL, Rodenberg TJ, Edmonds HJ, Burger CD. Acute mesenteric ischemia: a clinical review. Archives of Internal Medicine. 2004;164(10):1054–1062.

14 Ballian N, Brunicardi FC. Islet vasculature as a regulator of endocrine pancreas function. World Journal of Surgery. 2007;31(4):705–714.

15 Krejci V, Hiltebrand L, Banic A, Erni D, Wheatley AM, Sigurdsson GH. Continuous measurements of microcirculatory blood flow in gastrointestinal organs during acute haemorrhage. British Journal of Anaesthesia. 2000;84(4):468–475.

16 Phillips AR, Farrant GJ, Abu-Zidan FM, Cooper GJ, Windsor JA. A method using laser Doppler flowmetry to study intestinal and pancreatic perfusion during an acute intestinal ischaemic injury in rats with pancreatitis. European Surgical Research. 2001;33(5–6):361–369.

17 Saluja AK, Steer MLP. Pathophysiology of pancreatitis. Role of cytokines and other mediators of inflammation. Digestion. 1999;60 Suppl 1:27–33.

18 Bassi D, Kollias N, Fernandez-del Castillo C, Foitzik T, Warshaw AL, Rattner DW. Impairment of pancreatic microcirculation correlates with the severity of acute experimental pancreatitis. Journal of the American College of Surgeons. 1994;179(3):257–263.

19 Kelly DM, McEntee GP, McGeeney KF, Fitzpatrick JM. Microvasculature of the pancreas, liver, and kidney in cerulein-induced pancreatitis. Archives of Surgery. 1993;128(3):293–295.

20 Salomone T, Tosi P, Palareti G, Tomassetti P, Migliori M, Guariento A, et al. Coagulative disorders in human acute pancreatitis: role for the D-dimer. Pancreas. 2003;26(2):111–116.

21 Ranson JH, Lackner H, Berman IR, Schinella R. The relationship of coagulation factors to clinical complications of acute pancreatitis. Surgery. 1977;81(5):502–511.

22 Ceranowicz P, Dembinski A, Warzecha Z, Dembinski M, Cieszkowski J, Rembisz K, et al. Protective and therapeutic effect of heparin in acute pancreatitis. Journal of Physiology and Pharmacology 2008;59 Suppl 4:103–125.

23 Mimidis K, Papadopoulos V, Kartasis Z, Baka M, Tsatlidis V, Bourikas G, et al. Assessment of platelet adhesiveness and aggregation in mild acute pancreatitis using the PFA-100 system. Journal of the Pancreas. 2004;5(3):132–137.

24 Kinnala PJ, Kuttila KT, Gronroos JM, Havia TV, Nevalainen TJ, Niinikoski JH. Pancreatic tissue perfusion in experimental acute pancreatitis. European Journal of Surgery. 2001;167(9):689–694.

25 Spanier BWM, Nio Y, van der Hulst RWM, Tuynman HARE, Dijkgraaf MGW, Bruno MJ. Practice and yield of early CT scan in acute pancreatitis: a Dutch Observational Multicenter Study. Pancreatology. 2010;10(2–3):222–228.

26 Denham W, Norman J. The potential role of therapeutic cytokine manipulation in acute pancreatitis. Surgical Clinics of North America. 1999;79(4):767–781.

27 Klar E, Schratt W, Foitzik T, Buhr H, Herfarth C, Messmer K. Impact of microcirculatory flow pattern changes on the development of acute edematous and necrotizing pancreatitis in rabbit pancreas. Digestive Diseases and Sciences. 1994;39(12):2639–2644.

28 Norman J. The role of cytokines in the pathogenesis of acute pancreatitis. The American Journal of Surgery. 1998;175(1):76–83.

29 Merilainen S, Makela J, Anttila V, Koivukangas V, Kaakinen H, Niemela E, et al. Acute edematous and necrotic pancreatitis in a porcine model. Scandinavian Journal of Gastroenterology. 2008;43(10):1259–1268.

30 Besselink MG, van Santvoort HC, Boermeester MA, Nieuwenhuijs VB, van Goor H, Dejong CHC, et al. Timing and impact of infections in acute pancreatitis. British Journal of Surgery. 2009;96(3):267–273.

31 Petrov MS, Chong V, Windsor JA. Infected pancreatic necrosis: not necessarily a late event in acute pancreatitis. World Journal of Gastroenterology. 2011;17(27):3173–3176.

32 Buchler MW, Gloor B, Muller CA, Friess H, Seiler CA, Uhl W. Acute necrotizing pancreatitis: treatment strategy according to the status of infection. Annals of Surgery. 2000;232(5):619–626.

33 Isenmann R, Schwarz M, Rau B, Trautmann M, Schober W, Beger HG. Characteristics of infection with Candida species in patients with necrotizing pancreatitis. World Journal of Surgery. 2002;26(3):372–376.

34 Fernandez-del Castillo C, Rattner DW, Makary MA, Mostafavi A, McGrath D, Warshaw AL. Debridement and closed packing for the treatment of necrotizing pancreatitis. Annals of Surgery. 1998;228(5):676–684.

35 Howard TJ, Temple MB. Prophylactic antibiotics alter the bacteriology of infected necrosis in severe acute pancreatitis. Journal of the American College of Surgeons. 2002;195(6):759–767.

36 Brown LA, Hore TA, Phillips ARJ, Windsor JA, Petrov MS. A systematic review of the extra-pancreatic infectious complications in acute pancreatitis. Pancreatology. 2014;14(6):436–443.

37 Widdison AL, Karanjia ND, Reber HA. Routes of spread of pathogens into the pancreas in a feline model of acute pancreatitis. Gut. 1994;35(9):1306–1310.

38 Opie EL. The relation of cholelithiasis to disease of the pancreas and to fat necrosis. American Journal of the Medical Sciences. 1901;121(1):27–42.

39 Deitch EA, Berg R. Bacterial translocation from the gut: a mechanism of infection. The Journal of Burn Care & Rehabilitation. 1987;8(6):475–482.

40 Buchler MW, Uhl W, Malfertheiner P, Sarr MG. Diseases of the Pancreas: Acute pancreatitis, Chronic Pancreatitis, Neoplasms of the Pancreas. Basel, Switzerland: Karger Publishers; 2004.

41 Loveday BP. Infected Local Complications of Acute Pancreatitis: The Role of Lymphatics and Minimal Access Treatment. Auckland: The University of Auckland; 2012.

42 Loveday BPT, Phillips ARJ, Swirft S, Windsor JA. Does mesenteric lymph inhibit or promote bacterial growth? Pancreatology. 2014;14(3):S11.

43 Windsor JA, Fearon KC, Ross JA, Barclay GR, Smyth E, Poxton I, et al. Role of serum endotoxin and antiendotoxin core antibody levels in predicting the development of multiple organ failure in acute pancreatitis. British Journal of Surgery. 1993;80(8):1042–1046.

44 Bonham MJ, Abu-Zidan FM, Simovic MO, Windsor JA. Gastric intramucosal pH predicts death in

severe acute pancreatitis. British Journal of Surgery. 1997;84(12):1670–1674.

45 Kovacs GC, Telek G, Hamar J, Furesz J, Regoly-Merei J. Prolonged intestinal mucosal acidosis is associated with multiple organ failure in human acute pancreatitis: gastric tonometry revisited. World Journal of Gastroenterology. 2006;12(30):4892–4896.

46 Wang X, Gong Z, Wu K, Wang B, Yuang Y. Gastrointestinal dysmotility in patients with acute pancreatitis. Journal of Gastroenterology and Hepatology. 2003;18(1):57–62.

47 McClave SA. Nutrition support in acute pancreatitis. Gastroenterology Clinics of North America. 2007;36(1):65–74, vi.

48 Sautner T, Wessely C, Riegler M, Sedivy R, Gotzinger P, Losert U, et al. Early effects of catecholamine therapy on mucosal integrity, intestinal blood flow, and oxygen metabolism in porcine endotoxin shock. Annals of Surgery. 1998;228(2):239–248.

49 Hagiwara A, Miyauchi H, Shimazaki S. Predictors of vascular and gastrointestinal complications in severe acute pancreatitis. Pancreatology. 2008;8(2):211–218.

50 Camilleri M, Madsen K, Spiller R, Greenwood-Van Meerveld B, Verne GN. Intestinal barrier function in health and gastrointestinal disease. Neurogastroenterology & Motility. 2012;24(6):503–512.

51 Mittal R, Coopersmith CM. Redefining the gut as the motor of critical illness. Trends in Molecular Medicine. 2014;20(4):214–223.

52 Scaldaferri F, Pizzoferrato M, Gerardi V, Lopetuso L, Gasbarrini A. The gut barrier: new acquisitions and therapeutic approaches. Journal of Clinical Gastroenterology 2012;46 Suppl:S12-S17.

53 Wu LM, Sankaran SJ, Plank LD, Windsor JA, Petrov MS. Meta-analysis of gut barrier dysfunction in patients with acute pancreatitis. British Journal of Surgery. 2014;101(13):1644–1656.

54 Qin X, Caputo FJ, Xu D-Z, Deitch EA. Hydrophobicity of mucosal surface and its relationship to gut barrier function. Shock. 2008;29(3):372–376.

55 Sharpe SM, Qin X, Lu Q, Feketeova E, Palange DC, Dong W, et al. Loss of the intestinal mucus layer in the normal rat causes gut injury but not toxic mesenteric lymph nor lung injury. Shock. 2010;34(5):475–481.

56 Fishman JE, Levy G, Alli V, Zheng X, Mole DJ, Deitch EA. The intestinal mucus layer is a critical component of the gut barrier that is damaged during acute pancreatitis. Shock. 2014;42(3):264–270.

57 Caputo FJ, Rupani B, Watkins AC, Barlos D, Vega D, Senthil M, et al. Pancreatic duct ligation abrogates the trauma hemorrhage-induced gut barrier failure and the subsequent production of biologically active intestinal lymph. Shock. 2007;28(4):441–446.

58 Takala J. Determinants of splanchnic blood flow. British Journal of Anaesthesia.77(1):50–58.

59 van Wijck K, Lenaerts K, Grootjans J, Wijnands KAP, Poeze M, van Loon LJC, et al. Physiology and pathophysiology of splanchnic hypoperfusion and intestinal injury during exercise: strategies for evaluation and prevention. American Journal of Physiology: Gastrointestinal and Liver Physiology. 2012;303(2):G155-G168.

60 Hiltebrand LB, Krejci V, Banic A, Erni D, Wheatley AM, Sigurdsson GH. Dynamic study of the distribution of microcirculatory blood flow in multiple splanchnic organs in septic shock. Critical Care Medicine. 2000;28(9):3233–3241.

61 Reilly PM, Wilkins KB, Fuh KC, Haglund U, Bulkley GB. The mesenteric hemodynamic response to circulatory shock: an overview. Shock. 2001;15(5):329–343.

62 Mittal A, Hickey AJR, Chai CC, Loveday BPT, Thompson N, Dare A, et al. Early organ-specific mitochondrial dysfunction of jejunum and lung found in rats with experimental acute pancreatitis. Hepato Pancreato Biliary. 2011;13(5):332–341.

63 Chiu CJ, McArdle AH, Brown R, Scott HJ, Gurd FN. Intestinal mucosal lesion in low-flow states. I. A morphological, hemodynamic, and metabolic reappraisal. Archives of Surgery. 1970;101(4):478–483.

64 Biffl WL, Moore EE. Splanchnic ischaemia/reperfusion and multiple organ failure. British Journal of Anaesthesia. 1996;77(1):59–70.

65 Carden DL, Granger DN. Pathophysiology of ischaemia-reperfusion injury. The Journal of Pathology. 2000;190(3): 255–266.

66 Tian R, Tan JT, Wang RL, Xie H, Qian YB, Yu KL. The role of intestinal mucosa oxidative stress in gut barrier dysfunction of severe acute pancreatitis. European Review for Medical and Pharmacological Sciences. 2013;17(3):349–355.

67 Flint RS, Phillips ARJ, Power SE, Dunbar PR, Brown C, Delahunt B, et al. Acute pancreatitis severity is exacerbated by intestinal ischemia-reperfusion conditioned mesenteric lymph. Surgery. 2008;143(3):404–413.

68 Hernandez G, Velasco N, Wainstein C, Castillo L, Bugedo G, Maiz A, et al. Gut mucosal atrophy after a short enteral fasting period in critically ill patients. Journal of Critical Care. 1999;14(2):73–77.

69 Fukuyama K, Iwakiri R, Noda T, Kojima M, Utsumi H, Tsunada S, et al. Apoptosis induced by ischemia-reperfusion and fasting in gastric mucosa compared to small intestinal mucosa in rats. Digestive Diseases and Sciences. 2001;46(3):545–549.

70 Ammori BJ, Cairns A, Dixon MF, Larvin M, McMahon MJ. Altered intestinal morphology and immunity in patients with acute necrotizing pancreatitis. Journal of Hepato-Biliary-Pancreatic Surgery. 2002;9(4):490–496.

71 Menger MD, Bonkhoff H, Vollmar B. Ischemia-reperfusion-induced pancreatic microvascular injury. An intravital fluorescence microscopic study in rats. Digestive Diseases and Sciences. 1996;41(5):823–830.

72 Busing M, Hopt UT, Quacken M, Becker HD, Morgenroth K. Morphological studies of graft pancreatitis following pancreas transplantation. British Journal of Surgery. 1993;80(9):1170–1173.

73 Arumugam M, Raes J, Pelletier E, Le Paslier D, Yamada T, Mende DR, et al. Enterotypes of the human gut microbiome.[Erratum appears in Nature. 2011 Jun 30;474(7353):666]. Nature. 2011;473(7346):174–180.

74 Arrieta MC, Bistritz L, Meddings JB. Alterations in intestinal permeability. Gut. 2006;55(10):1512–1520.

75 Howard TJ. The role of antimicrobial therapy in severe acute pancreatitis. Surgical Clinics of North America. 2013;93(3):585–593.

76 Wang X, Andersson R, Soltesz V, Leveau P, Ihse I. Gut origin sepsis, macrophage function, and oxygen extraction associated with acute pancreatitis in the rat. World Journal of Surgery. 1996;20(3):299–307; discussion −8.

77 Leveau P, Wang X, Soltesz V, Ihse I, Andersson R. Alterations in intestinal motility and microflora in experimental acute pancreatitis. International Journal of Pancreatology. 1996;20(2):119–125.

78 Zhou H, Liu L, Bai Y, Wu W, Li G, Li J, et al. Damage of the interstitial cells of Cajal and myenteric neurons causing ileus in acute necrotizing pancreatitis rats. Surgery. 2011;149(2):262–275.

79 Chen D-c, Wang L. Mechanisms of therapeutic effects of rhubarb on gut origin sepsis. Chinese Journal of Traumatology. 2009;12(6):365–369.

80 Olah A, Belagyi T, Issekutz A, Gamal ME, Bengmark S. Randomized clinical trial of specific lactobacillus and fibre supplement to early enteral nutrition in patients with acute pancreatitis. British Journal of Surgery. 2002;89(9):1103–1107.

81 Marik PE, Zaloga GP. Meta-analysis of parenteral nutrition versus enteral nutrition in patients with acute pancreatitis. British Medical Journal. 2004;328(7453):1407.

82 Petrov MS, van Santvoort HC, Besselink MGH, van der Heijden GJMG, Windsor JA, Gooszen HG. Enteral nutrition and the risk of mortality and infectious complications in patients with severe acute pancreatitis: a meta-analysis of randomized trials. Archives of Surgery. 2008;143(11):1111–1117.

83 O'Keefe SJD, Ou J, Delany JP, Curry S, Zoetendal E, Gaskins HR, et al. Effect of fiber supplementation on the microbiota in critically ill patients. World Journal of Gastrointestinal Pathophysiology. 2011;2(6):138–145.

84 Moore EE, Moore FA, Franciose RJ, Kim FJ, Biffl WL, Banerjee A. The postischemic gut serves as a priming bed for circulating neutrophils that provoke multiple organ failure. Journal of Trauma. 1994;37(6):881–887.

85 Deitch EA, Xu D, Kaise VL. Role of the gut in the development of injury- and shock induced SIRS and MODS: the gut-lymph hypothesis, a review. Frontiers in Bioscience 2006;11:520–528.

86 Fanous MYZ, Phillips AJ, Windsor JA. Mesenteric lymph: the bridge to future management of critical illness. Journal of the Pancreas. 2007;8(4):374–399.

PART C: Pathophysiology of systemic inflammatory response syndrome and multiorgan dysfunction syndrome in acute pancreatitis

Pramod Kumar Garg

Department of Gastroenterology, All India Institute of Medical Sciences, New Delhi, India

Acute pancreatitis (AP) runs a severe course in 20–30% of patients with a mortality of up to 40% [1]. Severe pancreatitis is associated with systemic inflammation and remote organ dysfunction [2]. There is a correlation between the extent of pancreatic necrosis and organ failure [3, 4]. Although there has been a decline in mortality due to improved intensive and minimally invasive care [5], a substantial reduction in mortality will require a breakthrough in our understanding of the critical molecular pathways leading to severe AP.

It is helpful to recognize three phases in the evolution of AP: (i) initiation, (ii) perpetuation, and (iii) secondary escalation phases. The initiation phase starts in the pancreatic acinar cells leading to cellular injury and inflammation within the pancreas (Chapter 2a). The perpetuating events in the inflammatory process involve recruitment and activation of immune cells mainly leukocytes, in the pancreas and intestine (Chapter 2b). In the secondary escalation phase, infection of pancreatic necrosis leads to an accentuated systemic inflammatory response and organ dysfunction. The patterns of inflammation and its consequences are reasonably similar between different acute diseases, including AP, sepsis, burns, hemorrhage, and major trauma. In AP, inflammation is initiated from within the acinar cell, which leads to pancreatic and peripancreatic inflammation, and then to systemic inflammation and organ dysfunction. This chapter focuses on the pathophysiology of the systemic inflammatory response syndrome (SIRS) and multiple organ dysfunction syndrome (MODS) in AP.

Systemic inflammatory response syndrome

(SIRS) SIRS is a clinical syndrome comprising at least two of these four features: tachycardia, tachypnea, leukocytosis, and altered body temperature. The diagnostic criteria of SIRS are given in Table 2C.1. SIRS persisting for more than 48 h may indicate severe AP [6], and it is one of the predictors currently recommended for severity assessment [7].

Multiple organ dysfunction syndrome (MODS)

Severe systemic inflammation is associated with dysfunction of vital end organs, including the cardiovascular, respiratory, and renal systems. While the inflammatory and immune responses to acute disease can be protective, in the setting of severe AP, there is an out of proportion and dysregulated immune response and hyperinflammation, which can result in end-organ dysfunction and failure. This can occur at anytime during the course of AP, but it appears that early and late organ dysfunction result from different mechanisms. Early organ dysfunction occurs as a result of severe systemic inflammatory response. Pancreatitis with early organ failure developing within a few days of its onset, termed early severe acute pancreatitis (ESAP), carries a high mortality [8]. This is mainly due to sterile inflammation whereas late organ dysfunction

Pancreatitis: Medical and Surgical Management, First Edition.
David B. Adams, Peter B. Cotton, Nicholas J. Zyromski and John Windsor.
© 2017 John Wiley & Sons, Ltd. Published 2017 by John Wiley & Sons, Ltd.

Table 2C.1 Diagnostic criteria for systemic inflammatory response syndrome.

Body temperature	>38 °C (100.4 °F) or <36 °C (96.8 °F)
Heart rate	>90/min
Respiratory rate	>20 breaths/min or PaCO$_2$ <32 mmHg
Total leukocyte count	>12,000/cmm or <4,000/cmm or >10% immature cells

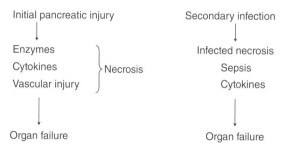

Figure 2C.1 Representation of different mechanisms of organ failure during early and late phases of acute pancreatitis due to sterile inflammation and sepsis, respectively.

follows secondary infection of pancreatic necrosis with sepsis. The pathophysiological mechanisms driving these phases of organ dysfunction in AP are different and not well understood (Figure 2C.1). As the pattern and consequences of SIRS and MODS are similar in sepsis, hemorrhage, and trauma, it is worth considering some of the insights gained from the study of these acute diseases. Organ dysfunction of at least grade 2 that persists for >48 h defines severe AP [9]. The modified Marshall's system has been recommended for scoring organ dysfunction in AP (Table 2C.2).

Activation of innate immune system

The innate immune system is activated by foreign (*nonself*) antigens particularly microbe-related peptides. Cells involved in innate immunity possess pattern recognition receptors (PRRs), which recognize what are termed as "pathogen-associated molecular patterns" (PAMPs) present on the microbes. There are four types of receptors: Toll-like receptors (TLRs), nucleotide-binding oligomerization domain (NOD)-like receptors (NLR), retinoic acid-inducible gene 1-like receptors, and C-type lectin receptors. The NLR act in concert with cytoplasmic protein complexes called inflammasomes. When stimulated by PAMPs through PRRs, the immune cells

(especially macrophages) become activated and secrete cytokines and chemokines, which lead to inflammation.

Similar to microbe-related PAMPs, there are certain *self* molecules that can stimulate immune cells. These molecules are normally not exposed to the immune cells but are released from dying cells (e.g., necrotic acinar cells in AP). These molecules also stimulate the innate immune cells through the same receptors, that is, PRRs. These self molecules are called "damage-associated molecular patterns" (DAMPs). Various molecules that act as DAMPs include high-mobility group (HMG) proteins particularly B1 (HMGB1), S100 proteins, extracellular double-stranded DNA (dsDNA), ATP, and many others. The subsequent activation of immune cells and inflammatory response are similar through the PAMP and DAMP pathways, that is, whether they follow microbial infection or sterile inflammatory diseases.

DAMPs, inflammation, and acute pancreatitis

Different DAMPs activate different PRRs on immune cells. For example, HMGB1 activates TLR-4 while dsDNA activates TLR-9. Following activation of the surface receptor, downstream signaling involves the NF-kB pathway to upregulate gene transcription of proinflammatory cytokines (e.g., pro-IL-1 and pro-IL-18) (Figure 2C.2). DAMP also mediates another signal, for example, ATP acting on the immune cell P2X7 surface receptor and NLRP3 cytoplasmic receptor complex "inflammasome." Activation of NLRP3 inflammasome releases caspase-1 that mediates the conversion of pro-IL-1 and pro-IL-18 to active IL-1 and IL-18. Caspase-1 activity has been correlated with the severity of sepsis. Inhibition of caspase-1 prevented acute kidney injury induced by endotoxin and acute lung injury in AP [10, 11]. HMGB1, a potent DAMP, has been found to be increased in patients with AP, and

Table 2C.2 Modified Marshall's scoring system for grading organ failure.

Organ system	Grade				
	0	1	2	3	4
Respiratory (PaO$_2$/FIO$_2$)	>400	301–400	201–300	101–200	≤101
Renal (serum creatinine, mg/dl)	<1.5	1.5–1.9	1.9–3.5	3.5–4.9	≥5
Cardiovascular (systolic blood pressure, mmHg)	>90	<90 Fluid responsive	<90 Not fluid responsive	<90, pH <7.3	<90, pH <7.2

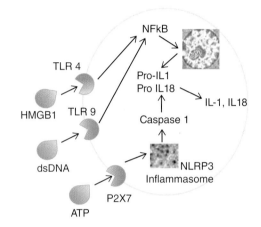

Figure 2C.2 Schematic representation of activation of immune cells by damage-associated molecular pattern (DAMP) through pattern recognition receptors (PRRs) and release of inflammatory mediators.

serum levels of HMGB1 correlate with disease severity [12, 13]. Inhibition of HMGB1 release from necrotic pancreatic tissue protects against systemic organ injury in experimental AP [9].

Consistent with the role of TLR-4 through which HMGB1 acts, it was shown that the severity of AP and associated lung injury was ameliorated in a TLR-4 knockout mouse model of experimental pancreatitis [14]. In experimental pancreatitis, ethyl pyruvate decreased the levels of HMGB1, TNF-α, and IL-1β, and this decreased the severity of AP and also reduced associated lung injury [15].

Serum levels of extracellular DNA are increased in experimental AP. Following activation of TLR-9 by mitochondrial DNA (ATP6 gene), there was a marked secretion of IL-1β, a mediator of inflammation [16]. Biochemical inhibition of TLR-9 resulted in decreased inflammation and severity of AP and subdued inflammation. Similar findings were noted in TLR-9 knockout animals [16].

Interestingly, TLR-4 and TLR-9 are expressed on pancreatic ductal cells and resident macrophages but not on acinar cells, which suggests that it is the immune cells and not acinar cells that produce the proinflammatory cytokines in response to DAMPs.

Escalation of systemic inflammation

After activation, immune cells secrete many proinflammatory cytokines, including TNF-α and IL-1. The initial inflammatory response by itself does not have significant clinical consequences, but it leads to the adherence, migration, and activation of leukocytes. The different types of leukocytes (i.e., neutrophils, monocytes, and lymphocytes) play important roles in escalating the local inflammation and promoting systemic inflammation and organ dysfunction.

The infiltration of leukocytes is an orderly process that requires upregulation of vascular endothelial adhesion molecules and interaction of activated leukocytes with these adhesion molecules via their ligands, namely, selectins and integrins [17]. P-selectin and E-selectin are upregulated in experimental pancreatitis. The interaction of endothelial and leukocyte selectins is involved in leukocyte attachment and rolling prior to their migration across the endothelium [18]. Blood levels of soluble P-selectin and E-selectin correlated with the severity of pancreatitis and lung injury, respectively, in a human study [19]. Upregulation of endothelial cell adhesion molecule ICAM-1 has been well studied in experimental AP [20]. Mac-1 and LFA-1 integrins act as intercellular ligands for the endothelial adhesion molecules facilitating leukocyte migration [21, 22]. Anti-ICAM-1 antibodies reduce the severity of experimental AP and its associated lung injury suggesting that leukocyte infiltration is an important event in determining the severity of AP [23].

The leukocytes have complimentary roles in promoting inflammation. The effects of the neutrophils are mediated through their enzymes such as MPO and proteases, that is, elastase. Neutrophilic elastase is considered responsible for tissue damage such as lung injury [24]. Monocytes also infiltrate the pancreas along with neutrophils. Monocytes secrete proinflammatory cytokines such as IL-1, IL-6, and TNF-α. Il-6 levels in the blood have been shown to correlate with organ injury and severe pancreatitis in humans [25]. Lymphocytes, mediator of the adaptive immune response, have also been shown to be involved in AP. CD4-positive cells are found within the pancreas within 6 h of caerulein-induced AP [26]. Serum levels of soluble CD4 receptors were significantly higher in patients with AP compared with healthy controls [27].

Inflammatory mediators in AP

Inflammatory cytokines are considered to play a central role in pathophysiology of AP, including the development and progression of MODS [28, 29]. Some are proinflammatory and others anti-inflammatory. Many inflammatory mediators have been studied in AP as risk factors, prognostic markers, and possible therapeutic targets. The array of proinflammatory cytokines has been described as a cascade, with multiple complimentary roles and significant redundancy. A description of the multiple roles of the numerous inflammatory cytokines is beyond the scope of this chapter. However, three key cytokines merit a brief description.

Interleukin-1 (IL-1) produced by activated macrophages mediates recruitment of neutrophils and other immune cells to promote inflammation. IL-1β has been most extensively studied for its role in AP. TNF-α is a proinflammatory cytokine that plays a pivotal role in AP. It is one of the earliest cytokines which is increased in AP. It can cause upregulation of other cytokines, synthesis of free radical species, cell death, and endothelial activation. It is an important determinant of the systemic progression and organ failure in AP [30, 31]. TNF-α and IL-1 augment inflammatory response by activating macrophages to release other inflammatory mediators (IL-6, IL-8, and MIF) and reactive oxygen and nitrogen species leading to organ dysfunction [32]. Injection of TNF-α and IL-1 causes a septic shock-like syndrome in experimental animals, which act synergistically [33]. IL-6 is another important and extensively studied molecule in AP. IL-6 levels rise subsequent to TNF-α and IL-1 release. IL-6 activates B and T lymphocytes and the coagulation system. In IL-6-knockout mice, lung inflammation was significantly less in a model of acute lung injury, and there was protection from organ failure in a model of acute peritoneal inflammation with decreased mortality [34]. Many studies have shown that levels of IL-6 correlate with organ failure and mortality [25, 35, 36].

Circulatory disturbances

Circulatory disturbances in AP contribute to systemic organ dysfunction. Both pancreatic microcirculation and systemic circulation are affected [37]. At the local level, microcirculatory changes include reduced pancreatic blood flow leading to pancreatic ischemia and increased capillary permeability [38]. Endothelial cell dysfunction leads to loss of barrier function that promotes capillary leakage, edema formation, and sequestration of activated immune cells into tissues. Increased vascular permeability is an important consequence of AP that results in edema and systemic effects such as pleural effusion and ascites [39]. It also exacerbates the systemic hemodynamic disturbances. Such changes in the circulation affect tissue oxygenation and lead to distant organ dysfunction. The relationship of circulatory changes with AP is bidirectional. Severe AP may cause profound adverse effect on systemic hemodynamic status that may result in circulatory failure with hypotension and acute renal failure. Myocardial contractility is suppressed by high levels of inflammatory mediators including NO [40]. Circulatory changes in turn may further exacerbate AP due to pancreatic ischemia.

Coagulopathy and systemic inflammation

The systemic inflammatory response is associated with coagulation abnormalities [41]. Intravascular coagulation may exacerbate pancreatitis by impairing the microcirculation, and microthrombi may be seen in AP [42]. Derangement in the coagulation might be due to a protease-mediated state of hypercoagulability and activation of fibrinolysis. Raised D-dimer serum levels on admission predict severe AP, the development of organ failure [41], and clinical outcome [43]. Heparin improves the microcirculation in experimental AP, particularly decreasing leukocyte–endothelium interactions. Both antithrombin III and heparin have been shown to reduce the severity of AP in animal models [44, 45]. A recent randomized controlled clinical trial from China showed that heparin improved survival over conventional treatment in severe AP [46].

Visceral adipose tissue and systemic inflammation

In addition to the pancreas, the intestine and adipose tissue also contribute to systemic inflammation (Figure 2C.3). The important role of the intestine in the pathophysiology of AP has been covered in the chapter 2B. Adipose tissue also has a role in promoting systemic inflammation. Clinical observations have consistently shown that obese patients have a more severe course of pancreatitis [47]. In a systematic review, obesity was found to be associated with an augmented inflammatory response and a worse outcome in AP [48]. Visceral adipose tissue appears to be the major culprit [49] and acts as an endocrine organ, releasing many proinflammatory cytokines and adipokines (including adiponectin and leptin). These correlate with the severity of AP and other prognostic markers such as APACHE II and serum CRP levels [50]. Another mechanism is lipolysis of adipose tissue by activated pancreatic enzymes that releases toxic lipids which act as proinflammatory mediators. In an

experimental study, unsaturated fatty acids from lipolysis of visceral fat by pancreatic lipases converted mild AP into severe AP in obese mice [51]. In another study, necrotic collections from patients with AP showed higher levels of fatty acids, IL-8, and IL-1β compared with pseudocyst fluid. In a rodent study, administration of free fatty acids and IL-1 resulted in more pancreatic necrosis, but administration of triolein caused more severe MODS and mortality [52]. In a clinical study, the increased volume of intrapancreatic adipocytes was associated with more pancreatic necrosis and MODS [53]. In a human study, it has been shown that the levels of proinflammatory cytokines were significantly higher in patients with central fat distribution and the levels correlated with the severity of AP [54]. Thus, there are experimental and clinical evidences to show that excess visceral adipose tissue contributes to a more marked systemic inflammatory response and organ dysfunction in AP.

Inflammation and organ dysfunction

An intense systemic inflammatory response is associated with an increased risk of organ dysfunction, failure, and death in patients with AP. The key pathophysiology events in the different end organs are (i) circulatory changes such as vasodilation, capillary leakage, and edema, (ii) tissue hypoxia due to hypotension and coagulation abnormality, and (iii) cellular injury mediated by inflammation and mitochondrial injury. These common manifestations of end-organ dysfunction in different diseases suggest common pathophysiological mechanisms. It is unlikely that systemic inflammation promoted by events in the pancreas, the intestine, and the adipose tissue are sufficient to explain the development MODS. There is emerging evidence that the altered composition of mesenteric lymph, draining from the pancreas, intestine, and adipose tissue may promote MODS, the so-called "gut lymph hypothesis" [55]. While there is evidence of migration of inflammatory cells (neutrophils and macrophages), increased capillary leak, and edema in end organs, there is surprisingly little apoptotic or necrotic cell death. Recovery of end-organ function is usually rapid and complete, which suggests that organ failure is more of a functional issue than tissue injury. This realization has increased the interest in the role of mitochondrial dysfunction in MODS.

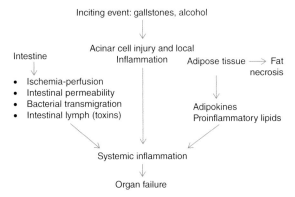

Figure 2C.3 Drivers of systemic inflammation in acute pancreatitis: apart from the pancreas itself, intestine and adipose tissue play major roles in the development of MODS.

Mitochondrial dysfunction in MODS

Mitochondria provide ATP for cellular processes, consume 98% of the body's oxygen, and generate reactive oxygen species (ROS). The excess production of ROS, NO, and other compounds cause direct damage to mitochondria [56]. Sustained opening of mitochondrial permeability transition pore, commonly referred to as the mitochondrial permeability transition (MPT), leads to loss of the chemiosmotic gradient generated across the inner mitochondrial membrane by proton pumping and the ability to produce ATP. When ATP generation is reduced to below a critical threshold, as with hypotension and microcirculatory disturbances, mitochondrial dysfunction may induce cellular necrosis. Apoptosis is also initiated through release of mitochondrial cytochrome *c* into the cytoplasm. Mitophagy is a process of degrading damaged mitochondria as a protective response. Increased oxidative stress and other processes can inactivate mitophagy. Mitophagy has been shown as a part of general autophagy (macroautophagy) in AP [57]. Impaired autophagy has been observed in a mouse model of AP [58]. Inadequate ATP production can also lead to a hibernation state [59]. The reduced cellular activity due to mitochondrial dysfunction may translate into organ dysfunction. Recovery of organs within days to weeks after controlling the infection or resolution of AP suggests that the cellular and possible mitochondrial dysfunction rather than cell death is the main driver of organ dysfunction.

Areas for future research

A complete understanding of the pathophysiology of AP is still far from clear. In experimental AP, the pancreatic injury is predictable and measurable, but the situation is different in humans. Patients with AP may have a wide range of causes, severities, and outcomes. Some patients may develop early severe or fulminant pancreatitis that is associated with a high mortality [2]. Further research is required to confirm preliminary data that suggest that genetic polymorphism of certain proinflammatory genes may confer additional risk of developing more severe pancreatitis [60, 61]. Another important area for research and one that is directly related to the outcome is developing specific treatments targeting systemic inflammation and organ dysfunction.

In experimental models, a variety of agents have been shown to reduce the severity of AP, especially when used prophylactically. However, these experimental treatments have failed in clinical settings. Examples include lexipafant (antiplatelet-activating factor), antioxidants, and probiotics [62, 63]. Anti-TNF-α and anti-IL-1 treatments have also failed in clinical trials for MODS secondary to sepsis. Reasons for this may include a relatively brief therapeutic window, the inability to provide prophylactic treatment in humans, and/or the redundancies in the cytokine pathways [64]. Blocking one cytokine is probably not enough as multiple pathways are involved and are mediated by a variety of cytokines and chemokines. Furthermore, the precise temporal relationship of various deranged pathways remains to be elucidated preventing intervention timed at the most effective time point in the evolution of AP. Further research is also required in understanding the way in which gut-derived factors transported in lymph might contribute to systemic inflammation and organ dysfunction.

In summary, great advances have taken place in our understanding of the pathophysiology of AP, including the drivers of SIRS and MODS. And although there appears to be an orderly sequence from initiation within the acinar cell, the development of local pancreatic inflammation, the elaboration of systemic inflammation, and the dysfunction in end organs, the underlying mechanisms are complex and not fully understood. Deciphering the molecular mechanisms at work is necessary if we are to develop targeted treatments that will have a meaningful impact on the clinical outcome of patients with AP.

References

1 Forsmark CE, Baillie J. AGA Institute technical review on acute pancreatitis. Gastroenterology 2007;132: 2022–2044.

2 Sharma, M, Banerjee D, Garg PK. Characterization of newer subgroups of fulminant and subfulminant pancreatitis associated with a high early mortality. The American Journal of Gastroenterology 2007;102:2688–2695.

3 Garg PK, Madan K, Pande GK, Khanna S, Sathyanarayan G, Bohidar NP, Tandon RK. Association of extent and infection of pancreatic necrosis with organ failure and death in acute necrotizing pancreatitis. Clinical Gastroenterology and Hepatology 2005;3:159–166.

4 Isenmann R, Rau B, Beger HG. Bacterial infection and extent of necrosis are determinants of organ failure in

patients with acute necrotizing pancreatitis. British Journal of Surgery 1999;86:1020–1024.

5 Werner J, Feuerbach S, Uhl W, et al. Management of acute pancreatitis: from surgery to interventional intensive care. Gut 2005;54:426–436.

6 Mofidi R, Duff MD, Wigmore SJ, Madhavan KK, Garden OJ, Parks RW Association between early systemic inflammatory response, severity of multiorgan dysfunction and death in acute pancreatitis. British Journal of Surgery 2006; 93:738–744.

7 Working Group IAP/APA Acute Pancreatitis Guidelines. IAP/APA evidence based guidelines for the management of acute pancreatitis. Pancreatology 2013;13(Suppl 2):e1-e15.

8 Isenmann R, Rau B, Beger HG. Early severe acute pancreatitis: characteristics of a new subgroup. Pancreas 2001;22:274–278.

9 Sawa H, Ueda T, Takeyama Y, et al. Blockade of high mobility group box-1 protein attenuates experimental severe acute pancreatitis. World Journal of Gastroenterology 2006; 12:7666–7670.

10 Wang W, Faubel S, Ljubanovic D, Mitra A, Falk SA, Kim J, et al. Endotoxemic acute renal failure is attenuated in caspase-1-deficient mice. American Journal of Physiology: Renal Physiology 2005; 288:F997– F1004.

11 Zhang XH, Zhu RM, Xu WA, Wan HJ, Lu H. Therapeutic effects of caspase-1 inhibitors on acute lung injury in experimental severe acute pancreatitis. World Journal of Gastroenterology 2007;13:623– 627.

12 Yasuda T, Ueda T, Takeyama Y, et al. Significant increase of serum high-mobility group box chromosomal protein 1 levels in patients with severe acute pancreatitis. Pancreas 2006; 33:359–363.

13 Kocsis AK, Szabolcs A, Hofner P, et al. Plasma concentrations of high-mobility group box protein 1, soluble receptor for advanced glycation end-products and circulating DNA in patients with acute pancreatitis. Pancreatology 2009;9:383–391.

14 Sharif R, Dawra R, Wasiluk K, et al. Impact of toll-like receptor 4 on the severity of acute pancreatitis and pancreatitis-associated lung injury in mice. Gut 2009;58:813–819.

15 Luan ZG, Zhang J, Yin XH, Ma XC, Guo RX.Ethyl pyruvate significantly inhibits tumour necrosis factor-α, interleukin-1β and high mobility group box 1 releasing and attenuates sodium taurocholate-induced severe acute pancreatitis associated with acute lung injury. Clinical & Experimental Immunology 2013;172:417–426.

16 Hoque R, Sohail M, Malik A, et al. TLR9 and the NLRP3 inflammasome link acinar cell death with inflammation in acute pancreatitis. Gastroenterology 2011;141:358–369

17 Telek G, Ducroc R, Scoazec JY, Pasquier C, Feldmann G, Roze C. Differential up-regulation of cellular adhesion molecules at the sites of oxidative stress in experimental acute pancreatitis. Journal of Surgical Research 2001;1:56–67.

18 Folch E, Salas A, Panes J, Gelpi E, Rosello-Catafau J, Anderson DC, et al. Role of P-selectin and ICAM-1 in pancreatitis induced lung inflammation in rats: significance of oxidative stress. Annals of Surgery 1999;6:792–798; discussion 798–799.

19 Powell JJ, Siriwardena AK, Fearon KC, Ross JA. Endothelial derived selectins in the development of organ dysfunction in acute pancreatitis. Critical Care Medicine 2001;3:567–572.

20 Hartwig W, Werner J, Warshaw AL, Antoniu B, Castillo CF, Gebhard MM, et al. Membrane-bound ICAM-1 is up-regulated by trypsin and contributes to leukocyte migration in acute pancreatitis. American Journal of Physiology: Gastrointestinal and Liver Physiology 2004;6:G1194–G1199.

21 Ostermann G, Weber KS, Zernecke A, Schroder A, Weber C. JAM-1 is a ligand of the β2-integrin LFA-1 involved in transendothelial migration of leukocytes. Nature Immunology 2002;2:151–158.

22 Santoso S, Sachs UJ, Kroll H, Linder M, Ruf A, Preissner KT, et al. The junctional adhesion molecule 3 (JAM-3) on human platelets is a counterreceptor for the leukocyte integrin Mac-1. The Journal of Experimental Medicine 2002;5:679–691.

23 Werner J, Z'Graggen K, Fernandez-del Castillo C, Lewandrowski KB, Compton CC, Warshaw AL. Specific therapy for local and systemic complications of acute pancreatitis with monoclonal antibodies against ICAM-1. Annals of Surgery 1999;6:834–840; discussion 841–832.

24 Dominguez-Munoz JE, Villanueva A, Larino J, Mora T, Barreiro M, Iglesias-Canle J, et al. Accuracy of plasma levels of polymorphonuclear elastase as early prognostic marker of acute pancreatitis in routine clinical conditions. European Journal of Gastroenterology & Hepatology 2006;1:79–83.

25 Sathyanarayan G, Garg PK, Prasad HK, Tandon RK. Elevated level of interleukin-6 predicts organ failure and severe disease in patients with acute pancreatitis. Journal of Gastroenterology and Hepatology 2007;22:550–554.

26 Demols A, Le Moine O, Desalle F, Quertinmont E, Van Laethem JL, Deviere J. CD4+ T cells play an important role in acute experimental pancreatitis in mice. Gastroenterology 2000;3:582–590.

27 Pezzilli R, Billi P, Gullo L, Beltrandi E, Maldini M, Mancini R, et al. Behavior of serum soluble interleukin-2 receptor, soluble CD8 and soluble CD4 in the early phases of acute pancreatitis. Digestion 1994;4:268–273.

28 Bhatia M, Neoptolemos JP, Slavin J. Inflammatory mediators as therapeutic targets in acute pancreatitis. Current Opinion in Investigational Drugs 2001; 2: 496–501

29 Zhang XP et al. The pathogenic mechanism of severe acute pancreatitis complicated with renal injury: a review of current knowledge. Digestive Diseases and Sciences2008; 3:297–306

30 Pooran N, Indaram A, Singh P, Bank S. Cytokines (IL-6, IL-8, TNF): early and reliable predictors of severe

acute pancreatitis. Journal of Clinical Gastroenterology 2003;37:263–266.

31 Chen CC, Wang SS, Lee FY, Chang FY, Lee SD. Proinflammatory cytokines in early assessment of the prognosis of acute pancreatitis. The American Journal of Gastroenterology 1999; 94: 213–218.

32 Cohen J. The immunopathogenesis of sepsis. Nature 2002;420:885–891.

33 Okusawa S, Gelfand JA, Ikejima T, Connolly RJ, DInarello CA. Interleukin 1 induces a shock-like state in rabbits. Synergism with tumor necrosis factor and the effect of cyclooxygenase inhibition. Journal of Clinical Investigation 1988;81:1162–1172.

34 Cuzzocrea S, De Sarro G, Costantino G et al. Role of interleukin-6 in a non-septic shock model induced by zymosan. European Cytokine Network 1999;10:191–203.

35 Dambrauskas Z, Giese N, Gulbinas A, et al. Different profiles of cytokine expression during mild and severe acute pancreatitis.World Journal of Gastroenterology 2010; 16:1845–1853.

36 Aoun E, Chen J, Reighard D, Gleeson FC, Whitcomb DC, Papachristou GI. Diagnostic accuracy of interleukin-6 and interleukin-8 in predicting severe acute pancreatitis: a meta-analysis. Pancreatology 2009;9:777–785

37 Cuthbertson CM, Christophi C. Disturbances of the microcirculation in acute pancreatitis. British Journal of Surgery 2006;93:518–530.

38 Pitkaranta P, Kivisaari L, Nordling S, Nuutinen P, Schroder T. Vascular changes of pancreatic ducts and vessels in acute necrotizing, and in chronic pancreatitis in humans. International Journal of Pancreatology 1991;8:13–22.

39 Foitzik T, Eibl G, Hotz HG, Faulhaber J, Kirchengast M, Buhr HJ. Endothelin receptor blockade in severe acute pancreatitis leads to systemic enhancement of microcirculation, stabilization of capillary permeability, and improved survival rates. Surgery 2000;128:399–407.

40 Rudiger A, Singer M. Mechanisms of sepsis-induced cardiac dysfunction. Critical Care Medicine 2007; 35:1599–1608; PMID:17452940

41 Salomone T, Tosi P, Palareti G, Tomassetti P, Migliori M, Guariento A et al. Coagulative disorders in human acute pancreatitis: role for the D-dimer. Pancreas 2003; 26: 111–116.

42 Nordback I, Lauslahti K. Clinical pathology of acute necrotising pancreatitis. Journal of Clinical Pathology 1986;39:68–74

43 Maeda K, Hirotas M, Ichihara A et al. Applicability of disseminated intravascular coagulation parameters in the assessment of the severity of acute pancreatitis. Pancreas 2006;32:87–92.

44 Bleeker WK, Agterberg J, Rigter G, Hack CE, Gool JV. Protective effect of antithrombin III in acute experimental pancreatitis in rats. Digestive Diseases and Sciences 1992; 37: 280–285.

45 Hackert T,Werner J, Gebhard MM, Klar E. Effects of heparin in experimental models of acute pancreatitis and post-ERCP pancreatitis. Surgery 2004; 135: 131–138.

46 Lu XS, Qiu F, Li YX et al. Effect of lower molecular weight heparin in the prevention of pancreatic encephalopathy in the patient with severe acute pancreatitis. Pancreas 2010;39:516–519.

47 Martínez J, Johnson CD, Sánchez-Payá J, de Madaria E, Robles-Díaz G, Pérez-Mateo M. Obesity is a definitive risk factor of severity and mortality in acute pancreatitis: an updated meta-analysis. Pancreatology. 2006; 6:206–209.

48 Premkumar R, Phillips AR, Petrov MS, Windsor JA. The clinical relevance of obesity in acute pancreatitis: targeted systematic reviews. Pancreatology 2015;15:25–33.

49 Yashima Y, Isayama H, Tsujino T et al. A large volume of visceral adipose tissue leads to severe acute pancreatitis. Journal of Gastroenterology 2011;46:1213–1218.

50 Karpavicius A, Dambrauskas Z, Sileikis A, Vitkus D, Strupas K. Value of adipokines in predicting the severity of acute pancreatitis: comprehensive review. World Journal of Gastroenterology 2012;18:6620–6627.

51 Patel K, Trivedi RN, Durgampudi C, et al. Lipolysis of visceral adipocyte triglyceride by pancreatic lipases converts mild acute pancreatitis to severe pancreatitis independent of necrosis and inflammation. American Journal of Pathology 2015;185:808–819.

52 Noel P, Patel K, Durgampudi C, et al. Peripancreatic fat necrosis worsens acute pancreatitis independent of pancreatic necrosis via unsaturated fatty acids increased in human pancreatic necrosis collections. Gut. 2016;65:100–111. (Epub ahead of publication). pii:gutjnl-2014-308043.

53 Navina S, Acharya C, DeLany JP, et al. Lipotoxicity causes multisystem organ failure and exacerbates acute pancreatitis in obesity. Science Translational Medicine 2011;3:107–110.

54 Park J, Chang JH, Park SH, et al. Interleukin-6 is associated with obesity, central fat distribution, and disease severity in patients with acute pancreatitis. Pancreatology. 2015;15:59–63.

55 Deitch EA. Gut-origin sepsis: evolution of a concept. The Surgeon 2012; 10: 350–356.

56 Brealey D, Brand M, Hargreaves I, et al. Association between mitochondrial dysfunction and severity and outcome of septic shock. Lancet 2002; 360:219–223;

57 Jacob TG, Vipin IS, Roy TS, Garg PK. Electron-microscopic evidence of mitochondriae containing macroautophagy in experimental acute pancreatitis: implications for cell death. Pancreatology 2014;14:433–435.

58 Mareninova OA, Hermann K, French SW, et al. Impaired autophagic flux mediates acinar cell vacuole formation and trypsinogen activation in rodent models of acute pancreatitis. Journal of Clinical Investigation 2009;119:3340–3355.

59 Singer M. The role of mitochondrial dysfunction in sepsis-induced multi-organ failure. Virulence 2014;5: 66–72.

60 Balog A, Gyulai Z, Boros LG, Farkas G, Takacs T, Lonovics J, Mandi Y. Polymorphism of the TNF-alpha, HSP70-2, and CD14 genes increases susceptibility to severe acute pancreatitis. Pancreas 2005;30:46–50.

61 Papachristou GI, Sass DA, Avula H, Lamb J, Lokshin A, Barmada MM et al. Is the monocyte chemotactic protein-1-2518 G allele a risk factor for severe acute pancreatitis? Clinical Gastroenterology and Hepatology 2005;3:475–481.

62 Johnson CD, Kingsnorth AN, Imrie CW, McMahon MJ, Neoptolemos JP, et al. Double blind, randomised, placebo controlled study of a platelet activating factor antagonist, lexipafant, in the treatment and prevention of organ failure in predicted severe acute pancreatitis. Gut 2001; 48: 62–69.

63 Besselink MG, van Santvoort HC, Buskens E, Boermeester MA, van Goor H, Timmerman HM et al. Probiotic prophylaxis in predicted severe acute pancreatitis: a randomised, double-blind, placebo-controlled trial. Lancet. 2008;371:651–659.

64 Parrish WR, Gallowitsch-Puerta M, Czura CJ, Tracey KJ. Experimental therapeutic strategies for severe sepsis: mediators and mechanisms. Annals of the New York Academy of Sciences, 2008;1144:210–236.

CHAPTER 3

Diagnosis, prediction, and classification

Efstratios Koutroumpakis & Georgios I. Papachristou

Division of Gastroenterology, Hepatology and Nutrition, University of Pittsburgh Medical Center, Pittsburgh, PA, USA

Introduction

Acute pancreatitis (AP) is an inflammatory disease of the pancreas with an increasing incidence over the last 20 years [1]. Currently, AP results in 270,000 hospital admissions per year in the United States, which is more than any other GI-related cause of hospitalization. This leads to a high economic burden, exceeding 2.5 billion dollars annually in the United States alone [2].

The majority of AP cases follow a mild course with inflammation and edema confined to the pancreatic gland. However, in about 20% of patients, the inflammation becomes more extensive resulting in local complications (e.g., inflammation, edema, necrosis of the pancreas and peripancreatic fat, and infection of local complications) and/or systemic complications (e.g., systemic inflammation and end-organ dysfunction/failure). Patients with local and systemic complication have a higher morbidity and mortality rate, reaching as high as 30%.

During the past two decades, intensive pancreatic research has led to better understanding of the pathophysiology of AP (Chapter 2). This in addition to advancements in imaging and management of AP has revealed a need for better definitions, predictors, and classification of severity. The aim of this chapter is to summarize the advances in these areas.

Diagnosis

The diagnosis of AP is established when two out of the three following criteria are present: (i) pancreatic-type abdominal pain, (ii) elevated serum amylase and/or lipase more than three times the upper limit of normal, and/or (iii) imaging findings consistent with AP [3, 4].

The diagnosis of AP should be considered when patients present with acute onset, severe, upper abdominal pain that often radiates to the back, and is associated with nausea and vomiting. Physical examination reveals epigastric tenderness but usually without peritoneal signs.

In patients with symptoms typical for AP, the measurement of elevated serum pancreatic enzymes (amylase and/or lipase) three times the upper limit of normal can confirm the diagnosis of AP. Studies have shown that the threefold elevation criteria are associated with a moderate sensitivity (55–100%) and a high specificity (93–99%) and that this is more accurate than lower cutoff values [5].

Among the pancreatic enzymes measured in clinical practice, there are certain limitations associated with the use of serum amylase. Amylase levels may remain normal in up to 20% of AP patients, especially in those with alcoholic and hypertriglyceridemic etiologies [6]. Furthermore, high serum amylase is not specific for AP as it can be found in patients with macroamylasemia, inflammation of the salivary glands, decreased glomerular filtration rate, and other intra-abdominal inflammatory processes. Although serum lipase has been recommended as a more specific diagnostic test [7], it also has limitations. Lipase levels may increase in certain extrapancreatic abdominal inflammatory processes such as appendicitis or cholecystitis, in renal disease, and in macrolipasemia, similarly to macroamylasemia. Additionally, diabetic patients appear to have higher median serum lipase levels [8], and a higher cutoff may be required for the diagnosis of AP in this population. Because of these limitations, clinicians should always correlate serum amylase/lipase levels with patient symptomatology [3].

Additionally, urinary trypsinogen-2 dipstick (positive if >50 ng/mL) is a fast bedside diagnostic test, which has been shown in several studies to be as accurate as the aforementioned criteria for amylase and lipase [5, 9]. Although urinary trypsinogen-2 dipstick has not been established in clinical practice, it may be an alternative test to serum pancreatic enzymes for the AP diagnosis given its convenience, as a blood sample is not required.

The diagnosis of AP is made in the majority of patients on the basis of characteristic abdominal pain and increased pancreatic enzyme levels. In such patients, there is no need to perform imaging for diagnostic purposes. However, there is a group of patients with either characteristic symptoms and enzyme levels less than three times the upper limit of normal (as in delayed presentations) or high enzymes levels in the absence of characteristic symptoms (as in patients with inability to give clear history), in which imaging is necessary to establish the diagnosis of AP. CT scan has more than 90% specificity and sensitivity for AP diagnosis [10]. In these settings CT and MRI scanning have an accuracy of more than 90% [10, 11], although CT is generally preferred due to its wide availability and lower cost. Ultrasound scanning has limited role in diagnosing AP, especially as bowel gas in associated intestinal ileus (i.e., "sentinel loop" seen on plain radiography) often obscures the view of the pancreas. Imaging is also important in the early diagnosis of etiological factors and local complications such as gallstones, pancreatic tumors, acute peripancreatic fluid collections, pancreatic necrosis, intestinal ischemia, and bleeding. As (peri)pancreatic necrosis develops over several days, the diagnosis of the extent of necrosis is best made by delaying contrast-enhanced imaging aiming for at least 72 hours after admission.

Prediction

AP is a highly variable inflammatory disease with a broad range of outcomes. This wide range covers mild self-limited disease to severe progressive complications and death. The local complications themselves may range from peripancreatic fat stranding, peripancreatic fluid collections, splanchnic vein thrombosis,

peripancreatic fat, and/or pancreatic gland necrosis to infection of pancreatic fluid collections and necrosis. This variability in disease course results in high variability in disease morbidity and mortality. Characteristically, it has been reported that mortality in the mild interstitial AP is less than 1% but increases to 17% when AP is complicated with pancreatic necrosis and may exceed 30% when multiple system organ failure develops [12–14]. Early identification of patients at risk of severe disease is important for the decision about patient triaging, transfer, and treatment to improve clinical outcomes. It is also important for accurate allocation to groups in randomized trials. Recognition of the importance of severity prediction has resulted in a significant body of research literature over several decades. Prediction of disease severity can be approached in three ways: identification of host risk factors, stratification of clinical risk, and determination of response to initial therapy [4].

1 Host risk factor identification

A thorough history is helpful not only for the diagnosis and etiology but also for severity prediction in AP patients. There are some demographic and environmental factors that relate to disease severity. Furthermore, there are pilot studies that support the role of genetic polymorphisms in predisposing to worse disease outcomes:

a) Demographic and environmental risk factors:

Demographic and environmental factors that increase the risk of more severe AP include older age, male sex, obesity, underlying comorbidities, and excessive alcohol consumption.

There are several studies reporting that older age predisposes to development of organ failure and early mortality. The age cutoff in the different reports ranges from 55 to 75 years [15, 16]. Male sex has been correlated with severe disease outcomes in some studies [16]; however, other reports have shown conflicting findings [17].

Obesity (BMI ≥30) has been studied thoroughly and established as an important risk factor for disease severity [18, 19]. In a meta-analysis of more than 700 patients, obesity was significantly associated with local complications, systemic complications, and mortality with odds ratios ranging between 2 and 4 [20].

Other preexisting chronic comorbidities including malignancy, heart failure, kidney, or liver disease have also been shown to be related with early death, likely because the reserves of vital organs in such patients are limited [16]. Finally, AP of alcoholic etiology has been shown to run a more complicated course. A recent report indicates that chronic alcohol consumption of two or more alcoholic drinks per day is a risk factor for severity regardless of AP etiology [21, 22].

b) Genetic risk factors:

Recent studies have suggested that host genetic factors can contribute to AP severity. A few single nucleotide polymorphisms (SNPs) mainly in genes coding inflammatory cytokines have been identified as disease severity modifiers. A small pilot study suggested that a polymorphism in the promoter region of the monocyte chemotactic protein-1 (MCP-1) gene (−2518 G allele) increases the risk for organ failure [23]. Expression-enhancing SNPs in areas −1031 and −863 of the promoter of tumor necrosis factor α (TNF-α) gene have been correlated with the development of multiorgan dysfunction syndrome [24]. Furthermore, the A/T heterozygosity in the −251 region of the interleukin-8 gene [25] and SNPs in the genes encoding human defensins 1 and 2 [26] have been associated with increased risk for severe disease. Genetic analysis may evolve into a critical tool for both susceptibility/severity stratification and eventually management of patients with pancreatic disorders, including AP.

2 Clinical risk stratification

Clinical and radiologic scoring systems and laboratory markers have been extensively studied and are in widespread use as predictive tools for disease severity in patients with AP.

Clinical scores

Ranson was the first to use clinical criteria to predict AP severity, and they have been widely used in clinical practice and research for four decades. The Ranson criteria comprise 11 variables that are scored at 2 time points, on admission and within 48 hours. A score of 3 or more is required for predicted severe AP and is usually associated with a worse outcome. Since the development of Ranson's score, several additional clinical scores for predicting severity have been developed. They incorporate clinical, laboratory, and occasionally radiographic findings and include in chronological order (i) the Glasgow criteria (also known as Imrie score), (ii) the

acute physiology and chronic health examination (APACHE) II score, (iii) the systemic inflammatory response syndrome (SIRS) score, (iv) the Panc 3 score, (v) the pancreatitis outcome prediction (POP) score, (vi) the bedside index for severity in acute pancreatitis (BISAP) score, (vii) the revised Japanese severity score (JSS), and (viii) the harmless acute pancreatitis score (HAPS) [27] (Table 3.1).

A recent large study that head-to-head compared all available clinical scores in a large cohort of prospectively enrolled AP patients and subsequently validated the results in an independent cohort showed that all perform with moderate accuracy (around 80%) and are comparable in predicting severe disease [27] (Table 3.2). One major limitation of the available scoring systems is that they mainly convert continuous into binary values of equal weight and thus fail to capture synergistic effects based on the interactions of interdependent systems [28]. It appears that the current clinical predictive scores have reached their maximum efficacy, and novel approaches for severity prediction are needed.

Pancreatic societies and expert recommendations have proposed SIRS as an easy-to-remember and easy-to-apply clinical predictive score, which is based on vital sign measurements and simple laboratory values [3, 4]. It involves four criteria and is positive when two or more of them are present: (i) heart rate >90 beats/min, (ii) core temperature <36 or >38 °C, (iii) white blood count <4000 or >12,000/mm^3, and (iv) respirations >20/min or PCO_2 <32 mmHg:

a) Radiologic scores

Since the early 1980s with the advent of computed tomography, several radiologic predictive scores have been developed. Balthazar's criteria were reported as early as 1985. It evaluated the pancreatic and peripancreatic inflammatory changes based on unenhanced imaging. Another score that focused only on changes in the pancreas gland is the "pancreatic size index" (PSI). Other scores, based on unenhanced CTs, that evaluate extrapancreatic complications are the "mesenteric edema and peritoneal fluid" (MOP) and the "extrapancreatic inflammation on CT" (EPIC) scores. In addition, radiologic scores based on contrast-enhanced CT (CECT) have been developed, namely, the "CT severity index" (CTSI), which has been widely studied, and the "modified CTSI" (MCTSI) which, in addition to

Table 3.1 Available clinical scoring systems predicting severity in chronological order.

Scores	Year	Cutoff	Variables assessed at admission and 48 hours
Ranson's	1974	3	Admission: age (>55 y), WBC (>16,000/mL), glucose (>200 mg/dL), LDH (>350 IU/mL), AST (>250 IU/mL) 48 hours: hematocrit (decrease >10%), BUN (increase >5 mg/dL), calcium (<8 mg/dL), PaO_2 (<60 mmHg), base deficit (>4 mEq/L), fluid sequestration (>6 L)
Glasgow	1984	2	Age (>55 y), WBC (>15,000/mL), glucose (>180 mg/dL), BUN (>45 mg/dL), PaO_2 (<60 mmHg), calcium (<8 g/dL), albumin (<3.2 g/dL), LDH (>600 IU/L)
APACHE-II	1989	8	Age, temperature, MAP, heart rate, respiratory rate, A-aPaO_2 or PaO_2, arterial pH or HCO_3, sodium, potassium, creatinine, hematocrit, WBC, Glasgow Coma Score, chronic health problems[a]
SIRS	2006	2	Temperature (<36 °C or >38 °C), heart rate (>90/min), respiratory rate (>20/min or $PaCO_2$ <32 mmHg), WBC (<4000/mm^3, >12,000/mm^3 or >10% bands)
Panc 3	2007	1	Hematocrit (>44%), BMI (>30 kg/m^2), pleural effusion
POP	2007	9	Age, MAP, PaO_2:FiO_2, arterial pH, BUN, calcium[a]
BISAP	2008	2	BUN (>25 mg/dL), impaired mental status (Glasgow Coma Score <15), SIRS (≥2), age (>60 y), pleural effusion
JSS	2009	2	Base excess (≤3 mEq/L), PaO_2 (≤60 mmHg or respiratory failure), BUN (≥40 mg/dL) or Cr (≥2 mg/dL), LDH (≥2× upper limit of normal), platelet (≤100,000/mm^3), calcium (≤7.5 mg/dL), CRP (≥15 mg/dL), SIRS (≥3), age (≥70 y)
HAPS	2009	1	Abdominal tenderness, hematocrit (>43% for men or >39.6% for women), creatinine (>2 mg/dL)

WBC: white blood cell count, LDH: lactate dehydrogenase, AST: aspartate aminotransferase, BUN: blood urea nitrogen, BMI: body mass index, MAP: mean arterial pressure, CRP: C-reactive protein, FiO_2: fraction of inspired oxygen.
[a]Cutoff values were not indicated for APACHE-II and POP variables since instead of cutoffs they utilize value ranges for each variable (but overall they did use cutoffs).
Mounzer 2012 [27]. Reproduced with permission of Elsevier.

Table 3.2 Performance of clinical scoring systems on admission in predicting persistent organ failure; prospective data from a large tertiary US center.

Scoring system	Sensitivity	Specificity	Accuracy
Ranson	0.66 (±0.09)	0.78 (±0.10)	0.72 (±0.06)
Glasgow	0.85 (±0.08)	0.83 (±0.07)	0.84 (±0.06)
APACHE-II	0.84 (±0.11)	0.71 (±0.06)	0.77 (±0.07)
SIRS	0.70 (±0.18)	0.71 (±0.04)	0.70 (±0.10)
Panc 3	0.76 (±0.15)	0.52 (±0.05)	0.64 (±0.06)
POP	0.57 (±0.15)	0.76 (±0.06)	0.67 (±0.09)
BISAP	0.61 (±0.20)	0.84 (±0.04)	0.72 (±0.10)
JSS	0.59 (±0.13)	0.92 (±0.05)	0.76 (±0.07)
HAPS	0.70 (±0.11)	0.53 (±0.21)	0.62 (±0.06)

Scoring systems are presented in chronological order.
Values in parentheses represent standard deviations.
Mounzer 2012 [27]. Reproduced with permission from Elsevier.

(peri)pancreatic inflammatory changes in CTSI, also assesses extrapancreatic complications [29].

Although all of these scores have been correlated with disease morbidity and mortality, they have shown only moderate predictive accuracy. Studies comparing the radiologic scores with the clinical scores have shown that they both perform similarly [28, 29].

The major limitation of radiologic scores is that they predominantly focus on local pancreatic complications and because these are best assessed after a delay of at least 72 hours. Therefore, the radiologic scores have no routine role in early prediction of AP severity. Considering the higher cost, radiation exposure, and moderate predictive accuracy, it is recommended that CECT scan in AP patients be used early when there is diagnostic uncertainty or when there is the suspicion of acute abdominal complications (e.g., bowel ischemia, perforation, bleeding) or local pancreatic complications (e.g., acute pancreatic fluid collections and (peri)pancreatic necrosis) [29].

b) **Laboratory markers**

Several individual measures of inflammation have been studied as markers of severe disease. These include C-reactive protein, interleukins 1, 6, and 8, procalcitonin, polymorphonuclear elastase, and trypsinogen activation peptide. With the exception of CRP, none of the aforementioned markers has become established in clinical practice and probably because it is routinely available from laboratories. Three other more widely available laboratory markers, namely, hematocrit, blood urea nitrogen (BUN), and creatinine have also been investigated as predictors of AP severity.

Elevated hematocrit levels on admission have been associated with development of pancreatic necrosis [30, 31]. Furthermore, low hematocrit levels have shown a high negative predictive value for necrosis [32]. This association has been attributed to the fact that systemic inflammation leads to vascular leak, third-space fluid loss, and hemoconcentration, which impacts pancreatic microcirculation and contributes to the formation of necrosis [33, 34]. Increased admission hematocrit levels have also been correlated with development of organ failure, prolonged hospitalization, and ICU stay [31, 32]. The cutoff values of hematocrit proposed in the different studies range from 44% to 47%.

There are two large studies reporting that early BUN levels represent an independent predictor of mortality in patients with AP. The first study utilized large hospital databases and suggested that with each 5 mg/dL increase in BUN, the odds ratio for mortality in AP increases by 2.2. The same study showed that BUN is the most accurate predictor of in-hospital mortality when compared to other routine labs to include calcium, hemoglobin, creatinine, white blood cell count, and glucose levels [35]. The second study was a multicenter international study of prospectively enrolled patients, where BUN ≥20 mg/dL was associated with a 4.6 odds ratio for mortality and BUN levels were comparable to admission creatinine and APACHE-II in predicting mortality [36].

The role of creatinine as a predictor of severity was examined in a recent prospective study where it was found that increased creatinine levels was associated with development of pancreatic necrosis. More specifically, peak creatinine >1.8 mg/dL during the first 2 days from hospital admission had the highest odds ratio for development of necrosis (OR = 35) when compared to admission hematocrit and BUN levels [37]. However, a follow-up study did not reproduce impressive results, and this was attributed to the heterogeneity of the patient population in the two studies [38, 39].

CRP levels have also been studied as a predictor of AP severity. In a recent retrospective study, CRP levels at 48 hours predicted organ failure, pancreatic necrosis development, and mortality with moderate efficacy at cutoff values of 190, 190, and 170 mg/L, respectively [40]:

3 **Determining response to initial treatment**

A third strategy for the prediction of severity is to evaluate the patient's response to initial treatment. There are several laboratory markers used to assess response to initial therapy, guide further management, and predict prognosis.

This has been demonstrated by the change in the acute physiology component of the APACHE-II score in response to initial intensive care treatment. It was highly predictive of mortality, although less so in patients with low and very high scores (Flint et al. [41]). More recently the failure of hematocrit to decrease within the first 24 hours in response to fluid therapy has been associated with development of pancreatic necrosis and organ failure [30, 31]. Furthermore, failure of BUN levels to decrease within the first 2 days has been correlated with increased mortality [36]. As mentioned earlier, an increase in creatinine within the first 48 hours has been strongly associated with pancreatic necrosis development [37].

In summary, numerous scoring systems and markers have been investigated for the prediction of AP early in the disease course, but all perform with only moderate accuracy. While they are valued in analyzing groups of patients, they are not accurate enough in the management of individual patients. This means that we are still in search of the Holy Grail – a simple, inexpensive, and accurate predictive tool.

Classification

In contrast to prediction, which is about predicting severity sometime in the future, the classification of severity is about grading severity at a particular time. And this might be any time during the disease course or it might be applied to the time when severity peaks. The classification of severity is useful for clinical and research purposes.

Although mild and severe pancreatitis had been distinguished for over 100 years, it was the Atlanta classification in 1992 which brought it into widespread clinical usage [42]. This was a breakthrough consensus that has proven useful to clinicians and researchers for more than 20 years. However, the original Atlanta classification has several limitations. The definition of severe disease is broad and even includes two predictive scoring systems, Ranson's and APACHE-II. Furthermore, all local complications are included in the severe disease group. It is currently clear that the clinical significance of an acute nonnecrotic pancreatic fluid collection is significantly less than extensive pancreatic necrosis. Through the last 10 years, our increased knowledge and better understanding of the pathophysiology and natural course of AP, along with the advancements in diagnostic imaging, have rendered the binary classification of mild and severe disease simplistic. In particular, it has become apparent that the severe category, as classified, comprised subgroups with different clinical courses.

Two new severity classification systems for AP were published recently, the determinant-based classification (2012) and the revised Atlanta classification (2013). They were developed by different processes, which account for their differences. The revised Atlanta classification defines three grades of severity. Severe AP is defined by the presence of persistent organ failure, moderate severity by transient organ failure (less than 48 hours), local complications, including infected pancreatic necrosis, and/or exacerbation of existing comorbidities, and mild severity when the aforementioned features are absent [12]. The determinant-based classification defines four severity categories based on local and systemic complications. Critical is defined by the presence of both infected pancreatic necrosis and persistent organ failure, severe by infected pancreatic necrosis or persistent organ failure, moderate by sterile pancreatic necrosis and/or transient organ failure, and finally the rest of the cases are classified as mild [13] (Table 3.3).

Recent studies comparing these two severity classifications showed that they perform similarly in clinical practice [45, 46]. The key difference is the importance ascribed to infected pancreatic necrosis. The revised Atlanta classification does not define it as a feature of severe AP, whereas the determinant-based classification does. Further research is required to further improve the classification of severity.

Conclusion

The diagnosis, prediction, and classification of the severity of AP are practical issues that affect the clinical management of cases. Diagnosis is based on the presence of two out of three simple and well-established criteria. There are many scoring systems and markers to predict the severity of AP, but they all perform with only moderate accuracy. The recent consensus is that the SIRS score should be used for the early prediction of severity, but greater accuracy is required in the care of individual patients. The classification of severity is also important and two recent approaches have been proposed. Both the determinant-based classification (four categories) and the revised Atlanta classification (three grades) reflect a better understanding of the pathophysiology of AP and are reasonably equivalent in

Table 3.3 Classification systems for AP severity.

Atlanta 1992	Mild AP	Severe AP		
Local[a] complications	No	Yes		
		And/or		
Organ failure[b]	No	Yes		
		And/or		
APACHE-II ≥8 or Ranson's ≥3	No	Yes		
RAC	Mild AP	Moderately severe AP	Severe AP	
Local[c] or comorbidities[d]	No	Yes		
		And/or		
Organ failure[e]	No	Transient	Persistent	
DBC	Mild AP	Moderate AP	Severe AP	Critical AP
(Peri)pancreatic necrosis	No	Sterile	Infected	Infected
	And	And/or	Or	And
Organ failure[f]	No	Transient	Persistent	Persistent

AP: acute pancreatitis, RAC: revised Atlanta classification, DBC: determinant-based classification.

[a]Local: acute fluid collection, pancreatic necrosis, pseudocyst, and pancreatic abscess.

[b]Cardiovascular: systolic BP <90 mmHg, respiratory failure: PaO_2 ≤60 mmHg, renal failure: creatinine ≥2 mg/dL, and/or gastrointestinal bleeding >500 mL/24 hours.

[c]Local: acute peripancreatic fluid collection, pseudocyst, acute necrotic collection, and walled-off necrosis.

[d]Exacerbation of preexisting comorbidity.

[e]Organ failure is defined as a score ≥2 in modified Marshall score which evaluates cardiovascular, respiratory, and renal systems [43].

[f]Organ failure is defined as either a score ≥2 in the sepsis-related organ failure (SOFA) score [44] or based on the following parameters: cardiovascular, requirement for inotropic support; respiratory, PaO_2/FiO_2 ≥300 mmHg; and renal, creatinine ≥2 mg/dL. Nawaz 2013 [45]. Reproduced with permission from Nature Publishing Group.

their ability to discriminate subgroups of patients with different outcomes.

References

1 Fagenholz PJ, Castillo CF, Harris NS, et al. Increasing United States hospital admissions for acute pancreatitis, 1988–2003. Annals of Epidemiology 2007;17:491–497.

2 Peery AF, Dellon ES, Lund J, et al. Burden of gastrointestinal disease in the United States: 2012 update. Gastroenterology 2012;143:1179–1187. e1–3

3 Tenner S, Baillie J, DeWitt J, et al. American College of Gastroenterology guideline: management of acute pancreatitis. The American Journal of Gastroenterology 2013;108:1400–1415.

4 Working Group IAP/APA Acute Pancreatitis Guidelines. IAP/APA evidence-based guidelines for the management of acute pancreatitis. Pancreatology 2013;13:e1–e15.

5 Kemppainen EA, Hedstrom JI, Puolakkainen PA, et al. Rapid measurement of urinary trypsinogen-2 as a screening test for acute pancreatitis. The New England Journal of Medicine 1997;336:1788–1793.

6 Winslet M, Hall C, London NJ, et al. Relation of diagnostic serum amylase levels to aetiology and severity of acute pancreatitis. Gut 1992;33:982–986.

7 UK Working Party on Acute Pancreatitis. UK guidelines for the management of acute pancreatitis. Gut 2005;54 (Suppl 3):iii1–iii9.

8 Steinberg WM, Nauck MA, Zinman B, et al. LEADER 3-lipase and amylase activity in subjects with type 2 diabetes: baseline data from over 9000 subjects in the LEADER trial. Pancreas 2014;43:1223–1231.

9 Mayumi T, Inui K, Maetani I, et al. Validity of the urinary trypsinogen-2 test in the diagnosis of acute pancreatitis. Pancreas 2012;41:869–875.

10 Balthazar EJ. Acute pancreatitis: assessment of severity with clinical and CT evaluation. Radiology 2002;223:603–613.

11 Stimac D, Miletic D, Radic M, et al. The role of nonenhanced magnetic resonance imaging in the early assessment of acute pancreatitis. The American Journal of Gastroenterology 2007;102:997–1004.

12 Banks PA, Bollen TL, Dervenis C, et al. Classification of acute pancreatitis–2012: revision of the Atlanta classification and definitions by international consensus. Gut 2013;62:102–111.

13 Dellinger EP, Forsmark CE, Layer P, et al. Determinant-based classification of acute pancreatitis severity: an international multidisciplinary consultation. Annals of Surgery 2012;256:875–880.

14 de Beaux AC, Palmer KR, Carter DC. Factors influencing morbidity and mortality in acute pancreatitis; an analysis of 279 cases. Gut 1995;37:121–126.

15 Gardner TB, Vege SS, Chari ST, et al. The effect of age on hospital outcomes in severe acute pancreatitis. Pancreatology 2008;8:265–270.

16 Frey C, Zhou H, Harvey D, et al. Co-morbidity is a strong predictor of early death and multi-organ system failure among patients with acute pancreatitis. Journal of Gastrointestinal Surgery 2007;11:733–742.

17 Lankisch PG, Assmus C, Lehnick D, et al. Acute pancreatitis: does gender matter? Digestive Diseases and Sciences 2001;46:2470–2474.

18 Papachristou GI, Papachristou DJ, Avula H, et al. Obesity increases the severity of acute pancreatitis: performance of APACHE-O score and correlation with the inflammatory response. Pancreatology 2006;6:279–285.

19 Hong S, Qiwen B, Ying J, et al. Body mass index and the risk and prognosis of acute pancreatitis: a meta-analysis. European Journal of Gastroenterology & Hepatology 2011;23:1136–1143.

20 Martinez J, Johnson CD, Sanchez-Paya J, et al. Obesity is a definitive risk factor of severity and mortality in acute pancreatitis: an updated meta-analysis. Pancreatology 2006;6:206–209.

21 Papachristou GI, Papachristou DJ, Morinville VD, et al. Chronic alcohol consumption is a major risk factor for pancreatic necrosis in acute pancreatitis. The American Journal of Gastroenterology 2006;101:2605–2610.

22 Lankisch PG, Assmus C, Pflichthofer D, et al. Which etiology causes the most severe acute pancreatitis? International Journal of Pancreatology 1999;26:55–57.

23 Papachristou GI, Sass DA, Avula H, et al. Is the monocyte chemotactic protein-1-2518 G allele a risk factor for severe acute pancreatitis? Clinical Gastroenterology and Hepatology 2005;3:475–481.

24 Bishehsari F, Sharma A, Stello K, et al. TNF-alpha gene (TNFA) variants increase risk for multi-organ dysfunction syndrome (MODS) in acute pancreatitis. Pancreatology 2012;12:113–118

25 Hofner P, Balog A, Gyulai Z, et al. Polymorphism in the IL-8 gene, but not in the TLR4 gene, increases the severity of acute pancreatitis. Pancreatology 2006;6:542–548.

26 Tiszlavicz Z, Szabolcs A, Takacs T, et al. Polymorphisms of beta defensins are associated with the risk of severe acute pancreatitis. Pancreatology 2010;10:483–490.

27 Mounzer R, Langmead CJ, Wu BU, et al. Comparison of existing clinical scoring systems to predict persistent organ failure in patients with acute pancreatitis. Gastroenterology 2012;142:1476–1482; quiz e15–16.

28 Papachristou GI, Muddana V, Yadav D, et al. Comparison of BISAP, Ranson's, APACHE-II, and CTSI scores in predicting organ failure, complications, and mortality in acute pancreatitis. The American Journal of Gastroenterology 2010;105:435–441; quiz 442.

29 Bollen TL, Singh VK, Maurer R, et al. A comparative evaluation of radiologic and clinical scoring systems in the early prediction of severity in acute pancreatitis. The American Journal of Gastroenterology 2012;107:612–619.

30 Baillargeon JD, Orav J, Ramagopal V, et al. Hemoconcentration as an early risk factor for necrotizing pancreatitis. The American Journal of Gastroenterology 1998;93:2130–2134.

31 Brown A, Orav J, Banks PA. Hemoconcentration is an early marker for organ failure and necrotizing pancreatitis. Pancreas 2000;20:367–372.

32 Lankisch PG, Mahlke R, Blum T, et al. Hemoconcentration: an early marker of severe and/or necrotizing pancreatitis? A critical appraisal. The American Journal of Gastroenterology 2001;96:2081–2085.

33 Knoefel WT, Kollias N, Warshaw AL, et al. Pancreatic microcirculatory changes in experimental pancreatitis of graded severity in the rat. Surgery 1994;116:904–913.

34 Klar E, Schratt W, Foitzik T, et al. Impact of microcirculatory flow pattern changes on the development of acute edematous and necrotizing pancreatitis in rabbit pancreas. Digestive Diseases and Sciences 1994;39:2639–2644.

35 Wu BU, Johannes RS, Sun X, et al. Early changes in blood urea nitrogen predict mortality in acute pancreatitis. Gastroenterology 2009;137:129–135.

36 Wu BU, Bakker OJ, Papachristou GI, et al. Blood urea nitrogen in the early assessment of acute pancreatitis: an international validation study. Archives of Internal Medicine 2011;171:669–676.

37 Muddana V, Whitcomb DC, Khalid A, et al. Elevated serum creatinine as a marker of pancreatic necrosis in acute pancreatitis. The American Journal of Gastroenterology 2009;104:164–170.

38 Lankisch PG, Weber-Dany B, Maisonneuve P, et al. High serum creatinine in acute pancreatitis: a marker for pancreatic necrosis? The American Journal of Gastroenterology 2010;105:1196–1200.

39 Papachristou GI, Muddana V, Yadav D, et al. Increased serum creatinine is associated with pancreatic necrosis in acute pancreatitis. The American Journal of Gastroenterology 2010;105:1451–1452.

40 Cardoso FS, Ricardo LB, Oliveira AM, et al. C-reactive protein prognostic accuracy in acute pancreatitis: timing of measurement and cutoff points. European Journal of Gastroenterology & Hepatology 2013;25:784–789.

41 Flint R, et al. The physiological response to intensive care: a clinically relevant predictor in severe acute pancreatitis. Archives of Surgery 2004;139:438–443.

42 Bradley EL, 3rd. A clinically based classification system for acute pancreatitis. Summary of the International Symposium on Acute Pancreatitis, Atlanta, GA, September 11 through 13, 1992. Archives of Surgery 1993;128:586–590.

43 Marshall JC, Cook DJ, Christou NV, et al. Multiple organ dysfunction score: a reliable descriptor of a complex clinical outcome. Critical Care Medicine 1995;23:1638–1652.

44 Vincent JL, Moreno R, Takala J, et al. The SOFA (Sepsis-related Organ Failure Assessment) score to describe organ dysfunction/failure. On behalf of the Working Group on Sepsis-Related Problems of the European Society of Intensive Care Medicine. Intensive Care Medicine 1996;22:707–710.

45 Nawaz H, Mounzer R, Yadav D, et al. Revised Atlanta and determinant-based classification: application in a prospective cohort of acute pancreatitis patients. The American Journal of Gastroenterology 2013;108:1911–1917.

46 Acevedo-Piedra NG, Moya-Hoyo N, Rey-Riveiro M, et al. Validation of the determinant-based classification and revision of the Atlanta classification systems for acute pancreatitis. Clinical Gastroenterology and Hepatology 2014;12:311–316.

CHAPTER 4

Medical treatment

Andree H. Koop & Timothy B. Gardner

Department of Medicine, Geisel School of Medicine at Dartmouth, Hanover, NH, USA

Introduction

Acute pancreatitis (AP) is a common inflammatory condition of the pancreas with significant morbidity, mortality, and health-care costs [1]. In 2009, it was the single most common inpatient gastrointestinal diagnosis with over 270,000 hospitalizations and estimated inpatient costs over 2.6 billion dollars [2]. It is well known that the incidence of AP is increasing despite continued advancements in medical therapy, with an overall mortality rate of approximately 5%, but as high as 30% in severe cases [3–6]. Originally published in 1992 and updated in 2012, the Atlanta classification subdivides AP into two types: mild pancreatitis and severe AP. Mild pancreatitis, also known as interstitial edematous pancreatitis, is defined as pancreatic inflammation without necrosis or organ failure and is generally self-limited, resolving within 1 week. Severe AP is less common, occurring in approximately 20% of cases, and is defined by organ failure and complications such as pancreatic necrosis, abscess, and pseudocyst. This category is further subdivided into moderate and severe pancreatitis according to the persistence of organ failure for more than 48 hours [7]. This chapter focuses on the initial medical treatment of AP, specifically the importance of intravenous fluid resuscitation and the evidence for pharmacologic and antibiotic therapy. Further treatment regarding nutritional management and the local and systemic complications of AP are presented in other chapters.

The importance of underlying etiology

The diagnosis of AP is made if two of the following three features are present: (i) characteristic abdominal pain, (ii) elevation of pancreatic specific enzymes, and/or (iii) characteristic findings on cross-sectional imaging [7]. During the initial diagnosis, it is critical to identify the etiology of disease to determine those causes that may affect acute management and those that may be eliminated to prevent recurrent disease [8]. The most common causes of AP are gallstones and heavy alcohol consumption. Less common etiologies include post-endoscopic retrograde cholangiopancreatography (ERCP), hypertriglyceridemia, hypercalcemia, postsurgery, and malignancy and can be HIV related and medication induced [3, 6]. Patients should be questioned about their history of biliary disease, alcohol consumption, medication and drug intake, known hyperlipidemia, abdominal trauma, recent invasive procedures such as ERCP, weight loss and symptoms suggesting malignancy, and a family history of pancreatitis suggesting a hereditary cause of disease. In addition to physical exam, minimum work-up within the first 24 hours should include laboratory serum tests with liver enzymes, calcium, and triglycerides and imaging such as right upper quadrant ultrasound [9, 10]. Should any causative abnormality be found, for example, biliary disease or hypertriglyceridemia, it should be treated prior to discharge. Treatment of AP involves correction of these underlying etiologies and

Pancreatitis: Medical and Surgical Management, First Edition.
David B. Adams, Peter B. Cotton, Nicholas J. Zyromski and John Windsor.
© 2017 John Wiley & Sons, Ltd. Published 2017 by John Wiley & Sons, Ltd.

control of the inflammatory process to prevent severe complications such as multiorgan failure and infected pancreatic necrosis [11].

The pancreatic microcirculation

Alterations to the pancreatic microcirculation play a central role in the pathophysiology and treatment of AP, specifically intravenous fluid resuscitation. Branches of the celiac and superior mesenteric arteries divide to form an intricate network of capillaries that supply the pancreatic acinus with a rich blood supply, referred to as the pancreatic microcirculation [12]. This microcirculation is susceptible to ischemia which may promote the development of pancreatitis [13]. Additionally, evidence suggests that disrupted perfusion of the pancreatic microcirculation is an important factor in the transition from mild interstitial edematous pancreatitis to severe necrotizing pancreatitis [14–16]. Several causes are implicated in disrupting the pancreatic microcirculation in AP including hypovolemia, increased capillary permeability, hypercoagulability with microthrombi, and endothelial damage from oxidative free radicals [12]. Regardless of the underlying pathophysiologic etiology, these disruptions increase the degree of pancreatic ischemia, the release of cytokines and inflammatory mediators, and local vasodilatation and vascular permeability. This can lead to the systemic inflammatory response syndrome (SIRS) and multiorgan failure and increase the risk for severe AP with pancreatic necrosis.

Fluid resuscitation

Long underappreciated intravenous fluid resuscitation is now recognized as the cornerstone of medical treatment for AP [17]. The goal of fluid resuscitation is to adequately perfuse the pancreatic microcirculation to prevent pancreatic ischemia and hopefully limit progression to pancreatic necrosis, SIRS, and multiorgan failure. Perfusion to the pancreatic and intestinal microcirculation is also important to prevent intestinal ischemia and translocation of enteric bacteria with secondary infection of pancreatic necrosis [18]. Additionally, patients with AP are at risk for underlying hypovolemia and require fluid replacement as they

commonly present clinically with vomiting, diaphoresis, and fever [9, 11].

Laboratory markers of intravascular volume depletion, specifically hematocrit, creatinine, and BUN, have been shown to predict the severity of AP. Two studies have demonstrated that an elevated hematocrit at admission or a failure to decrease hematocrit 24 hours after admission is a risk factor for the development of pancreatic necrosis [19, 20]. Another study found that the development of pancreatic necrosis was strongly associated with an increase in serum creatinine within 48 hours of admission [21]. Finally, in a meta-analysis published in 2011 analyzing 1043 cases of AP, a BUN level of 20 mg/dL or greater at admission and BUN rise within 24 hours of hospitalization were associated with an odds ratio of 4.6 and 4.3, respectively, for increased mortality and death [22]. These simple laboratory markers illustrate the importance of intravascular volume in the progression of AP.

The evidence for intravenous fluid resuscitation in AP continues to grow; studies are listed in Table 4.1. Inadequate fluid resuscitation has been associated with the development of acute necrotizing pancreatitis [28]. Recent studies have shown the importance of early fluid resuscitation. A retrospective study of 35 patients with severe AP studied patients in early and late resuscitation groups. Early fluid resuscitation was defined as receiving greater than one-third of the total first 72 hour fluid volume administered within the first 24 hours, and late resuscitation as receiving less than one-third. The investigators found that patients in the early resuscitation group experienced less mortality than those in the late resuscitation group. Although they advocate early fluid resuscitation, they did not suggest a specific fluid volume to be infused [23]. Following this study, a retrospective analysis of 436 patients with AP similarly examining early versus late fluid resuscitation found that early resuscitation was associated with decreased SIRS, decreased organ failure at 72 hours, a lower rate of admission to the intensive care unit, and a decreased length of hospital stay [24].

Despite widespread acceptance that fluid resuscitation is critical in the treatment of AP, no standard guidelines specify the optimal fluid type, volume, rate, and duration of treatment. Further randomized controlled trials are needed to determine standardized recommendations [29]. Regardless of the lack of specific guidelines, most experts recommend starting infusion

Table 4.1 Studies of fluid resuscitation in acute pancreatitis.

Study type	No. of patients	Comparison	Outcome
Retrospective [23]	45	Early versus late fluid resuscitation	Greater mortality in the late resuscitation group
Retrospective [24]	434	Early versus late fluid resuscitation	Less SIRS and organ failure, fewer ICU admissions, and a shorter length of hospital stay in the early resuscitation group. No difference in mortality
Randomized controlled trial [25]	40	Resuscitation with lactated Ringer's solution versus normal saline	Decreased SIRS and CRP levels in patients resuscitated with lactated Ringer's solution
Retrospective [26]	99	Fluid resuscitation with greater than 4 L of fluid versus less than 4 L within the first 24 hours of admission	Patients receiving >4 L of fluid had more respiratory complications and a greater need for intensive care
Randomized controlled trial [27]	115	Fast hemodilution versus slow hemodilution with a goal hematocrit below and above 35%, respectively, within 48 hours of treatment onset	A higher incidence of sepsis, an earlier onset of sepsis, and a lower survival rate in the fast hemodilution group
Prospective cohort study [66]	247	Patients were stratified into three groups, those receiving <3.1 L (low volume), 3.1–4.1 L (intermediate volume), or >4.1 L (high volume) of fluid volume in the first 24 hours of admission	The high-volume group had the highest risk of persistent organ failure (OR 9.1) and acute collections (OR 2.3). The low-volume group had a moderately reduced risk of organ failure (OR 4.1). The intermediate volume group had the best outcomes

in AP with a rate between 250 and 300 mL/h or enough to produce a urine output of at least 0.5 mL/kg [30]. This infusion follows a 1–2 L fluid bolus given to the patient in the emergency department. A total fluid infusion of 2.5–4 L in the first 24 hours will generally suffice to reach resuscitation goals [10]. Initial adjustments in the rate of fluid administration should be made based on the patient's age, weight, physical exam findings, and comorbid conditions. The adequacy of fluid resuscitation should be monitored with vital signs and urinary output, and a Foley catheter is generally not required if fluid intake and output can be accurately recorded. As discussed previously, laboratory markers including hematocrit, BUN, and creatinine are indirect measures of intravascular fluid volume and perfusion of the pancreatic microcirculation and should be measured at admission and at 12 hour intervals to guide fluid management. Symptoms and signs of pulmonary edema should also be monitored [17].

In 2011, Wu et al. published the first randomized controlled trial on early fluid resuscitation in AP. The

trial compared the outcomes of fluid resuscitation with two different crystalloid fluids, lactated Ringer's solution versus normal saline, during the first 24 hours of hospitalization in 40 consecutive patients with AP. They found a significant reduction in systemic inflammation with lactated Ringer's solution compared to normal saline as measured by SIRS and CRP [25]. It is well known that large volume saline infusion is associated with hyperchloremic metabolic acidosis, and studies have shown that acidosis and an acidic extracellular environment may play a key role in the pathophysiology of AP [31–33]. The investigators concluded that the more pH-balanced lactated Ringer's solution may provide improved pH and electrolyte homeostasis when compared to normal saline, leading to less pancreatic and systemic inflammation [25]. Further randomized controlled trials are needed to evaluate fluid management in AP, but lactated Ringer's solution in initial fluid resuscitation may be preferable to normal saline.

Two studies in patients with severe AP have concluded that aggressive fluid resuscitation is potentially harmful, although these conclusions are limited by study design. The first study was a retrospective analysis of 99 patients with severe AP. This study found that patients receiving 4 L or more of fluids in the first 24 hours following admission developed more respiratory complications and had a greater need of intensive care than patients who received less than 4 L of fluid. The respiratory complications were unspecified although no patients developed pulmonary edema [26].

The second study included 115 patients with severe AP in China randomized to slow and fast hemodilution groups. Patients with rapid hemodilution had a goal hematocrit below 35% at 48 hours after admission, and patients with slow hemodilution had a goal hematocrit of 35% or above at 48 hours from admission. They found more sepsis and mortality in the rapid hemodilution group. Fluids were administered over 72 hours in this study, with the majority in the second 24 hour period. As discussed previously, evidence suggests that the best clinical outcomes are obtained by administering more than one-third of the total 72 hour fluid volume in the first 24 hours after admission. All participants were also treated with antibiotics and somatostatin, controversial treatments in AP, as well as Chinese traditional and herbal medicines [27].

There is strong evidence that intravenous fluid resuscitation is important in the medical treatment of AP, and more studies are required before we can conclude that it may be harmful.

Targeted pharmacologic therapy

Despite thousands of animal studies and numerous human trials published on the treatment of AP, there are still no proven pharmacological therapies [34, 35]. Several drugs have been evaluated that specifically target the pathophysiologic process of AP with no benefit in important outcomes in randomized controlled trials [34]. A list of failed major pharmacologic trials is shown in Table 4.2.

These agents include those directed at reducing pancreatic secretions – specifically atropine, glucagon, cimetidine, somatostatin, and its long-acting analog octreotide [34]. A meta-analysis published in 2002 of five randomized controlled trials evaluating cimetidine in AP showed that cimetidine is not more effective than placebo in reducing complications or pain, but in fact

may increase them [49]. Somatostatin and octreotide have had similarly poor results. A randomized controlled trial in 1994 of 302 patients with AP treated with octreotide showed no significant difference in mortality or development of complications when compared with controls [44].

Antiproteases such as gabexate mesilate and aprotinin, hypothesized to inhibit the autodigestive process from proteases in AP, are also ineffective in treatment [34, 50, 51]. Lexipafant is an antagonist targeted against platelet-activating factor, an inflammatory mediator increased in AP, but treatment in randomized controlled trials has shown no significant decrease in mortality [51, 52]. There is no evidence that other pharmacologic therapies such as antioxidants, nitroglycerin, nonsteroidal anti-inflammatory drugs, corticosteroids, IL-10, or TNF-α antibodies are effective in the treatment of AP [34].

Although no medications are proven to be effective in treating AP, randomized controlled trials have validated indomethacin and sublingual nitroglycerin in preventing post-ERCP pancreatitis in high-risk individuals. It is unclear if these interventions benefit all patients undergoing ERCP; in fact, preliminary data from a large multicenter trial at lead by our center indicates that indomethacin may even be harmful in non-high-risk patients. No other medications are proven effective in the prevention or treatment of post-ERCP pancreatitis [53, 54].

Antibiotics

In patients who survive the early phase of AP, the most common cause of death is infection of pancreatic necrosis by enteric bacteria. Patients with pancreatic necrosis have an especially high risk of infection which occurs in 50–70% of cases. Although only 5% of patients with AP develop infected pancreatic necrosis, this complication may account for up to 70% of all deaths [3, 6]. Therefore, there has been much interest in the use of prophylactic antibiotics to prevent these infections in patients and reduce morbidity, mortality, and health-care costs. Antibiotic treatment in AP is a subject of considerable debate with conflicting studies and no clear guidelines. The use of prophylactic antibiotics in severe AP to prevent pancreatic infection is currently not recommended [9].

Table **4.2** Randomized controlled trials in the pharmacological management of acute pancreatitis.

Target	Treatment group	No. of patients	Trial	Outcomes
Antisecretory agents	Atropine [36]	51	RCT	No difference in days of fever, amylase elevation, or length of hospital stay
	Glucagon [37]	66	DBT	No difference in abdominal pain, analgesia, laboratory values including amylase, length of hospital stay, or mortality
	Glucagon [38]	22	DBT	No difference in abdominal pain, laboratory values including amylase, serious complications, or mortality
	Cimetidine [39]	27	DBT	The mean daily serum amylase was higher in the cimetidine group on hospital days 1 and 2. No difference in abdominal pain, analgesia, or other laboratory values
	Cimetidine [40]	60	DBT	No difference in abdominal pain, analgesia, serum amylase, or complications
	Cimetidine [41]	116	RCT	No difference in length of hospital stay, fever, hyperamylasemia, analgesia, complications, or death
	Cimetidine [42]	45	DBT	The cimetidine group had higher mean serum amylase at 48 and 72 hours and serum lipase at 48 hours, slower return of urine amylase to normal, and longer duration of abdominal pain
	Cimetidine [43]	88	RCT	No difference in abdominal pain, analgesia, laboratory values including amylase and lipase, or length of hospital stay
	Octreotide [44]	302	DBT	No difference in mortality, complications, abdominal pain, surgical interventions, or length of hospital stay
	Octreotide [45]	58	RCT	No difference in mortality or complications
	Somatostatin [46]	46	RCT	No difference in the length of hospital stay or mortality but the somatostatin group required fewer overall surgical interventions
Antiproteases	Gabexate [47]	223	DBT	No difference in mortality or complications.
Platelet-activating factor antagonists	Lexipafant [48]	290	DBT	Fewer patients in the lexipafant group developed pseudocysts and systemic sepsis. No difference in new organ failure, mortality, adverse events, length of hospital stay, or overall development of local complications

RCT: randomized controlled trial; DBT: randomized double-blind controlled trial.

Earlier meta-analyses of antibiotic treatment in AP showed that broad-spectrum antibiotics may improve outcomes and reduce mortality. Thus, in the past, use of antibiotics in all patients with acute necrotizing pancreatitis was recommended and widespread [51]. One of these meta-analyses, published in 2001, evaluated three randomized controlled trials comparing antibiotic prophylaxis versus no prophylaxis in 160 cases of acute necrotizing pancreatitis. In patients treated with prophylactic antibiotics, they found a significant reduction in sepsis and mortality by 21.1% and 12.3%, respectively, but no difference in the incidence of local pancreatic infection [55]. Subsequent meta-analyses have had conflicting results.

An updated meta-analysis was published in 2008, which included the same three trials and also four new randomized controlled trials comparing prophylactic antibiotics versus controls with a total of 467 patients. They found no difference in the rates of infected pancreatic necrosis or mortality between the antibiotic and control groups [56]. A Cochrane review of the same seven trials published in 2010 did not find a significant difference in mortality, but did find a significant difference in pancreatic infection when imipenem was used alone in treatment [57].

The most recent meta-analysis was published in 2011 and evaluated 14 randomized controlled trials with a total of 841 patients. They found no significant difference between antibiotic and control groups in mortality, incidence of infected pancreatic necrosis, nonpancreatic infections, and surgical interventions [58]. Furthermore, antibiotic use may be associated with an increased risk of pancreatic fungal infections [59]. As a result of these most recent meta-analyses, prophylactic antibiotics are not recommended for use in AP and should not be used in the first 24 hours of treatment unless there is a suspected or documented infection. As evidence continues to accumulate, antibiotics are appearing less helpful in the treatment of AP.

Probiotic prophylaxis, as shown in a meta-analysis in 2009, is not recommended for treating AP as it does not reduce the risk of infected pancreatic necrosis or decrease mortality [60]. In one randomized controlled trial, probiotics were actually associated with an increase in mortality [61]. Selective gut decontamination, which involves oral administration of antibiotics to eliminate enteric Gram-negative rods and reduce the risk of bacterial translocation from the intestine to the pancreas, may be beneficial in preventing infected pancreatic necrosis, but further studies are necessary. Only one randomized controlled trial in 1995 evaluated this treatment, which showed improvement in mortality [62].

It is important to note that in the initial hospital course of patients with severe AP and pancreatic necrosis, they may appear septic with SIRS and/or multiorgan failure. If infection or sepsis is suspected, treatment with antibiotics is appropriate while conducting a thorough evaluation for infection including blood cultures and cultures of a fine-needle aspirate from the site of pancreatic necrosis. If the infectious work-up is negative, antibiotics should be stopped [9].

Enteral feeding

Although not the primary topic of this chapter, enteral feeding is important in the medical management of AP. In mild AP, enteral feeding is generally started within 1 week of hospitalization following reduction in abdominal pain, absence of nausea and vomiting, cessation of parenteral analgesics, return of bowel sounds, and improvement in the overall clinical picture [9]. It can be started with a low-fat diet, and nutritional support is generally not required [63].

In severe AP or predicted severe pancreatitis, enteral feeding via tube feedings should be started within 72 hours of hospitalization. Multiple studies have shown that enteral feeding is superior to parenteral feeding in severe AP as it maintains the gut barrier. In a meta-analysis published in 2012 of 381 patients

with severe AP randomized to total parenteral nutrition versus total enteral nutrition, total enteral nutrition was superior regarding mortality, infectious complications, organ failure, and lower surgical intervention rate [64]. Although historically nasojejunal feeding has been preferred, nasogastric feeding may be just as effective [65].

If it is clear that the patient is not meeting nutritional goals within the first week of hospitalization with enteral feeding, parenteral nutrition should be initiated. However, enteral feeding should be continued even at low rates to maintain gut barrier function and prevent bacterial translocation.

Conclusion

In summary, despite high morbidity, mortality, and health-care costs, the medical treatment of AP remains largely supportive with no pharmacologic therapies verified to improve important clinical outcomes. Intravenous fluid resuscitation, especially within the first 24 hours of presentation, is the cornerstone of treatment and critical to maintaining the microcirculation of the pancreas to prevent progression from mild to severe AP and complications such as SIRS, multiorgan failure, and pancreatic necrosis. Further randomized controlled trials are needed to create specific guidelines on the optimal type, volume, and rate of intravenous fluid resuscitation. Antibiotics are not recommended in the prevention of infected pancreatic necrosis as they have shown no benefit in overall mortality in multiple meta-analyses.

References

1 Neoptolemos JP, Raraty M, Finch M, et al. Acute pancreatitis: the substantial human and financial costs. Gut 1998; 42:886–891.

2 Peery AF, Dellon ES, Lund J, et al. Burden of gastrointestinal disease in the United States: 2012 update. Gastroenterology 2012; 132:1179–1187.

3 Mann DV, Hershman MJ, Hittinger R, et al. Multicentre audit of death from acute pancreatitis. British Journal of Surgery 1994; 81:890–893.

4 Russo MW, Wei JT, Thiny MT, et al. Digestive and liver disease statistics, 2004. Gastroenterology 2004; 126:1448–1453.

5 Fagenholz PJ, Castillo CF, Harris NS, et al. Increasing United States hospital admissions for acute pancreatitis, 1988–2003. Annals of Epidemiology 2007; 17:491–497.

6 Appelros S, Lindgren S, Borgström A. Short and long term outcome of severe acute pancreatitis. European Journal of Surgery 2001; 167:281–286.

7 Banks PA, Bollen TL, Dervenis C, et al. Classification of acute pancreatitis 2012: revision of the Atlanta classification and definitions by international consensus. Gut 2013; 62:102–111.

8 Phillip V, Steiner JM, Algül H. Early phase of acute pancreatitis: assessment and management. World Journal of Gastrointestinal Pathophysiology 2014; 5(3):158–168.

9 Banks PA, Freeman ML. Practice guidelines in acute pancreatitis. American Journal of Gastroenterology 2006; 101:2379–2400

10 Besselink M, van Santvoort H, Freeman M, et al. IAP/APA evidence-based guidelines for the management of acute pancreatitis. Pancreatology 2013; 13:e1-e15.

11 Cruz-Santamaria DM, Taxonera C, Giner M. Update on pathogenesis and clinical management of acute pancreatitis. World Journal of Gastrointestinal Pathophysiology 2012; 3:60–70.

12 Cuthbertson CM, Christophi C. Disturbances of the microcirculation in acute pancreatitis. British Journal of Surgery 2006; 93:518–530.

13 Warshaw AL, O'Hara PJ. Susceptibility of the pancreas to ischemic injury in shock. Annals of Surgery 1978; 188:197–201.

14 Knoefel WT, Kollias N, Warshaw AL, et al. Pancreatic microcirculatory changes in experimental pancreatitis of graded severity in the rat. Surgery 1994; 116:904–913.

15 Strate T, Mann O, Kleinhans H, et al. Microcirculatory function and tissue damage is improved after therapeutic injection of bovine hemoglobin in severe acute rodent pancreatitis. Pancreas 2005; 30:254–259.

16 Bassi D, Kollias N, Fernandez-del Castillo C, et al. Impairment of pancreatic microcirculation correlates with the severity of acute experimental pancreatitis. Journal of the American College of Surgeons 1994; 179:257–263.

17 Fisher JM, Gardner TB. The "golden hours" of management in acute pancreatitis. American Journal of Gastroenterology 2012; 107:1146–1150.

18 Hotz HG, Foitzik T, Rohweder J, et al. Intestinal microcirculation and gut permeability in acute pancreatitis: early changes and therapeutic implications. Journal of Gastrointestinal Surgery 1998; 2:518–525.

19 Baillargeon JD, Orav J, Ramaqopal V, et al. Hemoconcentration as an early risk factor for necrotizing pancreatitis. American Journal of Gastroenterology 1998; 93:2130–2134.

20 Brown A, Orav J, Banks PA. Hemoconcentration is an early marker for organ failure and necrotizing pancreatitis. Pancreas 2000; 20:367–372.

21 Muddana V, Whitcomb DC, Khalid A, et al. Elevated serum creatinine as a marker of pancreatic necrosis in acute pancreatitis. American Journal of Gastroenterology 2009; 104:164–170.

22 Wu BU, Bakker OJ, Papachristou GI, et al. Blood urea nitrogen in the early assessment of acute pancreatitis. Archives of Internal Medicine 2011; 171:669–676.

23 Gardner TB, Vege SS, Chari ST, et al. Faster rate of initial fluid resuscitation in severe acute pancreatitis diminishes in-hospital mortality. Pancreatology 2009; 9:770–776.

24 Warndorf MG, Kurtzman JT, Bartel MJ, et al. Early fluid resuscitation reduces morbidity among patients with acute pancreatitis. Clinical Gastroenterology and Hepatology 2011; 9:705–709.

25 Wu BU, Hwang JQ, Gardner TH, et al. Lactated ringer's solution reduces systemic inflammation compared with saline in patients with acute pancreatitis. Clinical Gastroenterology and Hepatology 2011; 9:710–717.

26 Eckerwall G, Olin H, Andersson B, et al. Fluid resuscitation and nutritional support during severe acute pancreatitis in the past: what we have learned and how we can do better? Clinical Nutrition 2006; 25:497–504.

27 Mao EQ, Fei J, Peng YB, et al. Rapid hemodilution is associated with increased sepsis and mortality among patients with severe acute pancreatitis. Chinese Medical Journal (England) 2010; 123:1639–1644.

28 Brown A, Baillargeon JD, Hughes MD, et al. Can fluid resuscitation prevent pancreatic necrosis in severe acute pancreatitis? Pancreatology 2002; 2:104–107.

29 Nasr JY, Papachristou GI. Early fluid resuscitation in acute pancreatitis: a lot more than just fluids. Clinical Gastroenterology and Hepatology 2011; 9:633–634.

30 Talukdar R, Vege SS. Early management of severe acute pancreatitis. Current Gastroenterology Reports 2011; 13:123–130.

31 Kellum JA. Saline-induced hyperchloremic metabolic acidosis. Critical Care Medicine 2002; 30:259–261.

32 Noble MD, Romac J, Vigna SR, et al. A pH-sensitive, neurogenic pathway mediates disease severity in a model of post-ERCP pancreatitis. Gut 2008; 57:1566–1571

33 Bhoomagoud M, Jung T, Atladottir J, et al. Reducing extracellular pH sensitizes the acinar cell to secretagogue-induced pancreatitis responses in rats. Gastroenterology 2009; 137:1083–1092.

34 Bang UC, Semb S, Nojgaard C, et al. Pharmacological approach to acute pancreatitis. World Journal of Gastroenterology 2008; 14:2968–2976.

35 Fantini L, Tomassetti P, Pezzilli R. Management of acute pancreatitis: current knowledge and future perspectives. World Journal of Emergency Surgery 2006; doi:10.1186/1749-7922-1-16

36 Cameron JL, Mehigan D, Zuidema GD. Evaluation of atropine in acute pancreatitis. Surgery, Gynecology & Obstetrics 1979; 148(2):206–208.

37 Debas HT, Hancock RJ, Soon-Shiong P, et al. Glucagon therapy in acute pancreatitis: prospective randomized double-blind study. Canadian Journal of Surgery 1980; 23:578–580.

38 Kronborg O, Bulow S, Joergensen PM. A randomized double-blind trial of glucagon in treatment of first attack of severe acute pancreatitis without associated biliary disease. American Journal of Gastroenterology 1980; 73:423–425.

39 Meshkinpour H, Molinari MD, Gardner L, et al. Cimetidine in the treatment of acute alcoholic pancreatitis. A randomized, double-blind study. Gastroenterology 1979; 77:687–690.

40 Sillero C, Perez-Mateo M, Vazquez N, et al. Controlled trial of cimetidine in acute pancreatitis. European Journal of Clinical Pharmacology 1981; 21:17–21.

41 Broe PJ, Zinner MJ, Cameron JL. A clinical trial of cimetidine in acute pancreatitis. Surgery, Gynecology & Obstetrics 1982; 154:13–16.

42 Loiudice TA, Lang J, Mehta H. Treatment of acute alcoholic pancreatitis: the roles of cimetidine and nasogastric suction. American Journal of Gastroenterology 1984; 79:553–558.

43 Navarro S, Ros E, Aused R, et al. Comparison of fasting, nasogastric suction and cimetidine in the treatment of acute pancreatitis. Digestion 1984; 30:224–230.

44 Uhl W, Buchler MW, Malfertheiner P, et al. A randomized, double blind, multicentre trial of octreotide in moderate to severe acute pancreatitis. Gut 1999; 45:97–104.

45 McKay C, Baxter T, Imrie C. A randomized, controlled trial of octreotide in the management of patients with acute pancreatitis. International Journal of Pancreatology 1997; 21:13–19.

46 Planas M, Pérez A, Iglesias R, et al. Severe acute pancreatitis: treatment with somatostatin. Intensive Care Medicine 1998; 24:37–39.

47 Büchler M, Malfertheiner P, Uhl W et al. Gabexate mesilate in human acute pancreatitis. German Pancreatitis Study Group. Gastroenterology 1993; 104:1165–1170.

48 Johnson CD, Kingsnorth AN, Imrie CW, et al. Double blind, randomised, placebo controlled study of a platelet activating factor antagonist, lexipafant, in the treatment and prevention of organ failure in predicted severe acute pancreatitis. Gut 2001; 48:62–69.

49 Morimoto T, Noguchi Y, Sakai T, et al. Acute pancreatitis and the role of histamine-2 receptor antagonists: a meta-analysis of randomized controlled trials of cimetidine. European Journal of Gastroenterology & Hepatology 2002; 14:679–686.

50 Andriulli A, Leandro G, Clemente R, et al. Meta-analysis of somatostatin, octreotide and gabexate mesilate in the therapy of acute pancreatitis. Alimentary Pharmacology & Therapeutics 1998; 12:237–245.

51 Heinrich S, Schäfer M, Rousson V, et al. Evidence-based treatment of acute pancreatitis: a look at established paradigms. Annals of Surgery 2006; 243:154–168.

52 Imrie CW, McKay CJ. The possible role of platelet-activating factor antagonist therapy in the management of severe acute pancreatitis. Baillieres Best Practice & Research Clinical Gastroenterology 1999; 13:357–364.

53 Elmunzer BJ, Scheiman JM, Lehman GA, et al. A randomized trial of rectal indomethacin to prevent post-ERCP pancreatitis. New England Journal of Medicine 2012; 366:1414–1422.

54 Sotoudehmanesh R, Eloubeidi MA, Asgari AA, et al. A randomized trial of rectal indomethacin and sublingual nitrates to prevent post-ERCP pancreatitis. American Journal of Gastroenterology 2014; 109:903–909.

55 Sharma VK, Howden CW. Prophylactic antibiotic administration reduces sepsis and mortality in acute necrotizing pancreatitis: a meta-analysis. Pancreas 2001; 22:28–31.

56 Bai Y, Gao J, Zou DW, et al. Prophylactic antibiotics cannot reduce infected pancreatic necrosis and mortality in acute necrotizing pancreatitis: evidence from a meta-analysis of randomized controlled trials. American Journal of Gastroenterology 2008; 103:104–110.

57 Villatoro E, Mulla M, Larvin M. Antibiotic therapy for prophylaxis against infection of pancreatic necrosis in acute pancreatitis. Cochrane Database of Systematic Reviews 2010; (5):CD002941.

58 Wittau M, Mayer B, Scheele J, et al. Systematic review and meta-analysis of antibiotic prophylaxis in severe acute pancreatitis. Scandinavian Journal of Gastroenterology 2011; 46:261–270.

59 Trikudanathan G, Navaneethan U, Vege SS. Intra-abdominal fungal infections complicating acute pancreatitis: a review. American Journal of Gastroenterology 2011; 106:1188–1192.

60 Sun S, Yang K, He X, et al. Probiotics in patients with severe acute pancreatitis: a meta-analysis. Langenbeck's Archives of Surgery 2009; 394:171–177.

61 Besselink MGH, van Santvoort HC, Buskens E, et al. Probiotic prophylaxis in predicted severe acute pancreatitis: a randomized, double-blind, placebo-controlled trial. Lancet 2008; 371:651–659.

62 Luiten EJ, Hop WC, Lange JF, et al. Controlled clinical trial of selective decontamination for the treatment of severe acute pancreatitis. Annals of Surgery 1995; 222:57–65.

63 Jacobson BC, Vander Vliet MB, Hughes MD, et al. A prospective, randomized trial of clear liquids versus low-fat solid diet as the initial meal in mild acute pancreatitis. Clinical Gastroenterology and Hepatology 2007; 5:946–951.

64 Yi F, Ge L, Zhao J, et al. Meta-analysis: total parenteral nutrition versus total enteral nutrition in predicted severe acute pancreatitis. Internal Medicine 2012; 51:523–530.

65 Eatock FC, Chong P, Menezes N, et al. A randomized study of early nasogastric versus nasojejunal feeding in severe acute pancreatitis. American Journal of Gastroenterology 2005; 100:432–439.

66 de-Madaria E, Soler-Sala G, Sánchez-Payá J, et al. Influence of fluid therapy on the prognosis of acute pancreatitis: a prospective cohort study. American Journal of Gastroenterology 2011; 106(10):1843–50.

CHAPTER 5

Nutritional treatment in acute pancreatitis

Maxim S. Petrov

Department of Surgery, University of Auckland, Auckland, New Zealand

Introduction

The last half-century has seen several advances in the early management of acute pancreatitis. These include emergence of randomized controlled trials on fluid resuscitation and analgesia, more data (albeit conflicting) on the prophylactic use of antibiotics, and restriction of indications for early therapeutic endoscopic retrograde cholangiopancreatography to patients with coexisting acute cholangitis. However, the most notable and consistent improvement in outcomes has come from the use of nutrition in patients with acute pancreatitis [1–4].

Type of nutrition

The importance of providing nutritional support in patients with acute pancreatitis has been known since the 1970s. Parenteral nutrition was regarded as the standard of nutritional management for nearly four decades due to the advocacy of the "pancreatic rest" concept [5–7]. The rationale for this concept was to rest the inflamed pancreas, thereby preventing stimulation of exocrine function and release of proteolytic enzymes. However, critics argued that, in addition to cost- and catheter-related sepsis, parenteral nutrition might lead to electrolyte and metabolic disturbances, gut barrier alteration, and increased intestinal permeability [8–13]. Comparison of total parenteral nutrition and total enteral nutrition in patients with predicted severe acute pancreatitis was the subject of several randomized controlled trials (Table 5.1) [14–21]. The results were statistically aggregated in a number of meta-analyses, all

of which demonstrated the benefits of enteral over parenteral nutrition [22–26]. In particular, a meta-analysis of high-quality randomized controlled trials only has shown a significant twofold reduction in the risk of total and pancreatic infectious complications and a 2.5-fold reduction in the risk of death in patients receiving total enteral nutrition [25].

Despite the evident clinical benefits of enteral over parenteral nutrition in terms of the reduction in risk of infectious complications and mortality, the exact mechanism of its favorable effect remains unclear [27–29]. It is believed that enteral nutrition may prevent or attenuate the mucosal barrier breakdown and subsequent bacterial translocation that is thought to play a pivotal role in the development of infectious complications in the course of severe acute pancreatitis. When monitoring mucosal barrier function, permeability of the structural mucosal barrier is the usual parameter measured. Unfortunately, there is no consistency in the clinical studies with regard to gut permeability. On the one hand, three clinical studies of acute pancreatitis showed increased intestinal permeability to both micromolecules and macromolecules in patients with predicted severe acute pancreatitis when compared with those with predicted mild acute pancreatitis and healthy volunteers [30, 31]. On the other hand, the randomized controlled trial by Powell and colleagues, in which patients with predicted severe acute pancreatitis were randomized to receive either enteral nutrition or no artificial nutritional support, showed significantly increased intestinal permeability by day 4 in patients allocated to the enteral nutrition group [32]. Similarly, the randomized controlled trial of nasogastric versus parenteral feeding in predicted severe patients by

Pancreatitis: Medical and Surgical Management, First Edition.
David B. Adams, Peter B. Cotton, Nicholas J. Zyromski and John Windsor.
© 2017 John Wiley & Sons, Ltd. Published 2017 by John Wiley & Sons, Ltd.

Table 5.1 Randomized controlled trials of total enteral versus total parenteral nutrition in patients with predicted severe acute pancreatitis.

Reference	Setting	Patients (n)		Allocation concealment	Reduction of infectious complications and mortality
		Enteral nutrition	Parenteral nutrition		
Kalfarentzos et al. [14]	Greece	18	20	Open label	Significantly lower rate of pancreatic infection in the total enteral nutrition group
Gupta et al. [15]	United Kingdom	8	9	Open label	Nonsignificantly lower rate of pancreatic infection in the total enteral nutrition group
Louie et al. [16]	Canada	10	18	Open label	Nonsignificantly lower rate of pancreatic infection in the total enteral nutrition group
Eckerwall et al. [17]	Sweden	23	25	Open label	No significant difference in outcomes
Petrov et al. [18]	Russia	35	34	Open label	Significantly lower rate of pancreatic infection and mortality in the total enteral nutrition group
Casas et al. [19]	Spain	11	11	Open label	Nonsignificantly lower rate of pancreatic infection in the total enteral nutrition group
Doley et al. [20]	India	25	25	Open label	No significant difference in the outcomes
Wu et al. [21]	China	53	54	Open label	Significantly lower rate of pancreatic infection and mortality in the total enteral nutrition group

Eckerwall and colleagues demonstrated impaired gut permeability on day 3 in the enteral nutrition group [17]. It should be noted that both randomized controlled trials included patients with mild acute pancreatitis (11 of 27 and 26 of 48, respectively), in whom intestinal permeability is not likely to change.

Furthermore, concentrations of antiendotoxin core antibodies for immunoglobulin M were also used as an indirect marker for intestinal permeability. Results of the randomized controlled trial from the United Kingdom showed that serum immunoglobulin M antibodies decreased significantly following 7 days of enteral nutrition when compared with the parenteral nutrition group ($P < 0.05$) [9]. Similarly, the randomized controlled trial by Gupta and colleagues demonstrated that immunoglobulin M antibodies fell significantly in the enteral nutrition group ($P = 0.03$) and tended to rise in the parenteral nutrition group over the week of treatment [15]. Conversely, the randomized controlled trial by Eckerwall and colleagues found decreasing levels of immunoglobulin M antibodies in both the enteral nutrition and parenteral nutrition groups, with no significant difference at any time point during 10 days of observation [17]. The mechanism of the beneficial effect of enteral nutrition in acute pancreatitis warrants further investigation, and more studies on the use and effect of enteral nutrition in patients with acute pancreatitis are needed.

Route of enteral nutrition

The previous section has demonstrated that enteral nutrition is preferred to parenteral nutrition because it leads to significantly better clinical outcomes. With these benefits apparent, the next important question to discuss is: what is the optimal site to deliver enteral nutrition? The usual options are postpyloric (mainly, nasojejunal) and prepyloric (nasogastric) tube placement. The former usually requires the assistance of an endoscopist or a radiologist, and this may result in a delay in commencing enteral nutrition. This delay may have an impact on the clinical outcome because it is now believed that enteral nutrition should commence as soon as possible after adequate fluid resuscitation in order to maximize clinical benefit. In contrast, a nasogastric feeding tube can usually be inserted immediately allowing prepyloric feeding to start without delay [33–36].

The question of optimal site of enteral feeding in acute pancreatitis also relates to the "pancreatic rest" concept. The central tenet of this concept is that enteral nutrition delivered into any part of the upper gastrointestinal tract other than the jejunum stimulates pancreatic secretion and, consequently, exacerbates the severity of acute pancreatitis [35]. Given that this concept remained unchallenged for decades, the majority of clinical studies in the field of acute pancreatitis were conducted using nasojejunal tube feeding. However, accumulating evidence from other fields, particularly critical care medicine, suggests that nasogastric feeding may be as safe and effective as nasojejunal feeding, at least in some patients. Thus, there is a need and justification for exploring questions concerning the optimal route of enteral nutrition delivery to be used in patients with acute pancreatitis.

A number of randomized controlled trials and a meta-analysis have demonstrated the equivalence of nasogastric and nasojejunal tube feeding in terms of safety and tolerance in critically ill patients [37–40]. While this may be true for this group of patients, it is recognized that patients with acute pancreatitis are particularly prone to gastric ileus because of the subjacent inflamed pancreas. This has been given as a reason for preferentially providing enteral nutrition into the jejunum [34]. Another reason given is to avoid the provision of enteral nutrition proximal to the jejunum where there is concern that it might induce exocrine pancreatic stimulation and consequently a risk of increasing the severity of acute pancreatitis. Most studies in patients with acute pancreatitis have employed nasojejunal tube feeding, but there are some studies that employed nasogastric tube feeding, and they were systematically reviewed to determine the safety and tolerance of nasogastric tube feeding alone and to assess the relative efficacy of nasogastric versus nasojejunal feeding in patients with acute pancreatitis [40]. Table 5.2 demonstrates the characteristics of studies included in this review.

Nasogastric feeding-related outcomes, including safety and tolerance, are presented in Table 5.3. Full tolerance was achieved in 107 of 131 (82%) patients who did not require temporary reduction, stoppage, or withdrawal of nasogastric feeding. The 24 patients who had a modification of the nasogastric tube feeding regimen presented signs of gastric ileus ($n = 7$) and troublesome diarrhea ($n = 14$) or repeatedly removed their feeding tube ($n = 3$).

Table 5.2 Characteristics of studies of nasogastric tube feeding.

Reference	Setting	Design	Control group	APACHE II Score	Feeding start	Feeding formulation	Duration of nutrition
Eatock et al. [9]	United Kingdom	Cohort study	N/A	10 (4–28)[a]	<48 hours of admission	Semielemental	Not stated
Eatock et al. [37]	United Kingdom	RCT	Nasojejunal	10 (7–18)[a]	72 (24–72) hours after onset	Semielemental	5 days
Kumar et al. [38]	India	RCT	Nasojejunal	10.5 ± 3.8[b]	48–72 hours of admission	Semielemental	7 days
Eckerwall et al. [17]	Sweden	RCT	Parenteral	10 (8–13)[a]	<24 hours of admission	Polymeric	6 (5–9)[a] days
Singh et al. [39]	India	RCT	Nasojejunal	8.5 (2–19)[a]	10 (4–23)[a] days after onset	Semielemental	7 days

APACHE, acute physiology and chronic health evaluation; RCT, randomized controlled trial; N/A, not available.

[a]Values are median (range).

[b]Values are mean ± standard deviation.

Table 5.3 Safety and tolerance of nasogastric tube feeding in acute pancreatitis.

Reference	Total patients	Troublesome diarrhea, n (%)	Tube removal, n (%)	Gastric retention, n (%)	Exacerbation of pain following feeding, n (%)	Achievement of nutritional goal	Full tolerance of feeding, n (%)[a]
Eatock et al. [9]	26	3 (11.5)	1 (3.8)	3 (11.5)	0 (0)	Not stated	19 (73.1)
Eatock et al. [37]	27	3 (11.1)	1 (3.7)	0 (0)	2 (7.4)	21 patients (78%) after 60 hours	23 (85.1)
Kumar et al. [38]	16	4 (25)	1 (6.3)	0 (0)	1 (6.3)	16 patients (100%) by day 7[b]	11 (68.8)
Eckerwall et al. [17]	23	0 (0)	0 (0)	3 (13)	Not stated	15 patients (66%) by day 7	20 (86.9)
Singh et al. [39]	39	4 (10.4)	0 (0)	1 (2.5)	3 (7.7.)	Not stated	34 (85.6)
Total	131	14 (10.7)	3 (2.3)	7 (5.3)	6 (4.5)	N/A	107 (82.0)

N/A, not available.
[a]Did not require temporary reduction, stoppage, or withdrawal of feeding.
[b]Six patients were supplemented by parenteral nutrition during the commencement of feeding.

The meta-analysis was restricted to randomized studies of nasogastric versus nasojejunal feeding [37–39]. In three eligible trials, a total of 82 patients received enteral nutrition via the nasogastric route and 75 patients via the nasojejunal route. The use of nasogastric feeding resulted in a nonsignificant reduction in the risk of death (relative risk: 0.71; 95% confidence interval: 0.38–1.32; $P = 0.28$). The number of nutrition-associated adverse events was similar between the two groups. As a consequence, nasogastric feeding was associated with a nonsignificant increase in the risk of troublesome diarrhea (relative risk 1.39; 95% confidence interval 0.57–3.36; $P = 0.47$) and a nonsignificant decrease in the risk of pain relapse following feeding (relative risk 0.84; 95% confidence interval 0.27–2.59; $P = 0.76$). Overall, patients in both groups did not differ significantly in terms of intolerance to feeding (relative risk 1.23; 95% confidence interval 0.59–2.55; $P = 0.57$). There was no heterogeneity between the study results for all comparisons ($I^2 = 0\%$).

This systematic review demonstrated the safety and tolerance of nasogastric tube feeding in at least four out of five patients with acute pancreatitis [40]. The study population was limited to patients with a predicted severe acute pancreatitis and the clinical outcomes were within the expected range for this category of patients. Nasogastric tube feeding-related problems occurred in less than 20% of patients; they were relatively minor, and there were no recorded cases of aspiration pneumonia.

Three randomized controlled trials included in the meta-analysis consistently yielded no tangible difference between nasogastric and nasojejunal feeding in terms of safety and tolerance [37–39]. It should be acknowledged that the trials had some flaws. In particular, it was argued that it is likely that jejunal feeding in the trial from Glasgow was actually duodenal (because true jejunal placement would have been difficult with the types of feeding tubes and placement techniques used), meaning that both feeding arms may have caused equivalent stimulation of pancreatic secretion [37]. The shortcoming of the randomized controlled trial by Kumar and colleagues was that there was a considerable delay (7.8 ± 6.5 and 5.7 ± 4.7 days after symptom onset in the nasogastric and nasojejunal groups, respectively) and that enteral nutrition was commenced late [38]. In addition, the authors observed a high mortality (31% and 29% in the nasogastric and nasojejunal groups, respectively) which might reflect the tendency toward conservative management of patients with infected pancreatic necrosis. The randomized controlled trial by Singh and colleagues suffered from the same shortcoming, that is, the feeding protocol in both groups was commenced relatively late (10 [4–23] and

11 [3–48] days after symptom onset in the nasogastric and nasojejunal groups, respectively) [39]. Apart from these concerns, the three randomized controlled trials were insufficiently powered individually to detect any difference or to demonstrate equivalence between the studied groups in terms of mortality. An adequately powered randomized controlled trial would need to enroll nearly 200 patients per arm in order to show a decrease in mortality from 14% (average rate in the nasogastric group in the present review) to 6% (best results in the nasojejunal group of randomized controlled trials on enteral vs. parenteral nutrition) with 80% power and $\alpha = 0.05$ (two sided). Such a sample size is appreciably large, even for a multicenter study.

Another relevant issue in considering nasogastric tube feeding is the effect on exocrine pancreatic function. It was shown by O'Keefe and colleagues that all forms of enteral nutrition stimulate pancreatic secretion [41, 42]. In particular, when compared with placebo saline, an oral liquid polymeric diet resulted in a significantly higher level of amylase ($P < 0.01$) and lipase ($P < 0.01$); a duodenal polymeric enteral formula led to increased levels of amylase ($P < 0.01$), lipase ($P < 0.01$), and trypsin ($P < 0.01$); and a duodenal elemental feeding formula resulted in an elevated level of lipase ($P < 0.05$). The same research group also compared the pancreatic secretory response to tube feeding delivered into the duodenum and the mid (40–60 cm distal to the ligament of Treitz) and distal (100–120 cm distal to the ligament of Treitz) jejunum [40, 42]. Even though the authors did not find a direct relationship between the decrease in enzyme secretion and distance down the mid–distal jejunum, they demonstrated significantly lower secretion of trypsin ($P < 0.01$) and lipase ($P < 0.05$) in response to the elemental formula delivered into the jejunum (40 cm or more distal to the ligament of Treitz) in comparison with the duodenum. Moreover, the trypsin and lipase secretory response in the mid–distal jejunum group was as low as in the control group (fasting).

However, it should be noted that these studies of the effects of enteral feeding on exocrine pancreatic function were in healthy subjects. There is now convincing evidence that patients with acute pancreatitis have significantly lower rates of enzyme secretion compared with healthy subjects [41, 43]. Furthermore, when patients with mild to moderate acute pancreatitis were compared with those with severe acute pancreatitis, a lower secretion of trypsin (sixfold), amylase (22-fold), and lipase (42-fold) was found in the latter group, suggesting that pancreatic enzyme secretion is inversely related to the severity of acute pancreatitis. In line with this finding, another study showed an 86% rate of pancreatic exocrine insufficiency (measured by fecal pancreatic elastase-1) in patients recovering from severe attacks of acute pancreatitis. Moreover, the severity of pancreatic exocrine insufficiency correlated with the extent of pancreatic necrosis. These data suggest that injured acinar cells are not able to respond fully to the physiological stimuli of secretion which may go some way toward explaining the findings of this study that, contrary to popular belief, nasogastric tube feeding does not appear to aggravate the severity of acute pancreatitis.

Enteral nutrition formulations

There are more than 100 different enteral nutrition formulations available [44]. These can be broadly classified into the following categories:

- Elemental – comprising amino acids or oligopeptides, maltodextrins, and medium-chain and long-chain triglycerides
- Polymeric – comprising nonhydrolyzed proteins, maltodextrins and oligofructosaccharides, as well as long-chain triglycerides
- Immune enhancing – comprising substrates that have been hypothesized to modulate the activity of the immune system, for example, immunonutrition (glutamine, arginine, and omega-3 fatty acids), probiotics, fiber-enriched formulation)

A comprehensive systematic literature review has compared the safety, tolerance, and efficacy of all enteral nutrition formulations used in randomized controlled trials of patients with acute pancreatitis [45]. A total of 20 randomized controlled trials, encompassing 1070 patients, met all the inclusion criteria. Patients received an elemental formulation in eight arms of the included trials, a polymeric formulation in seven arms, a fiber-enriched enteral formulation in six arms, enteral nutrition supplemented with probiotics in four arms, and immunonutrition (glutamine, arginine, and omega-3 fatty acids) in three arms (Table 5.4).

One randomized controlled trial directly compared an elemental formulation with a polymeric formulation in

Table 5.4 Characteristics of randomized controlled trials of various enteral nutrition formulations.

Reference	Intervention group	Control group	Number of patients	
			Intervention group	Control group
McClave et al. [48]	Semielemental EN	PN	15	15
Kalfarentzos et al. [14]	Semielemental EN	PN	18	20
Windsor et al. [49]	Polymeric EN	PN	16	18
Powell et al. [32]	Polymeric EN	NN	13	14
Hallay et al. [50]	EN with fiber + glutamine + arginine	EN with fiber	11	8
Olah et al. [51]	Elemental EN	PN	41	48
Abou-Assi et al. [52]	Elemental EN	PN	26	27
Olah et al. [51]	EN with fiber + probiotics	EN with fiber	22	23
Gupta et al. [15]	Polymeric EN	PN	8	9
Louie et al. [16]	Semielemental EN	PN	10	18
Lasztity et al. [53]	Polymeric EN + n-3 PUFAs	Polymeric EN	14	14
Pearce et al. [54]	EN with fiber + glutamine + arginine + omega-3 fatty acids	EN with fiber	15	16
Tiengou et al. [55]	Semielemental EN	Polymeric EN	15	15
Eckerwall et al. [17]	Polymeric EN	PN	23	25
Petrov et al. [18]	Semielemental EN	PN	35	34
Casas et al. [19]	Semielemental EN	PN	11	11
Olah et al. [56]	EN with fiber + probiotics	EN with fiber	33	29
Karakan et al. [57]	EN with fiber	Polymeric EN	15	15
Besselink et al. [58]	EN with fiber + probiotics	EN with fiber	152	144
Qin et al. [59]	Semielemental EN + probiotics	PN	36	38

EN, enteral nutrition; PN, parenteral nutrition; PUFA, polyunsaturated fatty acid.

30 patients with mild or severe acute pancreatitis. Given that direct meta-analysis was not possible, the two formulations were compared using the methodology of indirect adjusted meta-analysis. A total of 10 randomized controlled trials comprising 428 patients compared elemental and polymeric formulations indirectly, using parenteral nutrition as a reference treatment. In all patients with acute pancreatitis, the use of an elemental formulation did not result in a significant difference in risk of infectious complications (indirectly estimated relative risk 0.48; 95% confidence interval 0.06–3.76; $P = 0.482$) and death (indirectly estimated relative risk 0.63; 95% confidence interval 0.04–9.86; $P = 0.741$). The risk of feeding intolerance did not differ significantly between the two formulations (indirectly estimated relative risk 0.62; 95% confidence interval 0.10–3.97; $P = 0.611$).

A total of three randomized controlled trials comprising 403 patients directly compared a fiber-enriched formulation supplemented with probiotics and a fiber-enriched formulation only. In all patients with acute pancreatitis, the use of probiotics did not result in a significant difference in the risk of infectious complications (relative risk 0.71; 95% confidence interval 0.40–1.27; p = 0.250) or death (relative risk 0.85; 95% confidence interval 0.18–4.14; $P = 0.850$). The risk of feeding intolerance did not differ significantly between the two formulations (relative risk 0.69; 95% confidence interval 0.43–1.09; $P = 0.110$).

The major finding of this systematic literature review was that the use of a polymeric, in comparison with an elemental, enteral nutrition formulation was not associated with a statistically significant difference in tolerance of feeding or risk of infectious complications and mortality. In addition, it showed that a fiber-enriched formulation may be safely administered in patients with acute pancreatitis, and its supplementation with immunonutrition or probiotics does not improve clinically meaningful outcomes [46, 47].

Conclusion

Nutritional treatment of patients with acute pancreatitis rapidly evolves. The findings presented in this chapter highlight the importance of enteral nutrition in the management of acute pancreatitis. There is ample evidence in the literature that the use of nasojejunal tube feeding improves outcomes in patients with predicted severe course of acute pancreatitis. Several studies have demonstrated the safety and efficacy of nasogastric tube feeding in these patients. Lastly, optimal enteral feeding formulations have been determined based on the best available data.

References

1 O'Keefe SJ, Lee RB, Anderson FP, et al. Physiological effects of enteral and parenteral feeding on pancreaticobiliary secretion in humans. American Journal of Physiology: Gastrointestinal and Liver Physiology 2003;284(1):G27–G36.

2 Banks PA, Freeman ML. Practice guidelines in acute pancreatitis. American Journal of Gastroenterology 2006;101(10):2379–2400.

3 Gianotti L. Nutrition and infections Surgical Infections (Larchmt) 2006;7 Suppl 2:S29–S32.

4 Petrov MS. To feed or not to feed early in acute pancreatitis: still depend on severity? Clinical Nutrition 2008;27(2):317–318.

5 Hyde D, Floch MH. The effect of peripheral nutritional support and nitrogen balance in acute pancreatitis. Gastroenterology 1984;86:1119.

6 Ranson JH. Acute pancreatitis: pathogenesis, outcome and treatment. Clinical Gastroenterology 1984;13(3):843–863.

7 Sax HC, Warner BW, Talamini MA, et al. Early total parenteral-nutrition in acute-pancreatitis – lack of beneficial-effects. American Journal of Surgery 1987;153(1):117–124.

8 Fernandez-Banares F, Cabre E, Esteve-Comas M, Gassull MA. How effective is enteral nutrition in inducing clinical remission in active Crohn's disease? A meta-analysis of the randomized clinical trials. Journal of Parenteral and Enteral Nutrition 1995;19(5):356–364.

9 Eatock FC, Brombacher GD, Steven A, Imrie CW, McKay CJ, Carter R. Nasogastric feeding in severe acute pancreatitis may be practical and safe. International Journal of Pancreatology 2000;28(1):23–29.

10 Zhao G, Wang CY, Wang F, Xiong JX. Clinical study on nutrition support in patients with severe acute pancreatitis. World Journal of Gastroenterology 2003;9(9):2105–2108.

11 Makola D, Krenitsky J, Parrish C, et al. Efficacy of enteral nutrition for the treatment of pancreatitis using standard enteral formula. American Journal of Gastroenterology 2006;101(10):2347–2355.

12 Petrov MS. Enteral nutrition: goody or good-for-nothing in acute pancreatitis? American Journal of Gastroenterology 2007;102(8):1828–1829; author reply 1829–1830.

13 Petrov MS, Pylypchuk RD, Emelyanov NV. Systematic review: nutritional support in acute pancreatitis. Alimentary Pharmacology & Therapeutics 2008;28:704–712.

14 Kalfarentzos F, Kehagias J, Mead N, Kokkinis K, Gogos CA. Enteral nutrition is superior to parenteral nutrition in severe acute pancreatitis: results of a randomized prospective trial. British Journal of Surgery 1997;84(12):1665–1669.

15 Gupta R, Patel K, Calder PC, Yaqoob P, Primrose JN, Johnson CD. A randomised clinical trial to assess the effect of total enteral and total parenteral nutritional support on metabolic, inflammatory and oxidative markers in patients with predicted severe acute pancreatitis (APACHE II > or =6). Pancreatology 2003;3(5):406–413.

16 Louie BE, Noseworthy T, Hailey D, Gramlich LM, Jacobs P, Warnock GL. 2004 MacLean-Mueller prize enteral or parenteral nutrition for severe pancreatitis: a randomized controlled trial and health technology assessment. Canadian Journal of Surgery 2005;48(4):298–306.

17 Eckerwall GE, Axelsson JB, Andersson RG. Early nasogastric feeding in predicted severe acute pancreatitis: a clinical, randomized study. Annals of Surgery 2006;244(6):959–965, discussion 965–957.

18 Petrov MS, Kukosh MV, Emelyanov NV. A randomized controlled trial of enteral versus parenteral feeding in patients with predicted severe acute pancreatitis shows a significant reduction in mortality and in infected pancreatic complications with total enteral nutrition. Digestive Surgery 2006;23(5–6):336–344; discussion 344–335.

19 Casas M, Mora J, Fort E, et al. Total enteral nutrition vs. total parenteral nutrition in patients with severe acute pancreatitis. Revista Espanola de Enfermedades Digestivas 2007;99(5):264–269.

20 Doley RP, Yadav TD, Wig JD, et al. Enteral nutrition in severe acute pancreatitis. Journal of the Pancreas 2009;10(2):157–162.

21 Wu XM, Ji KQ, Wang HY, Li GF, Zang B, Chen WM. Total enteral nutrition in prevention of pancreatic necrotic infection in severe acute pancreatitis. Pancreas 2010;39(2):248–251.

22 Dervenis C. Enteral nutrition in severe acute pancreatitis: future development. Journal of the Pancreas 2004;5(2):60–63.

23 Al-Omran M, Albalawi ZH, Tashkandi MF, Al-Ansary LA. Enteral versus parenteral nutrition for acute pancreatitis. Cochrane Database of Systematic Reviews 2010(1):CD002837.

24 Petrov MS, Zagainov VE. Influence of enteral versus parenteral nutrition on blood glucose control in acute

pancreatitis: a systematic review. Clinical Nutrition 2007;26(5):514–523.

25 Petrov MS, van Santvoort HC, Besselink MG, van der Heijden GJ, Windsor JA, Gooszen HG. Enteral nutrition and the risk of mortality and infectious complications in patients with severe acute pancreatitis: a meta-analysis of randomized trials. Archives of Surgery 2008;143(11):1111–1117.

26 Marik PE, Zaloga GP. Meta-analysis of parenteral nutrition versus enteral nutrition in patients with acute pancreatitis. British Medical Journal 2004;328(7453):1407.

27 Maykel JA, Bistrian BR. Is enteral feeding for everyone? Critical Care Medicine 2002;30(3):714–716.

28 Yazdanpanah Y, Sissoko D, Egger M, Mouton Y, Zwahlen M, Chene G. Clinical efficacy of antiretroviral combination therapy based on protease inhibitors or non-nucleoside analogue reverse transcriptase inhibitors: indirect comparison of controlled trials. British Medical Journal 2004;328(7434):249.

29 Kaushik N, Pietraszewski M, Holst JJ, O'Keefe SJ. Enteral feeding without pancreatic stimulation. Pancreas 2005;31(4):353–359.

30 Ammori BJ, Leeder PC, King RF, et al. Early increase in intestinal permeability in patients with severe acute pancreatitis: correlation with endotoxemia, organ failure, and mortality. Journal of Gastrointestinal Surgery 1999;3(3):252–262.

31 Juvonen PO, Alhava EM, Takala JA. Gut permeability in patients with acute pancreatitis. Scandinavian Journal of Gastroenterology 2000;35(12):1314–1318.

32 Powell JJ, Murchison JT, Fearon KC, Ross JA, Siriwardena AK. Randomized controlled trial of the effect of early enteral nutrition on markers of the inflammatory response in predicted severe acute pancreatitis. British Journal of Surgery 2000;87(10):1375–1381.

33 Tanguy M, Seguin P, Malledant Y. Bench-to-bedside review: Routine postoperative use of the nasogastric tube – utility or futility? Critical Care 2007;11(1):201.

34 Witting MD. "You wanna do what?!" Modern indications for nasogastric intubation. Journal of Emergency Medicine 2007;33(1):61–64.

35 O'Keefe SJ. Physiological response of the human pancreas to enteral and parenteral feeding. Current Opinion in Clinical Nutrition & Metabolic Care 2006;9(5):622–628.

36 O'Keefe SJ, McClave SA. Feeding the injured pancreas. Gastroenterology 2005;129(3):1129–1130.

37 Eatock FC, Chong P, Menezes N, et al. A randomized study of early nasogastric versus nasojejunal feeding in severe acute pancreatitis. American Journal of Gastroenterology 2005;100(2):432–439.

38 Kumar A, Singh N, Prakash S, Saraya A, Joshi YK. Early enteral nutrition in severe acute pancreatitis: a prospective randomized controlled trial comparing nasojejunal and nasogastric routes. Journal of Clinical Gastroenterology 2006;40(5):431–434.

39 Singh N, Sharma B, Sharma M, et al. Evaluation of early enteral feeding through nasogastric and nasojejunal tube in severe acute pancreatitis: a noninferiority randomized controlled trial. Pancreas 2011; 41: 153–159.

40 Petrov MS, Correia MI, Windsor JA. Nasogastric tube feeding in predicted severe acute pancreatitis. A systematic review of the literature to determine safety and tolerance. Journal of the Pancreas 2008;9(4):440–448.

41 O'Keefe S J, Lee RB, Li J, Zhou W, Stoll B, Dang Q. Trypsin and splanchnic protein turnover during feeding and fasting in human subjects. American Journal of Physiology: Gastrointestinal and Liver Physiology 2006;290(2):G213–G221.

42 O'Keefe SJ, Lee RB, Li J, Stevens S, Abou-Assi S, Zhou W. Trypsin secretion and turnover in patients with acute pancreatitis. American Journal of Physiology: Gastrointestinal and Liver Physiology 2005;289(2):G181–G187.

43 Petrov MS, Whelan K. Comparison of complications attributable to enteral and parenteral nutrition in predicted severe acute pancreatitis: a systematic review and meta-analysis. British Journal of Nutrition 2010;103(9):1287–1295.

44 Silk DB. Formulation of enteral diets. Nutrition 1999;15(7–8):626–632.

45 Petrov MS, Savides TJ. Systematic review of endoscopic ultrasonography versus endoscopic retrograde cholangiopancreatography for suspected choledocholithiasis. British Journal of Surgery 2009;96(9):967–974.

46 Petrov MS, Atduev VA, Zagainov VE. Advanced enteral therapy in acute pancreatitis: is there a room for immunonutrition? A meta-analysis. International Journal of Surgery 2008;6(2):119–124.

47 Heyland DK, Novak F, Drover JW, Jain M, Su X, Suchner U. Should immunonutrition become routine in critically ill patients? A systematic review of the evidence. Journal of the American Medical Association. 2001;286(8):944–953.

48 McClave SA, Greene LM, Snider HL, et al. Comparison of the safety of early enteral vs parenteral nutrition in mild acute pancreatitis. Journal of Parenteral and Enteral Nutrition. 1997;21(1):14–20.

49 Windsor AC, Kanwar S, Li AG, et al. Compared with parenteral nutrition, enteral feeding attenuates the acute phase response and improves disease severity in acute pancreatitis. Gut. 1998;42(3):431–435.

50 Hallay J, Kovacs G, Kiss Sz S, et al. Changes in the nutritional state and immune-serological parameters of esophagectomized patients fed jejunally with glutamine-poor and glutamine-rich nutriments. Hepatogastroenterology. 2002;49(48):1555–1559.

51 Olah A, Belagyi T, Issekutz A, Gamal ME, Bengmark S. Randomized clinical trial of specific lactobacillus and fibre supplement to early enteral nutrition in patients with acute pancreatitis. British Journal of Surgery. 2002;89(9):1103–1107.

52 Abou-Assi S, Craig K, O'Keefe SJ. Hypocaloric jejunal feeding is better than total parenteral nutrition in acute pancreatitis: results of a randomized comparative study. American Journal of Gastroenterology. 2002;97(9):2255–2262.

53 Lasztity N, Hamvas J, Biro L, et al. Effect of enterally administered n-3 polyunsaturated fatty acids in acute pancreatitis – a prospective randomized clinical trial. Clinical Nutrition. 2005;24(2):198–205.

54 Pearce CB, Sadek SA, Walters AM, et al. A double-blind, randomised, controlled trial to study the effects of an enteral feed supplemented with glutamine, arginine, and omega-3 fatty acid in predicted acute severe pancreatitis. Journal of the Pancreas. 2006;7(4):361–371.

55 Tiengou LE, Gloro R, Pouzoulet J, et al. Semi-elemental formula or polymeric formula: is there a better choice for enteral nutrition in acute pancreatitis? Randomized comparative study. Journal of Parenteral and Enteral Nutrition. 2006;30(1):1–5.

56 Olah A, Belagyi T, Poto L, Romics L, Jr, Bengmark S. Synbiotic control of inflammation and infection in severe acute pancreatitis: a prospective, randomized, double blind study. Hepatogastroenterology. 2007;54(74):590–594.

57 Karakan T, Ergun M, Dogan I, Cindoruk M, Unal S. Comparison of early enteral nutrition in severe acute pancreatitis with prebiotic fiber supplementation versus standard enteral solution: a prospective randomized double-blind study. World Journal of Gastroenterology. 2007;13(19):2733–2737.

58 Besselink MG, van Santvoort HC, Buskens E, et al. Probiotic prophylaxis in patients with predicted severe acute pancreatitis: a randomised, double-blind, placebo-controlled trial. Nederlands Tijdschrift voor Geneeskunde. 2008;152(12):685–696. Dutch.

59 Qin HL, Zheng JJ, Tong DN, et al. Effect of Lactobacillus plantarum enteral feeding on the gut permeability and septic complications in the patients with acute pancreatitis. European Journal of Clinical Nutrition. 2008;62(7):923–930.

CHAPTER 6

Gallstone pancreatitis: diagnosis and treatment

Marsela Sina[1] & Gregory A. Coté[2]

[1] *University Clinic of Gastrohepatology, University Hospital Center Mother Theresa, Tirana, Albania*
[2] *Division of Gastroenterology, Hepatology, and Nutrition, Department of Medicine, Medical University of South Carolina, Charleston, SC, USA*

Abbreviations

ALT   alanine transaminase
AP   acute pancreatitis
CBD   common bile duct
CCY   cholecystectomy
CT   computed tomography
ERCP   endoscopic retrograde cholangiopancreatography
ES   endoscopic sphincterotomy
EUS   endoscopic ultrasound
IOC   intraoperative cholangiogram
MRCP   magnetic resonance cholangiopancreatography
SIRS   systemic inflammatory response syndrome
TUS   transabdominal ultrasound
US   ultrasound

Summary

Acute pancreatitis (AP) is the leading gastrointestinal disorder requiring hospitalization in the United States, and gallstone disease is the most common etiologic factor worldwide [1]. Recurrence and complications of gallstone pancreatitis may be avoidable with proper diagnosis and treatment. Clinical history coupled with laboratory and imaging is accurate in diagnosing gallstone disease, particularly with the advent of magnetic resonance cholangiopancreatography (MRCP) and endoscopic ultrasound (EUS). While less utilized as a diagnostic test, endoscopic retrograde cholangiopancreatography (ERCP) remains the preferred approach for the treatment of choledocholithiasis and concomitant cholangitis or biliary obstruction in the setting of severe AP. When performed in a timely manner, cholecystectomy (CCY) is highly effective in preventing recurrent gallstone pancreatitis. Among poor operative candidates, ERCP with biliary sphincterotomy is a reasonable surrogate. This chapter reviews the current evidence for diagnosing and treating acute gallstone pancreatitis.

Introduction

Gallstone disease represents the single leading cause of acute pancreatitis (AP), accounting for approximately 50% of cases in the Western world [2, 3]. The majority of AP patients will experience a benign course and rapid recovery with supportive management. However, up to 20% develop severe pancreatitis with systemic (organ failure) or local complications that may result in mortality, with rates quoted as high as 15% [4]. Although there is a definite correlation between gallstones and AP, the precise pathophysiology of gallstone (a.k.a., biliary) pancreatitis remains unclear. The most important purported mechanisms include (i) transient or sustained occlusion of the pancreatic duct leading to an increase in intraductal pressure and (ii) bile reflux into the pancreatic duct [5].

When a patient presents with AP, the clinician often jumps to the conclusion that the underlying cause is alcohol or gallstones. While there are numerous alternative etiologies that will be discussed in other chapter(s), our discussion is organized by several key

Pancreatitis: Medical and Surgical Management, First Edition.
David B. Adams, Peter B. Cotton, Nicholas J. Zyromski and John Windsor.
© 2017 John Wiley & Sons, Ltd. Published 2017 by John Wiley & Sons, Ltd.

questions that should be considered by the treating physician:

1 How is gallstone pancreatitis diagnosed?
2 What tests are available to evaluate for common bile duct (CBD) stones?
3 For patients with gallstone pancreatitis, what is the role of ERCP in the acute setting?
4 What is the impact of CCY for the prevention of recurrent gallstone pancreatitis, and when should it be performed?
5 What is the benefit of ERCP for patients who are poor candidates for CCY?

In this chapter, we review the definition of gallstone pancreatitis and the methods by which gallstones may be implicated as the cause. We underscore the indications for ERCP and CCY and alternative strategies to attenuate the disease course and prevent its recurrence.

How is gallstone pancreatitis diagnosed?

Once a diagnosis of AP is established, identifying gallstones as the underlying cause is crucial since complications and recurrence may be avoidable with interventions such as CCY and ERCP (Figure 6.1) [6]. CCY is highly effective in preventing recurrent episodes of AP, but only when the etiology is gallstones [7]. Therefore, gallstone pancreatitis should be confirmed by documenting gallbladder stones on cross-sectional imaging, transient fluctuation in liver chemistries >3× upper limit of normal, or both. If neither is present, the benefit of empiric CCY is unproven [8].

Laboratories

An early clue that gallstones are the primary etiology is the relative elevation of serum amylase, which is often disproportionately higher in comparison to other etiologies [9]. However, amylase levels tend to drop rapidly and even normalize within 24 hours. In contrast, lipase remains elevated for a longer period; among patients who present several days after symptom onset, the amylase may have normalized/near-normalized while the lipase remains elevated [10]. Serum lipase is more sensitive and specific than amylase for establishing the diagnosis of AP since lipase persists longer than amylase, and there are fewer nonpancreatic etiologies for elevations in serum lipase (Table 6.1) [11].

Beyond characterizing the pattern of pancreatic chemistry elevation, marked increases (>3× upper limit of normal) in liver chemistries are useful for distinguishing gallstones from alternative etiologies. Alanine transaminase (ALT) is probably the single most reliable test, having a positive predictive value of 93% for a biliary cause when elevated threefold [12, 13]. However, up to 15% of patients with biliary pancreatitis have normal liver chemistries at presentation, and any cause for AP may induce elevation of these parameters simply by extrinsic compression of the extrahepatic biliary tree [14].

Cross-sectional imaging

Given its wide availability, lack of ionizing radiation, low cost, minimal interoperator variability, and high sensitivity/specificity (>95%) for gallbladder stones, transabdominal ultrasound (TUS) is the preferred initial imaging modality for patients with suspected gallstone pancreatitis [15]. However, in the setting of AP, the sensitivity is reduced to approximately 60% due to bowel distension and poor patient compliance with the examination: deep probing of the upper abdomen with the ultrasound (US) transducer is rarely feasible in such individuals. In addition, the sensitivity for diagnosing bile duct stones is even lower (20–50%), particularly in the setting of obesity. Moreover, the lack of biliary dilation does not rule out a biliary etiology during the first 48 hours [16].

Compared to TUS, computed tomography (CT) is marginally better for detecting CBD stones. While useful for diagnosing local complications of AP, CT during the first 48 hours of AP should be reserved for uncertain diagnoses, since iodinated contrast may precipitate renal failure or even pancreatic necrosis [17].

Although sonographic characteristics of gallstones are the same when detected by TUS or EUS, the latter has a higher sensitivity (85–100%) in diagnosing gallbladder stones (especially small stones and sludge) due to the proximity of the US transducer to the gallbladder [18]. MRCP is also more sensitive than TUS and can identify local complications of AP and pancreatic ductal anatomy at the same time [19].

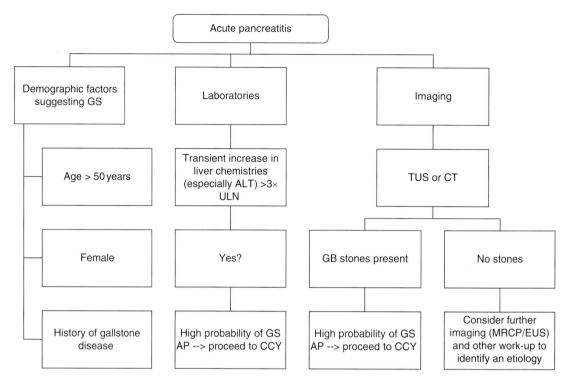

Figure 6.1 Confirming a diagnosis of gallstone pancreatitis. TUS, transabdominal ultrasound; CT, computed tomography; CCY, cholecystectomy; GS, gallstone; GB, gallbladder; MRCP, magnetic resonance cholangiopancreatography; EUS, endoscopic ultrasound; ULN, upper limit normal; AP, acute pancreatitis; ALT, alanine transaminase.

Table 6.1 Nonpancreatic etiologies for elevation in serum amylase or lipase.

Causes	Amylase	Lipase
Abdominal pathology	Peptic ulcer disease Mesenteric ischemia Acute appendicitis Cholecystitis Intestinal obstruction Gynecological disorders	Peptic ulcer disease Mesenteric ischemia Acute appendicitis
Extra-abdominal pathology	Salivary gland disease Pneumonia Head injury	Bone fractures Crush injury Fat embolism
Metabolic disorders	Renal failure Liver failure Diabetic ketoacidosis Anorexia nervosa and Bulimia	Renal failure
Others	HIV Macroamylasemia Cigarette smoking Neoplasms: lung, gastric, breast, and myeloma	

Since there are fewer causes for elevation in serum lipase (specificity), and it remains elevated longer than serum amylase (sensitivity), lipase is considered more specific and sensitive for the diagnosis of acute pancreatitis.

What tests are available to evaluate for common bile duct stones?

While CCY is highly effective in preventing recurrent bouts of gallstone pancreatitis, unrecognized CBD stones are likely to cause additional complications – including AP – even following CCY. In all cases of gallstone pancreatitis, the possibility of choledocholithiasis must be considered in any management algorithm (Figure 6.2). Usually, gallstone pancreatitis is

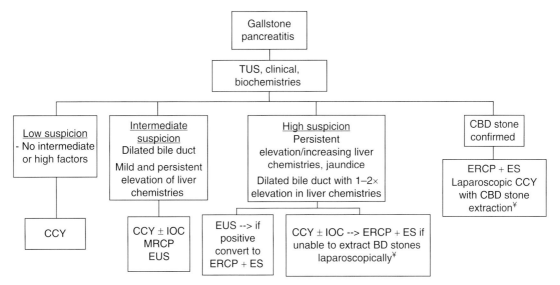

Figure 6.2 Recommended algorithm for diagnosing choledocholithiasis. TUS, transabdominal ultrasound; CCY, cholecystectomy; IOC, intraoperative cholangiogram; MRCP, magnetic resonance cholangiopancreatography; ERCP, endoscopic retrograde cholangiopancreatography; EUS, endoscopic ultrasound; CBD, common bile duct. IOC is an option; the CBD should be imaged by some modality, that is, MRCP, ERCP, and IOC. ¥Being highly operator dependent, the best strategy between laparoscopic and endoscopic stone extraction will be determined by the availability of local expertise and technology.

caused by the spontaneous passage of a CBD stone into the duodenum. Since the majority of patients do not have retained CBD stones, diagnostic testing should be titrated to the level of clinical suspicion (Figure 6.2).

ERCP

ERCP is the gold standard for diagnosing CBD stones, but its risk profile [20] and the advent of less invasive imaging modalities have significantly reduced its utility as a purely diagnostic test. Furthermore, cholangiography may miss small gallstones [21]; in cases where there is a very high suspicion for or prior confirmation of CBD stones, ERCP with endoscopic sphincterotomy (ES) and balloon sweep is typically performed. If available, laparoscopic surgical expertise with CBD stone extraction actually appears preferential to an ERCP-first strategy; in this scenario, the surgeon performs a CCY and attempts to clear the CBD laparoscopically, using ERCP with sphincterotomy only if unsuccessful. Even when the pretest probability of CBD stones approaches 100%, an intraoperative cholangiography (IOC)-first as opposed to ERCP-first strategy is more cost effective [22]. In our experience, most surgeons prefer to have the CBD cleared preoperatively via ERCP when this is readily available so as to minimize the morbidity of CCY.

Regardless of local expertise, ERCP should no longer be considered a diagnostic test for bile duct stones. The availability of EUS and MRCP, lower risk and highly sensitive imaging modalities for suspected choledocholithiasis, has relegated ERCP to a therapeutic intervention when stones are present assuredly.

Intraoperative cholangiography (IOC)

In the United States, IOC is performed in approximately 30% of individuals undergoing CCY. Its sensitivity varies from 59% to 100% and specificity from 93% to 100% in detecting CBD stones and is highly operator dependent [23, 24]. In patients with mild gallstone pancreatitis but no ongoing biliary obstruction, the optimal approach to clearing the CBD is to perform CCY with IOC first using ERCP to clear stones that are retained postoperatively [25]. Since most stones have already passed into the duodenum and only a minority of patients have CBD stones at the time of CCY, ERCP is unnecessary for most patients presenting with acute gallstone pancreatitis [26, 27]. By performing IOC first, fewer patients undergo unnecessary ERCP (and other diagnostics), and the length of hospitalization can be shortened.

However, many surgeons perform IOC infrequently – and fewer are comfortable with laparoscopic removal of bile duct stones [22, 25, 28–32]. Some surgeons have proposed laparoscopic CBD exploration as an excellent single-step approach for CBD stone clearance [33, 34], but this technique is infrequently performed [35]. The single-stage laparoendoscopic treatment (a.k.a., "rendezvous technique") is an alternative to laparoscopic stone extraction. During IOC, a guidewire can be advanced under fluoroscopic guidance and in an antegrade manner across the sphincter of Oddi. A duodenoscope is advanced *per os* to the major papilla, where the wire is grasped and the bile duct accessed without the need for traditional cannulation maneuvers [36]. This results in high rates of BD stone clearance during CCY and is less invasive and costly than sequential CCY followed by ERCP under a second sedative. This combination approach has not been widely accepted since laparoscopic and ERCP expertise usually obligates two physicians, creating a logistical conundrum [37]. For these reasons, EUS and MRCP have been increasingly utilized in these cases of gallstone pancreatitis with question of retained CBD stones [38, 39].

MRCP

MRCP has high sensitivity (81–100%) and specificity (92–100%) for the diagnosis of choledocholithiasis [40]. However, the sensitivity of MRCP is directly related to the size of gallstones, so its diagnostic yield is lowest for small (<5 mm) stones and sludge [41, 42]. This means that a negative MRCP cannot always exclude gallstones as the etiology since small stones are often the cause of AP [16]. In addition, patients must be able to hold their breath for approximately 20 seconds to acquire images of reasonable quality. However, MRCP has the advantage of being noninvasive, more widely available, and less operator dependent than EUS [43].

EUS

Several studies have shown that EUS is highly sensitive (>90%) for detecting choledocholithiasis when conventional imaging is negative [18, 44]. EUS is comparable or superior to cholangiography in detecting biliary stones [45, 46], and its performance is not influenced by stone size or bile duct diameter [21]. In an economic evaluation, an EUS-based approach was superior to ERCP with ES in severe biliary AP (costing C$742 less per patient) and only slightly more expensive in the setting of nonsevere biliary AP; using an EUS-first as opposed to ERCP-first approach was associated with fewer complications (3% fewer cases of post-ERCP pancreatitis) [47]. Moreover, in a meta-analysis comparing EUS to ERCP in patients with acute biliary pancreatitis, EUS avoided unnecessary ERCP in up to 71% of cases (another reminder that most patients with gallstone pancreatitis pass the CBD stone spontaneously) [48]. In the appropriate setting, patients with a moderate suspicion of CBD stones may be consented for EUS and ERCP in the same setting. An EUS should be performed initially, and if a CBD stone is identified, the procedure may be converted to ERCP with ES during the same session (Table 6.2).

Table 6.2 Cross-sectional imaging for gallstone disease.

Modality	Sensitivity/accuracy		Risk profile	Cost
	CBD stones	GB stones		
TUS	+	+++	−	+
CT	++	++	−	++
EUS	++++[a]	++++[b]	+	+++
MRCP	++++	++++[b]	+	+++
ERCP	++++	++	+++	+++

CBD, common bile duct; GB, gallbladder; TUS, transabdominal ultrasound; CT, computed tomography; EUS, endoscopic ultrasound; MRCP, magnetic resonance cholangiopancreatography; ERCP, endoscopic retrograde cholangiopancreatography.
[a]EUS has a better sensitivity than MRCP and ERCP in detecting small stones (<5 mm) and sludge.
[b]Although the sensitivity of EUS and MRCP is higher than the sensitivity of TUS in identifying gallstones, they are rarely used as a first-line technique due to their cost, availability, and slightly higher risk profile.

In summary, the decision to perform an MRCP, EUS, ERCP, or IOC depends on pretest probability and local expertise. In cases of low to intermediate suspicion, where the probability of a bile duct stone is approximately 30% or less, laparoscopic CCY with IOC first is probably the most expeditious and cost-effective strategy, assuming local surgical expertise. If a stone is identified during IOC and it cannot be extracted or flushed through the sphincter of Oddi during laparoscopy, then ERCP with ES within 24 hours is appropriate. In cases of higher suspicion or known choledocholithiasis preoperatively, EUS with a plan to convert to ERCP during the same session is the preferred approach. In these cases, next-day laparoscopic CCY would result in the shortest hospitalization [49]. MRCP is an excellent and minimally invasive tool to guide management when laparoscopic IOC and EUS expertise are lacking.

For patients with acute gallstone pancreatitis, what is the role for ERCP in the acute setting?

At this point, the clinician has established a diagnosis of gallstone pancreatitis and the probability of chole-docholithiasis. In specific cases, early ERCP – typically defined as within 72 hours of clinical presentation – may impact the disease course. In a nutshell, early ERCP reduces the complications of AP when patients have concomitant acute cholangitis or predicted severe AP with biliary obstruction (Figure 6.3). There are a variety of scoring systems to assess disease severity, including Ranson's criteria, APACHE-II score, BISAP score, Balthazar CT severity index, and the systemic inflammatory response syndrome (SIRS) score [50–54]. Due to their simplicity and reasonable predictive value, we prefer to couple clinical judgment with SIRS, serum blood urea nitrogen, and hematocrit at the time of admission and after 24–48 hours to make this determination [55–58].

Ample evidence supports performing early ERCP (<72 hours) with or without ES, in patients with gallstone pancreatitis and concurrent signs or symptoms of cholangitis (typically fever, jaundice, sepsis physiology, and rigors, among others) [59, 60]. In a meta-analysis of seven randomized controlled trials including 757 patients, Tse et al. confirmed a significant reduction in mortality (relative risk (RR) 0.20, 95% CI 0.06–0.68) and local (RR 0.45, 95% CI 0.20–0.99) and systemic complications (RR 0.37, 95% CI 0.18–0.78) using an early ERCP strategy for patients with AP and concomitant acute cholangitis [61]. There were no differences in outcome between individuals undergoing ERCP within 24 or 72 hours. However, in patients with acute cholangitis, we advocate urgent ERCP [6, 55]. Individuals with predicted severe gallstone AP and coexisting biliary obstruction (a conjugated bilirubin level >5 mg/dL) also benefit from early ERCP [3, 62]. This strategy can reduce the frequency of local (RR 0.53, 95% CI 0.26–1.07) and systemic (RR 0.56 95% CI 0.30–1.02) complications [61]. In the absence of cholangitis or biliary obstruction, the role of urgent ERCP remains controversial even in predicted severe AP [60].

Stone removal may not always be accomplished especially in the setting of suppurative acute cholangitis or in cases of large (>1.5 cm) or multiple CBD stones. In these situations, placing a bridging plastic stent is a reasonable temporizing measure in order to achieve short-term biliary drainage [63, 64]. Moreover, stent placement may help by softening or fracturing large CBD stones. Studies have shown that stones are smaller and occasionally even absent several weeks after stent placement [65, 66]. Whenever possible, multiple stents should be placed since the rate of stent occlusion and secondary cholangitis is smaller compared to one stent [67]. Stents with a double pigtail configuration, as opposed to flanged stents, probably have a lower risk of migration below retained stones.

In addition to CBD stone extraction and assuring bile duct drainage, there are limited data suggesting the benefit of early pancreatic duct stent placement to assure pancreatic duct drainage/decompression. In a pilot study of 27 patients, Fejes and colleagues evaluated the feasibility and safety of urgent ERCP with pancreatic stent placement in patients with biliary AP [68]. The authors observed a significantly lower rate of local (pancreatic necrosis, phlegmon, pseudocyst, abdominal fluid collections) and systemic complications (sepsis and shock) and organ failure in those who underwent PD stent placement (7%) than in controls who underwent ERCP with ES alone (25%); mortality rates (0% vs. 7%, respectively) also favored pancreatic stent placement, although this did not reach statistical significance. These data have been supported by two other small studies [69] [70]. However, in all three reports, pancreatic stent placement

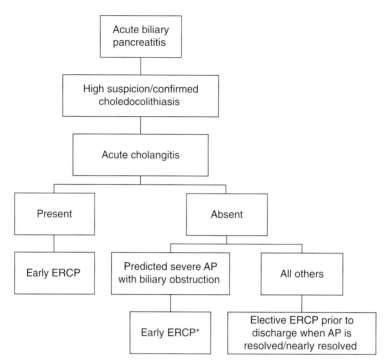

Figure 6.3 Indications and timing of ERCP in acute biliary pancreatitis. *Early ERCP is defined as ERCP within 72 hours of clinical presentation. AP, acute pancreatitis; ERCP, endoscopic retrograde cholangiopancreatography.

was performed only in individuals considered high risk (difficult sphincterotomies) for post-ERCP pancreatitis. The role of urgent PD stent placement as an intervention to attenuate the disease course for patients with gallstone (or other causes) pancreatitis requires further investigation, as there are inherent potential hazards of applying ERCP to this population.

What is the impact of cholecystectomy on the prevention of recurrent gallstone pancreatitis, and when should it be performed?

Once the patient recovers from an episode of mild gallstone pancreatitis, laparoscopic CCY should be performed during the same hospitalization to prevent the recurrence of gallstone-related complications [6, 55, 71]. If the gallbladder is left *in situ*, pancreatitis may recur in 30–50% [72]. The risk is higher in the first month following index gallstone AP [73, 74]. In contrast, when early CCY is performed, the risk can be reduced to <5%; the reasons for recurrence

following CCY include inadequate clearance of the CBD at the time of initial presentation and incorrectly attributing gallstones as the underlying etiology for AP [75, 76]. Same-stay CCY is preferred to a postdischarge strategy based on several studies including a systematic review that included 998 patients, which found higher readmission rates (18% vs. 0%, $P < 0.0001$) in those who did not undergo same-stay CCY [77]. Additionally, early CCY is associated with reduced length of stay and total hospital charges [78].

Among patients who are good operative candidates, CCY following ERCP with ES is superior to ES alone for the prevention of recurrent gallstone AP [79, 80]. In a cohort of 4682 patients admitted with their first episode of acute gallstone AP, the rate of recurrent AP was significantly lower for those who had ES + CCY (1.2%) as compared to those who underwent CCY alone (4.4%, $P < 0.05$) or ES alone (6.7%, $P = 0.0001$) [7]. Additionally, while ES significantly decreases the rate of recurrent gallstone AP (compared to medical management), ES alone does not prevent other complications of retained gallbladder stones [77].

In patients with severe gallstone AP and evolving local complications such as fluid collections, laparoscopic CCY during the index admission is technically difficult and has greater morbidity, particularly from postoperative infection [81, 82]. In these cases, CCY should be delayed until peripancreatic fluid collections/necrosis resolve or if they persist at least 6 weeks, at which time CCY can be safely performed as part of the surgical management of organized pancreatic necrosis [55].

What is the benefit of ERCP for patients who are poor candidates for cholecystectomy?

In patients who are poor candidates for CCY, such as those with Child class B or C cirrhosis, ERCP with ES is an acceptable therapeutic alternative to CCY, irrespective of the presence of CBD stones [7, 83]. Hwang et al. found that the probability of developing recurrent attacks of pancreatitis after 1, 2, and 5 years among individuals with gallstone pancreatitis and gallbladder *in situ* was significantly lower in patients who underwent ERCP (5%, 7% and 11%, respectively) compared to those who did not (11%, 16%, and 23%; hazard ratio 0.45 [95% CI, 0.30–0.69]; $P < 0.01$) [84]. However, it is worth reiterating that other complications related to gallstone disease such as cholecystitis and/or biliary pain may still occur [75].

Summary

Gallstones represent one of few etiologies of AP where appropriate and timely intervention may significantly impact the patient's short- and long-term prognosis. While confirming the diagnosis of gallstone pancreatitis is fairly straightforward, it is inappropriate to assume gallstones as the underlying etiology without supporting evidence, since CCY and ES have no proven benefit for individuals with AP secondary to other etiologies. With improvements in laparoscopy, EUS, and MRCP, diagnostic ERCP should be avoided almost without exception. A multidisciplinary approach to patients with known or suspected gallstone AP should include the input of surgeons, gastroenterologists, and radiologists in deciding the need for and appropriate sequence of imaging and interventions. With rare exception, gallstone pancreatitis is now a curable disease.

References

1 Yadav D, Lowenfels AB. The epidemiology of pancreatitis and pancreatic cancer. Gastroenterology 2013;144: 1252–1261.
2 Johnson C, Levy P. Detection of gallstones in acute pancreatitis: when and how? Pancreatology 2010;10:27–32.
3 Fogel EL, Sherman S. ERCP for gallstone pancreatitis. New England Journal of Medicine 2014;370:150–157.
4 van Santvoort HC, Bakker OJ, Bollen TL, et al. A conservative and minimally invasive approach to necrotizing pancreatitis improves outcome. Gastroenterology 2011; 141:1254–1263.
5 Lerch MM, Gorelick FS. Models of acute and chronic pancreatitis. Gastroenterology 2013;144:1180–1193.
6 Tenner S, Baillie J, DeWitt J, et al. American College of Gastroenterology guideline: management of acute pancreatitis. American Journal of Gastroenterology 2013;108:1400–1415; 1416.
7 Mustafa A, Begaj I, Deakin M, et al. Long-term effectiveness of cholecystectomy and endoscopic sphincterotomy in the management of gallstone pancreatitis. Surgical Endoscopy 2014;28:127–133.
8 Trna J, Vege SS, Pribramska V, et al. Lack of significant liver enzyme elevation and gallstones and/or sludge on ultrasound on day 1 of acute pancreatitis is associated with recurrence after cholecystectomy: a population-based study. Surgery 2012;151:199–205.
9 Alexakis N, Lombard M, Raraty M, et al. When is pancreatitis considered to be of biliary origin and what are the implications for management? Pancreatology 2007;7:131–141.
10 Gomez D, Addison A, De Rosa A, et al. Retrospective study of patients with acute pancreatitis: is serum amylase still required? British Medical Journal Open 2012;2.
11 Koizumi M, Takada T, Kawarada Y, et al. JPN Guidelines for the management of acute pancreatitis: diagnostic criteria for acute pancreatitis. Journal of Hepato-Biliary-Pancreatic Surgery 2006;13:25–32.
12 Levy P, Boruchowicz A, Hastier P, et al. Diagnostic criteria in predicting a biliary origin of acute pancreatitis in the era of endoscopic ultrasound: multicentre prospective evaluation of 213 patients. Pancreatology 2005;5:450–456.
13 Liu CL, Fan ST, Lo CM, et al. Clinico-biochemical prediction of biliary cause of acute pancreatitis in the era of endoscopic ultrasonography. Alimentary Pharmacology & Therapeutics 2005;22:423–431.
14 Dholakia K, Pitchumoni CS, Agarwal N. How often are liver function tests normal in acute biliary pancreatitis? Journal of Clinical Gastroenterology 2004;38:81–83.
15 Benarroch-Gampel J, Boyd CA, Sheffield KM, et al. Overuse of CT in patients with complicated gallstone

disease. Journal of the American College of Surgeons 2011;213:524–530.

16 Fogel EL, Sherman S. Acute biliary pancreatitis: when should the endoscopist intervene? Gastroenterology 2003;125:229–235.

17 Arvanitakis M, Delhaye M, De Maertelaere V, et al. Computed tomography and magnetic resonance imaging in the assessment of acute pancreatitis. Gastroenterology 2004;126:715–723.

18 O'Neill DE, Saunders MD. Endoscopic ultrasonography in diseases of the gallbladder. Gastroenterology Clinics of North America 2010;39:289–305; ix.

19 Hou LA, Van Dam J. Pre-ERCP imaging of the bile duct and gallbladder. Gastrointestinal Endoscopy Clinics of North America 2013;23:185–197.

20 Freeman ML. Adverse outcomes of ERCP. Gastrointestinal Endoscopy 2002;56:S273–S282.

21 Ney MV, Maluf-Filho F, Sakai P, et al. Echo-endoscopy versus endoscopic retrograde cholangiography for the diagnosis of choledocholithiasis: the influence of the size of the stone and diameter of the common bile duct. Arquivos de Gastroenterologia 2005;42:239–243.

22 Rogers SJ, Cello JP, Horn JK, et al. Prospective randomized trial of LC+LCBDE vs ERCP/S+LC for common bile duct stone disease. Archives of Surgery 2010;145:28–33.

23 Maple JT, Ben-Menachem T, Anderson MA, et al. The role of endoscopy in the evaluation of suspected choledocholithiasis. Gastrointestinal Endoscopy 2010;71:1–9.

24 Orenstein SB, Marks JM, Hardacre JM. Technical aspects of bile duct evaluation and exploration. Surgical Clinics of North America 2014;94:281–296.

25 Brown LM, Rogers SJ, Cello JP, et al. Cost-effective treatment of patients with symptomatic cholelithiasis and possible common bile duct stones. Journal of the American College of Surgeons 2011;212:1049–1060; e1–e7.

26 Tabone LE, Conlon M, Fernando E, et al. A practical cost-effective management strategy for gallstone pancreatitis. American Journal of Surgery 2013;206:472–477.

27 Iranmanesh P, Frossard JL, Mugnier-Konrad B, et al. Initial cholecystectomy vs sequential common duct endoscopic assessment and subsequent cholecystectomy for suspected gallstone migration: a randomized clinical trial. Journal of the American Medical Association 2014;312:137–144.

28 Sanjay P, Tagolao S, Dirkzwager I, et al. A survey of the accuracy of interpretation of intraoperative cholangiograms. Hepato Pancreato Biliary (Oxford) 2012;14:673–676.

29 Videhult P, Sandblom G, Rasmussen IC. How reliable is intraoperative cholangiography as a method for detecting common bile duct stones? A prospective population-based study on 1171 patients. Surgical Endoscopy 2009;23:304–312.

30 Dasari BV, Tan CJ, Gurusamy KS, et al. Surgical versus endoscopic treatment of bile duct stones. Cochrane Database of Systematic Reviews 2013;9:CD003327.

31 Lu J, Cheng Y, Xiong XZ, et al. Two-stage vs single-stage management for concomitant gallstones and common bile duct stones. World Journal of Gastroenterology 2012;18:3156–3166.

32 Bencini L, Tommasi C, Manetti R, et al. Modern approach to cholecysto-choledocholithiasis. World Journal of Gastrointestinal Endoscopy 2014;6:32–40.

33 Hanif F, Ahmed Z, Samie MA, et al. Laparoscopic transcystic bile duct exploration: the treatment of first choice for common bile duct stones. Surgical Endoscopy 2010;24:1552–1556.

34 Bansal VK, Misra MC, Rajan K, et al. Single-stage laparoscopic common bile duct exploration and cholecystectomy versus two-stage endoscopic stone extraction followed by laparoscopic cholecystectomy for patients with concomitant gallbladder stones and common bile duct stones: a randomized controlled trial. Surgical Endoscopy 2014;28:875–885.

35 Sheffield KM, Han Y, Kuo YF, et al. Variation in the use of intraoperative cholangiography during cholecystectomy. Journal of the American College of Surgeons 2012;214:668–679; discussion 679–681.

36 Tommasi C, Bencini L, Bernini M, et al. Routine use of simultaneous laparoendoscopic approach in patients with confirmed gallbladder and bile duct stones: fit for laparoscopy fit for "rendezvous". World Journal of Surgery 2013;37:999–1005.

37 La Greca G, Barbagallo F, Di Blasi M, et al. Laparoendoscopic "Rendezvous" to treat cholecysto-choledocolithiasis: Effective, safe and simplifies the endoscopist's work. World Journal of Gastroenterology 2008;14:2844–2850.

38 Ragulin-Coyne E, Witkowski ER, Chau Z, et al. Is routine intraoperative cholangiogram necessary in the twenty-first century? A national view. Journal of Gastrointestinal Surgery 2013;17:434–442.

39 Buddingh KT, Hofker HS, ten Cate Hoedemaker HO, et al. Safety measures during cholecystectomy: results of a nationwide survey. World Journal of Surgery 2011;35:1235–1241; discussion 1242–1243.

40 Hallal AH, Amortegui JD, Jeroukhimov IM, et al. Magnetic resonance cholangiopancreatography accurately detects common bile duct stones in resolving gallstone pancreatitis. Journal of the American College of Surgeons 2005;200:869–875.

41 Srinivasa S, Sammour T, McEntee B, et al. Selective use of magnetic resonance cholangiopancreatography in clinical practice may miss choledocholithiasis in gallstone pancreatitis. Canadian Journal of Surgery 2010;53:403–407.

42 Kondo S, Isayama H, Akahane M, et al. Detection of common bile duct stones: comparison between endoscopic ultrasonography, magnetic resonance cholangiography, and helical-computed-tomographic cholangiography. European Journal of Radiology 2005;54:271–275.

43 Aube C, Delorme B, Yzet T, et al. MR cholangiopancreatography versus endoscopic sonography in suspected common

bile duct lithiasis: a prospective, comparative study. American Journal of Roentgenology 2005;184:55–62.

44 Zhan X, Guo X, Chen Y, et al. EUS in exploring the etiology of mild acute biliary pancreatitis with a negative finding of biliary origin by conventional radiological methods. Journal of Gastroenterology and Hepatology 2011;26:1500–1503.

45 Sivak MV, Jr., EUS for bile duct stones: how does it compare with ERCP? Gastrointestinal Endoscopy 2002;56:S175–S177.

46 Scheiman JM, Carlos RC, Barnett JL, et al. Can endoscopic ultrasound or magnetic resonance cholangiopancreatography replace ERCP in patients with suspected biliary disease? A prospective trial and cost analysis. American Journal of Gastroenterology 2001;96:2900–2904.

47 Romagnuolo J, Currie G, Calgary Advanced Therapeutic Endoscopy Center study g. Noninvasive vs. selective invasive biliary imaging for acute biliary pancreatitis: an economic evaluation by using decision tree analysis. Gastrointestinal Endoscopy 2005;61:86–97.

48 De Lisi S, Leandro G, Buscarini E. Endoscopic ultrasonography versus endoscopic retrograde cholangiopancreatography in acute biliary pancreatitis: a systematic review. European Journal of Gastroenterology & Hepatology 2011;23:367–374.

49 Arguedas MR, Dupont AW, Wilcox CM. Where do ERCP, endoscopic ultrasound, magnetic resonance cholangiopancreatography, and intraoperative cholangiography fit in the management of acute biliary pancreatitis? A decision analysis model. American Journal of Gastroenterology 2001;96:2892–2899.

50 Ranson JH, Rifkind KM, Roses DF, et al. Prognostic signs and the role of operative management in acute pancreatitis. Surgery, Gynecology & Obstetrics 1974;139:69–81.

51 Larvin M, McMahon MJ. APACHE-II score for assessment and monitoring of acute pancreatitis. Lancet 1989;2:201–205.

52 Wu BU, Johannes RS, Sun X, et al. The early prediction of mortality in acute pancreatitis: a large population-based study. Gut 2008;57:1698–1703.

53 Balthazar EJ, Robinson DL, Megibow AJ, et al. Acute pancreatitis: value of CT in establishing prognosis. Radiology 1990;174:331–336.

54 Bone RC. Sepsis, sepsis syndrome, and the systemic inflammatory response syndrome (SIRS). Gulliver in Laputa. Journal of the American Medical Association 1995;273:155–156.

55 Working Group IAP/APA Acute Pancreatitis Guidelines. IAP/APA evidence-based guidelines for the management of acute pancreatitis. Pancreatology 2013;13:e1–e15.

56 Wu BU, Bakker OJ, Papachristou GI, et al. Blood urea nitrogen in the early assessment of acute pancreatitis: an international validation study. Archives of Internal Medicine 2011;171:669–676.

57 Cote GA, Sagi SV, Schmidt SE, et al. Early measures of hemoconcentration and inflammation are predictive of prolonged hospitalization from post- endoscopic retrograde cholangiopancreatography pancreatitis. Pancreas 2013;42:850–854.

58 Mounzer R, Langmead CJ, Wu BU, et al. Comparison of existing clinical scoring systems to predict persistent organ failure in patients with acute pancreatitis. Gastroenterology 2012;142:1476–1482; quiz e15–e16.

59 Moretti A, Papi C, Aratari A, et al. Is early endoscopic retrograde cholangiopancreatography useful in the management of acute biliary pancreatitis? A meta-analysis of randomized controlled trials. Digestive and Liver Disease 2008;40:379–385.

60 van Geenen EJ, van Santvoort HC, Besselink MG, et al. Lack of consensus on the role of endoscopic retrograde cholangiography in acute biliary pancreatitis in published meta-analyses and guidelines: a systematic review. Pancreas 2013;42:774–780.

61 Tse F, Yuan Y. Early routine endoscopic retrograde cholangiopancreatography strategy versus early conservative management strategy in acute gallstone pancreatitis. Cochrane Database of Systematic Reviews 2012;5:CD009779.

62 Folsch UR, Nitsche R, Ludtke R, et al. Early ERCP and papillotomy compared with conservative treatment for acute biliary pancreatitis. The German Study Group on Acute Biliary Pancreatitis. New England Journal of Medicine 1997;336:237–242.

63 Katanuma A, Maguchi H, Osanai M, et al. Endoscopic treatment of difficult common bile duct stones. Digestive Endoscopy 2010;22 Suppl 1:S90–S97.

64 Maple JT, Ikenberry SO, Anderson MA, et al. The role of endoscopy in the management of choledocholithiasis. Gastrointestinal Endoscopy 2011;74:731–744.

65 Jain SK, Stein R, Bhuva M, et al. Pigtail stents: an alternative in the treatment of difficult bile duct stones. Gastrointestinal Endoscopy 2000;52:490–493.

66 Hong WD, Zhu QH, Huang QK. Endoscopic sphincterotomy plus endoprostheses in the treatment of large or multiple common bile duct stones. Digestive Endoscopy 2011;23:240–243.

67 Stefanidis G, Christodoulou C, Manolakopoulos S, et al. Endoscopic extraction of large common bile duct stones: a review article. World Journal of Gastrointestinal Endoscopy 2012;4:167–179.

68 Fejes R, Kurucsai G, Szekely A, et al. Feasibility and safety of emergency ERCP and small-caliber pancreatic stenting as a bridging procedure in patients with acute biliary pancreatitis but difficult sphincterotomy. Surgical Endoscopy 2010;24:1878–1885.

69 Dubravcsik Z, Hritz I, Fejes R, et al. Early ERCP and biliary sphincterotomy with or without small-caliber pancreatic stent insertion in patients with acute biliary pancreatitis: better overall outcome with adequate pancreatic drainage. Scandinavian Journal of Gastroenterology 2012;47:729–736.

70 Ding G, Qin M, Cai W, et al. The safety and utility of pancreatic duct stents in the emergency ERCP of acute biliary pancreatitis but difficult sphincterotomy. Hepatogastroenterology 2012;59:2374–2376.

71 Working Party of the British Society of Gastroenterology, Association of Surgeons of Great Britain and Ireland, Pancreatic Society of Great Britain and Ireland, et al. UK guidelines for the management of acute pancreatitis. Gut 2005;54 Suppl 3:iii1–iii9.

72 Heider TR, Brown A, Grimm IS, et al. Endoscopic sphincterotomy permits interval laparoscopic cholecystectomy in patients with moderately severe gallstone pancreatitis. Journal of Gastrointestinal Surgery 2006;10:1–5.

73 Ammori BJ, Davides D, Vezakis A, et al. Laparoscopic cholecystectomy: are patients with biliary pancreatitis at increased operative risk? Surgical Endoscopy 2003; 17:777–780.

74 Wilson CT, de Moya MA. Cholecystectomy for acute gallstone pancreatitis: early vs delayed approach. Scandinavian Journal of Surgery 2010;99:81–85.

75 Kaw M, Al-Antably Y, Kaw P. Management of gallstone pancreatitis: cholecystectomy or ERCP and endoscopic sphincterotomy. Gastrointestinal Endoscopy 2002;56:61–65.

76 Ito K, Ito H, Whang EE. Timing of cholecystectomy for biliary pancreatitis: do the data support current guidelines? Journal of Gastrointestinal Surgery 2008;12:2164–2170.

77 van Baal MC, Besselink MG, Bakker OJ, et al. Timing of cholecystectomy after mild biliary pancreatitis: a systematic review. Annals of Surgery 2012;255:860–866.

78 Morris S, Gurusamy KS, Patel N, et al. Cost-effectiveness of early laparoscopic cholecystectomy for mild acute gallstone pancreatitis. British Journal of Surgery 2014;101:828–835.

79 van Geenen EJ, van der Peet DL, Mulder CJ, et al. Recurrent acute biliary pancreatitis: the protective role of cholecystectomy and endoscopic sphincterotomy. Surgical Endoscopy 2009;23:950–956.

80 Boerma D, Rauws EA, Keulemans YC, et al. Wait-and-see policy or laparoscopic cholecystectomy after endoscopic sphincterotomy for bile-duct stones: a randomised trial. Lancet 2002;360:761–765.

81 Sanjay P, Yeeting S, Whigham C, et al. Endoscopic sphincterotomy and interval cholecystectomy are reasonable alternatives to index cholecystectomy in severe acute gallstone pancreatitis (GSP). Surgical Endoscopy 2008;22:1832–1837.

82 Nealon WH, Bawduniak J, Walser EM. Appropriate timing of cholecystectomy in patients who present with moderate to severe gallstone-associated acute pancreatitis with peripancreatic fluid collections. Annals of Surgery 2004;239:741–749; discussion 749–751.

83 Banks PA, Freeman ML, Practice Parameters Committee of the American College of Gastroenterology. Practice guidelines in acute pancreatitis. American Journal of Gastroenterology 2006;101:2379–2400.

84 Hwang SS, Li BH, Haigh PI. Gallstone pancreatitis without cholecystectomy. Journal of the American Medical Association Surgery 2013;148:867–872.

CHAPTER 7

Treatment of local complications

Stefan A.W. Bouwense[1], Thomas L. Bollen[2], Paul Fockens[3] & Marc G.H. Besselink[4] for the Dutch Pancreatitis Study Group

[1] Department of Surgery, Radboudumc, Nijmegen, the Netherlands
[2] Department of Radiology, St. Antonius Hospital, Nieuwegein, the Netherlands
[3] Department of Gastroenterology and Hepatology, Academic Medical Center, Amsterdam, the Netherlands
[4] Department of Surgery, Academic Medical Center, Amsterdam, the Netherlands

Introduction

The recently revised Atlanta classification addresses the clinical presentation, types, and (clinical and morphologic) complications of acute pancreatitis [1]. This revised classification aims to clarify terminology and stimulate the use of uniform definitions and standardized reporting in patients with acute pancreatitis. Local complications are peripancreatic fluid collections, pancreatic and peripancreatic necrosis (sterile or infected), pseudocyst, and walled off necrosis (WON; sterile or infected) (Table 7.1).

About 80% of patients with acute pancreatitis have mild disease and symptoms that usually resolve within 1 week with basic supportive care [1, 2]. The remainder of the 20% of patients develops a severe form of pancreatitis (moderately severe or severe acute pancreatitis) with usually persistent organ failure and pancreatic or peripancreatic tissue necrosis (necrotizing pancreatitis). In this group of patients, the first 1–2 weeks are marked by a persisting systemic inflammatory response syndrome and/or (multiple) organ failure. Mortality is high despite maximal supportive care in the intensive care unit [3, 4].

In at least 30% of patients with necrotizing pancreatitis, the necrosis becomes infected [5]. This group of patients is at risk for major morbidity with a mortality of around 32% [6]. Infected necrosis should be suspected when clinical and biochemical deterioration is present after an initial period of clinical improvement or when patients fail to show clinical improvement from their systemic inflammatory response syndrome and/or organ failure. In these clinical scenarios, a contrast-enhanced computed tomography (CECT) is indicated, which may show acute necrotic collection(s) or WON [1, 2]. Gas bubbles in collections are pathognomonic for infected necrosis and are caused by gas-forming bacteria or fistulas between the collection and intestines [7]. If the diagnosis of infected necrosis is unclear, fine-needle aspiration (FNA) of the collection can be obtained but is usually not required. One has to bear in mind that up to 20% of FNAs may be false negative [8].

In the case of proven or suspected infected necrosis, intravenous broad-spectrum antibiotics should be started. Positive cultures of infected collections usually result in a switch from broad-spectrum antibiotics to narrow-spectrum antibiotics specifically aimed at those microorganisms [2]. At present, there is no evidence for prophylactic antibiotics [9]. Recovery with antibiotics has been described in some patients with infected necrosis [5]. But in the vast majority of patients, antibiotics should be regarded as supportive care during the disease course, where drainage and necrosectomy of necrotic collections are regarded as definitive treatment.

Traditionally, major surgery was performed early in the clinical course of necrotizing pancreatitis. Nowadays, interventions are postponed whenever feasible until WON is present on CECT, a process that usually takes 3–4 weeks [7]. During this period, antibiotics should be continued and patients should be stabilized on the intensive care unit if needed. Delayed intervention, until the stage of complete encapsulation of collections, probably reduces morbidity and mortality compared with an early laparotomy in the first 2 weeks [5, 10].

Table 7.1 Collections as defined in the revised Atlanta classification.

Definition	Description
Acute fluid collection (less than 4 weeks after onset)	• Homogenous fluid density • Confined by normal peripancreatic fascial planes • No definable wall encapsulating the collection • Adjacent to pancreas (not intrapancreatic)
Pseudocyst (usually more than 4 weeks after onset)	• Well circumscribed, usually round/oval • Homogenous fluid density • Well-defined wall and completely encapsulated • Adjacent to pancreas (not intrapancreatic)
Acute necrotic collection (less than 4 weeks after onset)	• Heterogeneous and nonliquid density • No definable wall encapsulating the collection • Location: intrapancreatic and/or extrapancreatic
Walled-off necrosis (usually more than 4 weeks after onset)	• Heterogeneous and nonliquid density • Well-defined wall and completely encapsulated • Location: intrapancreatic and/or extrapancreatic

Revised definitions of morphological features of acute pancreatitis [1].

In the acute phase, there is no indication for intervention to treat sterile collections. These collections tend to have a mild clinical course and are usually absorbed within weeks to months [2]. Performing interventions for sterile collections carries a risk of introducing infection, thereby increasing morbidity and mortality [11]. However, in rare cases, interventions for sterile collections may be needed. Such indications include obstruction of the biliary or gastrointestinal tract, long-lasting pain, and collections resulting from a disrupted pancreatic duct [2].

Invasive treatment

Open necrosectomy

Laparotomy with complete necrosectomy has long been the standard intervention in patients with necrotizing pancreatitis who showed clinical deterioration. Morbidity (up to 95%) and mortality (11–39%) for this procedure were high [12, 13]. Recent studies have shown that the success rate of open necrosectomy has improved significantly (11–19%), probably due to better supportive care on the intensive care unit and optimal timing of surgery [14, 15].

The indications for laparotomy have sharply diminished in recent years due to minimally invasive procedures, which have improved outcome in these patients [10, 15, 16]. Albeit rare, some acute abdominal complications in acute pancreatitis still require laparotomy. Bowel ischemia, bowel perforation, and abdominal compartment syndrome have high rates of mortality and usually require emergency laparotomy [5, 17–19]. When a laparotomy is performed, it is recommended not to explore the retroperitoneum, because the retroperitoneal collections may not be infected at that time.

Minimally invasive intervention

Several minimally invasive intervention strategies are available for drainage and/or debridement of infected necrotizing pancreatitis. Instead of complete removal of all nonviable tissue by laparotomy [20], the first step of minimally invasive interventions is to drain the infected collections. If needed, the next step is necrosectomy of nonadherent necrotic tissue. This approach reduces the risk of iatrogenic damage and hemorrhage. Less surgical injury accelerates patient recovery and decreases complications in an already critically ill patient population.

Percutaneous catheter drainage [21], percutaneous necrosectomy [22], video-assisted retroperitoneal debridement (VARD) [23], laparoscopic necrosectomy [24], and endoscopic transluminal drainage and necrosectomy [25] are all examples of minimally invasive interventions.

Percutaneous catheter drainage and video-assisted retroperitoneal debridement

The concept of percutaneous catheter drainage is to drain "pus under pressure" in the necrotic collection for sepsis control and to serve as a bridge to definitive surgery. First described by Freeny et al. [21], it is the least invasive procedure and the most widely available technique.

Success rates of percutaneous catheter drainage up to 50% have been described [26, 27]. Success is defined as full recovery with percutaneous catheter drainage alone without additional necrosectomy (Figure 7.1). In the Dutch randomized multicenter PANTER trial, patients with (suspected) infected pancreatic necrosis were randomized between open necrosectomy (by laparotomy) and a surgical step-up approach, which consisted of percutaneous catheter drainage first, followed, if no improvement was present after 72 hours [15], by VARD. In this trial, success rate of percutaneous catheter

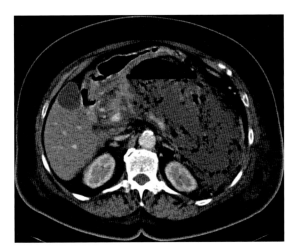

Figure 7.1 Contrast-enhanced CT scan of a patient with infected necrotizing pancreatitis. A single large percutaneous drain was placed through the left retroperitoneum. The patient recovered fully after the drainage procedure without additional drainage procedures and without necrosectomy.

drainage only was 35%, and reversal of sepsis after percutaneous catheter drainage occurred in 62–84%. The latter was important because this created a time interval where collections could become more encapsulated and necrosis could mature, facilitating the effectiveness of necrosectomy.

Nearly all peripancreatic collections can be reached percutaneously either via the retroperitoneal or transperitoneal route [15, 28]. However, the retroperitoneal route is preferred because it is associated with less complications. Also, it prevents the advancement of infection to the intraperitoneal space, and it can be used as guidance for minimally invasive retroperitoneal necrosectomy (Figure 7.2).

Data on the impact of drain size and management on outcome are scarce. One study described a success rate of 43% without necrosectomy in 80 patients who were drained with 8–24 French drains [30]. In the PANTER trial, the minimal drain size was 12 French, and drains were irrigated 4 times daily with 250 cc normal saline to keep the drains open. Aggressive lavage of the necrotic cavity with multiple drains has been advocated by some authors although the evidence for this approach is (yet) limited [31]. Placement of additional drains and drain upsizing are methods to deal with inadequately drained collections.

In a systematic review of percutaneous drainage including 384 patients, complication rates of 20% were reported [26]. Most common complications were the formation of pancreaticocutaneous and pancreaticoenteric fistula, which usually can be treated nonoperatively. Catheter dislodgement, abdominal pain, and pneumothorax are less common complications. Rare life-threatening complications are bowel perforations and vascular damage, necessitating immediate intervention.

If additional intervention is needed after percutaneous catheter drainage, a VARD procedure can be performed as part of the surgical step-up approach [15]. Because percutaneous catheter drainage only can prevent necrosectomy in 35–50% of patients, it is recommended that VARD should always be preceded by percutaneous catheter drainage [2, 26]. The VARD procedure was first described by Horvath et al. in the United States in 2001 [23]. Under general anesthesia, the patient is placed in the right lateral position. A subcostal incision of a few centimeters is made near the exit of the drain. Guided by the drain and imaging,

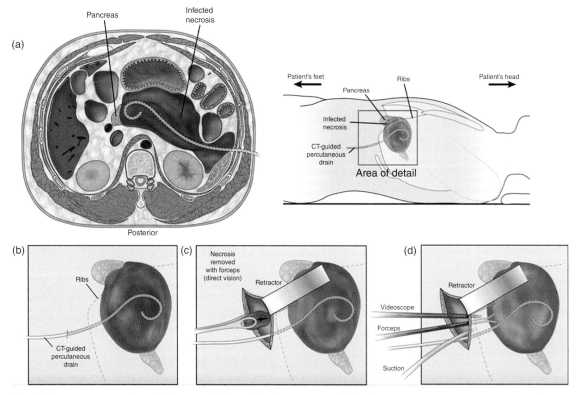

Figure 7.2 Percutaneous catheter drainage and video-assisted retroperitoneal debridement. (a) A transverse cross-sectional image as can be seen on a contrast-enhanced CT image of a patient with necrotizing pancreatitis. The preferred route for catheter drainage is through the left side of the retroperitoneum. (b) More detail on the drained area. (c) A small subcostal incision is made near the puncture site of the percutaneous drain. The drain is used as a guide through the retroperitoneum to the necrotic collection. All visible necrosis is removed directly. (d) A videoscope is introduced and further debridement is performed with laparoscopic instruments. Reprinted from: van Brunschot S, Bakker OJ, Besselink MG, et al. Treatment of necrotizing pancreatitis. Clinical Gastroenterology and Hepatology: The Official Clinical Practice journal of the American Gastroenterological Association 2012;10:1190–1201, with permission from Elsevier [29].

the route is chosen through the retroperitoneum to the necrotic collection. When the collection is entered, visible nonadherent necrosis is removed with grasping forceps. A 0° videoscope is introduced in the cavity and, if needed, CO_2 can be inflated through the drain. With laparoscopic instruments only loosely adherent necrosis is removed, to reduce the risk of bleeding from viable underlying tissue. Subsequently, all drains and instruments are removed, and two large catheters are placed in the cavity for postoperative lavage (up to 10 L per 24 hours). Finally, the fascia and skin are closed (Figure 7.2).

The PANTER trial showed that the surgical step-up approach is superior to primary open necrosectomy [15]. The step-up approach showed a significant lower rate of the combined endpoint of mortality and major complications (40% vs. 69%, $P=0.006$). Other complications of the step-up approach also compared favorably with open necrosectomy: pancreatic fistula formation (28% vs. 38%, $P=0.33$), incisional hernia (7% vs. 24%, $P=0.03$), and new-onset diabetes (16% vs. 38%, $P=0.02$). Overall, patients treated with the step-up approach had significantly less new-onset of multiple organ failure and less need for interventions including necrosectomies. In only three patients, the step-up approach was technically not successful because the retroperitoneal collection could not be reached. In these cases, laparotomy was needed.

There are numerous variations of the VARD procedure, that is, single-port, three-port, and flexible endoscope necrosectomy. In small series, all show similar results compared with VARD [32–34].

Sinus tract necrosectomy

Originally described by the group of Carter et al. from Glasgow, sinus tract necrosectomy was one of the first minimally invasive procedures in infected necrosis [22]. Prior to surgery, a CT-guided retroperitoneal drain is placed in the necrotic collection. The tract is stepwise dilated until 30 French, which is used as an entry for a nephroscope to enter the collection during surgery. With grasping forceps only loosely adherent necrosis is removed. After surgery the cavity is continuously rinsed with fluids. Success of a single procedure is limited. However, necrosectomy can be repeated and usually three to four procedures are needed [35, 36]. In up to a quarter of patients, conversion to an open procedure was needed. Fistula formation (4–22%) and bleeding (10–17%) are common procedure-related complications. Mortality of patients treated with sinus tract necrosectomy is reported to be between 9% and 19% [35–37].

Laparoscopic necrosectomy

Laparoscopic cystogastrostomy is the most frequently described minimally invasive transperitoneal approach [24]. With this technique, instruments are introduced in the abdominal cavity, and an anterior gastrostomy is performed. Subsequently, the necrotic collection is located and entered through a posterior gastrostomy. A wide cystogastrostomy is created with an endoscopic stapling device, and necrosectomy is performed. After the debridement, only the anterior gastrostomy is closed, either with sutures or by staples.

Scientific evidence on this approach is limited. Some retrospective studies suggest that this laparoscopic approach is associated with low morbidity and mortality rates [24, 38–41]. However, the quality of these studies is difficult to assess since important baseline characteristics such as preoperative disease severity are often missing. A recent retrospective study of 76 patients compared laparoscopic necrosectomy with open necrosectomy and found the laparoscopic approach superior regarding the rate of postoperative complications [42].

Endoscopic drainage and necrosectomy

In the past decade, endoscopic transgastric drainage and necrosectomy of pancreatic necrosis have gained popularity [25, 43, 44]. Comparable with the surgical step-up approach, a step-up approach can also be applied endoscopically: endoscopic transluminal catheter drainage followed, if needed, by endoscopic transluminal necrosectomy. When an infected pancreatic collection lies close to the duodenum or stomach, endoscopic transluminal drainage can be considered. The patient is placed in left lateral position under deep sedation or general anesthesia (in case of high risk of aspiration or preference of the anesthesiologist). Endoscopic ultrasound is used to examine the size, content, and relation to other structures of the collection [45]. The optimal puncture site of gastric wall or the duodenum to the collection is chosen by endoscopic ultrasound. Endoscopic drainage without ultrasound is possible, but the technical success is inferior compared with ultrasound-guided drainage procedures [46, 47].

A 19-gauge FNA needle is used to access the collection through the intestinal wall. Aspiration of the content and injection of contrast into the cavity can be used to check the proper location. A sample of the fluid in the collection is always sent for culture. Under fluoroscopic guidance, a guidewire is introduced and looped in the collection [48]. By using electrocauterization and/or balloon dilatation, a larger fistula tract is created between the collection and the intestinal lumen. Initial dilation is usually performed up to 8–12 mm, and two double pigtails and a nasocystic catheter are placed into the cavity. Specially designed metal stents are used progressively as they have the advantage of creating and maintaining a larger opening (1 cm or more) [49, 50] (Figure 7.3). Alternatively, self-expandable metallic stents from 16×30 mm up to 23×105 mm have been placed in the fistula tract during the first procedure [51]. Through these stents future endoscopic interventions could be performed. Initial reports showed that a mean of five interventions per patient were needed and a success rate of 88% with low morbidity and mortality [49, 51]. The use of stents seems promising regarding the ease of the endoscopic procedure and drainage of the cavity. Further prospective trials are necessary to assess the indication and effectiveness of stenting, together with stent choice and duration of stenting.

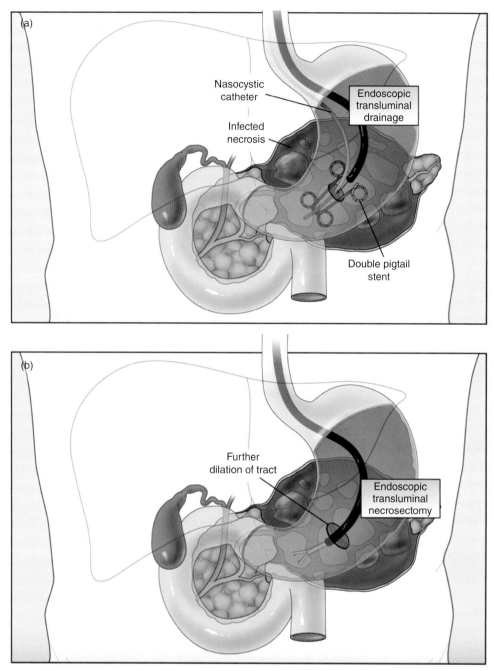

Figure 7.3 Endoscopic transluminal drainage and endoscopic transluminal necrosectomy. Endoscopic transluminal intervention through the posterior wall of the stomach. (a) The necrotic collection is punctured through the stomach wall, and a guidewire is placed in the collection, if needed under the guidance of endoscopic ultrasound. The tract is balloon dilated over the guidewire. Two pigtail drains and a nasocystic catheter are placed into the collection for continuous lavage. (b) The cystogastrostomy is further dilated and the collection is entered by an endoscope. Under direct vision a necrosectomy can be performed. Reprinted from: van Brunschot S, Bakker OJ, Besselink MG, et al. Treatment of necrotizing pancreatitis. Clinical Gastroenterology and Hepatology: The Official Clinical Practice journal of the American Gastroenterological Association 2012;10:1190–1201, with permission from Elsevier [29].

The nasocystic catheter is used to flush the contents of the collection into the stomach (1 L per 24 hours). Noncommunicating collections can be drained by multiple cystogastrostomies. Drainage of WON by multiple cystogastrostomies or combined endoscopic and percutaneous drainage has shown good results, but these results need to be confirmed in well-designed trials [52–54].

Comparable with the surgical step-up approach, an endoscopic necrosectomy is performed if a patient does not improve within 72 hours after drainage. The fistula tract is dilated up to 15–18 mm with a forward-viewing endoscope. After dilation, the endoscope is advanced into the collection, and with endoscopic accessories (i.e., snares, baskets, nets, and forceps), necrosectomy is performed through this tract, leaving the debris in the stomach. After removing the loosely adherent necrosis, pigtails and again a nasocystic catheter are left into the cavity to leave the fistula tract open [48, 55, 56]. Endoscopic necrosectomy is repeated every 48 hours until most necrotic material is removed.

Clinical success rate up to 91% with a 97% technical success rate in 1134 cases of pancreatic fluid collections [45]. A systematic review of 455 patients found that clinical recovery with endoscopic necrosectomy only was achieved in 81% of patients [57]. Infected necrosis was diagnosed in 57% of all patients, and overall morbidity was 36% with 8% mortality. Major complications were bleeding (18%), pancreatic fistula (5%), and spontaneous perforation of a hollow organ (4%). Rare complications such as air embolisms have been described, and hence CO_2 insufflation is recommended although this is not 100% protective since endoscopes insufflate without pressure control.

Combined techniques

To reduce pancreaticocutaneous fistula, the group from Seattle developed a "dual-modality drainage" combining both percutaneous and endoscopic drainage [53, 54, 58]. Compared with percutaneous drainage only, this dual-modality drainage reduced hospital stay. In 117 patients, outcomes were promising with low rates of additional necrosectomy, pancreaticocutaneous fistula, and mortality. Prospective data, however, are awaited.

Which technique to choose?

Currently, there is lack of definitive evidence regarding the optimal technique for necrosectomy. The most recent studies suggest that minimally invasive procedures are superior to open necrosectomy. However, there are no trials directly comparing open necrosectomy with minimally invasive necrosectomy. Even in the PANTER trial, there was no head-to-head comparison between open necrosectomy and VARD, because a VARD was always preceded by percutaneous drainage.

When comparing sinus tract necrosectomy with VARD, it seems that in sinus tract necrosectomy, more procedures are needed [35, 36]. This is explained by the fact that in VARD the 3–5 cm incision facilitates necrosectomy, but incisional hernias are reported in up to 7% of patients [15]. Overall, sinus tract necrosectomy and VARD seem comparable with regard to complications and mortality.

The PENGUIN trial was a pilot study comparing VARD with endoscopic transluminal necrosectomy in 22 patients with infected necrosis. The postoperative proinflammatory response was significantly more reduced after endoscopic necrosectomy than after VARD. Also, the combined endpoint of major complications and death was in favor of the endoscopic approach [59]. These data suggest the superiority of an endoscopic necrosectomy over VARD. A large randomized controlled multicenter trial, the TENSION trial (ISRCTN09186711), is currently comparing endoscopic step-up approach with the surgical step-up approach regarding major morbidity and mortality [60]. At present, endoscopic necrosectomy is comparable to VARD regarding morbidity (36% vs. 28–50%) and mortality (6% vs. 3–19%) [15, 57, 61].

IAP/APA guideline

In 2013, the IAP/APA evidence-based guideline for the management for acute pancreatitis was published [2]. Experts from around the world formed 12 multidisciplinary review groups that performed systematic literature reviews to answer predefined clinical questions. Subsequently, a joint meeting was held to finalize all the discussions and come to overall agreement. The following recommendations were made regarding interventions in necrotizing pancreatitis [2]:

A. Indications for intervention in necrotizing pancreatitis are (i) clinical suspicion or documented infected necrotizing pancreatitis with clinical deterioration and (ii) ongoing organ failure for several weeks after the disease onset in the absence of documented infected necrotizing pancreatitis.

B. Indications for intervention in sterile necrotizing pancreatitis are (i) ongoing gastric outlet, intestinal, or biliary obstruction due to mass effect of WON (i.e., arbitrarily more then 4–8 weeks after onset of acute pancreatitis), (ii) persistent debilitating symptoms in patients with WON without signs of infection (i.e., arbitrarily more than 8 weeks after onset of acute pancreatitis), and (iii) disconnected duct syndrome with persisting symptoms (e.g., pain and obstruction) collection(s) with WON.

C. For patients with proven or suspected infected necrotizing pancreatitis, invasive intervention should be preferably delayed until at least 4 weeks after initial presentation to allow collections to become "walled-off."

D. The optimal interventional strategy for patients with suspected or confirmed infected necrotizing pancreatitis is initial image-guided percutaneous (retroperitoneal) catheter drainage or endoscopic transluminal drainage, followed, if necessary, by endoscopic or surgical necrosectomy.

References

1 Banks PA, Bollen TL, Dervenis C, et al. Classification of acute pancreatitis--2012: revision of the Atlanta classification and definitions by international consensus. Gut 2013;62:102–111.

2 Working Group IAP/APA Acute Pancreatitis Guidelines. IAP/APA evidence-based guidelines for the management of acute pancreatitis. Pancreatology 2013;13:e1–e15.

3 Johnson CD, Abu-Hilal M. Persistent organ failure during the first week as a marker of fatal outcome in acute pancreatitis. Gut 2004;53:1340–1344.

4 Mofidi R, Duff MD, Wigmore SJ, Madhavan KK, Garden OJ, Parks RW. Association between early systemic inflammatory response, severity of multiorgan dysfunction and death in acute pancreatitis. British Journal of Surgery 2006;93:738–744.

5 van Santvoort HC, Bakker OJ, Bollen TL, et al. A conservative and minimally invasive approach to necrotizing pancreatitis improves outcome. Gastroenterology 2011;141:1254–1263.

6 Petrov MS, Shanbhag S, Chakraborty M, Phillips AR, Windsor JA. Organ failure and infection of pancreatic necrosis as determinants of mortality in patients with acute pancreatitis. Gastroenterology 2010;139:813–820.

7 Bollen TL. Imaging of acute pancreatitis: update of the revised Atlanta classification. Radiologic clinics of North America 2012;50:429–445.

8 van Baal MC, Bollen TL, Bakker OJ, et al. The role of routine fine-needle aspiration in the diagnosis of infected necrotizing pancreatitis. Surgery 2014;155:442–448.

9 Wittau M, Mayer B, Scheele J, Henne-Bruns D, Dellinger EP, Isenmann R. Systematic review and meta-analysis of antibiotic prophylaxis in severe acute pancreatitis. Scandinavian Journal of Gastroenterology 2011;46:261–270.

10 Besselink MG, Verwer TJ, Schoenmaeckers EJ, et al. Timing of surgical intervention in necrotizing pancreatitis. Archives of Surgery 2007;142:1194–1201.

11 Besselink MG, Van Santvoort HC, Bakker OJ, Bollen TL, Gooszen HG. Draining sterile fluid collections in acute pancreatitis? Primum non nocere! Surgical Endoscopy 2010;25:331–332.

12 Howard TJ, Patel JB, Zyromski N, et al. Declining morbidity and mortality rates in the surgical management of pancreatic necrosis. Journal of Gastrointestinal Surgery 2007;11:43–49.

13 Rau B, Bothe A, Beger HG. Surgical treatment of necrotizing pancreatitis by necrosectomy and closed lavage: changing patient characteristics and outcome in a 19-year, single-center series. Surgery 2005;138:28–39.

14 Rodriguez JR, Razo AO, Targarona J, et al. Debridement and closed packing for sterile or infected necrotizing pancreatitis: insights into indications and outcomes in 167 patients. Annals of Surgery 2008;247:294–299.

15 van Santvoort HC, Besselink MG, Bakker OJ, et al. A step-up approach or open necrosectomy for necrotizing pancreatitis. New England Journal of Medicine 2010;362:1491–1502.

16 Hartwig W, Maksan SM, Foitzik T, Schmidt J, Herfarth C, Klar E. Reduction in mortality with delayed surgical therapy of severe pancreatitis. Journal of Gastrointestinal Surgery 2002;6:481–487.

17 De Waele JJ, Hoste E, Blot SI, Decruyenaere J, Colardyn F. Intra-abdominal hypertension in patients with severe acute pancreatitis. Critical Care 2005;9:R452–R457.

18 Mentula P, Hienonen P, Kemppainen E, Puolakkainen P, Leppaniemi A. Surgical decompression for abdominal compartment syndrome in severe acute pancreatitis. Archives of Surgery 2010;145:764–769.

19 Takahashi Y, Fukushima J, Fukusato T, et al. Prevalence of ischemic enterocolitis in patients with acute pancreatitis. Journal of Gastroenterology 2005;40:827–832.

20 Beger HG, Buchler M, Bittner R, Oettinger W, Block S, Nevalainen T. Necrosectomy and postoperative local lavage in patients with necrotizing pancreatitis: results

of a prospective clinical trial. World Journal of Surgery 1988;12:255–262.

21 Freeny PC, Hauptmann E, Althaus SJ, Traverso LW, Sinanan M. Percutaneous CT-guided catheter drainage of infected acute necrotizing pancreatitis: techniques and results. American Journal of Roentgenology 1998;170:969–975.

22 Carter CR, McKay CJ, Imrie CW. Percutaneous necrosectomy and sinus tract endoscopy in the management of infected pancreatic necrosis: an initial experience. Annals of Surgery 2000;232:175–180.

23 Horvath KD, Kao LS, Wherry KL, Pellegrini CA, Sinanan MN. A technique for laparoscopic-assisted percutaneous drainage of infected pancreatic necrosis and pancreatic abscess. Surgical Endoscopy 2001;15:1221–1225.

24 Gibson SC, Robertson BF, Dickson EJ, McKay CJ, Carter CR. 'Step-port' laparoscopic cystogastrostomy for the management of organized solid predominant post-acute fluid collections after severe acute pancreatitis. HPB: The Official Journal of the International Hepato Pancreato Biliary Association 2014;16:170–176.

25 Seifert H, Wehrmann T, Schmitt T, Zeuzem S, Caspary WF. Retroperitoneal endoscopic debridement for infected peripancreatic necrosis. Lancet 2000;356:653–655.

26 van Baal MC, van Santvoort HC, Bollen TL, et al. Systematic review of percutaneous catheter drainage as primary treatment for necrotizing pancreatitis. British Journal of Surgery 2011;98:18–27.

27 Mouli VP, Sreenivas V, Garg PK. Efficacy of conservative treatment, without necrosectomy, for infected pancreatic necrosis: a systematic review and meta-analysis. Gastroenterology 2013;144:333–340 ;e2.

28 Besselink MG, Van Santvoort HC, Schaapherder AF, Van Ramshorst B, van Goor H, Gooszen HG. Feasibility of minimally invasive approaches in patients with infected necrotizing pancreatitis. British Journal of Surgery 2007;94:604–608.

29 van Brunschot S, Bakker OJ, Besselink MG, et al. Treatment of necrotizing pancreatitis. Clinical Gastroenterology and Hepatology: The Official Clinical Practice Journal of the American Gastroenterological Association 2012;10:1190–1201.

30 Bruennler T, Langgartner J, Lang S, et al. Outcome of patients with acute, necrotizing pancreatitis requiring drainage-does drainage size matter? World Journal of Gastroenterology 2008;14:725–730.

31 Zerem E, Imamovic G, Susic A, Haracic B. Step-up approach to infected necrotising pancreatitis: a 20-year experience of percutaneous drainage in a single centre. Digestive and Liver Disease 2011;43:478–483.

32 Castellanos G, Pinero A, Doig LA, Serrano A, Fuster M, Bixquert V. Management of infected pancreatic necrosis using retroperitoneal necrosectomy with flexible endoscope: 10 years of experience. Surgical Endoscopy 2013;27:443–453.

33 Sileikis A, Beisa V, Simutis G, Tamosiunas A, Strupas K. Three-port retroperitoneoscopic necrosectomy in management of acute necrotic pancreatitis. Medicina 2010;46:176–179.

34 Tang C, Wang B, Xie B, Liu H, Chen P. Treatment of severe acute pancreatitis through retroperitoneal laparoscopic drainage. Frontiers of Medicine 2011;5:302–305.

35 Ahmad HA, Samarasam I, Hamdorf JM. Minimally invasive retroperitoneal pancreatic necrosectomy. Pancreatology 2011;11:52–56.

36 Raraty MG, Halloran CM, Dodd S, et al. Minimal access retroperitoneal pancreatic necrosectomy: improvement in morbidity and mortality with a less invasive approach. Annals of Surgery 2010;251:787–793.

37 Connor S, Raraty MG, Howes N, et al. Surgery in the treatment of acute pancreatitis–minimal access pancreatic necrosectomy. Scandinavian Journal of Surgery 2005;94:135–142.

38 Bucher P, Pugin F, Morel P. Minimally invasive necrosectomy for infected necrotizing pancreatitis. Pancreas 2008;36:113–119.

39 Parekh D. Laparoscopic-assisted pancreatic necrosectomy: a new surgical option for treatment of severe necrotizing pancreatitis. Archives of Surgery 2006;141:895–902; discussion 902–903.

40 Melman L, Azar R, Beddow K, et al. Primary and overall success rates for clinical outcomes after laparoscopic, endoscopic, and open pancreatic cystogastrostomy for pancreatic pseudocysts. Surgical Endoscopy 2009;23:267–271.

41 Palanivelu C, Senthilkumar K, Madhankumar MV, et al. Management of pancreatic pseudocyst in the era of laparoscopic surgery–experience from a tertiary centre. Surgical Endoscopy 2007;21:2262–2267.

42 Tan J, Tan H, Hu B, et al. Short-term outcomes from a multicenter retrospective study in China comparing laparoscopic and open surgery for the treatment of infected pancreatic necrosis. Journal of Laparoendoscopic & Advanced Surgical Techniques Part A 2012;22:27–33.

43 Working Party of the British Society of Gastroenterology, Association of Surgeons of Great Britain and Ireland, Pancreatic Society of Great Britain and Ireland, et al. UK guidelines for the management of acute pancreatitis. Gut 2005;54 Suppl 3:iii1–iii9.

44 Isaji S, Takada T, Kawarada Y, et al. JPN Guidelines for the management of acute pancreatitis: surgical management. Journal of Hepato-Biliary-Pancreatic Surgery 2006;13:48–55.

45 Fabbri C, Luigiano C, Maimone A, Polifemo AM, Tarantino I, Cennamo V. Endoscopic ultrasound-guided drainage of pancreatic fluid collections. World Journal of Gastrointestinal Endoscopy 2012;4:479–488.

46 Park DH, Lee SS, Moon SH, et al. Endoscopic ultrasound-guided versus conventional transmural drainage for pancreatic pseudocysts: a prospective randomized trial. Endoscopy 2009;41:842–848.

47 Varadarajulu S, Christein JD, Tamhane A, Drelichman ER, Wilcox CM. Prospective randomized trial comparing EUS and EGD for transmural drainage of pancreatic pseudocysts (with videos). Gastrointestinal Endoscopy 2008;68:1102–1111.

48 Rana SS, Bhasin DK, Rao C, Gupta R, Singh K. Non-fluoroscopic endoscopic ultrasound-guided transmural drainage of symptomatic non-bulging walled-off pancreatic necrosis. Digestive Endoscopy 2013;25:47–52.

49 Yamamoto N, Isayama H, Kawakami H, et al. Preliminary report on a new, fully covered, metal stent designed for the treatment of pancreatic fluid collections. Gastrointestinal Endoscopy 2013;77:809–814.

50 Moon JH, Choi HJ, Kim DC, et al. A newly designed fully covered metal stent for lumen apposition in EUS-guided drainage and access: a feasibility study (with videos). Gastrointestinal Endoscopy 2014;79:990–995.

51 Sarkaria S, Sethi A, Rondon C, et al. Pancreatic necrosectomy using covered esophageal stents: a novel approach. Journal of Clinical Gastroenterology 2014;48:145–152.

52 Bang JY, Wilcox CM, Trevino J, et al. Factors impacting treatment outcomes in the endoscopic management of walled-off pancreatic necrosis. Journal of Gastroenterology and Hepatology 2013;28:1725–1732.

53 Ross AS, Irani S, Gan SI, et al. Dual-modality drainage of infected and symptomatic walled-off pancreatic necrosis: long-term clinical outcomes. Gastrointestinal Endoscopy 2014;79:929–935.

54 Bang JY, Holt BA, Hawes RH, et al. Outcomes after implementing a tailored endoscopic step-up approach to walled-off necrosis in acute pancreatitis. British Journal of Surgery 2014;101:1729–1738.

55 Freeman ML, Werner J, van Santvoort HC, et al. Interventions for necrotizing pancreatitis: summary of a multidisciplinary consensus conference. Pancreas 2012;41:1176–1194.

56 Gardner TB. Endoscopic management of necrotizing pancreatitis. Gastrointestinal Endoscopy 2012;76:1214–1223.

57 van Brunschot S, Fockens P, Bakker OJ, et al. Endoscopic transluminal necrosectomy in necrotising pancreatitis: a systematic review. Surgical Endoscopy 2014;28:1425–1438.

58 Gluck M, Ross A, Irani S, et al. Endoscopic and percutaneous drainage of symptomatic walled-off pancreatic necrosis reduces hospital stay and radiographic resources. Clinical Gastroenterology and Hepatology 2010;8:1083–1088.

59 Bakker OJ, van Santvoort HC, van Brunschot S, et al. Endoscopic transgastric vs surgical necrosectomy for infected necrotizing pancreatitis: a randomized trial. Journal of the American Medical Association 2012;307:1053–1061.

60 van Brunschot S, van Grinsven J, Voermans RP, et al. Transluminal endoscopic step-up approach versus minimally invasive surgical step-up approach in patients with infected necrotising pancreatitis (TENSION trial): design and rationale of a randomised controlled multicenter trial [ISRCTN09186711]. BMC Gastroenterology 2013;13:161.

61 Horvath K, Freeny P, Escallon J, et al. Safety and efficacy of video-assisted retroperitoneal debridement for infected pancreatic collections: a multicenter, prospective, single-arm phase 2 study. Archives of Surgery 2010;145:817–825.

CHAPTER 8

Treatment of systemic complications and organ failure

Alexsander K. Bressan[1] & Chad G. Ball[2]

[1] Department of Surgery, Foothills Medical Centre and the University of Calgary, Calgary, AB, Canada
[2] Departments of Surgery and Oncology, Foothills Medical Centre and the University of Calgary, Calgary, AB, Canada

Introduction

Approximately 80% of all patients with acute pancreatitis present with self-limiting organ inflammation. These cases typically resolve within the first week by engaging in only medical treatment. The remainder is characterized by a more severe disease course that is associated with an exacerbated inflammatory response, local and systemic complications, and increased mortality.

Mortality is classically described by a bimodal distribution curve. Up to half of all deaths occur within the first week, secondary to an overactive systemic inflammatory response and subsequent multiple organ dysfunction. Mortality after the second week results from local complications, infection, and/or sepsis. In both scenarios, organ failure is a major determinant of disease severity and a common final event directly associated with the majority of deaths.

Initial retrospective studies outlining organ system dysfunction in acute pancreatitis date to the 1970s [1–3]. Respiratory dysfunction remains the most common extrapancreatic organ failure, reported in up to 25% of cases. More specifically, early deaths most often result from progressive respiratory deterioration followed by cumulative involvement of renal and cardiovascular systems. Despite the lack of uniform diagnostic criteria among early studies, organ system dysfunction has been long recognized as a major prognostic factor in acute pancreatitis.

The prognostic value of organ dysfunction was contemplated in the 1992 Atlanta severity classification system for acute pancreatitis [4]. Severe disease was defined by the occurrence of either organ failure or local complications. Definitions for specific local complications and organ failure were also proposed. It became the most widely employed classification system for acute pancreatitis.

In the mid-2000s, the importance surrounding the time of onset and duration of organ failure was further explored [5–7]. Mortality in severe acute pancreatitis was reported as 11–14%. Furthermore, early organ failure was found in 44–60% of patients with severe acute pancreatitis. Organ dysfunction persisting more than 48 hours was associated with higher mortality (34.9–67%) compared with transient organ failure (0–8.3%). In comparison, mortality in severe acute pancreatitis *without* early organ failure was only 2.6–3.2%. These deaths occurred secondary to local complications and systemic infection. As a whole, it became clear then that persistent organ failure is a major determinant of disease severity.

Revision of the Atlanta classification system was concluded in 2012. The goal of this project was to refine the severity classification, as well as to review and clarify definitions of local and systemic complications [8]. A new intermediate severity group (moderately severe acute pancreatitis) was described by the presence of either transient organ failure (<48 hours) or local

Pancreatitis: Medical and Surgical Management, First Edition.
David B. Adams, Peter B. Cotton, Nicholas J. Zyromski and John Windsor.
© 2017 John Wiley & Sons, Ltd. Published 2017 by John Wiley & Sons, Ltd.

Table 8.1 Revised Atlanta classification (2012).

Mild acute pancreatitis
- No organ failure
- No local systemic complications

Moderately severe acute pancreatitis
- Organ failure that resolves within 48 hours (transient organ failure)
- Local or systemic complications without organ failure

Severe acute pancreatitis
- Persistent organ failure (<48 hours)
  - Single organ failure
  - Multiple organ failure

Modified Marshall scoring system for acute pancreatitis
Respiratory   Pa O$_2$/Fi O$_2$
Renal   Serum Cr
Cardiovascular   Systolic BP

complications. Consequently, the definition of "severe disease" was limited to patients with organ failure persisting beyond 48 hours. The multiple organ dysfunction score, also known as Marshall score [9], was also used to simplify and standardize the clinical assessment of organ dysfunction (Table 8.1).

The Marshall scoring system was originally developed to quantify multiple organ dysfunction syndrome within critical illnesses. Scoring of respiratory, renal, hepatic, cardiovascular, hematologic, and neurologic dysfunction is based on objective and reproducible physiologic measures. Score stratification correlates with mortality on admission to the ICU and during follow-up [10]. A modified version of the Marshall score limited to the respiratory, renal, and cardiovascular systems was proposed by the 2012 revised Atlanta classification. It can be engaged on admission and repeated daily and is also applicable for patients managed outside the critical care unit. Stratification of organ dysfunction severity based on this score is also possible but was not included in the Atlanta classification system.

Similar to the Marshall score, the sequential organ failure assessment (SOFA) score [11] is another system used to quantify organ dysfunction. The same six organ systems were originally included, but the descriptor for the cardiovascular system reflects requirement for vasopressor support, instead of physiologic parameters. The SOFA score was recommended for the assessment of respiratory, renal, and cardiovascular dysfunction by the determinant-based classification of acute pancreatitis [12]. The determinant-based system is a severity classification system proposed almost simultaneously to the 2012 revised Atlanta version, with an additional higher risk category characterized by both organ failure and infected necrosis (critical acute pancreatitis).

Physiological scoring systems have also been proposed to predict persistent organ failure in acute pancreatitis. Since the initial publication by Ranson in 1974, multiple scoring systems based on combinations of clinical, biochemical, and radiologic parameters have been proposed to predict varied clinical outcomes (local complications, systemic complications, ICU length of stay, mortality). Unfortunately, accuracy to predict persistent organ failure at admission is merely modest [13]. Furthermore, a recent systematic review found that the use of scoring systems within 48 hours of admission to predict persistent organ failure is not justifiable based on current evidence [14].

Respiratory dysfunction

Pulmonary complications occur in up to 55% of patients with acute pancreatitis [15] and typically fall within the spectrum of acute respiratory distress syndrome. Respiratory failure is reported in 10–25% of all cases [16], but variable diagnostic criteria based on respiratory rate, hypoxemia levels, and/or treatment-related parameters have been classically employed. Marshall and SOFA scores are currently recommended to define respiratory dysfunction in acute pancreatitis and are based on oxygen exchange assessment as determined by PaO$_2$/FiO$_2$ ratio.

Respiratory distress also represents the earliest extrapancreatic organ dysfunction with an incidence that is directly related to the magnitude of the systemic inflammatory response. Mortality usually results from cumulative involvement of other organ systems due to a persistently overactive inflammatory cascade or a secondary insult (most often infection). Respiratory failure accounts for approximately 60% of all deaths from acute pancreatitis [17].

Acute lung injury within acute pancreatitis is characterized by diffuse lung inflammation. The initial exudative phase results from increased permeability of epithelial and endothelial pulmonary membranes leading to interstitial and alveolar infiltration with exudate and inflammatory cells. Systemic release of pancreatic proteases also appears to contribute to the inflammatory lung injury [18]. Edema and diffuse damage to respiratory membranes cause impaired oxygen exchange and hypoxemic respiratory failure, typically in the absence of increased cardiac filling pressure.

During the subsequent fibroproliferative phase, resolution of the systemic inflammatory response allows lung repair through proliferation of fibroblasts and type II pneumocytes. At this stage, however, a second insult, such as ventilator-induced lung injury, pneumonia, bacterial translocation, or catheter-associated infection, can rapidly accentuate respiratory dysfunction and lead to multiple organ failure.

Chest radiographs reveal nonspecific alveolar infiltrate in 10–26% of patients [15]. Pleural effusion has been reported in up to 17% of cases [19], most commonly left sided, and occasionally amylase-rich effusions. Large left-sided pleural effusion may also be associated with subdiaphragmatic collections.

The optimal treatment of respiratory failure relies on ventilatory support using low tidal volumes, limitation of plateau pressures, and appropriate PEEP to minimize ventilator-induced pulmonary injury [20]. Despite the inflammatory nature of lung damage, no benefit from specific systemic agents has been demonstrated in severe acute pancreatitis. Clinical trials utilizing anticytokine therapy have also failed to decrease associated mortality.

Cardiovascular dysfunction

A hyperdynamic circulatory state is present during the initial inflammatory phase of acute pancreatitis. Despite the myocardial depression associated with the systemic inflammatory state, an increase in the cardiac index dominates, secondary to a low peripheral vascular resistance and concurrent tachycardia [21, 22]. Focal and transient stress-induced contractility abnormalities in the absence of structural damage have also been reported [23].

Metabolic and electrolyte abnormalities are also common in the early phase of severe pancreatitis. Hyperglycemia, hypocalcemia, and acidosis within 48 hours of admission are classic prognostic factors contemplated in Ranson's criteria. Such metabolic imbalances can further compromise cardiac rhythm and function.

Low calcium levels occur in 30–60% of patients with acute pancreatitis [24]. However, only ionized calcium level, low in less than one-third of patients [25], affects myocardial function. Decreased contractility and electrocardiographic changes (prolongation of the QT interval and changes in the ST segment) can result from low levels of ionized calcium. Hypomagnesemia is often associated with hypocalcemia in acute pancreatitis [26] and can precipitate myriad electrocardiographic disturbances.

Alcohol abuse, one of the most important etiological factors for acute pancreatitis, is also associated with phosphate deficiency, which can adversely affect myocardial contractility and the oxygen dissociation curve. Dilated cardiomyopathy and vitamin deficiencies (thiamine, pyridoxine, folic acid, cyanocobalamin, and others) must also be considered as possible causes of cardiovascular dysfunction in alcohol-dependent patients.

Fluid resuscitation and correction of electrolyte and metabolic abnormalities are the basis for cardiovascular supportive treatments in patients with severe acute pancreatitis.

Acute kidney injury

The reported prevalence of acute kidney injury in acute pancreatitis ranges from 14% to 42% [27–30]. Such wide variability is partly explained by the use of heterogeneous diagnostic criteria, most often based on serum creatinine values. A major advance over the past decade included the development of consensus definitions for acute kidney injury overall [31], as well as specifically in the context of acute pancreatitis [9, 11].

Depletion of intravascular volume is the leading cause of kidney injury and begins before hospital admission. Experimental models in the 1960s demonstrated that up to a 40% loss of circulating plasma volume occurs due to extensive abdominal fluid sequestration [24]. Resultant hypovolemia, in conjunction with impaired control of glomerular perfusion due to inflammatory microcirculation abnormalities, leads to ischemic renal damage. Acute kidney injury also results from increased levels of phospholipase A2 in the blood filtrate causing tubular deposits and direct injury to the nephrons [32].

Renal hypoperfusion may also result from intra-abdominal hypertension, an early complication secondary to extensive intra- and retroperitoneal fluid sequestration, paralytic ileus, and possibly excessive fluid resuscitation. Abdominal compartment syndrome is reported in up to 27% of patients [33] and has recently been considered to be associated with early aggressive fluid resuscitation. This syndrome is intimately linked with both respiratory and renal failure [34]. Goal-directed hydration based on periodic monitoring of physiologic parameters has therefore gained more popularity in the past decade [35].

Treatment of established renal failure in acute pancreatitis is based upon supportive measures, ultimately involving renal replacement therapy. The use of continuous hemodiafiltration or veno-venous hemofiltration to balance fluid replacement and remove proinflammatory cytokines has also been considered outside the renal failure scenario. This therapy is still investigational and lacks appropriate quality evidence to be applied in routine clinical practice.

Coagulation abnormalities

Consumption coagulopathy in acute pancreatitis has been repeatedly demonstrated in both animal models and small cohorts of patients since the early 1980s [36–38]. Decreased platelet counts, low values of coagulation factors, and exhaustion of the fibrinolytic system are directly related to the magnitude of the acute pancreatitis [39]. Variable clinical manifestations may result from vascular thrombosis to disseminated intravascular coagulation.

Although coagulation abnormalities are not included in contemporary severity classification systems, the coagulation system is actively involved in the pathogenesis of severe acute pancreatitis. Endothelial production of platelet-activating factor (PAF) in response to inflammatory mediators is known to amplify cytokine production and activate inflammatory cells and platelets, leveraging the inflammatory response to a systemic level.

The resulting combination of a hypercoagulable state and systemic inflammation may accelerate progression to multiple organ dysfunction and death. Unfortunately,

the use of PAF antagonist (lexipafant) in acute pancreatitis did not prevent adverse outcomes in clinical trials [40]. In the absence of specific therapies targeting the coagulation system and inflammatory response, appropriate treatment of coagulation abnormalities in acute pancreatitis relies on early supportive measures. Close monitoring for both thrombotic events and coagulopathy is crucial to prevent additional complications in patients with severe disease.

Gut barrier dysfunction

Gut barrier dysfunction is characterized by increased permeability of the intestinal barrier allowing translocation of intraluminal bacteria and their toxic products and inflammatory compounds produced within the intestinal wall into the portal blood and mesenteric lymph. Disruption of structural and functional components of this barrier in critical illnesses results mainly from inflammation and ischemia/reperfusion injury and is intensified by prolonged fasting and mucosal atrophy.

Translocation of intestinal bacteria is implicated in the pathogenesis of secondary infection of pancreatic necrosis, sepsis, and progression to multiple organ failure. A recent meta-analysis including 44 prospective series using a variety of noninvasive tests identified gut barrier dysfunction in 59% of patients with acute pancreatitis [41]. Unfortunately, precise association of gut barrier dysfunction, disease severity, and mortality is still unclear.

The role of enteral nutrition to prevent gut barrier dysfunction in acute pancreatitis is also unclear, but a reduction in mortality compared with parenteral nutrition is extensively supported in the literature [42]. Possible mechanisms include prevention of intestinal mucosa atrophy and stimulation of gut motility to avoid intestinal bacterial overgrowth. Early enteral nutrition, started within 48 hours of admission, is also associated with reduced risk of multiple organ failure and infectious complications compared with delayed onset of enteral nutrition after the first week [43].

The preferential route for enteral nutrition, nasogastric, or nasojejunal is still debated [44]. Despite the convenience of nasogastric feeding, arguments against this route include a potentially increased risk of pulmonary aspiration and worsening of local inflammation by stimulating pancreatic secretions. A recent meta-analysis including 157 patients from three randomized clinical trials comparing nasogastric and nasojejunal feeding found no significant differences in mortality, tracheal aspiration, or exacerbation of pain between the two groups [45].

Conclusion

Acute pancreatitis represents a unique model of systemic inflammatory response, sepsis, and multiple organ dysfunction syndrome where the patient often presents early in the disease course. Progression from localized inflammation to multiple organ dysfunction remains difficult to predict. Early and precise resuscitation measures require continuous monitoring of respiratory, cardiovascular, and renal systems. Timely and appropriate fluid resuscitation and correction of electrolyte abnormalities represent the basic initial measures to prevent organ failure.

Persistent organ dysfunction after 48 hours is associated with a significant increase in mortality. No specific systemic therapy is proven to be beneficial, and current treatment of organ failure in severe acute pancreatitis consists of supportive measures often involving ventilatory and cardiovascular support and renal replacement therapy. Additional recommendations to prevent second-insult organ dysfunction include early enteral nutrition, judicious use of antibiotics, and close monitoring for thromboembolic events.

References

1 Imrie CW, Ferguson JC, Murphy D, Blumgart LH. Arterial hypoxia in acute pancreatitis. British Journal of Surgery. 1977;64(3):185–188.

2 Gordon D, Calne RY. Renal failure in acute pancreatitis. British Medical Journal. 1972;3(5830):801–802.

3 Lefer AM, Glenn TM, O'Neill TJ, Lovett WL, Geissinger WT, Wangensteen SL. Inotropic influence of endogenous peptides in experimental hemorrhagic pancreatitis. Surgery. 1971;69(2):220–228.

4 Bradley EL, 3rd., A clinically based classification system for acute pancreatitis. Summary of the International Symposium on Acute Pancreatitis, Atlanta, GA, September 11 through 13, 1992. Archives of Surgery. 1993;128(5):586–590.

5 Lytras D, Manes K, Triantopoulou C, Paraskeva C, Delis S, Avgerinos C, et al. Persistent early organ failure: defining the high-risk group of patients with severe acute pancreatitis? Pancreas. 2008;36(3):249–254.

6 Johnson CD, Abu-Hilal M. Persistent organ failure during the first week as a marker of fatal outcome in acute pancreatitis. Gut. 2004;53(9):1340–1344.

7 Mofidi R, Duff MD, Wigmore SJ, Madhavan KK, Garden OJ, Parks RW. Association between early systemic inflammatory response, severity of multiorgan dysfunction and death in acute pancreatitis. British Journal of Surgery. 2006;93(6):738–744.

8 Banks PA, Bollen TL, Dervenis C, Gooszen HG, Johnson CD, Sarr MG, et al. Classification of acute pancreatitis–2012: revision of the Atlanta classification and definitions by international consensus. Gut. 2013;62(1):102–111.

9 Marshall JC, Cook DJ, Christou NV, Bernard GR, Sprung CL, Sibbald WJ. Multiple organ dysfunction score: a reliable descriptor of a complex clinical outcome. Critical Care Medicine. 1995;23(10):1638–1652.

10 Halonen KI, Pettila V, Leppaniemi AK, Kemppainen EA, Puolakkainen PA, Haapiainen RK. Multiple organ dysfunction associated with severe acute pancreatitis. Critical Care Medicine. 2002;30(6):1274–1279.

11 Vincent JL, Moreno R, Takala J, Willatts S, De Mendonca A, Bruining H, et al. The SOFA (Sepsis-related Organ Failure Assessment) score to describe organ dysfunction/failure. On behalf of the Working Group on Sepsis-Related Problems of the European Society of Intensive Care Medicine. Intensive Care Medicine. 1996;22(7):707–710.

12 Dellinger EP, Forsmark CE, Layer P, Levy P, Maravi-Poma E, Petrov MS, et al. Determinant-based classification of acute pancreatitis severity: an international multidisciplinary consultation. Annals of Surgery. 2012; 256(6):875–880.

13 Mounzer R, Langmead CJ, Wu BU, Evans AC, Bishehsari F, Muddana V, et al. Comparison of existing clinical scoring systems to predict persistent organ failure in patients with acute pancreatitis. Gastroenterology. 2012; 142(7):1476–1482; quiz e15–e16.

14 Yang CJ, Chen J, Phillips AR, Windsor JA, Petrov MS. Predictors of severe and critical acute pancreatitis: a systematic review. Digestive and Liver Disease. 2014;46(5):446–451.

15 Pastor CM, Matthay MA, Frossard JL. Pancreatitis-associated acute lung injury: new insights. Chest. 2003; 124(6):2341–2351.

16 Elder AS, Saccone GT, Dixon DL. Lung injury in acute pancreatitis: mechanisms underlying augmented secondary injury. Pancreatology. 2012;12(1):49–56.

17 Shields CJ, Winter DC, Redmond HP. Lung injury in acute pancreatitis: mechanisms, prevention, and therapy. Current Opinion in Critical Care. 2002;8(2):158–163.

18 Friess H, Shrikhande S, Riesle E, Kashiwagi M, Baczako K, Zimmermann A, et al. Phospholipase A2 isoforms in acute pancreatitis. Annals of Surgery. 2001;233(2):204–212.

19 Basran GS, Ramasubramanian R, Verma R. Intrathoracic complications of acute pancreatitis. British Journal of Diseases of the Chest. 1987;81(4):326–331.

20 Koh Y. Update in acute respiratory distress syndrome. Journal of Intensive Care. 2014;2(1):2.

21 Beger HG, Bittner R, Buchler M, Hess W, Schmitz JE. Hemodynamic data pattern in patients with acute pancreatitis. Gastroenterology. 1986;90(1):74–79.

22 Wilson PG, Manji M, Neoptolemos JP. Acute pancreatitis as a model of sepsis. Journal of Antimicrobial Chemotherapy 1998;41(Suppl A):51–63.

23 Patel J, Movahed A, Reeves WC. Electrocardiographic and segmental wall motion abnormalities in pancreatitis mimicking myocardial infarction. Clinical Cardiology. 1994;17(9):505–509.

24 Anderson MC, Schoenfeld FB, Iams WB, Suwa M. Circulatory changes in acute pancreatitis. The Surgical Clinics of North America. 1967;47(1):127–140.

25 Weir GC, Lesser PB, Drop LJ, Fischer JE, Warshaw AL. The hypocalcemia of acute pancreatitis. Annals of Internal Medicine. 1975;83(2):185–189.

26 Ryzen E, Rude RK. Low intracellular magnesium in patients with acute pancreatitis and hypocalcemia. Western Journal of Medicine. 1990;152(2):145–148.

27 Ljutic D, Piplovic-Vukovic T, Raos V, Andrews P. Acute renal failure as a complication of acute pancreatitis. Renal Failure. 1996;18(4):629–633.

28 Kes P, Vucicevic Z, Ratkovic-Gusic I, Fotivec A. Acute renal failure complicating severe acute pancreatitis. Renal Failure. 1996;18(4):621–628.

29 Company L, Saez J, Martinez J, Aparicio JR, Laveda R, Grino P, et al. Factors predicting mortality in severe acute pancreatitis. Pancreatology. 2003;3(2):144–148.

30 Herrera Gutierrez ME, Seller Perez G, de La Rubia De Gracia C, Chaparro Sanchez MJ, Nacle Lopez B. Acute renal failure profile and prognostic value in severe acute pancreatitis. Medicina Clinica (Barcelona). 2000;115(19):721–725.

31 Bellomo R, Ronco C, Kellum JA, Mehta RL, Palevsky P. Acute renal failure – definition, outcome measures, animal models, fluid therapy and information technology needs: the Second International Consensus Conference of the Acute Dialysis Quality Initiative (ADQI) Group. Critical Care. 2004;8(4):R204-R212.

32 Gronroos JM, Hietaranta AJ, Nevalainen TJ. Renal tubular cell injury and serum phospholipase A2 activity in acute pancreatitis. British Journal of Surgery. 1992; 79(8):800–801.

33 Trikudanathan G, Vege SS. Current concepts of the role of abdominal compartment syndrome in acute pancreatitis – an opportunity or merely an epiphenomenon. Pancreatology. 2014;14(4):238–243.

34 Aggarwal A, Manrai M, Kochhar R. Fluid resuscitation in acute pancreatitis. World Journal of Gastroenterology. 2014;20(48):18092–18103.

35 Bortolotti P, Saulnier F, Colling D, Redheuil A, Preau S. New tools for optimizing fluid resuscitation in acute pancreatitis. World Journal of Gastroenterology. 2014;20(43):16113–16122.

36 Feldman BF, Attix EA, Strombeck DR, O'Neill S. Biochemical and coagulation changes in a canine model of acute necrotizing pancreatitis. American Journal of Veterinary Research. 1981;42(5):805–809.

37 Lasson A, Ohlsson K. Consumptive coagulopathy, fibrinolysis and protease–antiprotease interactions during acute human pancreatitis. Thrombosis Research. 1986; 41(2):167–183

38 Aasen AO, Kierulf P, Ruud TE, Godal HC, Aune S. Studies on pathological plasma proteolysis in patients with acute pancreatitis. A preliminary report. Acta Chirurgica Scandinavica. Supplementum. 1982;509:83–87.

39 Radenkovic D, Bajec D, Karamarkovic A, Stefanovic B, Milic N, Ignjatovic S, et al. Disorders of hemostasis during the surgical management of severe necrotizing pancreatitis. Pancreas. 2004;29(2):152–156.

40 Johnson CD, Kingsnorth AN, Imrie CW, McMahon MJ, Neoptolemos JP, McKay C, et al. Double blind, randomised, placebo controlled study of a platelet activating factor antagonist, lexipafant, in the treatment and prevention of organ failure in predicted severe acute pancreatitis. Gut. 2001;48(1):62–69.

41 Wu LM, Sankaran SJ, Plank LD, Windsor JA, Petrov MS. Meta-analysis of gut barrier dysfunction in patients with acute pancreatitis. British Journal of Surgery. 2014; 101(13):1644–1656.

42 Yi F, Ge L, Zhao J, Lei Y, Zhou F, Chen Z, et al. Meta-analysis: total parenteral nutrition versus total enteral nutrition in predicted severe acute pancreatitis. Internal Medicine. 2012;51(6):523–530.

43 Sun JK, Mu XW, Li WQ, Tong ZH, Li J, Zheng SY. Effects of early enteral nutrition on immune function of severe acute pancreatitis patients. World Journal of Gastroenterology. 2013;19(6):917–922.

44 Olah A, Romics L, Jr., Enteral nutrition in acute pancreatitis: a review of the current evidence. World Journal of Gastroenterology. 2014;20(43):16123–16131.

45 Chang YS, Fu HQ, Xiao YM, Liu JC. Nasogastric or nasojejunal feeding in predicted severe acute pancreatitis: a meta-analysis. Critical Care. 2013;17(3):R118.

CHAPTER 9

Specific treatment for acute pancreatitis

Li Wen[1,2], Muhammad A. Javed[1,2], Kiran Altaf[1,2], Peter Szatmary[1,2] & Robert Sutton[1,2]

[1] NIHR Liverpool Pancreas Biomedical Research Unit, Institute of Translational Medicine, Royal Liverpool University Hospital, Liverpool, UK
[2] Institute of Translational Medicine, University of Liverpool, Liverpool, UK

Introduction

Acute pancreatitis (AP) is a leading cause of emergency hospitalization for gastrointestinal (GI) disease that results in substantial morbidity, mortality, and financial burden on health-care services [1]. The mortality of AP rises to ~30% in the patients with persistent organ failure with or without infected necrosis [2]. The incidence and the rates of hospitalization continue to increase, and yet AP is without specific, licensed drug therapy. Pancreatic necrosis and organ failure are two key determinants of the severity and outcome of AP [3], both of which often take several days to develop and might be targeted by specific drug treatment. In this chapter, we discuss the current understanding of the pathogenesis of AP and discuss preclinical and clinical studies undertaken in the light of this. We also highlight potential novel therapeutic targets and make proposal for future clinical trial design that may contribute to the successful development of effective therapies.

Pathogenesis of acute pancreatitis

The initial injury occurs within pancreatic acinar cells (PACs; [4]), which make up the bulk of the organ, and pancreatic ductal cells (PDCs; [2]). Sustained elevation of cytosolic Ca^{2+} concentration ($[Ca^{2+}]_i$) is the earliest intracellular event in response to pancreatitis-associated toxins (bile acids, alcohol metabolites, hyperstimulation; [4]). After Ca^{2+} release from endoplasmic reticulum (ER) via second messenger Ca^{2+} release channels, there is activation in Ca^{2+} influx through store-operated Ca^{2+} entry (SOCE) channels on the plasma membrane,

maintenance of which is a critical rate-limiting step of initial PAC injury [4]. While Ca^{2+} release from the ER and uptake by mitochondrial is essential for normal ATP production such that in PACs stimulus–secretion coupling is matched by stimulus–metabolism coupling, the excessive Ca^{2+} release induced by toxins and sustained by continued Ca^{2+} entry overwhelms mitochondria [5]. As a result normal mitochondrial synthesis and supply of ATP is impaired and mitochondria may respond by shutting down the cell through apoptosis, an energy-dependent process, or necrosis [5]. The severity of AP correlates directly with the extent of necrosis and inversely with apoptosis in experimental AP (EAP; [6]). Mitochondrial dysfunction is a key determinant of disease severity during EAP [7]. Most recently, programmed necrotic cell death (necroptosis) has been implicated in the pathogenesis of AP [8].

Other early intracellular events, notably trypsinogen activation and nuclear factor-kappaB (NF-κB) activation, also contribute to AP pathogenesis and severity [9–11]. Intracellular digestive enzyme activation has long been considered the hallmark of AP [9, 10], and while this is an important component, the early events within PACs described earlier have been identified as critical upstream determinants [4]. NF-κB activation within injured PACs causes the release of cytokines to drive innate and adaptive immunity [11]. Tumor necrosis factor-alpha (TNF-α) is foremost among the cytokines in promoting recruitment of inflammatory cells into the pancreas that exacerbate the initial injury and cause this to spread systemically [12]. Damage-associated molecular patterns (DAMPs), including extracellular ATP, high-mobility group box 1 (HMGB1), and S100A, are released from dying or dead cells and bind to

Pancreatitis: Medical and Surgical Management, First Edition.
David B. Adams, Peter B. Cotton, Nicholas J. Zyromski and John Windsor.
© 2017 John Wiley & Sons, Ltd. Published 2017 by John Wiley & Sons, Ltd.

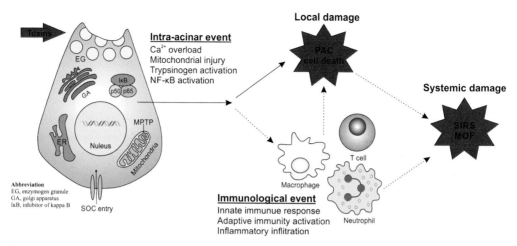

Figure 9.1 Pathogenesis of acute pancreatitis. In response to pancreatitis-associated toxins the release of Ca^{2+} from endoplasmic reticulum (ER) causes a delayed activation of sustained Ca^{2+} influx through store-operated Ca^{2+} entry (SOCE) channels and cytosolic Ca^{2+} overload. Mitochondrial injury characterized as $\Delta\Psi_m$ depletion and impaired ATP production is the key determinant of AP severity, mediated through mediating cell death pathway activation. Intracellular trypsinogen and nuclear factor-κB (NF-κB) are activated independently and in parallel at an early stage during AP. Injured pancreatic acinar cells (PACs) activate innate and adaptive immunity. The release of inflammatory mediators prompts inflammatory infiltration that causes further local damage, release of multiple cytokines and danger-associated molecular patterns (DAMPs) from PACs and infiltrating inflammatory cells, leading to systemic inflammatory response syndrome (SIRS) and multiple organ failure (MOF).

specific sensors on/in inflammatory cells, subsequently leading to sterile inflammation that contributes to local and systemic injury in AP [13, 14]. These intra-acinar and immunological events are two key synergistic components that contribute to AP initiation, severity, progression, and resolution (Figure 9.1).

Lessons from animal experiments

There are many preclinical studies reported that have tested a large range of agents in rodent EAP, the majority of which reported protective effects in at least one model of EAP [15]. Disappointingly, none of these agents have been successfully developed as clinical therapies (see Table 9.1; [16–25]), for which there are several possible explanations. First, it must be noted that many of the agents have not been tested clinically, either because the evidence has not been considered sufficiently compelling, there has been a lack of interest from expert teams, there has been no suitable agent developed, there has been insufficient resource, or there have been other obstacles to undertaking clinical trials in AP. Specifically, there have been no trials of agents that block Ca^{2+} entry, inhibit Ca^{2+} release, prevent

mitochondria-mediated cell death, or inhibit cytokine release or actions. Second, many of these agents have been administered prophylactically (i.e., before the induction of EAP) rather than therapeutically. This does not represent the majority of clinical scenarios that patients present at hospitals with AP, when therapy can only be given hours or even days after the onset of the symptoms. Nevertheless, prophylactic agents may be useful in the prevention of AP from endoscopic retrograde cholangiopancreatography. Third, the majority of the preclinical studies have tested agents in only one model, limiting the generalizability of potential treatments. With the addition of likely publication bias, such incomplete preclinical assessment may provide misleading data for potential clinical development. Fourth, EAP does not represent all aspects of clinical AP, and caution is required in the extrapolation of findings in animals to humans [15]. The most widely used model is hyperstimulation with caerulein, which is reproducible and noninvasive, but hyperstimulation is a rare cause as in organophosphate insecticide poisoning and *Tityus* spp. scorpion bites [26]. Amino acid-induced pancreatitis such as induced by L-arginine is another relatively easy and noninvasive model but of limited clinical relevance. Only a small number of inborn errors

Table 9.1 Selected agents tested in EAP but have not translated to clinical trials.

Agents	Species	EAP model	Preclinical outcome	References
Secretion inhibitors				
Somatostatin	Rat	Pancreatic duct ligation	Reduce disease severity	Berthet *et al.* [16]
Octreotide	Rat	Cerulein IV infusion glycodeoxycholic acid pancreatic duct + cerulein IV infusion	Reduced disease severity in less severe form	Küçüktülü *et al.* [17]
Protease inhibitors				
Camostat mesilate	Mouse	Taurocholate pancreatic duct injection CDE-diet	Reduced disease severity given prophylactically and at the beginning of disease induction	Lankisch *et al.* [18]
Ulinastatin	Mouse	Pancreatic duct obstruction + cerulein + systemic hypotension	Reduced disease severity given both prophylactically and therapeutically	Hirano *et al.* [19]
Antioxidant				
NAC	Mouse	Cerulein IP	Reduced disease severity given prophylactically, but not therapeutically	Demols *et al.* [20]
Selenium	Rat	l-Arginine IP	Reduced disease severity	Hardman *et al.* [21]
Inflammatory modulators				
PAF antagonist	Mouse	Cerulein IP	Reduced disease severity given therapeutically in mild form	Lane *et al.* [22]
Pentoxifylline	Rat	Taurocholate pancreatic duct injection	Reduced disease severity	de Campos *et al.* [23]
Others				
Heparin	Rat	Cerulein IV infusion Glycodeoxycholic acid pancreatic duct + cerulein IV infusion Pancreatic duct obstruction	Reduced disease severity given prophylactically	Hackert *et al.* [24]
APC	Rat	Taurocholate pancreatic duct injection	Reduced disease severity given 6 h after induction	Yamanel *et al.* [25]

EAP, experimental acute pancreatitis; IV, intravenously; CDE, choline-deficient ethionine-supplemented; NAC, *N*-acetylcysteine; IP, intraperitoneally; APC, activated protein C.

of amino acid metabolism, which are rare, cause AP. The models that mimic biliary and alcohol-associated AP, such as those induced by duct ligation/infusion [27] or intraperitoneal ethanol and fatty acid [28] may be more valuable for preclinical evaluation of agents that might subsequently be tested in patients with AP.

Potential novel therapeutic targets

There are several criteria that can help define a potentially effective therapeutic target: (i) the target is upstream in the pathogenesis of the disease, close to the first initiating event; (ii) the target has a key role in a rate-limiting step in the disease process; (iii) modulation of the target does not have a major impact on physiological processes or exacerbate other diseases; (iv) the target is not uniformly expressed throughout the body; (v) potential side effects can be favorably predicted according to phenotype data; (vi) a target and/or disease-specific biomarker exists to monitor therapeutic efficacy [29, 30]. Not all of these features are needed to ensure success but at least one key feature is desirable. All the aforementioned criteria apply to the development of any potential drug for AP, principal features of which are pancreatic injury and the immunological response that follows.

Store-operated Ca²⁺ entry (SOCE) channels

SOCE channels on the plasma membrane, notably Ca^{2+} release-activated Ca^{2+} (CRAC) channels, meet several of the criteria listed earlier for a potential therapeutic target. The criteria met are that SOCE channels are upstream in the initiation of the disease, are rate-limiting in Ca^{2+}-dependent PAC injury, and have enriched expression in non-excitable cells, including PACs and immune cells [31]. The CRAC channel and transient receptor potential canonical (TRPC) channels are two main SOCE channels present on PACs. These channels work interdependently [32] and are gated by stromal interacting molecule 1 (STIM1; [33]), although this gating applies particularly to Orai channels (discussed later). STIM1, an ER sensor protein, responds to Ca^{2+} ER store depletion by eliciting Ca^{2+} influx following translocation to the plasma membrane to form the puncta with Ca^{2+} entry channels [34]. Orai has three isoforms – Orai1, Orai2, and Orai3; Orai proteins shared no homology with any other known ion channel protein [35]. Orai1 was first identified as a key molecular component of CRAC channels in two distinct ways: (i) by genotyping and analyzing cells from patients with hereditary severe combined immune deficiency (SCID) syndrome and (ii) by genome-wide RNA interference (RNAi) screening followed by secondary patch-clamp screening [36, 37]. PACs contain

two pools of Orai1: an apical pool that colocalizes and interacts with IP_3Rs and a basal pool that interacts with STIM1 following Ca^{2+} store depletion [38]. GSK-7975A is a novel molecular entity developed by GSK, which blocks Orai1 and Orai3 channels with an IC_{50} of approximately 4.1 and 3.8 µM, respectively [39]. Inhibition of Orai by GSK-7975A was shown to prevent Ca^{2+} entry in a concentration-dependent manner, by more than 90%, and markedly reduce both murine and human PAC necrosis *in vitro* [31, 39]. Orai inhibition with GSK-7975A dramatically reduced EAP severity in three clinically representative models [31]. Although GSK-7975A is not being taken forward for clinical development, Calcimedica's compound CM_128 has the same actions and is being taken forward for clinical development [31] (Figure 9.2a). Furthermore, unlike GSK-7975A, CM_128 does not lose efficacy at high concentrations [31]. Both GSK-7975A and CM_128 were found to be significantly more effective in aborting AP if given within an hour in comparison with 6 hours after induction of AP [31]. Some of the effects of targeting Orai may be mediated by inhibition of inflammatory cell function; inhibition of Orai or STIM has been found

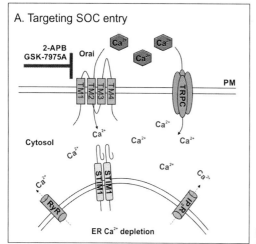
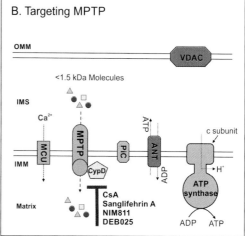

Figure 9.2 Novel drug targets for acute pancreatitis. (a) Following endoplasmic reticulum (ER) Ca^{2+} release through inositol $(1,4,5)$-triphosphate receptor (IP_3R) and ryanodine receptor (RyR) Ca^{2+} channels, the ER Ca^{2+} sensor protein-stromal interacting molecule 1 (STIM1) translocates to below the plasma membrane and forms puncta with SOCE channels. Sustained Ca^{2+} influx from the external environment is the rate-limiting step of cytosolic Ca^{2+} overload. Ca^{2+} release-activated Ca^{2+} (CRAC) channels, namely Orai and transient receptor potential canonical (TPRC) channels, are the principal SOCE channels in PACs. (b) In response to cytosolic Ca^{2+} overload, the mitochondrial Ca^{2+} uniporter takes up Ca^{2+} to buffer high cytosolic Ca^{2+} concentrations. Ca^{2+} overload of the mitochondrial matrix leads to mitochondrial permeability transition pore (MPTP) opening and cell death pathway activation. The exact molecular components of MPTP are not clearly defined. Cyclophilin (Cyp D) is a mitochondrial matrix protein with peptidyl-prolyl *cis–trans* isomerase activity encoded by the *Ppif* gene, a critical regulator of MPTP opening.

to reduce neutrophil activation and ROS production and migration [40]. The same effects on both PACs and immune cells might be achieved through the inhibition of second messenger Ca^{2+} release channels, notably inositol trisphosphate receptor channels, but there is considerable medicinal chemistry required as the best lead is caffeine that is limited by neurotoxicity [41].

A further possible approach to SOCE in PACs could be to inhibit TRPC channels, as PACs express TRPC1, TRPC3, and TRPC6 [42]. Genetic depletion ($Trpc3^{-/-}$) and pharmacological inhibition of TRPC3 using pyrazole 3 resulted in ~50% reduction of Ca^{2+} influx and ~50% reduction of pancreatic injury, notably hyperstimulation EAP, although the model used was mild with four injections of caerulein [43]. Nevertheless, the experimental data targeting TRPC channels do confirm proof of principle that targeting SOCE could lead to development of an effective therapy for AP.

Mitochondrial permeability transition pore (MPTP)

The MPTP is a multiprotein channel that forms at contact sites between the OMM and IMM, allowing through solutes of up to 1500 Da. Two open conformations of the MPTP have been proposed, the first being a low-conductance mode contributing to normal regulation of Ca^{2+} homeostasis [44]. The switch to the second high-conductance mode is considered an irreversible process dependent on mitochondrial Ca^{2+} ± reactive oxygen species (ROS) overload, resulting in loss of mitochondrial membrane potential and of ATP production, followed by necrotic cell death pathway activation [44]. A number of proteins have been proposed to make up the MPTP, including the adenine nucleotide translocator (ANT), voltage-dependent anion channel (VDAC), peptidyl-prolyl isomerase F (cyclophilin D (Cyp D) encoded by the *Ppif* gene), and phosphate carrier (PiC) [45]. Genetic deletion studies have not confirmed that any are structurally essential to the MPTP, although there are many data demonstrating that the mitochondrial matrix protein Cyp D is a key regulator [45]. Further studies indicate that the F_0F_1 ATP synthase forms the MPTP [46], regulated by Cyp D. Cyp D-deficient ($Ppif^{-/-}$) mice are viable, fertile, and have little abnormal phenotype, although older mice have obesity and learning defects [47]. PACs from $Ppif^{-/-}$ mice have significantly less necrosis when exposed to pancreatitis toxins and $Ppif^{-/-}$ mice develop markedly

less severe forms of AP in response to pancreatitis toxins [48, 49]. These findings are born out in other organs as $Ppif^{-/-}$ mice are protected against necrosis induced by Ca^{2+}-overload and oxidative stress, resulting in significantly reduced disease severity in ischemic/reperfusion (I/R) injury *in vivo* models [50]. Cyp D inhibitors, such a cyclosporine A (CsA), sanglifehrin A, and NIM811 protect against cardiac I/R injury *in vitro* and *in vivo* [45]. Moreover, a proof-of-concept clinical trial with 58 acute ST-elevation myocardial infarction patients showed that the administration of CsA resulted in smaller infarct size compared to a placebo group [51]. CsA also binds to Cyp A, then complexing with calcineurin to greatly inhibit immune responses, which could be deleterious in AP as infection is a major contributor to morbidity and mortality [2]. The immunosuppressive actions of CsA may be avoided, however, by using analogs that are not immunosuppressive, for example, Debio-025 [49], which has been in clinical trials for other indications [52]. Thus, Cyp D meets more than one criterion as a suitable drug target for AP and there are agents that could be applied clinically; furthermore, new agents are under development for acute tissue injury (e.g., Cypralis) that might be suitable for AP (Figure 9.2b).

Immune signaling pathways

Despite the concern that profound, generalized immunosuppression would be deleterious in AP, inhibition of specific pathways may have a role. TNF-α is released in AP by injured PACs to initiate immune responses in which TNF-α has a central role [12, 53], driving many deleterious inflammatory cascades [54–58]. The central role of TNF-α has been shown in animal AP models, with marked amelioration from anti-TNF treatment [53]. TNF-α rises in human AP for a week or more, proportional to disease severity [54–57], and anti-TNF treatment used for other indications reduces the incidence of AP to less than one-tenth of that without anti-TNF treatment [58]. Anti-TNF therapy has been documented to abrogate human AP [59]. Also, TNF-α expression-enhancing −1031C and −863A alleles significantly increase the risk of organ dysfunction in AP [60]. TNF-α, therefore, meets more than one criterion of a suitable drug target for AP. A pilot trial of pentoxifylline, which has anti-TRF effects, found the administration of this agent to be associated with reduced admission to and length of intensive care, although no disease parameter was modified [61], suggesting the requirement of more powerful anti-TNF therapy. Biologics have been in use for two decades, including those targeting TNF-α signaling, as well as other specific inflammatory pathways implicated in AP, including that mediated by interleukin-6 (IL-6; [62]). There is significant opportunity, therefore, for trials of biologics that target TNF-α and, potentially, IL-6.

Lessons from clinical trials

There have been >300 clinical trials published evaluating drug therapy in AP, including late-phase clinical trials (see Table 9.2; [63–68]), but results have been disappointing and no therapy has been licensed specifically for AP. Consideration of the possible causes of failure may inform and guide us toward improved study designs. First, the choice of agent may have been unsatisfactory. There has been a lack of trials of anti-inflammatory agents and there have been no trials of biologics, for example, anti-TNF or anti-IL-6

therapies. Second, almost all the clinical trials have restricted recruitment to patients with predicted severe AP, who comprise up to one-third of patients. This is predicated on the use of mortality or new organ failure as the primary outcome measure, as these end points do not occur in two-thirds of patients with AP and their inclusion would greatly increase the necessary sample size required to demonstrate efficacy. Nevertheless, milder forms of AP are responsible for significant health service costs, affecting the majority of AP patients with inpatient stays of up to a week or more. Were there to be an effective therapy that was shown to abort mild AP, a major impact would be made on this disease. It is of note in this regard that milder forms of EAP are easier to ameliorate than more severe forms [2, 15]. Third, trial treatment has been initiated after some delay, randomization typically being conducted within 72–120 hours after the onset of symptoms or admission to hospital. This is partly because the typical investigations required to predict severity are more accurate if conducted on the second rather than first day. Initiation of treatment

Table 9.2 Selected drugs from phase II/III clinical trials of AP.

Drugs	Patients (sample size)	Intervention duration	Primary endpoint	Outcome	References
Secretion inhibitors					
Octreotide	Moderate to severe AP within 96 h after the onset of symptoms (302)	Three times daily for 7 days	Mortality 15 complications	No benefit	Uhl et al. [63]
Protease inhibitors					
Gabexate mesilate	Severe AP (223)	Once daily for 7 days	Mortality 14 complications	No benefit	Büchler et al. [64]
Antioxidant (N-acetylcysteine, selenium, vitamin C)					
Combined antioxidant	Severe AP within 48 h of admission (43)	Once daily for 7 days	Presence of organ dysfunction at day 7	No benefit	Siriwardena et al. [65]
Inflammatory modulators					
PAF antagonist	Severe AP within 72 h after the onset of symptoms (290)	Once daily for 7 days	Reduction rate of complication	No benefit	Johnson et al. [66]
Others					
APC	AP with one or more organ failure less than 48 h (32)	Once daily for 5 days	The change in SOFA during day 0–day 5	No benefit	Pettilä et al. [67]
	Severe AP (44)	Continuous IV infusion for 24 h	The occurrence of a serious bleeding event	No significant benefit	Miranda et al. [68]

AP, acute pancreatitis; PAF, platelet-activating factor; APC, activated protein C; SOFA, sequential organ failure assessment; IV, intravenous.

by this time may be too late for a significant impact on the disease, in particular to prevent organ dysfunction and/or pancreatic necrosis. Fourth, heterogeneous patient populations with different AP etiologies may influence responses to treatment.

Future clinical trial design

In view of the issues highlighted, we propose that future clinical trials in AP should (i) test agents for which there is sound rationale as targeting central pathways in AP in line with the criteria listed earlier, whether new or repositioned drugs; (ii) administer trial treatments as early as possible in the course of AP, in line with acute treatments for other medical emergencies, and at the very latest within 24 hours; (iii) administer trial treatments to establish rapid bioavailability and avoid failure of GI absorption, usually by an intravenous route; (iv) develop biomarkers and/or scoring systems that facilitate recruitment of all patients with AP, representative of the whole natural history and outcome of AP, rather than restricting recruitment to predicted severe AP, which may slow down trial entry and depends on prediction methods that have inaccuracies. Such biomarkers would preferably be linked to the drug target and its modulation by any trial treatment.

As discussed, agents are either in development or are available now for repositioning. Taking this forward depends on collaborations between academia, the pharmaceutical and biotechnology sectors, regulators, patients, and the public. The means to pursue these collaborations include national and international initiatives such as the International Pancreatitis Study Group [69] and the Scientific Advisory Board of the International Association of Pancreatology.

References

1 Peery AF, Crockett SD, Barritt AS, Dellon ES, Eluri S, Gangarosa LM, Jensen ET, Lund JL, Pasricha S, Runge T, Schmidt M, Shaheen NJ, Sandler RS. Burden of gastrointestinal, liver, and pancreatic diseases in the United States. Gastroenterology 2015;149:1731–1741.

2 Pandol SJ, Saluja AK, Imrie CW, Banks PA. Acute pancreatitis: bench to the bedside. Gastroenterology. 2007; 132:1127–1151.

3 Dellinger EP, Forsmark CE, Layer P, Levy P, Maravi-Poma E, Petrov MS, et al. Determinant-based classification of acute pancreatitis severity: an international multidisciplinary consultation. Annals of Surgery 2012;256:875–880.

4 Petersen OH, Sutton R. Ca²⁺ signalling and pancreatitis: effects of alcohol, bile and coffee. Trends in Pharmacological Sciences 2006;27:113–120.

5 Mukherjee R, Criddle DN, Gukovskaya A, Pandol S, Petersen OH, Sutton R. Mitochondrial injury in pancreatitis. Cell Calcium 2008;44:14–23.

6 Kaiser AM, Saluja AK, Sengupta A, Saluja M, Steer ML. Relationship between severity, necrosis, and apoptosis in five models of experimental acute pancreatitis. American Journal of Physiology 1995;269:C1295–C1304.

7 Maleth J, Rakonczay Z, Jr., Venglovecz V, Dolman NJ, Hegyi P. Central role of mitochondrial injury in the pathogenesis of acute pancreatitis. Acta Physiologica 2013;207:226–235.

8 He S, Wang L, Miao L, Wang T, Du F, Zhao L, et al. Receptor interacting protein kinase-3 determines cellular necrotic response to TNF-alpha. Cell. 2009;137(6):1100–1111.

9 Dawra R, Sah RP, Dudeja V, Rishi L, Talukdar R, Garg P, et al. Intra-acinar trypsinogen activation mediates early stages of pancreatic injury but not inflammation in mice with acute pancreatitis. Gastroenterology 2011; 141:2210–2217.

10 Gaiser S, Daniluk J, Liu Y, Tsou L, Chu J, Lee W, et al. Intracellular activation of trypsinogen in transgenic mice induces acute but not chronic pancreatitis. Gut 2011;60:1379–1388.

11 Rakonczay Z, Jr.,, Hegyi P, Takacs T, McCarroll J, Saluja AK. The role of NF-kappaB activation in the pathogenesis of acute pancreatitis. Gut 2008;57:259–267.

12 Gukovskaya AS, Gukovsky I, Zaninovic V et al. Pancreatic acinar cells produce, release, and respond to tumor necrosis factor-alpha. Role in regulating cell death and pancreatitis. Journal of Clinical Investigation 1997; 100: 1853–1862.

13 Hoque R, Malik AF, Gorelick F, Mehal WZ. Sterile inflammatory response in acute pancreatitis. Pancreas 2012;41:353–357.

14 Chen GY, Nunez G. Sterile inflammation: sensing and reacting to damage. Nature Reviews Immunology 2010;10:826–837.

15 Lerch MM, Gorelick FS. Models of acute and chronic pancreatitis. Gastroenterology 2013;144:1180–1193.

16 Berthet B, Guillou N, Brioche MI, Choux R, Viret P, Ledoray V, Billardon M, Assadourian R. Influence of somatostatin on acute pancreatitis in rats. European Journal of Surgery 1998;164:785–790.

17 Küçüktülü U, Alhan E, Erçin C, Cinel A, Calik A. Effects of octreotide on acute pancreatitis of varying severity in rats. European Journal of Surgery 1999;165:891–896.

18 Lankisch PG, Pohl U, Göke B, Otto J, Wereszczynska-Siemiatkowska U, Gröne HJ, Rahlf G. Effect of FOY-305 (camostate) on severe acute pancreatitis in two experimental animal models. Gastroenterology 1989;96:193–199.

19 Hirano T, Manabe T. Human urinary trypsin inhibitor, urinastatin, prevents pancreatic injuries induced by pancreaticobiliary duct obstruction with cerulein stimulation

and systemic hypotension in the rat. Archives of Surgery 1993;128:1322–1329; discussion 1329.

20 Demols A, Van Laethem JL, Quertinmont E, Legros F, Louis H, Le Moine O, Devière J. N-acetylcysteine decreases severity of acute pancreatitis in mice. Pancreas 2000;20:161–169.

21 Hardman J, Jamdar S, Shields C, McMahon R, Redmond HP, Siriwardena AK. Intravenous selenium modulates L-arginine-induced experimental acute pancreatitis. Journal of the Pancreas 2005;6:431–437.

22 Lane JS, Todd KE, Gloor B, Chandler CF, Kau AW, Ashley SW, Reber HA, McFadden DW. Platelet activating factor antagonism reduces the systemic inflammatory response in a murine model of acute pancreatitis. Journal of Surgical Research 2001;99:365–370.

23 de Campos T, Deree J, Martins JO, Loomis WH, Shenvi E, Putnam JG, Coimbra R. Pentoxifylline attenuates pulmonary inflammation and neutrophil activation in experimental acute pancreatitis. Pancreas 2008;37:42–49.

24 Hackert T, Werner J, Gebhard MM, Klar E. Effects of heparin in experimental models of acute pancreatitis and post-ERCP pancreatitis. Surgery 2004;135:131–138.

25 Yamanel L, Mas MR, Comert B, Isik AT, Aydin S, Mas N, Deveci S, Ozyurt M, Tasci I, Unal T. The effect of activated protein C on experimental acute necrotizing pancreatitis. Critical Care 2005;9:R184–R190.

26 Gallagher S, Sankaran H, Williams JA. Mechanism of scorpion toxin-induced enzyme secretion in rat pancreas. Gastroenterology 1981;80:970–973.

27 Laukkarinen JM, Van Acker GJ, Weiss ER, Steer ML, Perides G. A mouse model of acute biliary pancreatitis induced by retrograde pancreatic duct infusion of Na-taurocholate. Gut 2007;56:1590–1598.

28 Huang W, Booth DM, Cane MC, Chvanov M, Javed MA, Elliott VL, Armstrong JA, Dingsdale H, Cash N, Li Y, Greenhalf W, Mukherjee R, Kaphalia BS, Jaffar M, Petersen OH, Tepikin AV, Sutton R, Criddle DN. Fatty acid ethyl ester synthase inhibition ameliorates ethanol-induced Ca^{2+}-dependent mitochondrial dysfunction and acute pancreatitis. Gut 2014;63:1313–1324.

29 Simmons DL. What makes a good anti-inflammatory drug target? Drug Discovery Today 2006;11:210–219.

30 Gashaw I, Ellinghaus P, Sommer A, Asadullah K. What makes a good drug target? Drug Discovery Today 2011;16:1037–1043.

31 Wen L, Voronina S, Javed MA, Awais M, Szatmary P, Latawiec D, Chvanov M, Collier D, Huang W, Barrett J, Begg M, Stauderman K, Roos J, Grigoryev S, Ramos S, Rogers E, Whitten J, Velicelebi G, Dunn M, Tepikin AV, Criddle DN, Sutton R. Inhibitors of ORAI1 prevent cytosolic calcium-associated injury of human pancreatic acinar cells and acute pancreatitis in 3 mouse models. Gastroenterology 2015;149:481–492.

32 Liao Y, Erxleben C, Yildirim E, Abramowitz J, Armstrong DL, Birnbaumer L. Orai proteins interact with TRPC channels and confer responsiveness to store depletion. Proceedings of the National Academy of Sciences of the United States of America 2007;104:4682–4687.

33 Lee KP, Yuan JP, Hong JH, So I, Worley PF, Muallem S. An endoplasmic reticulum/plasma membrane junction: STIM1/Orai1/TRPCs. FEBS Letters 2010;584:2022–2027.

34 Park CY, Hoover PJ, Mullins FM, Bachhawat P, Covington ED, Raunser S, Walz T, Garcia KC, Dolmetsch RE, Lewis RS. STIM1 clusters and activates CRAC channels via direct binding of a cytosolic domain to Orai1. Cell 2009;136:876–890.

35 Roberts-Thomson SJ, Peters AA, Grice DM, Monteith GR. ORAI-mediated calcium entry: mechanism and roles, diseases and pharmacology. Pharmacology & Therapeutics 2010;127:121–130.

36 Feske S, Gwack Y, Prakriya M, Srikanth S, Puppel SH, Tanasa B, et al. A mutation in Orai1 causes immune deficiency by abrogating CRAC channel function. Nature 2006;441:179–185.

37 Prakriya M, Feske S, Gwack Y, Srikanth S, Rao A, Hogan PG. Orai1 is an essential pore subunit of the CRAC channel. Nature 2006;443:230–233.

38 Lur G, Sherwood MW, Ebisui E, Haynes L, Feske S, Sutton R, Burgoyne RD, Mikoshiba K, Petersen OH, Tepikin AV. InsP(3)receptors and Orai channels in pancreatic acinar cells: co-localization and its consequences. Biochemical Journal 2011;436:231–239.

39 Gerasimenko JV, Gryshchenko O, Ferdek PE, Stapleton E, Hebert TO, Bychkova S, Peng S, Begg M, Gerasimenko OV, Petersen OH. Ca2+ release-activated Ca2+ channel blockade as a potential tool in antipancreatitis therapy. Proceedings of the National Academy of Sciences of the United States of America 2013;110:13186–13191.

40 Clemens RA, Lowell CA. Store-operated calcium signaling in neutrophils. Journal of Leukocyte Biology 2015;98:497–502.

41 Huang W, Cane MC, Mukherjee R, Szatmary P, Zhang X, Elliott V, Ouyang Y, Chvanov M, Latawiec D, Wen L, Booth DM, Haynes AC, Petersen OH, Tepikin AV, Criddle DN, Sutton R. Caffeine protects against experimental acute pancreatitis by inhibition of inositol 1,4,5-trisphosphate receptor-mediated Ca^{2+} release. Gut 2015. [Epub ahead of print]

42 Parekh AB, Putney JW, Jr., Store-operated calcium channels. Physiological Reviews 2005;85:757–810.

43 Kim MS, Lee KP, Yang D, Shin DM, Abramowitz J, Kiyonaka S, Birnbaumer L, Mori Y, Muallem S. Genetic and pharmacologic inhibition of the Ca^{2+} influx channel TRPC3 protects secretory epithelia from Ca^{2+}-dependent toxicity. Gastroenterology 2011;140:2107–2115.

44 Ichas F, Mazat JP. From calcium signaling to cell death: two conformations for the mitochondrial permeability transition pore. Switching from low- to high-conductance state. Biochimica et Biophysica Acta 1998;1366:33–50.

45 Fayaz SM, Raj YV, Krishnamurthy RG. CypD: the key to the death door. CNS & Neurological Disorders Drug Targets 2015;14:654–663.

46 Giorgio V, von Stockum S, Antoniel M, Fabbro A, Fogolari F, Forte M, Glick GD, Petronilli V, Zoratti M, Szabó I, Lippe G, Bernardi P. Dimers of mitochondrial ATP synthase form the permeability transition pore. Proceedings of the National Academy of Sciences of the United States of America. 2013;110(15):5887–5892.

47 Luvisetto S, Basso E, Petronilli V, Bernardi P, Forte M. Enhancement of anxiety, facilitation of avoidance behavior, and occurrence of adult-onset obesity in mice lacking mitochondrial cyclophilin D. Neuroscience 2008;155:585–596.

48 Shalbueva N, Mareninova OA, Gerloff A, Yuan J, Waldron RT, Pandol SJ, et al. Effects of oxidative alcohol metabolism on the mitochondrial permeability transition pore and necrosis in a mouse model of alcoholic pancreatitis. Gastroenterology 2013;144:437–446.

49 Mukherjee R, Mareninova OA, Odinokova IV, Huang W, Murphy J, Chvanov M, Javed MA, Wen L, Booth DM, Cane MC, Awais M, Gavillet B, Pruss RM, Schaller S, Molkentin JD, Tepikin AV, Petersen OH, Pandol SJ Gukovsky I, Criddle DN, Gukovskaya AS, Sutton R, NIHR Pancreas Biomedical Research Unit. Mechanism of mitochondrial permeability transition pore induction and damage in the pancreas: inhibition prevents acute pancreatitis by protecting production of ATP. Gut 2016;65:1333–1346.

50 Baines CP, Kaiser RA, Purcell NH, Blair NS, Osinska H, Hambleton MA, et al. Loss of cyclophilin D reveals a critical role for mitochondrial permeability transition in cell death. Nature 2005;434:658–662.

51 Piot C, Croisille P, Staat P, Thibault H, Rioufol G, Mewton N, Elbelghiti R, Cung TT, Bonnefoy E, Angoulvant D, Macia C, Raczka F, Sportouch C, Gahide G, Finet G, André-Fouët X, Revel D, Kirkorian G, Monassier JP, Derumeaux G, Ovize M. Effect of cyclosporine on reperfusion injury in acute myocardial infarction. New England Journal of Medicine 2008;359:473–481.

52 Naoumov NV. Cyclophilin inhibition as potential therapy for liver diseases. Journal of Hepatology 2014;61: 1166–1174.

53 Malleo G, Mazzon E, Siriwardena AK et al. Role of tumor necrosis factor-alpha in acute pancreatitis: from biological basis to clinical evidence. Shock 2007;28:130–140.

54 Ho YP, Chiu CT, Sheen IS et al. Tumor necrosis factor-α and interleukin-10 contribute to immunoparalysis in patients

with acute pancreatitis. Human Immunology 2011; 72: 18–23.

55 Malmstrøm ML, Hansen MB, Andersen AM et al. Cytokines and organ failure in acute pancreatitis: inflammatory response in acute pancreatitis. Pancreas 2012; 41: 271–277.

56 Shen Y, Cui NQ. Clinical observation of immunity in patients with secondary infection from severe acute pancreatitis. Inflammation Research 2012; 61: 743–748.

57 Fisic E, Poropat G, Bilic-Zulle L et al. The role of IL-6, 8, and 10, sTNFr, CRP, and pancreatic elastase in the prediction of systemic complications in patients with acute pancreatitis. Gastroenterology Research and Practice 2013; 2013: 282645.

58 Stobaugh DJ, Deepak P. Effect of tumor necrosis factor-α inhibitors on drug-induced pancreatitis in inflammatory bowel disease. Annals of Pharmacotherapy 2014; 48: 1282–1287.

59 Clayton H, Flatz L, Vollenweider-Roten S et al. Anti-TNF therapy in the treatment of psoriasis in a patient with acute-on-chronic pancreatitis. Dermatology 2013; 227: 193–196.

60 Bishehsari F, Sharma A, Stello K et al. TNF-alpha gene (TNFA) variants increase risk for multi-organ dysfunction syndrome (MODS) in acute pancreatitis. Pancreatology 2012; 12: 113–118.

61 Vege SS, Atwal T, Bi Y et al. Pentoxifylline treatment in severe acute pancreatitis: a pilot, double-blind, placebo-controlled, randomized trial. Gastroenterology 2015; 149; 318–320.

62 Zhang H, Neuhöfer P, Song L, Rabe B, Lesina M, Kurkowski MU, Treiber M, Wartmann T, Regnér S, Thorlacius H, Saur D, Weirich G, Yoshimura A, Halangk W, Mizgerd JP, Schmid RM, Rose-John S, Algül H. IL-6 trans-signaling promotes pancreatitis-associated lung injury and lethality. Journal of Clinical Investigation 2013;123:1019–1031.

63 Uhl W, Büchler MW, Malfertheiner P, Beger HG, Adler G, Gaus W. A randomised, double blind, multicentre trial of octreotide in moderate to severe acute pancreatitis. Gut 1999;45:97–104.

64 Büchler M, Malfertheiner P, Uhl W, Schölmerich J, Stöckmann F, Adler G, Gaus W, Rolle K, Beger HG. Gabexate mesilate in human acute pancreatitis. German Pancreatitis Study Group. Gastroenterology 1993;104: 1165–1170.

65 Siriwardena AK, Mason JM, Balachandra S, Bagul A, Galloway S, Formela L, Hardman JG, Jamdar S. Randomised, double blind, placebo controlled trial of intravenous antioxidant (n-acetylcysteine, selenium, vitamin C) therapy in severe acute pancreatitis. Gut 2007;56:1439–1444.

66 Johnson CD, Kingsnorth AN, Imrie CW, McMahon MJ, Neoptolemos JP, McKay C, Toh SK, Skaife P, Leeder PC, Wilson P, Larvin M, Curtis LD. Double blind, randomised, placebo controlled study of a platelet activating factor antagonist, lexipafant, in the treatment and prevention of organ failure in predicted severe acute pancreatitis. Gut 2001;48:62–69.

67 Pettilä V, Kyhälä L, Kylänpää ML, Leppäniemi A, Tallgren M, Markkola A, Puolakkainen P, Repo H, Kemppainen E. APCAP--activated protein C in acute pancreatitis: a double-blind randomized human pilot trial. Critical Care 2010;14:R139.

68 Miranda CJ, Mason JM, Babu BI, Sheen AJ, Eddleston JM, Parker MJ, Pemberton P, Siriwardena AK. Twenty-four hour infusion of human recombinant activated protein C (Xigris) early in severe acute pancreatitis: The XIG-AP 1 trial. Pancreatology 2015;15:635–641.

69 Afghani E, Pandol SJ, Shimosegawa T, Sutton R, Wu BU, Vege SS, Gorelick F, Hirota M, Windsor J, Lo SK, Freeman ML, Lerch MM, Tsuji Y, Melmed GY, Wassef W, Mayerle J. Acute pancreatitis – Progress and challenges: a report on an international symposium. Pancreas 2015;44:1195–1210

CHAPTER 10

Sequelae of acute pancreatitis

Nicholas J. Zyromski & Lucas McDuffie

Department of Surgery, Indiana University School of Medicine, Indianapolis, IN, USA

Introduction

Contemporary management of patients with severe acute pancreatitis (SAP) has evolved dramatically over the past decade. Improved overall understanding of the acute pancreatitis (AP) disease process has led to the adoption of properly timed and more minimally invasive intervention to treat acute complications such as infected peripancreatic and pancreatic necrosis [1–4]. Judicious use of antibiotic treatment and advances in critical care medicine improve the support to patients with pancreatitis through the initial severe phase as well as the second more chronic phase of disease. The overall mortality of SAP patients surviving the initial storm of multiple organ dysfunction appears to be decreasing [3, 4]. Nevertheless, AP (particularly in its severe form) remains a formidable problem and is accompanied by numerous complications ("sequelae"). Remarkably few data are available particularly cataloging those complications seen in the longer term. This chapter provides a brief review of individual complications, highlighting diagnosis and therapy.

Sequelae of mild acute pancreatitis

In the United States alone, each year over 270,000 patients are hospitalized with the primary ICD-9 diagnosis 577.0 – "Acute Pancreatitis (AP)" [5]. More than 80% of these patients will manifest a relatively mild disease course, with spontaneous resolution of pain and the inflammatory process. Sequelae of mild AP include exocrine and endocrine insufficiency; data regarding pancreatic function after mild AP are scant.

The primary sequelae of mild AP must be considered to be recurrent AP.

Population-based studies estimate the incidence of recurrent AP to range from 25% to 45% [6–11]. A recent thorough analysis of nearly 7500 Pennsylvania residents documented a 22% incidence of recurrent AP after initial insult; smoking and alcohol were significant independent predictors of a recurrent pancreatitis episode [6]. These authors' data also confirmed the well-documented increased risk of recurrent biliary AP with delay of cholecystectomy – 29.5% increased risk when cholecystectomy was delayed past 6 months.

Clinicians caring for AP patients must be aware of and work to address the underlying pathology. These treatments include timely cholecystectomy for biliary pancreatitis, promoting alcohol or tobacco cessation programs, and aggressive management of metabolic conditions such as hypertriglyceridemia and hypercalcemia. In older patients with idiopathic pancreatitis, the clinician will do well to consider cystic pancreatic disease (intraductal papillary mucinous neoplasm – usually obvious on imaging study) or small solid malignant neoplasm (often more subtle on imaging study, occasionally presenting as mild pancreatic duct (PD) stricture) as causative agents.

Sequelae of severe acute pancreatitis/necrotizing pancreatitis (SAP/NP)

SAP is accompanied by mortality of approximately 20%. A large proportion of SAP/necrotizing pancreatitis (NP) mortality is observed within the first 48 hours

Pancreatitis: Medical and Surgical Management, First Edition.
David B. Adams, Peter B. Cotton, Nicholas J. Zyromski and John Windsor.

and is related to multiple organ failure in patients who lack the physiologic reserve to withstand this massive inflammatory insult [12]. Those patients surviving the early phase of SAP/NP may experience myriad complications related to the inflammatory process, mass effect from acute or walled-off pancreatic/peripancreatic collections or as a consequence of intervention aimed toward treating these collections. Complications may arise during the acute phase of disease or months to years remote from the initial disease insult. Anticipating these sequelae permits prompt recognition, expeditious treatment, and optimal patient outcomes.

Disconnected pancreatic duct syndrome

Kozarek coined the term "disconnected pancreatic duct syndrome" (DPDS) to describe the situation of upstream viable pancreatic tail in the setting of pancreatic neck/body necrosis that completely disrupts the main PD (Figure 10.1) [13]. This situation has also been termed the disconnected pancreatic tail syndrome and disconnected left pancreatic remnant and occurs in 30–50% of patients suffering an episode of NP [14, 15]. The pancreatic neck is a relative vascular "watershed" between the pancreaticoduodenal arcades supplying the head and the transverse pancreatic arterial branches from the splenic artery that supply the body and tail [16]. As such, the neck is susceptible to insult from hypotension, which may perpetuate parenchymal necrosis.

Complete PD disruption may be suspected clinically early in the patient's course by the pattern of necrosis observed on contrast-enhanced cross-sectional imaging and by the observation of enlarging peripancreatic collections during the first few weeks following the initial insult of pancreatitis (Figure 10.1).

The DPDS anatomy with necrosis/fluid collection localized to the lesser sac lends itself ideally to transgastric drainage. This approach may be either endoscopic or surgical depending on the volume of solid necrosis, need for cholecystectomy (favors surgical), and local expertise. External drainage of the disconnected tail – either percutaneous or operative – will result in pancreatic fistula. Proper management of pancreaticocutaneous fistula in these cases is challenging. Some suggest simply removing the drain and that most of these fistulae will heal spontaneously (likely working their way into a loop of adjacent intestine). Our experience has been that these problems are not solved so easily. Our approach

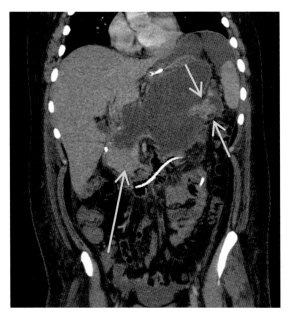

Figure 10.1   Disconnected pancreatic duct syndrome (DPDS) – typical computed tomography finding (coronal) of patient with DPDS 4 weeks into the course of severe acute pancreatitis. Note large peripancreatic collection in lesser sac with viable pancreatic head (long arrow) and small disconnected pancreatic tail (two short arrows).

has been to offer patients internal drainage into a Roux limb of jejunum if they have a large enough remnant, or tail remnant resection for those with smaller remnants and left-sided portal hypertension [14, 17].

Importantly, early enthusiasm for drainage into the fistula track (as opposed to the pancreatic remnant itself) has been tempered with time. This operation (fistula tract-jejunostomy) is easier technically than formal pancreaticojejunostomy; however, not surprisingly, the narrow, nonepithelialized tracks tend to close and the patients present with recurrent pancreatitis or pseudocyst [18]. South American pancreatic surgeons call the DPDS "el Diablo" – this devilish problem is exemplified by patients with a small pancreatic remnant that will not make enough exocrine secretion to keep a track open and may present with recurrent pain (typically left upper quadrant) and intra-abdominal collections. Resection is most appropriate in these cases.

Pseudocyst/pancreatic duct stricture

Pseudocysts by definition are related to PD disruption and contain mostly fluid with minimal amount of necrotic material. Clarity of terminology is important and stressed in the revised Atlanta criteria [19]. Most peripancreatic collections in early AP are just "acute fluid collections" and not "pseudocysts." Many acute collections resolve without intervention or with simple aspiration of the fluid. It is critically important not to confuse walled-off necrosis with a "pseudocyst" as the treatment of these two entities is different. True pseudocysts occur later in the course of SAP and may even present years after the initial insult (Figure 10.2). Most pseudocysts are discovered as a consequence of patient symptoms such as pain, early satiety, or progressive bloating. Proper therapy of pseudocyst is directed by understanding the underlying pancreatic ductal anatomy [20]. Drainage into the alimentary tract may be accomplished endoscopically or surgically. The durability of endoscopic drainage and optimal timing of endoscopic stent removal are currently unknown. Other important considerations are how much pancreatic parenchyma remains and the presence of venous collateral formation. Small-volume remnant pancreas produces less pancreatic secretion and has less of a chance to keep the enteral connection open. The presence of venous collateral disease complicates surgical drainage; resection may be more prudent in this situation [14].

PD strictures as a consequence of SAP typically manifest within the first few years of the initial insult [21]. Presenting symptoms are commonly recurrent pancreatitis attacks, though PD stricture may also present as pseudocyst. Interestingly, patients with PD

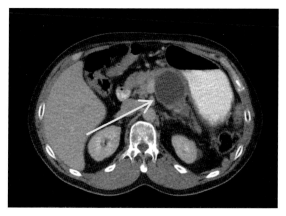

Figure 10.2 Symptomatic pseudocyst (arrow) in a patient 7 years after "definitive" treatment of necrotizing pancreatitis including debridement of peripancreatic necrosis.

stricture in the tail often report more left-sided or left upper quadrant abdominal pain (as opposed to the classic epigastric pain of AP). Treatment of PD stricture depends largely on anatomic location and local expertise. Endoscopic (transpapillary) stricture treatment becomes harder with strictures further out the body and tail of the gland. Isolated neck or body strictures may be amenable to middle segment pancreatectomy [22], while strictures with PD dilation upstream toward the tail may be best approached by lateral pancreatico-jejunostomy. Multidisciplinary input from experienced endoscopists and surgeons is important in treatment planning.

Recurrent retroperitoneal collection/abscess

Classic surgical reports from the era of open pancreatic debridement document a 10–30% incidence of recurrent intra-abdominal and retroperitoneal collections following operative debridement [4, 23]. In the contemporary era, a parallel is seen in patients treated with percutaneous drainage or the "step-up" approach, many (most) of whom require more than one drain and/or upsizing of the drains to achieve definitive drainage [24]. Retroperitoneal collections may be related to persistent leak of pancreatic digestive juice or may be abscess of infectious origin.

Recurrent retroperitoneal collections should be considered in a patient whose recovery plateaus or deteriorates after a period of recuperation (particularly after intervention). These collections are easily diagnosed by cross-sectional imaging and are largely amenable to drainage by the percutaneous approach.

Understanding the underlying pancreatic ductal anatomy is an essential tenet in treating SAP/NP patients in general; this knowledge is particularly important in treating those with recurrent retroperitoneal collections. Leakage of pancreatic juice from small branch ducts may cause problems in the anatomic distribution of either the head or the tail. These side branch leaks may not be obvious from computed tomography (CT) or even magnetic resonance cholangiopancreatography (MRCP) and may only be diagnosed by ERCP. ERCP may prove to be therapeutic as well as diagnostic; PD strictures may be dilated and stented, and some PD disruptions may be amenable to bridging with a stent. Alternatively, ERCP may diagnose complete PD disruption, in which case management should proceed

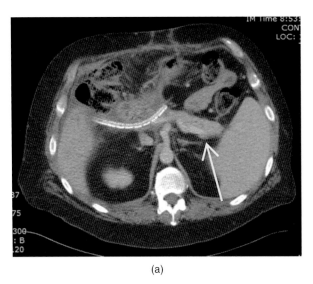
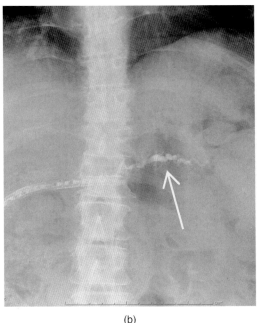

(a)   (b)

Figure 10.3 (a) Computed tomography shows surgical drain adjacent to disconnected tail (arrow). (b) Sinogram through drain illuminates pancreatic duct in the body and tail (arrow).

along the pathway described earlier for the DPDS. Performing sinogram through an existing catheter is an inexpensive and simple diagnostic test that is often overlooked (Figure 10.3). Sinogram may diagnose communication with pancreatic ductal system; on the other hand, a "negative" sinogram does not necessarily rule out PD disruption.

Many retroperitoneal collections are related to leak from the disrupted PD, though other collections may simply be abscess secondary to infected pancreatic necrosis. Treatment of retroperitoneal abscess is almost always possible with percutaneous drainage; systemic antibiotic therapy should be tailored to the cultured organism(s). After source control has been achieved, the optimal duration of antibiotic treatment is poorly defined. The clinician must be aware that drug pharmacokinetic distribution into the retroperitoneum is different from that in the peritoneal cavity and that discontinuing antibiotics too soon may lead to recurrent abscess. We have found that a 7–10-day course is typically sufficient *after source control has been achieved*. Pancreatic and peripancreatic collections may become infected by resistant organisms such as methicillin-resistant *Staphylococcus aureus* (MRSA),

vancomycin-resistant *Enterococcus* (VRE), and other multidrug-resistant strains (*E. coli, Pseudomonas,* etc.). These resistant organisms are particularly difficult to clear from the retroperitoneum – recurrent abscess is relatively common, and protracted courses of systemic antibiotic treatment may be necessary to achieve bacterial clearance.

Ischemic colon

From 10% to 27% of patients with SAP/NP may develop some form of colonic complication – stricture, perforation, fistula, or ischemia [25, 26]. Colonic ischemia is an important but underrecognized problem in SAP/NP patients. The true incidence of colonic ischemia is difficult to estimate for several reasons: this problem is commonly reported in conjunction with other colonic problems and in some cases may occur as a consequence of pancreatic debridement. The pathophysiology of *de novo* (as opposed to perioperative) colonic ischemia is most likely due to venous thrombosis secondary to local inflammatory effect. The ischemic process may be initiated or perpetuated by an episode of hypotension.

Colonic ischemia is notoriously challenging to diagnose preoperatively but should be suspected in patients who suddenly deteriorate after a stable clinical course. A large systematic review found the median time to presentation of colonic ischemia to be 25 days [27]. Unfortunately, no imaging test is completely accurate to either rule in or rule out colonic ischemia; the diagnosis must be secured at the time of laparotomy. It is worth mentioning that even at laparotomy, the profound inflammatory response accompanying NP may make diagnosis of ischemic colon difficult.

Treatment of ischemic colon is by resection of the affected colon with proximal diversion. Some authors have advocated diverting ileostomy while leaving the affected colon *in situ*; our feeling is that ischemic organs should be removed unless the patient's physiologic condition and/or the density of inflammatory response absolutely prohibits resection.

Not surprisingly, NP patients with colonic complications have significantly worse outcomes compared to those without colon problems. Review of 344 NP patients treated at our institution identified 37 requiring colectomy. Colectomy patients had longer length of stay, higher readmission rate, and 19% mortality compared to 5% mortality in a control group.

Enteric fistula

Fistulae from the stomach, small bowel, colon, or pancreas typically arise after intervention for complications of NP, but may also present later – even months after "resolution" of initial disease. Interestingly, the inflammatory response surrounding peripancreatic collections (walled-off necrosis) not uncommonly creates internal fistulae, particularly to the proximal small bowel under the overhanging transverse mesocolon. These fistulae may be suspected when a large volume of gas becomes apparent in the walled-off necrosis.

The incidence of postoperative enteric fistulae ranges from 9% to 22% after open pancreatic debridement [3, 28–30]. Enteric fistulae may also occur after retroperitoneal debridement and percutaneous drainage of pancreatic collections (Figure 10.4), though robust data describing their true incidence have yet to accrue.

Diagnosis of enterocutaneous fistula is usually straightforward when succus entericus is visualized in drain effluent or draining through an incision. Cross-sectional imaging provides information about the portion of bowel involved as well as any adjacent residual inflammatory collections (which may delay or prevent spontaneous fistula closure). Anatomical information is supplemented by enteric contrast studies and sinogram through existing fistula. Predictors of spontaneous closure are similar to those for enteric fistulae arising in other settings – long fistula tract, resolution of local inflammation, and absence of distal obstruction. Optimizing nutritional status is also important; few fistulae close spontaneously in a catabolic patient.

Should operative correction be required, proper timing of surgery is a critical consideration. Delaying operation as long as possible from primary debridement permits softening of intra-abdominal adhesive disease. On the other hand, the clinician must be acutely aware of the patient's nutritional state – experienced judgment will identify a patient who has reached optimal condition. High-volume fistulae (arbitrarily >500 mL/day) and those with little (or no) track length between the fistula and the atmosphere are unlikely to close spontaneously and place a tremendous metabolic demand on the patient. Such patients will never be "perfect" for operation; the clinical judgment lies in selecting appropriate time for operative repair before the fistula atrophies the patient's underlying physiologic state.

A special note regarding duodenal fistulae is worthwhile, as these patients often present a formidable management challenge. Duodenal fistula may be extremely high volume; these patients have high electrolyte, fluid, and protein loss and can become metabolically wasted in a very short time. In some circumstances, complete diversion of biliopancreatic secretion by percutaneous transhepatic drain placement may facilitate spontaneous closure [31]. This interventional radiology procedure is often quite challenging in the setting of a nondilated intrahepatic biliary tree. Refeeding biliopancreatic secretions distally in the intestine via jejunostomy tube simplifies fluid and electrolyte management and prevents the high protein loss associated with external bile drainage.

Biliary stricture

Biliary stricture is typically a consequence of SAP/NP involving the pancreatic head. The true incidence of bile duct stricture complicating NP is unknown; in fact, the medical literature contains only sporadic case reports describing this problem. In clinical practice, biliary obstruction may present either early or relatively late in the disease process.

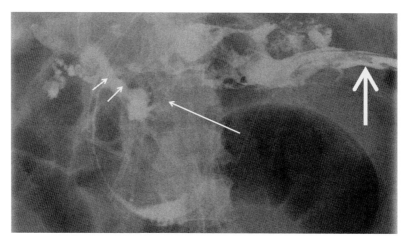

Figure 10.4 Sinogram through drain (arrowhead) illuminates duodenum (long arrow) and biliary tree (short arrows).

Biliary obstruction presenting in the first few weeks of SAP/NP is easily diagnosed by clinical examination (jaundice) and confirmed by the finding of elevated bilirubin and alkaline phosphatase on laboratory analysis. Hepatic transaminases are also typically elevated. Endoscopic biliary stenting is the treatment of choice, although endoscopic access to the major papilla may prove difficult because of duodenal or papillary edema. In this case, percutaneous transhepatic drainage (PTD) may be necessary. It is prudent to correct aberrant coagulation parameters prior to intervention (either endoscopic sphincterotomy or PTD); vitamin K and/or intravenous plasma administration is typically effective. If the patient does NOT have pancreatic head necrosis, endobiliary stenting often provides durable treatment, and the biliary stents may be removed after the disease process has resolved (Figure 10.5).

Patients with pancreatic head necrosis present a more substantial problem in general. These patients may manifest biliary obstruction either early or later (months) in the disease course. Unfortunately, biliary stenting in this setting is much less effective as a durable therapy due to the dense fibrotic process involving the pancreatic head. Surgical biliary bypass is often required, but is a challenging technical exercise. Pancreatic head necrosis is commonly associated with thrombosis of the superior mesenteric vein (SMV) and/or portal vein (PV) with subsequent collateral venous development around the pancreatic head. This so-called cavernous transformation in the porta hepatis increases operative complexity

dramatically. In the setting of cavernous venous transformation, side-to-side choledochoenterostomy may be a safer option than attempting to dissect the bile duct circumferentially. Suture ligation of the collateral veins at the periphery of planned choledochotomy minimizes hemorrhage.

Long-term follow-up of patients surviving an episode of SAP/NP should include periodic (annual) evaluation of liver chemistry tests. Early diagnosis of impending biliary stricture may be suspected by observing elevation of the serum alkaline phosphatase and/or bilirubin.

Duodenal stricture

Similar to biliary stricture, pancreatic head necrosis may lead to duodenal stricture. Duodenal strictures may present early or late in the disease course. Endoscopic duodenal stenting has emerged as an effective therapeutic option for patients with duodenal obstruction from malignancy. Experience with these endoscopic duodenal stents in the setting of NP is limited, but may effectively temporize a challenging clinical situation and permit accelerated recuperation by enhancing enteral nutritional intake. Surgical duodenal bypass is often required for definitive therapy; however, surgical gastrojejunostomy is notorious for poor efficacy. Gastric dysfunction in these situations is almost certainly multifactorial and includes gastric atony from long-standing obstruction and gastropathy related to left-sided portal hypertension. Prokinetic agents may be beneficial.

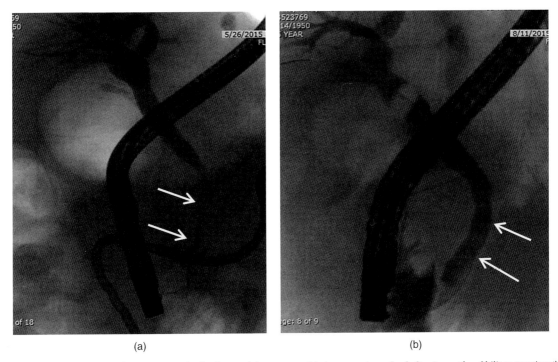

(a)   (b)

Figure 10.5 Biliary stricture during acute episode of necrotizing pancreatitis (a, arrows) resolved after 3 months of biliary stenting (b, arrows).

Venous thrombosis

Acute thrombosis of the SMV, PV, and splenic vein (SV) is a common complication of SAP/NP. These thromboses are most likely related to a combination of the inflammatory process and local mass effect of necrosis on the adjacent vascular structures. Contemporary analyses have documented 16–23% incidence of mesenteric venous thrombosis in AP patients, with substantially increased incidence in patients with pancreatic and peripancreatic necrosis [32–34]. Review of 171 NP patients at our institution identified 56% with venous thromboembolism (including splanchnic, central, and extremity veins), 38% with SMV/PV thrombosis, and 41% with SV thrombosis (unpublished data). Based on these data, periodic ultrasound screening seems reasonable.

Cavernous transformation around the pancreatic head or porta hepatis in isolation typically does not cause measurable clinical consequence, though hormonal and absorptive perturbations related to relative extrahepatic portal hypertension are difficult to quantitate. Less commonly, these collateral veins may cause gastrointestinal hemorrhage that is challenging to diagnose and control. Isolated SV thrombosis causes left-sided "sinistral" portal hypertension from decompression through the short gastric veins around the gastric fundus and the epiploic veins. A recent systematic review of sinistral portal hypertension identified 23% incidence in AP patients [32]. Overall, 53% of patients developed gastric varices (including 805 patients with AP and chronic pancreatitis (CP); the overall incidence of gastrointestinal bleeding was 12%. Both sinistral portal hypertension and cavernous transformation complicate intervention (endoscopic and surgical), in some cases making intervention prohibitively hazardous. In rare cases, recanalization of the SMV/PV may be possible through the interventional radiology approach; these procedures should be performed by experienced clinicians (Figure 10.6).

Most authorities recommend no anticoagulation for acute SV thrombosis. No consensus exists regarding the utility of anticoagulation in the setting of acute SMV/PV thrombosis. In patients with persistent mass effect (necrosis/peripancreatic collection), these thrombi are unlikely to resolve. On the other hand, aggressive

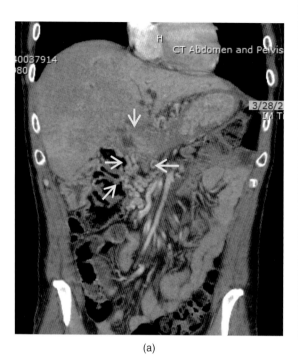

(a)

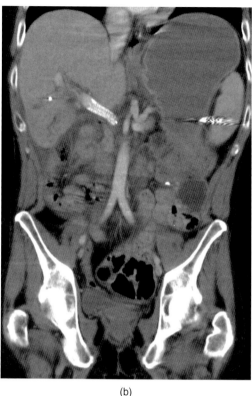

(b)

Figure 10.6 (a) Massive cavernous venous transformation (arrows) around pancreatic head in a survivor of SAP (necrosis originally involved pancreatic head). (b) Portal vein recannulation after transsplenic placement of SMV/PV stent.

anticoagulation of nonocclusive thrombi (or in an acute setting after treatment of the local collection) often leads to resolution and avoidance of problems related to cavernous transformation. Obviously, hemorrhagic risk must be weighed carefully in any decision to anticoagulate.

Visceral arterial pseudoaneurysm

Pseudoaneurysm (PSA) may arise from virtually any branch of the visceral arterial tree; this potentially life-threatening pathology must be taken seriously [35]. The most common presenting symptoms of PSA are significantly increased abdominal/back pain (in patients who have not had intervention), gastrointestinal bleeding, or the presence of blood in a surgically or radiologically placed drain. The suspicion of PSA should prompt evaluation by cross-sectional imaging such as contrast-enhanced CT, or ideally CT angiography. First-line therapy for any visceral PSA is angiographic

exclusion, either by coil embolization or by intra-arterial stent placement. These techniques successfully arrest hemorrhage in nearly all patients. The rare patient who presents with hemodynamic instability precluding radiological evaluation should undergo emergent operative exploration; in this situation, the surgeon should give strong consideration to "damage control" techniques with focus on hemostasis allowing time for resuscitation [36]. Mortality in patients who require operative repair of pseudoaneurysmal bleeding is extremely high.

Endocrine and exocrine insufficiency

Most data regarding the incidence of endocrine and exocrine insufficiency come from patients who have undergone intervention to debride pancreatic necrosis [37–40]. Overall, between 33% and 43% of patients will develop endocrine insufficiency after an episode of NP requiring intervention. Rates of exocrine insufficiency vary between 9% and 25%, possibly depending on the defining metric – symptoms of diarrhea, need for exocrine replacement enzymes, or documentation of decreased fecal pancreatic enzyme (elastase) concentration. The Mayo Clinic group performed early thorough analysis of their patients and described the correlation between greater amount of parenchymal necrosis and increased pancreatic insufficiency [37]. These investigators also highlighted the important point that pancreatic insufficiency develops and continues to progress with time beyond the initial disease treatment.

Ventral hernia

Not surprisingly, patients requiring surgical intervention to treat complications of SAP/NP have an extremely high rate of postoperative ventral hernia – as much as 42% in one large series [41]. These patients are subjected to operation under the terrible circumstances of local and systemic infection and ubiquitous malnutrition. Minimally invasive interventions most likely will decrease this hernia burden as they are more widely employed.

Intra-abdominal catastrophe/multivisceral transplant

SAP may lead to intra-abdominal catastrophe such as short gut or multiple and refractory enterocutaneous fistula in a "frozen" abdomen. Some patients will develop hepatic cirrhosis as a consequence of prolonged parenteral nutrition administration. In rare instances, multivisceral solid organ transplantation offers a lifesaving option for patients in these extreme circumstances.

Palliative care

Clinicians caring for SAP/NP patients are acutely aware of the fact that this disease process is not at all "benign." Advances in disease understanding and particularly in the treatment of critical illness and organ failure have enabled protracted support and patient salvage in what previously would have been fatal pancreatitis insults. Salvage of life for patients at the extreme end of the severe disease severity spectrum is often accompanied by a substantial negative impact on quality of life (QOL). Experienced and empathetic clinicians should keep in mind the end goals of reasonable QOL from early in the disease course. Open and frank dialogue with family members throughout the disease process facilitates difficult discussions regarding goals of treatment and end of life.

Recurrent acute pancreatitis

Currently, *chronic* pancreatitis is generally thought to develop along a spectrum of AP to recurrent AP to chronic pancreatitis. Multinational population-based data document an approximately 20% chance of recurrent AP among patients with an initial episode of mild AP. Most studies suggest that alcoholic etiology is associated with increased risk of recurrent AP. For example, Finnish population-based studies documented 25–45% recurrent AP after an initial attack of alcoholic AP [8]. More recent studies segregating patients by AP etiology have confirmed similar and significant numbers of patients (about 20%) experiencing recurrent AP after initial insult from ANY etiology [9–11]. Not surprisingly, delay in cholecystectomy was associated with increased incidence of recurrent AP in patients with biliary etiology [6].

A thorough population analysis from Allegheny County, Pennsylvania, took advantage of a unique data set linking longitudinal inpatient and outpatient data for 7456 patients at the individual patient level. These investigators found that readmission for recurrent AP was common – 22% for all etiology, 43% for alcoholic etiology, and 11% for biliary etiology. However, progression to chronic pancreatitis was generally rare; only 6% of patients with initial AP diagnosis were subsequently admitted with diagnosis of chronic pancreatitis.

Quality of life

QOL studies in AP patients are hampered in general by small sample size, nonstandard follow-up duration, and use of variable quality indices. A recent systemic review identified 10 different QOL instruments used in 16 studies, a situation that obviously challenges systematic analysis of outcomes [42].

Findings from published pancreatitis QOL studies are variable. Some reports suggest that patients surviving an episode of AP recuperate QOL similar to age- and sex-matched healthy individuals, while others document significantly decreased QOL after an episode of AP – particularly SAP.

The largest series in the literature queried 174 Finnish SAP patients treated over a 9-year period [39]. An outstanding 83% response rate provided data on

145 patients, who were surveyed with the validated RAND-36 QOL metric. When compared to age- and sex-matched control patients from the general population, the only difference was found in the category of "General Health." Pancreatitis patients had a statistically significantly decreased general health score; however, the z score was less than 2 and the difference between means was less than 10, leading the investigators to conclude that this statistical difference was not clinically significant. Sixty percent of pancreatitis survivors were able to return to work during the follow-up period of 5.5 years.

In contrast, a few other smaller studies have found significantly decreased QOL in pancreatitis patients, particularly in the short term. Wright and colleagues prospectively assessed pancreatitis survivors 3, 6, and 9 months after hospital discharge using the quality metric SF-36v2 Health Survey [43]. Seventeen of 21 survivors enrolled in the study, which included functional assessment by a 6-minute walk test. Over the year following hospital (ICU) discharge, significant improvement in physical function QOL was seen. However, at the study endpoint of 12 months, all QOL domains were significantly lower than would be expected based on national norms.

Clearly, an episode of AP affects QOL in the short term, and while many patients recuperate good physical functionality and QOL, some appear to have long-term decreased QOL. Future research will benefit from standardizing QOL metrics and evaluating larger patient populations including multicenter and multinational groups.

Summary

Treating patients with SAP remains a formidable challenge. Advances in understanding the disease process, intervention technique and timing, and care for the critically ill patient have improved survival of NP patients. With more NP patients surviving, long-term sequelae of the disease are encountered more frequently. Clinicians transitioning care of NP patients to primary care physicians should emphasize the need for routine follow-up to diagnose common sequelae such as endocrine and exocrine insufficiency. Pancreatic specialists should also be available to provide care for more complex problems such as enteric strictures, vascular pathology, and recurrent AP.

References

1 Working Group IAPAPAAPG. IAP/APA evidence-based guidelines for the management of acute pancreatitis. Pancreatology 2013;13:e1–e15.

2 van Santvoort HC, Besselink MG, Bakker OJ, et al. A step-up approach or open necrosectomy for necrotizing pancreatitis. The New England Journal of Medicine 2010;362:1491–1502.

3 Howard TJ, Patel JB, Zyromski N, et al. Declining morbidity and mortality rates in the surgical management of pancreatic necrosis. Journal of Gastrointestinal Surgery 2007;11:43–49.

4 Wormer BA, Swan RZ, Williams KB, et al. Outcomes of pancreatic debridement in acute pancreatitis: analysis of the nationwide inpatient sample from 1998 to 2010. American Journal of Surgery 2014;208:350–362.

5 Fagenholz PJ, Fernandez-del Castillo C, Harris NS, Pelletier AJ, Camargo CA, Jr., Direct medical costs of acute pancreatitis hospitalizations in the United States. Pancreas 2007;35:302–307.

6 Yadav D, O'Connell M, Papachristou GI. Natural history following the first attack of acute pancreatitis. The American Journal of Gastroenterology 2012;107:1096–1103.

7 Vipperla K, Papachristou GI, Easler J, et al. Risk of and factors associated with readmission after a sentinel attack of acute pancreatitis. Clinical Gastroenterology and Hepatology 2014;12:1911–1919.

8 Pelli H, Sand J, Laippala P, Nordback I. Long-term follow-up after the first episode of acute alcoholic pancreatitis: time course and risk factors for recurrence. Scandinavian Journal of Gastroenterology 2000;35:552–555.

9 Lankisch PG, Breuer N, Bruns A, Weber-Dany B, Lowenfels AB, Maisonneuve P. Natural history of acute pancreatitis: a long-term population-based study. The American Journal of Gastroenterology 2009;104:2797–2805; quiz 806.

10 Nojgaard C, Becker U, Matzen P, Andersen JR, Holst C, Bendtsen F. Progression from acute to chronic pancreatitis: prognostic factors, mortality, and natural course. Pancreas 2011;40:1195–1200.

11 Takeyama Y. Long-term prognosis of acute pancreatitis in Japan. Clinical Gastroenterology and Hepatology 2009;7:S15–S17.

12 Frey CF, Zhou H, Harvey DJ, White RH. The incidence and case-fatality rates of acute biliary, alcoholic, and idiopathic pancreatitis in California, 1994–2001. Pancreas 2006;33:336–344.

13 Kozarek RA, Ball TJ, Patterson DJ, Freeny PC, Ryan JA, Traverso LW. Endoscopic transpapillary therapy for disrupted pancreatic duct and peripancreatic fluid collections. Gastroenterology 1991;100:1362–1370.

14 Murage KP, Ball CG, Zyromski NJ, et al. Clinical framework to guide operative decision making in disconnected

left pancreatic remnant (DLPR) following acute or chronic pancreatitis. Surgery 2010;148:847–856; discussion 56–57.

15 Neoptolemos JP, London NJ, Carr-Locke DL. Assessment of main pancreatic duct integrity by endoscopic retrograde pancreatography in patients with acute pancreatitis. The British Journal of Surgery 1993;80:94–99.

16 Strasberg SM, McNevin MS. Results of a technique of pancreaticojejunostomy that optimizes blood supply to the pancreas. Journal of the American College of Surgeons 1998;187:591–596.

17 Fischer TD, Gutman DS, Hughes SJ, Trevino JG, Behrns KE. Disconnected pancreatic duct syndrome: disease classification and management strategies. Journal of the American College of Surgeons 2014;219:704–712.

18 Howard TJ, Rhodes GJ, Selzer DJ, Sherman S, Fogel E, Lehman GA. Roux-en-Y internal drainage is the best surgical option to treat patients with disconnected duct syndrome after severe acute pancreatitis. Surgery 2001;130:714–719; discussion 9–21.

19 Banks PA, Bollen TL, Dervenis C, et al. Classification of acute pancreatitis--2012: revision of the Atlanta classification and definitions by international consensus. Gut 2013;62:102–111.

20 Nealon WH, Bhutani M, Riall TS, Raju G, Ozkan O, Neilan R. A unifying concept: pancreatic ductal anatomy both predicts and determines the major complications resulting from pancreatitis. Journal of the American College of Surgeons 2009;208:790–799; discussion 9–801.

21 Howard TJ, Moore SA, Saxena R, Matthews DE, Schmidt CM, Wiebke EA. Pancreatic duct strictures are a common cause of recurrent pancreatitis after successful management of pancreatic necrosis. Surgery 2004;136:909–916.

22 Lavu H, Knuth JL, Baker MS, et al. Middle segment pancreatectomy can be safely incorporated into a pancreatic surgeon's clinical practice. Hepato Pancreato Biliary 2008;10:491–497.

23 Rodriguez JR, Razo AO, Targarona J, et al. Debridement and closed packing for sterile or infected necrotizing pancreatitis: insights into indications and outcomes in 167 patients. Annals of Surgery 2008;247:294–299.

24 Ross AS, Irani S, Gan SI, et al. Dual-modality drainage of infected and symptomatic walled-off pancreatic necrosis: long-term clinical outcomes. Gastrointestinal Endoscopy 2014;79:929–935.

25 Adams DB, Davis BR, Anderson MC. Colonic complications of pancreatitis. The American Surgeon 1994;60:44–49.

26 Van Minnen LP, Besselink MG, Bosscha K, Van Leeuwen MS, Schipper ME, Gooszen HG. Colonic involvement in acute pancreatitis. A retrospective study of 16 patients. Digestive Surgery 2004;21:33–38; discussion 9–40.

27 Mohamed SR, Siriwardena AK. Understanding the colonic complications of pancreatitis. Pancreatology 2008;8:153–158.

28 Ashley SW, Perez A, Pierce EA, et al. Necrotizing pancreatitis: contemporary analysis of 99 consecutive cases. Annals of Surgery 2001;234:572–579; discussion 9–80.

29 Gou S, Xiong J, Wu H, et al. Five-year cohort study of open pancreatic necrosectomy for necotizing pancreatitis suggests it is a safe and effective operation. Journal of Gastrointestinal Surgery 2013;17:1634–1642.

30 Ho HS, Frey CF. Gastrointestinal and pancreatic complications associated with severe pancreatitis. Archives of Surgery 1995;130:817–822; discussion 22–23.

31 Zarzour JG, Christein JD, Drelichman ER, Oser RF, Hawn MT. Percutaneous transhepatic duodenal diversion for the management of duodenal fistulae. Journal of Gastrointestinal Surgery 2008;12:1103–1109.

32 Butler JR, Eckert GJ, Zyromski NJ, Leonardi MJ, Lillemoe KD, Howard TJ. Natural history of pancreatitis-induced splenic vein thrombosis: a systematic review and meta-analysis of its incidence and rate of gastrointestinal bleeding. Hepato Pancreato Biliary 2011;13:839–845.

33 Easler J, Muddana V, Furlan A, et al. Portosplenomesenteric venous thrombosis in patients with acute pancreatitis is associated with pancreatic necrosis and usually has a benign course. Clinical Gastroenterology and Hepatology 2014,12:854 862.

34 Gonzelez HJ, Sahay SJ, Samadi B, Davidson BR, Rahman SH. Splanchnic vein thrombosis in severe acute pancreatitis: a 2-year, single-institution experience. Hepato Pancreato Biliary 2011;13:860–864.

35 Zyromski NJ, Vieira C, Stecker M, et al. Improved outcomes in postoperative and pancreatitis-related visceral pseudoaneurysms. Journal of Gastrointestinal Surgery 2007; 11:50–55.

36 Morgan K, Mansker D, Adams DB. Not just for trauma patients: damage control laparotomy in pancreatic surgery. Journal of Gastrointestinal Surgery 2010;14:768–772.

37 Tsiotos GG, Luque-de Leon E, Sarr MG. Long-term outcome of necrotizing pancreatitis treated by necrosectomy. The British Journal of Surgery 1998;85:1650–1653.

38 Connor S, Alexakis N, Raraty MG, et al. Early and late complications after pancreatic necrosectomy. Surgery 2005; 137:499–505.

39 Halonen KI, Pettila V, Leppaniemi AK, Kemppainen EA, Puolakkainen PA, Haapiainen RK. Long-term health-related quality of life in survivors of severe acute pancreatitis. Intensive Care Medicine 2003;29:782–786.

40 Reszetow J, Hac S, Dobrowolski S, et al. Biliary versus alcohol-related infected pancreatic necrosis: similarities and differences in the follow-up. Pancreas 2007;35:267–272.

41 Al-Azzawi HH, Kuhlenschmidt H, Howard TJ, et al. The burden of incisional hernia in necrotizing pancreatitis: how can we improve? American Journal of Surgery 2010;199:310–314; discussion 4.

42 Pendharkar SA, Salt K, Plank LD, Windsor JA, Petrov MS. Quality of life after acute pancreatitis: a systematic review and meta-analysis. Pancreas 2014;43:1194–1200.

43 Wright SE, Lochan R, Imrie K, et al. Quality of life and functional outcome at 3, 6 and 12 months after acute necrotising pancreatitis. Intensive Care Medicine 2009;35:1974–1978.

CHAPTER 11

History of chronic pancreatitis

Peter A. Banks[1,2]

[1] Department of Medicine, Harvard Medical School, Boston, MA, USA
[2] Center for Pancreatic Disease, Brigham and Women's Hospital, Boston, MA, USA

This international symposium on the Medical and Surgical Treatment of Chronic Pancreatitis has brought together more than 45 international thought leaders and specialists in chronic pancreatitis. Organized by David Adams, Peter Cotton, Horacio Rilo, and Nicholas Zyromski, the symposium includes thought leaders in medicine, surgery, psychology, physiology, pharmacology, and genetics. The goals of this symposium were to exchange ideas, to give thought to important unresolved issues in the medical and surgical treatment of chronic pancreatitis, and to plan future research.

The history of chronic pancreatitis is beautifully described in two outstanding books [1, 2]. The modern era is generally thought to date back to 1946, when Comfort and associates described the clinical course, pathology, and treatment of chronic relapsing pancreatitis and confirmed an association with excessive alcohol use [3]. Since then, the early features and natural history of chronic pancreatitis have been well described [4, 5]. There have been numerous efforts to classify and stage chronic pancreatitis [6–13] starting with the 1963 Marseille Meeting [6]. A listing of etiologic risk factors associated with chronic pancreatitis – the TIGAR-O Classification System – was outlined in 2010 [13]. This article defined chronic pancreatitis as "A continuing inflammatory disease of the pancreas characterized by irreversible morphologic changes that typically cause pain and/or permanent loss of function" [13].

Regarding etiologies of chronic pancreatitis, there has been considerable interest in tropical calcific pancreatitis [14], early- and late-onset idiopathic pancreatitis [15], autoimmune pancreatitis [16–19], and genetic predispositions [13, 20–28]. The association between chronic pancreatitis and pancreatic cancer has been firmly established [29]. The effect of alcohol and smoking on the development and severity of chronic pancreatitis has been well described [30, 31].

The pathophysiology of chronic pancreatitis initially focused on the importance of protein plugs within pancreatic ducts [32] and components of these plugs including GP2 [33]. More recently, emphasis has been placed on the activation of pancreatic stellate cells such as by ethanol [34, 35], the concept that sequential episodes of necrosis leads to fibrosis [3, 36, 37], and the sentinel acute pancreatitis event (SAPE) hypothesis model, which outlines the importance of metabolic and oxidative stress in the development of acute pancreatitis and the importance of activation of stellate cells which leads to fibrosis [22].

A variety of imaging techniques including abdominal ultrasound, CT scan, MRI, ERCP, and endoscopic ultrasound are now in use to support a diagnosis of chronic pancreatitis but thus far have not achieved sufficient accuracy to confirm a diagnosis of early chronic pancreatitis [13, 38–41].

Pancreatic function tests utilizing intravenous secretin with collection of pancreatic juice initially via a gastroduodenal tube and more recently via an endoscope have been utilized to identify a decrease in exocrine pancreatic function [41–43]. Fecal elastase test [44] has been shown to be significantly decreased in moderate to severe chronic pancreatitis but not mild chronic pancreatitis. The ^{13}C-mixed triglyceride breath test has been shown to be an accurate alternative to fecal fat quantification to detect fat maldigestion and to evaluate the effect of enzyme therapy on fat digestion [45].

The importance of pancreatic juice in digesting fat was demonstrated in 1856 by Bernard [46]. It was

Pancreatitis: Medical and Surgical Management, First Edition.
David B. Adams, Peter B. Cotton, Nicholas J. Zyromski and John Windsor.

established by DiMagno and associates in 1973 that steatorrhea does not occur until lipase output from the pancreas was 10% or less of normal [47]. The importance of curbing gastric acid output among patients who fail to respond to pancreatic enzymes replacement was established in 1977 [48]. Ways to improve efficiency of enzyme replacement therapy has recently been established [49].

In 1988, an analysis of nerves in chronic pancreatitis revealed evidence of edema in the nerve bundle and loss of barrier function by the perineural sheath [50]. In recent years, the neurobiology of pain in chronic pancreatitis has come under intense investigation [51–55]. In a recent randomized controlled trial, pregabalin reduced pain among patients with chronic pancreatitis [56].

Despite advances in our understanding of the neurobiology of chronic pancreatitis and despite numerous articles that report efficacy with a variety of treatments, effective therapies to relieve the pain of chronic pancreatitis are lacking. There have been two recent studies that have evaluated the efficacy of antioxidant therapy [57, 58]. One carried out in India mostly among patients with tropical pancreatitis reported a reduction in pain compared to the placebo [57]. The second among patients predominately with alcoholic chronic pancreatitis did not find a reduction in pain [58]. The use of pancreatic enzymes to reduce pain has been associated with uncertain benefit [59, 60]. Extracorporeal shock-wave lithotripsy of pancreatic calculi has been reported to decrease pain but has not been subjected to randomized prospective trials involving control patients who did not undergo shock-wave lithotripsy [61, 62]. Endoscopic ultrasound-guided celiac plexus block has not proven to be beneficial [63, 64]. Endoscopic therapy has been reported to relieve pain in chronic pancreatitis [65], but randomized prospective trials have suggested that surgical therapy is superior to endoscopic therapy for long-term pain reduction [66–68]. Several randomized prospective trials have compared surgical techniques to relieve pain associated with chronic pancreatitis and have determined that pain relief is comparable among the various techniques that were compared [69–75]. Total pancreatectomy with islet autotransplantation is now carried out in numerous medical centers. It has been pointed out that a multicenter registry will be very important to advance our knowledge of the efficacy of this technique and that well-designed clinical trials will be required to validate the benefit [76].

Despite a large number of recent articles on the diagnosis and treatment of chronic pancreatitis, many important questions remain unanswered, and many areas of research need to be addressed. Several are as follows:

- We need to be able to make an accurate diagnosis of early chronic pancreatitis. This will make possible the planning of randomized prospective trials on treatment options before the disease becomes firmly entrenched. It will also allow us to distinguish patients with early chronic pancreatitis from those with a chronic pain syndrome. Proteomic analysis of pancreatic fluid has identified candidate proteins that are being evaluated as possible biomarkers of early chronic pancreatitis [77].

- We need to have a better understanding of the natural history of chronic pancreatitis. At the present time, early intervention which may be ineffective may be altering the natural history of the disease such that it becomes impossible to distinguish changes in structure, function, and clinical features caused by the therapy itself versus the natural history of chronic pancreatitis. The Dutch Pancreatitis Study Group has undertaken a long-term prospective study of patients with chronic pancreatitis with active collaboration of 33 hospitals to study the natural history of the disease and the impact of treatment strategies [78].

- We need to have a better understanding of the impact of genetic mutations and ways to prevent and treat acute pancreatitis associated with these mutations.

- We need to improve our studies on the treatment of pain with emphasis on uniform criteria for the evaluation of pain and standardized reporting of patient outcomes [79, 80].

- We need rigorously designed controlled clinical trials to assess outcomes of treatment. Studies are needed to compare treatment alternatives such as medical versus surgical strategies.

- We need studies on the quality of life among patients with chronic pancreatitis and the impact of the disease on employment and other life domains affected by chronic pancreatitis [81].

- We need to identify new treatments of pain. New treatments may become available as a result of our better understanding of the neurobiology of pain.

- We need a better understanding of stellate cell function. A goal of this research would be to find ways to prevent and/or eliminate pancreatic fibrosis.

References

1 Howard JM, Hess W. History of the pancreas. Chapter 5, In: Chronic Pancreatitis, Including Pancreatic Lithiasis. Kluwer Academic/Plenum Publishers. NY. 2002. 261–316

2 Modlin IM, Kidd M. The paradox of the pancreas from Wirsung to Whipple. Solvay Pharmaceuticals.2003

3 Comfort MW, Gambill EE, Baggenstoss AH. Chronic relapsing in pancreatitis. Gastroenterology 1948; 6: 239–408

4 Ammann RW, Muellhaupt B, Zurich Pancreatitis Study Group. The natural history of pain in alcohol chronic pancreatitis. Gastroenterology 1999; 116: 1132–1140

5 Lankisch PG. Natural course of chronic pancreatitis. Pancreatology 2001; 1: 3–14

6 Sarles H Definitions and classifications of pancreatitis. Pancreas 1991; 6: 470–474

7 Chari ST, Singer MV. The problem of classification and staging of chronic pancreatitis. Proposals based on current knowledge of its natural history. Scandinavian Journal of Gastroenterology 1994; 29: 949–960

8 Ammann RW. A clinically based classification system for alcoholic chronic pancreatitis: summary of an international workshop on chronic pancreatitis. Pancreas 1997; 14: 215–221

9 Ramesh H Proposal for a new grading system for chronic pancreatitis. Journal of Clinical Gastroenterology 2002; 35: 67–70

10 Schneider A, Lohr JM, Singer MV. The M-ANNHEIM classification of chronic pancreatitis: introduction of a unifying classification system based on a review of previous classifications of the disease. Journal of Gastroenterology 2007; 42: 101–119

11 Kloppel G Toward a new classification of chronic panreatitis. Journal of Gastroenterology 2007; 42: 55–57

12 Buchler MW, Martignoni ME, Friess H, and Malfertheiner P. A proposal for a new clinical classification of chronic pancreatitis. BMC Gastroenterology 2009: 9: 93

13 Etemad B, Whitcomb DC. Chronic pancreatitis: diagnosis, classification and new genetic developments. Gastroenterology 2001; 120: 682–707

14 Geevarghese PJ. The differentiation of pancreatic and maturity-onset diabetes. Journal of the Indian Medical Association 1970; 54: 52–55

15 Layer P. Yamamoto H, Kalthoff L, et al. The different courses of early- and late-onset idiopathic and alcoholic chronic pancreatitis. Gastroenterology 1994; 107: 1481–1487

16 Zamboni G, Luttges J, Capelli P, Frulloni L. et al. Histopathological features of diagnostic and clinical relevance in autoimmune pancreatitis: a study of 53 resection specimens and 9 biopsy specimens. Virchows Archiv 2004; 445: 552–563

17 Okazak K, Sawa S, Kamisawa T, Naruse S, Tanaka S, et al. Clinical diagnostic criteria of autoimmune pancreatitis: revised proposal. Journal of Gastroenterology 2006; 41: 626–631

18 Chari ST, Kloeppel G, Zhang L, Notohara K, Lerch MM, et al. Histopathological and clinical subtypes of autoimmune pancreatitis. The Honolulu consensus document. Pancreas 2010; 39: 549–554

19 Kamisawa T, Chari ST, Giday SA, Kim MW, Chung JB, et al. Clinical profile of autoimmune pancreatitis and its histological subtypes. Pancreas 2011; 40: 809–814

20 Comfort MW, Steinberg A. Pedigree of a family with hereditary chronic relapsing pancreatitis. Gastro 1952; 21: 54–63

21 Whitcomb DC. Hereditary pancreatitis: new insights into acute and chronic pancreatitis. Gut 1999; 45: 317–322

22 Whitcomb DC. Value of genetic testing in the management of pancreatitis. Gut 2004; 53: 1710–1717

23 Rebours V, Bourtron-Rualt MC, Schnee M, Ferec C, LeMarechal C, et al. The natural history of hereditary pancreatitis: a national series. Gut 2009; 58: 97–103

24 Cohn JA, Friedman KJ, Noone PG, Knowles MR, et al. Relation between mutations of the cystic fibrosis gene and idiopathic pancreatitis. New England Journal of Medicine 1998; 339: 653–658

25 O Cy, Dorfman R, Cipolli M, Gonska T, Castellani C, et al. Type of CFTR mutation determines risk of pancreatitis in patients with cystic fibrosis. Gastroenterology 2011; 140: 153–161

26 Zhou J, Sahin-Toth M. Chymotrypsin C (CTRC) mutations in chronic pancreatitis. Journal of Gastroenterology and Hepatology 2011; 26: 1238–1246

27 Szabo A, Sahin-Toth M. Increased activation of hereditary pancreatitis-associated human cationic trypsinogen mutants in presence of Chymotryspin C. Journal of Biological Chemistry 2012; 287: 20701–20710

28 Whitcomb DC. Genetic risk factors for pancreatic disorders. Gastroenterology 2013; 144: 1292–1302

29 Lowenfels AB, Maisonneuve P, Cavallini G, Ammann RW, et al. Pancreatitis and the risk of pancreatic cancer. New England Journal of Medicine 1993; 328: 1433–1437

30 Yadav D, Whitcomb DC. The role of alcohol and smoking in pancreatitis. Nature Reviews Gastroenterology & Hepatology 2010; 1038: 1–15

31 Yen S, Hsieh CC, MacMahon B. Consumption of alcohol and tobacco and other risk factors for pancreatitis. American Journal of Epidemiology 1982; 116: 407–414

32 Provansal-Cheylan M, Mariani A, Bernard JP, Sarles H, Dupuy P Pancreatic stone protein: quantification in pancreatic juice by enzyme-linked immunosorbent assay and comparison with other methods. Pancreas 1989; 4: 680–689

33 Freedman SD, Sakamoto K, Venu RP. GP2, the homologue to the renal cast protein uromodulin, is a major component of intraductal plugs in chronic pancreatitis. Journal of Clinical Investigation 1993; 92: 83–90

34 Apte MV, Phillips PA, Fahmy RG, Darby SJ, et al. Does alcohol directly stimulate pancreatic fibrogenesis? Studies

with rat pancreatic stellate cells. Gastroenterology 2000; 118: 780–794

35 Witt H, Aptem V, Keim V, Wilson JS. Chronic pancreatitis: challenges and advances in pathogenesis, genetics, diagnosis, and therapy. Gastroenterology 2007; 132: 1557–1573

36 Kloppel G, Maillet B. Pathology of acute and chronic pancreatitis. Pancreas 1993; 8: 659–670

37 Ammann RW, Heitz PU, Kloppel G. Course of alcoholic chronic pancreatitis: a prospective clinic morphological long term study. Gastroenterology 1996; 111: 224–231

38 Conwell DL, Wu BU. Chronic pancreatitis: making the diagnosis. Clinical Gastroenterology and Hepatology 2012; 10: 1088–1095

39 Axon ATR, Classen M., Cotton PB, et al. Pancreatography in chronic pancreatitis: international definitions. Gut 1984; 25: 1107–1112

40 Catalano MF, Sahai A, Levy M, Romagnuolo J, Wiersema M, et al. EUS-based criteria for the diagnosis of chronic pancreatitis: the Rosemont classification. Gastrointestinal Endoscopy 2009; 69: 1251–1261

41 Conwell DL, Lee LL, Yadav D, Longnecker DS, et al. American pancreatic association practice guidelines in chronic pancreatitis. Pancreas 2014; 43: 1143–1162

42 Dreiling D, Hollander F. Studies in pancreatic function. Preliminary series of clinical studies with secretin test. Gastroenterology 1948; 11: 714–729

43 Conwell DL, Zuccaro G, Vargo J, Trolli PA, VanLente F, et al. An endoscopic pancreatic function test with synthetic porcine secretin for the evaluation of chronic abdominal pain and suspected chronic pancreatitis. Gastrointestinal Endoscopy 2003; 57: 37–40

44 Dominquez-Munoz JE, Hieronymus C, Sauerbruch T, et al. Fecal elastase test: evaluation of a new noninvasive pancreatic function test. American Journal of Gastroenterology 1995; 90: 1834–1837

45 Dominguez-Munoz JE, Iglesias-Garcia J, Vilarino-Insua M, et al. ^{13}C-mixed triglyceride breath test to assess oral enzyme substitution therapy in patients with chronic pancreatitis. Clinical Gastroenterology and Hepatology 2007; 5: 484–488

46 DiMagno EP. A short, eclectic history of exocrine pancreatic insufficiency and chronic pancreatitis. Gastroenterology 1993; 104: 1255–1262

47 DiMagno EP, Go VLW, Summerskill WHJ. Relations between pancreatic enzyme outputs and malabsorption in severe pancreatic insufficiency. New England Journal of Medicine 1973; 288: 813–815

48 Regan PT, Malagelada JR, DiMagno EP, et al. Comparative effects of antacids, cimetidine and enteric coating on the therapeutic response to oral enzymes in severe pancreatic insufficiency. New England Journal of Medicine 1977; 297: 854–858

49 Dominguez-Munoz JE. Pancreatic enzyme replacement therapy for pancreatic exocrine insufficiency: when it is

indicated, what is the goal and how to do it? Advances in Medical Sciences 2011; 56: 1–5

50 Bockman DE, Buchler M, Malfertheiner P, Berger HG. Analysis of nerves in chronic pancreatitis. Gastroenterology 1988; 94: 1459–1469

51 Friess H, Zhu ZW, diMola FF, Kulli C, et al. Nerve growth factor and its high-affinity receptor in chronic pancreatitis. Annals of Surgery 1999; 230: 615–624

52 Hoogerwerf WA, Shenoy M, Winston JH, et al. Trypsin mediates nociception via the proteinase-activated receptor 2: a potentially novel role in pancreatic pain. Gastroenterology 2004; 127: 883–891

53 Xu GY, Winston JH, Shenoy M, Yin H, et al. Transient receptor potential vanilloid 1 mediates hyperalgesia and is up-regulated in rats with chronic pancreatitis. Gastroenterol 2007; 133: 1282–1292

54 Dimcevski G, Sami SAK, Funch-Jensen P, LePera D, et al. Pain in chronic pancreatitis: the role of reorganization in the central nervous system. Gastroenterology 2007; 132: 1546–1556

55 Olesen SS, Brock C, Krarup AL, Funch-Jensen P, et al. Descending inhibitory pain modulation is impaired in patients with chronic pancreatitis. Clinical Gastroenterology and Hepatology 2010; 8: 724–730

56 Olesen SS, Bouwense SAW, Wilder-Smith OHG, et al. Pregabalin reduces pain in patients with chronic pancreatitis in a randomized, controlled study. Gastroenterology 2011; 141: 536–543

57 Bhardwaj P, et al. A randomized controlled trial of antioxidant supplementation for pain relief in patients with chronic pancreatitis. Gastroenterology 2009; 136: 149–159

58 Siriwardena AK, Mason JM, Sheen AJ, et al. Antioxidant therapy does not reduce pain in patients with chronic pancreatitis: the anticipate study. Gastroenterology 2012; 143: 655–663

59 Brown A, Hughes M, Tenner S, and Banks PA. Does pancreatic enzyme supplementation reduce pain in patients with chronic pancreatitis: A meta-analysis. American Journal of Gastroenterology 1997;92:2032–2035

60 Winstead NS, Wilcox CM. Clinical trials of pancreatic enzymes replacement for painful chronic pancreatitis – a review. Pancreatology 2009; 9: 344–350

61 Delhaye M, Vandermeeren A, Baize M, et al. Extracorporeal shock-wave lithotripsy of pancreatic calculi. Gastroenterology 1992; 102: 610–620

62 Dumonceau J-M, Costamagna G, Tringali A, Vahedi K, et al. Treatment for painful calcified chronic pancreatitis: extracorporeal shockwave lithotripsy versus endoscopic treatment: a randomized controlled trial. Gut 2007; 56: 545–552

63 Stevens T, Costanzo A, Lopez R, et al. Adding triamcinolone to endoscopic ultrasound-guided celiac plexus blockade does not reduce pain in patients with chronic pancreatitis. Clinical Gastroenterology and Hepatology 2012; 20: 186–191

64 Gress F, Schmitt C, Sherman S, Ciaccia D, et al. Endoscopic ultrasound-guided celiac plexus block for managing abdominal pain associated with chronic pancreatitis: a prospective single center experience. American Journal of Gastroenterology 2001; 96: 409–416

65 Clarke B, Slivka A, Tomizawa Y, Sanders M, Papachristou GI, et al. Endoscopic therapy is effective for patients with chronic pancreatitis. Clinical Gastroenterology and Hepatology 2012; 10: 795–802

66 Dite P, Ruzicka M, Zboril V, Novotny I. A prospective, randomized trial comparing endoscopic and surgical therapy for chronic pancreatitis. Endoscopy 2003; 35: 553–558

67 Cahen DL, Gouma DJ, Nio Y, et al. Endoscopic versus surgical drainage of the pancreatic duct in chronic pancreatitis. New England Journal of Medicine 2007; 356: 676–684

68 Cahen DL, Gouma DJ, Laramee PH, Nio Y, Rauws EAJ, et al. Long-term outcomes of endoscopic vs surgical drainage of the pancreatic duct in patients with chronic pancreatitis. Gastroenterology 2011; 141: 1690–1695

69 Izbicki JR, Bloechle C, Knoefel WT, et al. Duodenum-preserving resection of the head of the pancreas in chronic pancreatitis. Annals of Surgery 1995; 221: 350–358

70 Koninger J, Seiler CM, Sauerland S, et al. Duodenum-preserving pancreatic head resection – a randomized controlled trial comparing the original Beger procedure with Berne modification (ISRCTN No. 50638764). Surgery 2008; 143: 490–498

71 Muller MW, Friess H, Martin DJ, et al. Long term follow-up of a randomized clinical trial comparing Beger with pylorus-preserving Whipple procedure for chronic pancreatitis. British Journal of Surgery 2008; 95: 350–356

72 Strate T, Bachmann K, Busch P, Mann O, et al. Resection vs drainage in treatment of chronic pancreatitis: long-term results of randomized trial. Gastroenterology 2008; 134: 1406–1411

73 Keck T, Adam U, Makowiec F, et al. Short- and long-term results of duodenum preservation versus resection for the management of chronic pancreatitis: a prospective, randomized study. Surgery 2012; 152: S95–S102

74 Bachmann K, Tomkoetter L, Kutup A, et al. Is the Whipple procedure harmful for long-term outcome in treatment of chronic pancreatitis? Annals of Surgery 2013; 258: 815–821

75 Fernandez-del Castillo C, Warshaw AL. Surgical pioneers of the pancreas. American Journal of Surgery 2007; 194: S2–S5

76 Bellin MD, Gelrud A, Arreaza-Rubin G, Dunn TB, et al. Total pancreatectomy with islet autotransplantation. Pancreas 2014; 43: 1163–1171

77 Paulo JA, Kadiyala V, Lee LS, Banks PA, Conwell DL. Proteomic analysis (GeLC-MS/MS) of ePFT-collected pancreatic fluid in chronic pancreatitis. Journal of Proteome Research 2012; 11: 1897–1912

78 Ahmend Ali U, Issa Y, van Goor H, van Eijck CH, et al. Dutch chronic pancreatitis registry (CARE): design and rationale of a nationwide prospective evaluation and follow-up. Pancreatology 2015; 15: 46–52

79 Warshaw AL, Banks PA, Fernandez-Del CC. AGA technical review: treatment of pain in chronic pancreatitis. Gastroenterology 1998; 115: 765–776

80 Frey CF, Pitt HA, Yeo CJ, et al. A plea for uniform reporting of patient outcome in chronic pancreatitis. Archives of Surgery 1996; 131: 233–234

81 Gardner TB, Kennedy AT, Gelrud A, Banks PA, et al. Chronic pancreatitis and its effect on employment and health care experience. Results of a prospective American multicenter study. Pancreas 2010; 39: 498–501

CHAPTER 12

PART A: Epidemiology and pathophysiology: epidemiology and risk factors

Dhiraj Yadav & Julia Greer

Division of Gastroenterology & Hepatology, Department of Medicine, University of Pittsburgh Medical Center, Pittsburgh, PA, USA

Introduction

Chronic pancreatitis (CP) is a multifactorial disease characterized by long-standing inflammatory infiltration and destruction of pancreatic parenchyma, leading to glandular fibrosis, progressive endocrine, and exocrine failure. CP was first described in 1788 by Sir Thomas Cawley, when he remarked at autopsy that the pancreas of a diabetic patient was atrophied and full of calculi [1]. Further studies conducted in 1889 by Minkowski and von Mering demonstrated that removing the pancreas of various animals – including "dogs, cats, pigs, carnivorous birds, frogs, and turtles" – often resulted in permanent glycosuria similar to that seen in diabetics, and that death followed quickly for these animals [1].

Our understanding of the disease has grown significantly in the past few decades. How we define and characterize CP has also changed over the years. Terms that were previously used, such as chronic calcific pancreatitis, chronic obstructive pancreatitis, and relapsing alcoholic pancreatitis, have generally been replaced with "chronic pancreatitis" and "recurrent acute" or "acute recurrent pancreatitis." Advancements in medical imaging and endoscopy allow detailed evaluation of the morphology and functionality of the pancreas. CP is now more accurately diagnosed based on the widespread usage of computed tomography (CT), magnetic resonance imaging (MRI), magnetic resonance cholangiopancreatography (MRCP), and endoscopic ultrasound (EUS). The inception of thin slice, multidetector CT images provides excellent visual resolution for determining parenchymal and ductal changes as well as complications of CP. Population estimates of disease burden are now possible, due in large part to advances in computer technology and software programs that easily allow quantitative information to be captured and analyzed. Finally, advances in our understanding of genetic factors that increase the risk of pancreatitis, and ongoing molecular research hold promise into providing answers to the pathophysiology and course of this once considered enigmatic disease.

Changing epidemiology of chronic pancreatitis

Understanding the epidemiology can provide us with an understanding of disease estimates and trends, while elucidating risk factors and their respective degrees of disease association. Between the 1950 and 1990s, well-conducted, mostly single-center studies, consisting predominantly of male patients with alcoholic CP, defined the clinical presentation and natural course of CP [2–6]. A diagnosis of CP was established by imaging (abdominal X-ray, ultrasonography, or endoscopic retrograde cholangiopancreatography [ERCP] and CT scan in later years), functional testing or histology. Diagnosis was often possible only after substantial structural changes or functional alterations were detected. Although empiric data are not available, advancements in imaging technology, ability to study large populations, and performance of genetic testing in the past 2–3 decades have likely had an impact on the epidemiology of CP.

High-quality imaging studies enable the identification of subtle changes in pancreatic morphology and offer the ability to indirectly assess pancreatic function (secretin-stimulated MRCP). This may in turn lead to the detection of disease at a stage before the development of significant functional alterations. Imaging studies may also help to differentiate conditions that are not easily distinguishable from CP-related changes, such as cystic tumors of the pancreas (especially intraductal papillary mucinous neoplasms), or newly described entities such as autoimmune pancreatitis. Availability of population-based data provides a broader context of the distribution of risk factors and disease burden in a population and understanding of its natural history. Genetic discoveries provide insights into the mechanistic basis of disease, which can be studied through more focused evaluation of disease pathways.

It is also valuable to note that the epidemiology of CP may be modified by fluctuating predisposing factors at a population level in many regions of the world. Alcohol and cigarette smoking are becoming more common habits in less developed countries, resulting in rising rates of CP [7, 8]. With some exceptions, the per capita alcohol consumption in the Western countries is either stable or decreasing. In the United States, the per capita alcohol consumption has remained mostly constant but the habit of cigarette smoking is on the decline [9]. Adding to the medical literature, a growing number of studies that focus on unusual causes of CP, such as celiac disease and inflammatory bowel disease [10, 11], are being published.

Disease burden

Data on incidence and prevalence of CP are available from many populations [12–23] (Tables 12A.1 and 12A.2). The yearly incidence of CP ranges from 1.77 to 11.9 per 100,000 population and is generally higher in men when compared with women. The observed variability between studies and populations is related to definitions used for patient ascertainment, study design, and distribution of risk factors. As an example, a population-based cohort from Olmstead County, Minnesota, reported a yearly incidence rate from 1997 to 2006 to be 4.4 per 100,000 population [19]. Studies from Germany and the Czech Republic using a similar study design during roughly the same time period found

Table 12A.1 Incidence of chronic pancreatitis in population-based studies after 1985.

Population	Year(s) of study	Incidence per 100,000 population
Lunenburg County, Germany	1988–1995	6.4
Moravia, Czech Republic	1999	7.9
Olmsted County, Minnesota, USA	1997–2006	4.4
Japan	1994	5.4
Japan	2007	11.9
Japan	2011	14.0
Britain	1999–2000	8.6
USA	1988–2004	8.1
Netherlands	2000–2005	1.77
Netherlands	2004	8.4
Allegheny County, Pennsylvania, USA	1996–2005	7.8

Refs [12–15, 17–22].

Table 12A.2 Prevalence of chronic pancreatitis in population-based studies after 1985.

Population	Year(s) of study	Prevalence per 100,000 population
Japan	1994	28.5
Japan	2007	36.9
Japan	2011	52.4
France	2003	26.4
Olmsted County, USA	2006	41.8

Refs [14, 16, 19, 23].

incidence rates to be higher (6.4 and 7.9 per 100,000) [12, 15]. Within the United States, the incidence rate of CP varied from 4.4 to 7.8 and 8.1 per 100,000 depending on study design [18–20]. Based on the US reports, using a strict definition, there are an estimated 15,000–25,000 incident cases each year and between 150,000 and 200,000 prevalent cases of definite CP in the United States [19, 20, 23].

In Olmsted County, MN, the age- and gender-adjusted prevalence rate per 100,000 individuals was 41.76 (95% CI 30.21–53.32) [19]. An increase in the prevalence rate was noted in Japan over a 17-year period from

28.5 in 1994 to 52.4 per 100,000 population in 2011. An increase in the prevalence of CP was also described from 6 urban health-care regions and 22 hospitals in China from 1996 to 2003: 3.08, 3.91, 5.28, 7.61, 10.43, 11.92, 12.84, and 13.52 per 100,000 inhabitants [8].

Risk factors

Alcohol consumption

Heavy alcohol consumption is the most prominent risk factor for pancreatitis. However, the relationship between alcohol and pancreatitis is complex. While there is no doubt that the risk of both acute and chronic forms of pancreatitis is heightened by alcohol consumption, only ~5% alcoholics develop clinical pancreatitis [24, 25]. Studies have explored the reasons for this individual susceptibility in several ways, including the amount, style (e.g., binge drinking) [26], type of alcohol [27], role of cofactors, and genetic susceptibility.

The degree of statistical association with the amount of alcohol consumption is valuable information to know. Data from a sizeable cohort study, the Copenhagen Heart Study, noted that risk of pancreatitis increased in a dose-dependent manner [28]. Among their 17,905 male and female participants, hazard ratios (HRs) for pancreatitis associated with drinking 1–6, 7–13, 14–20, 21–34, 35–48, and >48 drinks/week were 1.1 (95% CI 0.8, 1.6), 1.2 (95% CI 0.8, 1.8), 1.3 (95% CI 0.8, 2.1), 1.3 (95% CI 0.7, 2.2), 2.6 (95% CI 1.4, 4.8), and 3.0 (95% CI 1.6, 5.7), respectively, compared with 0 drinks per week [P(trend) < 0.001]. An amply sized case–control study (416 cases, 555 controls) from the United States (NAPS2) found the risk of CP to increase at or beyond a threshold of approximately 5 drinks/day (odds ratio, 3.1) [29]. However, a systematic review and meta-analysis of 6 studies, including 146,517 individuals with 1671 cases of pancreatitis, found that CP risk was increased among individuals who drank 4 or more alcoholic beverages per day but not among lower drinking categories [30]. Finally, a recent study from Japan, not included in the systematic review and meta-analysis, also reported a dose-dependent increase in the risk of CP with alcohol consumption of ≥20 g/day [31].

A common environmental factor affiliated with alcohol consumption is cigarette smoking. Together, the risk of pancreatitis may be multiplicative in the presence of both behaviors [29]. Genetic susceptibility has been linked to polymorphisms in alcohol-metabolizing genes [32], and more recently to a factor identified on the X-chromosome at the *Claudin-2* locus, which may explain the heightened risk of alcoholic pancreatitis, especially in men [33].

Cigarette smoking

As early as 1982, it had been shown that cigarette smoking was associated with the development of chronic or recurrent pancreatitis, especially among males [34]. A decade later, a study that included 145 patients with CP noted that 94% were both smokers and drinkers and that the mean age at onset of pancreatitis was lower among smokers [35]. A 1999 Italian study noted that the risk of developing CP correlates with both alcohol intake and cigarette smoking, with a trend indicating higher risk with increasing levels of each factor; in addition, the authors of the study determined that alcohol and smoking are statistically independent risk factors for CP [36]. In the multi-institutional NAPS2 study, 47.3% of CP patients were current smokers, 24.1% were past smokers, and 28.6% reported being never smokers. The prevalence of smoking was noted to grow incrementally with the quantity of alcohol consumed, which reflects that these two habits often coexist [29].

In a meta-analysis of 10 case–control and 2 cohort studies that included 1705 patients, the pooled risk estimates of CP were 2.5 (95% CI, 1.3, 4.6) when the analysis was adjusted to control for alcohol consumption. Risk was more than doubled to 2.4 (95% CI, 0.9, 6.6) among participants who smoked <1 pack of cigarettes per day and increased to 3.3 (95% CI, 1.4 7.9) among those smoking ≥1 packs per day [37]. Smoking has been shown to increase the risk of developing CP independent of alcohol, although the pathologic impact of cigarette smoking appears to be greatest for patients with alcohol-related CP, providing evidence that it enhances the effects of alcohol consumption [29]. In a retrospective 5-country cohort study of 934 patients with chronic alcoholic pancreatitis where information on smoking was available, CP was diagnosed, on average, 4.7 years earlier in smokers than in non-smokers (P = 0.001) [38]. Tobacco smoking significantly increased the risk of pancreatic calcifications (HR 4.9 (95% CI 2.3, 10.5) for smokers vs. nonsmokers) and to a lesser extent the risk of diabetes (HR 2.3 (95% CI 1.2, 4.2)) during the course of pancreatitis [38].

There is high variability among physicians in the recognition of smoking as a risk factor for CP. In the NAPS2 study, among self-reported smokers, physicians recognized smoking to be a risk factor in only 45.3% ever, 53% current, and 49.8% heavy smokers and in 54.5% with alcohol etiology [39]. These findings highlight the need for educating physicians and the public on the potential benefits of smoking cessation. Although empiric data are not available, the effects of tobacco products other than cigarette smoking (e.g., tobacco chewing) could be similar to cigarette smoking. Counseling should also be extended to patients who indulge in these habits.

Genetic factors

One of the original reports on familial inheritance of pancreatitis was published over six decades ago [40]. It was only in 1996 that the genetic basis was first described when investigators traced the susceptibility to pancreatitis in multiple members of a large family to mutations in the cationic trypsinogen gene (*PRSS1*) in an autosomal dominant pattern [41]. This finding has been replicated from different parts of the world. Since then, several additional genes that affect susceptibility to pancreatitis have been identified (Table 12A.3) [42]. With ongoing research, many more genetic susceptibility factors are expected to be discovered.

Genetic causes are associated with an earlier age of disease onset and more often are noted among patients who do not have alcohol etiology. About one-fourth of patients with idiopathic CP are identified to have *CFTR* mutations. A 2010 study found that 242 of 411 (58.9%) CP patients at a tertiary care center in India had idiopathic chronic pancreatitis, with close to half of the individuals in this subgroup carrying a *SPINK1* N34S

Table 12A.3 Genetic factors associated with chronic pancreatitis.

Gene
Cationic trypsinogen (*PRSS1*, *PRSS2*)
Pancreatic secretory trypsin inhibitor (*SPINK1*), cystic fibrosis transmembrane conductance receptor (*CFTR*)
Chymotrypsin C (*CTRC*)
Calcium-sensing receptor (*CASR*)
Carboxypeptidase A1 (*CPA1*)
Claudin-2

mutation, while 50 patients carried either a mutation or polymorphism in the *CFTR* gene [43].

The mechanisms by which genetic mutations increase the risk of pancreatitis may involve trypsin activity or degradation (*PRSS1*, *SPINK1*, and *CTRC*), reduction of fluid secretion that may affect flushing of pancreatic enzymes from the ductal system (*CFTR*) or non-trypsin-dependent mechanisms (*CPA1*, *Claudin-2*). Clinical pancreatitis with *CFTR* mutations has been correlated with the degree of residual CFTR function. In an elegant study, the risk of clinical pancreatitis in patients with cystic fibrosis was correlated with the degree of residual CFTR function. In pancreas sufficient cystic fibrosis patients, the risk of clinical pancreatitis was noted to be ~25% (which is ~50-fold higher than the general population) [44]. More recently, a set of *CFTR* mutations previously considered to be benign were demonstrated to specifically affect bicarbonate transport, thereby increasing the risk of pancreatitis but not lung disease [45].

Anatomic abnormalities

Obstruction of the pancreatic duct can lead to changes of CP in the upstream segment. On pathology, CP changes are often described in surgical specimens from patients with pancreatic ductal adenocarcinoma, even when CP was not the predisposing factor. Changes of CP, including calcifications, can also be seen in patients with long-standing pancreatic duct strictures or from intermittent duct obstruction from mucin production in patients with intraductal papillary mucinous neoplasms [46]. Other uncommon causes would include anomalous pancreaticobiliary junction or annular pancreas.

The role of pancreas divisum and sphincter of Oddi dysfunction in the causation of CP remains uncertain. Physicians often consider these as potential etiologies in patients with otherwise unexplained pancreatitis. In a recent small study, the prevalence of *CFTR* mutations was noted to be significantly higher among patients with CP who also had pancreas divisum compared with controls and other forms of CP [47], suggesting that pancreas divisum may increase the risk of CP only in the presence of additional factors. These findings need to be replicated in a larger cohort and from other centers. In a large fraction of patients with recurrent acute pancreatitis, pancreatic sphincter pressures were noted to be high, raising the possibility that the increased pressure could be an effect of pancreatitis rather than its cause [48].

Other risk factors

Many nontraditional risk factors were identified in the TIGAR-O classification for pancreatitis proposed in 2001 [49]. Empiric data on the distribution of risk factors in a cohort of CP have been published in abstract form; formal results are anticipated to be published soon.

Etiology of chronic pancreatitis

Alcohol continues to be the most common etiology for CP in developed countries. With increasing affluence, the proportion of cases attributed to alcohol has also increased in other parts of the world. The etiologic spectrum of CP is broadening to recognize entities such as genetic, autoimmune, obstructive, and others. Data on the current etiologic distribution of CP published from select large studies in different regions are shown in Table 12A.4 [7, 8, 13, 50, 51]. Data have been collected in a nationwide registry from Netherlands the results of which will be forthcoming soon [52].

In the US, Italian, and Japanese studies, alcohol was considered to be the primary cause of CP in 43–67.5% of patients, while a sizeable fraction (17–28.6%) had idiopathic disease. Data from a multicenter study from India reported idiopathic disease to be most common (60.2%) followed by alcohol (38.7%). Only 3.8% of cases could be described as "tropical pancreatitis" using well-delineated criteria. In a multicenter study from China, alcohol and biliary causes were each attributed to about one-third cases, while 12.9% cases were diagnosed with idiopathic disease.

There are etiologic differences based on sex and age. Alcohol is the predominant etiology in men, and idiopathic is most common in women. The median age of diagnosis of CP is around 50–55 years. In patients with alcoholic etiology, symptoms typically begin between ages 40 and 50 years. Patients with genetic etiologies usually present between ages 10 and 30 years. Idiopathic CP can have a bimodal distribution. For reasons that have not been clearly defined, blacks have a two- to threefold higher risk of pancreatitis when compared with whites [18].

Natural history

The clinical course of patients with CP is highly variable and can include any combination of the following – episodes of acute pancreatitis, pain experience (none to severe, intermittent, or constant), endocrine and/or exocrine insufficiency, or local complications such as pseudocysts, compression of neighboring structures such as common bile duct or gastric outlet, and occlusion of peripancreatic vessels. The natural history of CP has been described for two broad etiologic subgroups: alcoholic and nonalcoholic [3, 53]. Patients with alcoholic CP have a more aggressive clinical course with development of calcifications, and exocrine and endocrine insufficiency over a period of few years. They have a higher chance of developing local complications. The majority of patients with early-onset idiopathic CP have abdominal pain and episodes of acute pancreatitis, but development of morphological changes, diabetes and exocrine insufficiency evolves slowly over a period

Table 12A.4 Etiology of chronic pancreatitis in selected recent large cross-sectional studies from different regions of the world.

%	USA (n = 539)	Italy (n = 893)	Japan (n = 1734)	China (n = 2008)	India (n = 1033)
Alcohol	44.5	34.0	67.5	35.11	38.7
Alcohol plus obstructive	-	9.0	-	-	-
Idiopathic	28.6	17.0	20.0	12.90	60.2
Obstructive	8.7	27.0	-	-	-
Genetic	8.7	4.0	0.3	7.22	-
Autoimmune	2.2	4.0	0.7	-	-
Other	7.2	6.0[a]	11.5	44.77[b]	1.1

[a]Dystrophy (6%).
[b]Biliary stone disease (34.36%), pancreatic trauma (10.41%).
Refs [7, 8, 13, 48, 50].

of two to three decades. Patients with late-onset idiopathic CP have a somewhat milder clinical course with less frequent abdominal pain and acute pancreatitis episodes when compared with early-onset and alcoholic CP. The clinical course of patients with specific nonalcoholic etiologies (e.g., genetic causes) generally mimics those with idiopathic CP.

CP has a profound effect on the physical quality of life and a significant effect on mental quality of life when compared with control subjects. Quality of life in CP patients is similar or worse when compared with many other chronic medical conditions. The NAPS2 study quantified the impact of CP on the physical and mental quality of life (a reduction of 12.02 and 4.24 points, respectively; a difference of 3 points of statistical significance) when compared with control subjects after accounting for demographic, lifestyle factors, and a limited number of medical comorbidities [54].

When compared with age- and sex- matched subjects in the general population, the lifespan of CP is significantly shorter. However, it is important to recognize that although CP has high morbidity, most patients die from causes other than CP [19]. CP increases the risk of pancreatic cancer, especially in patients with hereditary pancreatitis [55].

Evolution of chronic pancreatitis

There is growing recognition that acute, recurrent acute, and CP represent a disease continuum. In population studies, the risk of recurrence after the first episode of acute pancreatitis is about 20–25%. A similar fraction of patients with recurrent acute pancreatitis may transition to CP. The risk of progression is greater among patients with alcohol etiology when compared with nonalcoholic etiologies. In a Japanese study of 2533 patients with a first episode of moderate or severe acute pancreatitis, individuals who continued to drink at similar levels to what they drank prior to the acute event had a 41% chance of progressing to develop CP compared with 23% progression among those with decreased, but moderate, drinking; among patients who became abstinent to alcohol or only drank occasionally, the rate of progression to CP was only 14% [56]. Thus, decreasing the level of alcohol consumption diminishes the likelihood of disease progression. This observation is confirmed in a randomized controlled trial that enrolled

patients with a first episode of acute alcoholic pancreatitis. Subjects were randomized to repeated counseling every 6 months and compared with usual care after an initial counseling session. It was demonstrated that the risk of hospitalizations and recurrences of pancreatitis were significantly reduced in the intervention arm [57]. Smoking has also been associated with the risk of recurrent pancreatitis and progression of CP. Therefore, an important component of management should be to identify patients who may benefit from behavior modification and offer such services.

The risk of disease progression is high in patients with genetic etiologies, especially hereditary pancreatitis and subsets of patients with *CFTR* mutations. At present, there are no specific treatment options available to reduce the risk of disease progression in patients with genetic abnormalities.

Future directions

Many advances have been made in our understanding of the epidemiology of CP in the past few decades. Future studies in different populations should define disease estimates, evolution, and natural history more precisely. Studies that use information from genetic discoveries to identify disease mechanisms are needed to help design treatment strategies that may alter disease course.

Conflict of interest

The authors report no conflict of interest relevant to this manuscript.

References

1 Osler W, McCrae T. Modern Medicine: Its Theory and Practice, in Original Contributions by American and Foreign Authors, 1. Lea Brothers & Company, 1907.

2 Lankisch PG, Lohr-Happe A, Otto J, et al. Natural course in chronic pancreatitis. Pain, exocrine and endocrine pancreatic insufficiency and prognosis of the disease. Digestion. 1993;54(3):148–155.

3 Layer P, Yamamoto H, Kalthoff L, et al. The different courses of early- and late-onset idiopathic and alcoholic chronic pancreatitis. Gastroenterology. 1994;107(5):1481–1487.

4 Dani R, Mott CB, Guarita DR, et al. Epidemiology and etiology of chronic pancreatitis in Brazil: a tale of two cities. Pancreas. 1990;5(4):474–478.

5 Lowenfels AB, Maisonneuve P, Cavallini G, et al. Prognosis of chronic pancreatitis: an international multicenter study. International Pancreatitis Study Group. The American Journal of Gastroenterology. 1994 ;89(9):1467–1471.

6 Marks IN, Bank S, Louw JH. Chronic pancreatitis in the Western Cape. Digestion. 1973;9(5):447–453.

7 Balakrishnan V, Unnikrishnan AG, Thomas V, et al. Chronic pancreatitis. A prospective nationwide study of 1,086 subjects from India. Journal of the Pancreas.2008;9(5):593–600.

8 Wang LW, Li ZS, Li SD, et al. Prevalence and clinical features of chronic pancreatitis in China: a retrospective multicenter analysis over 10 years. Pancreas. 2009;38(3):248–254.

9 Trends in Current Cigarette Smoking Among High School Students and Adults, United States, 1965–2011. Smoking and Tobacco Use. The Centers for Disease Control and Prevention. Sourced from: Office on Smoking and Health, National Center for Chronic Disease Prevention and Health Promotion. http://www.cdc.gov/tobacco/data_statistics/tables/trends/cig_smoking/. Accessed December 19, 2014.

10 Barthet M, Hastier P, Bernard JP, et al. Chronic pancreatitis and inflammatory bowel disease: true or coincidental association? The American Journal of Gastroenterology. 1999;94(8):2141–2148.

11 Sadr-Azodi O, Sanders DS, Murray JA, et al. Patients with celiac disease have an increased risk for pancreatitis. Clinical Gastroenterology and Hepatology. 2012;10(10):1136–1142.

12 Dite P, Stary K, Novotny I, et al. Incidence of chronic pancreatitis in the Czech Republic. European Journal of Gastroenterology & Hepatology. 2001;13(6):749–750.

13 Hirota M, Shimosegawa T, Masamune A, et al. The seventh nationwide epidemiological survey for chronic pancreatitis in Japan: Clinical significance of smoking habit in Japanese patients. Pancreatology. 2014;14(6):490–496.

14 Hirota M, Shimosegawa T, Masamune A, et al. The sixth nationwide epidemiological survey of chronic pancreatitis in Japan. Pancreatology. 2012;12(2):79–84.

15 Lankisch PG, Assmus C, Maisonneuve P, et al. Epidemiology of pancreatic diseases in Luneburg County. A study in a defined German population. Pancreatology. 2002;2(5):469–477.

16 Levy P, Barthet M, Mollard BR, et al. Estimation of the prevalence and incidence of chronic pancreatitis and its complications. Gastroenterologie clinique et biologique. 2006;30(6–7):838–844.

17 Tinto A, Lloyd DA, Kang JY, et al. Acute and chronic pancreatitis--diseases on the rise: a study of hospital admissions in England 1989/90-1999/2000. Alimentary Pharmacology & Therapeutics. 2002;16(12):2097–2105.

18 Yadav D, Muddana V, O'Connell M. Hospitalizations for chronic pancreatitis in Allegheny county, Pennsylvania, USA. Pancreatology. 2011;11(6):546–552.

19 Yadav D, Timmons L, Benson JT, et al. Incidence, prevalence, and survival of chronic pancreatitis: a population-based study. The American Journal of Gastroenterology. 2011;106(12):2192–2199.

20 Yang AL, Vadhavkar S, Singh G, et al. Epidemiology of alcohol-related liver and pancreatic disease in the United States. Archives of Internal Medicine. 2008;168(6):649–656.

21 Spanier B, Bruno MJ, Dijkgraaf MG. Incidence and mortality of acute and chronic pancreatitis in the Netherlands: a nationwide record-linked cohort study for the years 1995–2005. World Journal of Gastroenterology. 2013;19(20):3018–3026.

22 Spanier BW, Dijkgraaf MG, Bruno MJ. Trends and forecasts of hospital admissions for acute and chronic pancreatitis in the Netherlands. European Journal of Gastroenterology & Hepatology. 2008;20(7):653–658.

23 Lin Y, Tamakoshi A, Matsuno S, et al. Nationwide epidemiological survey of chronic pancreatitis in Japan. Journal of gastroenterology. 2000;35(2):136–141.

24 Lankisch PG, Lowenfels AB, Maisonneuve P. What is the risk of alcoholic pancreatitis in heavy drinkers? Pancreas. 2002;25(4):411–412.

25 Yadav D, Eigenbrodt ML, Briggs MJ, et al. Pancreatitis: prevalence and risk factors among male veterans in a detoxification program. Pancreas. 2007;34(4):390–398.

26 Phillip V, Huber W, Hagemes F, et al. Incidence of acute pancreatitis does not increase during Oktoberfest, but is higher than previously described in Germany. Clinical Gastroenterology and Hepatology. 2011;9(11):995–1000.

27 Sadr Azodi O, Orsini N, Andren-Sandberg A, et al. Effect of type of alcoholic beverage in causing acute pancreatitis. British Journal of Surgery. 2011;98(11):1609–1616.

28 Kristiansen L, Gronbaek M, Becker U, et al. Risk of pancreatitis according to alcohol drinking habits: a population-based cohort study. American Journal of Epidemiology. 2008;168(8):932–937.

29 Yadav D, Hawes RH, Brand RE, et al. Alcohol consumption, cigarette smoking, and the risk of recurrent acute and chronic pancreatitis. Archives of Internal Medicine. 2009;169(11):1035–1045.

30 Irving HM, Samokhvalov AV, Rehm J. Alcohol as a risk factor for pancreatitis. A systematic review and meta-analysis. Journal of the Pancreas. 2009;10(4):387–392.

31 Kume K, Masamune A, Ariga H, et al. Alcohol consumption and the risk for developing pancreatitis: a case–control study in Japan. Pancreas. 2015;44(1):53–58.

32 Zhong Y, Cao J, Zou R, et al. Genetic polymorphisms in alcohol dehydrogenase, aldehyde dehydrogenase and alcoholic chronic pancreatitis susceptibility: a meta-analysis. Gastroenterology and Hepatology 2015 38(7):417–425.

33 Whitcomb DC, LaRusch J, Krasinskas AM, et al. Common genetic variants in the CLDN2 and PRSS1-PRSS2 loci alter risk for alcohol-related and sporadic pancreatitis. Nature Genetics. 2012;44(12):1349–1354.

34 Yen S, Hsieh CC, MacMahon B. Consumption of alcohol and tobacco and other risk factors for pancreatitis. American Journal of Epidemiology. 1982;116(3):407–414.

35 Bourliere M, Barthet M, Berthezene P, et al. Is tobacco a risk factor for chronic pancreatitis and alcoholic cirrhosis? Gut. 1991;32(11):1392–1395.

36 Talamini G, Bassi C, Falconi M, et al. Cigarette smoking: an independent risk factor in alcoholic pancreatitis. Pancreas. 1996;12(2):131–137.

37 Andriulli A, Botteri E, Almasio PL, et al. Smoking as a cofactor for causation of chronic pancreatitis: a meta-analysis. Pancreas. 2010;39(8):1205–1210.

38 Maisonneuve P, Lowenfels AB, Mullhaupt B, et al. Cigarette smoking accelerates progression of alcoholic chronic pancreatitis. Gut. 2005;54(4):510–514.

39 Yadav D, Slivka A, Sherman S, et al. Smoking is underrecognized as a risk factor for chronic pancreatitis. Pancreatology. 2010;10(6):713–719.

40 Comfort MW, Steinberg AG. Pedigree of a family with hereditary chronic relapsing pancreatitis. Gastroenterology. 1952;21(1):54–63.

41 Whitcomb DC, Gorry MC, Preston RA, et al. Hereditary pancreatitis is caused by a mutation in the cationic trypsinogen gene. Nature Genetics. 1996;14(2):141–145.

42 Whitcomb DC. Genetic risk factors for pancreatic disorders. Gastroenterology. 2013;144(6):1292–1302.

43 Midha S, Khajuria R, Shastri S, et al. Idiopathic chronic pancreatitis in India: phenotypic characterisation and strong genetic susceptibility due to SPINK1 and CFTR gene mutations. Gut. 2010;59(6):800–807.

44 Ooi CY, Dorfman R, Cipolli M, et al. Type of CFTR mutation determines risk of pancreatitis in patients with cystic fibrosis. Gastroenterology. 2011;140(1):153–161.

45 LaRusch J, Jung J, General IJ, et al. Mechanisms of CFTR functional variants that impair regulated bicarbonate permeation and increase risk for pancreatitis but not for cystic fibrosis. PLoS Genetics. 2014;10(7):e1004376.

46 Zapiach M, Yadav D, Smyrk TC, et al. Calcifying obstructive pancreatitis: a study of intraductal papillary mucinous neoplasm associated with pancreatic calcification. Clinical Gastroenterology and Hepatology. 2004;2(1):57–63.

47 Bertin C, Pelletier AL, Vullierme MP, et al. Pancreas divisum is not a cause of pancreatitis by itself but acts as a partner of genetic mutations. The American Journal of Gastroenterology. 2012;107(2):311–317.

48 Cote GA, Imperiale TF, Schmidt SE, et al. Similar efficacies of biliary, with or without pancreatic, sphincterotomy in treatment of idiopathic recurrent acute pancreatitis. Gastroenterology. 2012;143(6):1502–1509.

49 Etemad B, Whitcomb DC. Chronic pancreatitis: diagnosis, classification, and new genetic developments. Gastroenterology. 2001;120(3):682–707.

50 Frulloni L, Gabbrielli A, Pezzilli R, et al. Chronic pancreatitis: report from a multicenter Italian survey (PanCroInfAISP) on 893 patients. Digestive and Liver Disease. 2009;41(4):311–317.

51 Cote GA, Yadav D, Slivka A, et al. Alcohol and smoking as risk factors in an epidemiology study of patients with chronic pancreatitis. Clinical Gastroenterology and Hepatology. 2011;9(3):266–273.

52 Ahmed Ali U, Issa Y, van Goor H, et al. Dutch chronic pancreatitis registry (CARE): design and rationale of a nationwide prospective evaluation and follow-up. Pancreatology. 2014;15:46–52.

53 Ammann RW, Buehler H, Muench R, et al. Differences in the natural history of idiopathic (nonalcoholic) and alcoholic chronic pancreatitis. A comparative long-term study of 287 patients. Pancreas. 1987;2(4):368–377.

54 Amann ST, Yadav D, Barmada MM, et al. Physical and mental quality of life in chronic pancreatitis: a case–control study from the North American Pancreatitis Study 2 cohort. Pancreas. 2013;42(2):293–300.

55 Lowenfels AB, Maisonneuve P, DiMagno EP, et al. Hereditary pancreatitis and the risk of pancreatic cancer. International Hereditary Pancreatitis Study Group. Journal of the National Cancer Institute. 1997;89(6):442–446.

56 Takeyama Y. Long-term prognosis of acute pancreatitis in Japan. Clinical Gastroenterology and Hepatology. 2009;7(11 Suppl):S15-S17.

57 Nordback I, Pelli H, Lappalainen-Lehto R, et al. The recurrence of acute alcohol-associated pancreatitis can be reduced: a randomized controlled trial. Gastroenterology. 2009;136(3):848–855.

PART B: Epidemiology and pathophysiology: genetic insights into pathogenesis

David C. Whitcomb

Division of Gastroenterology, Hepatology and Nutrition, Departments of Medicine, Cell Biology & Physiology, and Human Genetics, University of Pittsburgh/UPMC, Pittsburgh, PA, USA

Introduction

Chronic pancreatitis (CP) is a clinical syndrome defined by the consequences of pancreatic injury, inflammation, morphologic changes, and dysfunction of the systems affecting the pancreas (acinar, duct, and islet), the immune system, the nervous system, and the regenerative processes. As discussed previously (Chapter 1), most clinical consensus reports define CP with a pragmatic approach as "a continuing inflammatory disease of the pancreas, characterized by irreversible morphological change, and typically causing pain and/or permanent loss of function" [1]. While this definition has practical utility in distinguishing more advanced cases from other gastrointestinal pathologies, it fails to capture early or variant cases, and provides no insight or guidance into etiology, trajectory, complications, or optimal treatment or (better yet) preventative approaches. This critique on the limitations of morphologic features does not mean that imaging has no value, but only that it must be interpreted within a larger context.

A fundamental limitation to both clinical and basic science investigations of the pancreatitis and resulting efforts to develop definitions, primary etiologies, and prognostic indicators of CP in the twentieth century was the medical paradigm of the germ theory of disease. The germ theory reduces diseases into *simple disorders* such as a specific microorganism causing a specific clinical syndrome. CP cannot be properly described and evaluated within this paradigm because it is a *complex disorder* caused by complex gene–environment, gene–gene, or multiple gene–environment interactions where the pathologic agents are neither necessary nor sufficient to cause the disorder. The challenges of evaluating and managing a complex disorder include developing a new way of thinking about the diagnosis and management of complex disorders. The new approach falls under the idea of complex gene–environment interactions, which is the basis of personalized medicine. This change reflects a paradigm shift, in which multiple factors related to the conceptual framework, data organization, predicted behavior within the paradigm, and other factors must all be changed at once. This is typically challenging, and there is always resistance to change. However, the failure of an early paradigm to address key issues, the availability of a new paradigm in which the failure is overcome, and a crisis to compel change from one paradigm to another is typically necessary for a paradigm shift. A paradigm shift in approaching CP is needed. Some of the factors that distinguish the germ theory and a complex gene–environment disease model of personalized medicine are given in Table 12B.1 to help understand the differences in structure, approach, and utility.

The practical application of the new paradigm to the study of CP is that the underlying mechanisms in many cases are not morphologic in nature; they are functional – with morphological changes coming as an eventual consequence in some cases, but not others. Thus, CP should be viewed as a broad "catch all" syndrome, which includes some simple etiologies, such as rare infections, duct obstruction, trauma, or catastrophic acute pancreatitis, and complex etiologies that are only understood in a new framework such as more complex genetics.

Pancreatitis: Medical and Surgical Management, First Edition.
David B. Adams, Peter B. Cotton, Nicholas J. Zyromski and John Windsor.
© 2017 John Wiley & Sons, Ltd. Published 2017 by John Wiley & Sons, Ltd.

Table 12B.1 Contrasting medical paradigms and disease models.

Domain	Germ theory and simple disorders	Complex gene-environment
Overarching goal	Treatment of disease	Prevention of disease
Enabling technology	Microscope, culture techniques, biopsies	NGS, biomarkers, computers
Paradigm-shifting force	Flexner Report of 1910	Economics
Education focus	Disease diagnosis and classification	Normal responses, assessment of variants
Scientific focus	Determine associations	Determine mechanisms
Scientific approach	Koch's postulates, global statistics	Modeling and simulation, performance characteristics
Disease classification	Tissue pathology, clinical syndromes	Genetic and environmental risks, surrogate endpoints
Disease time frame	Static, cross-sectional	Dynamic, longitudinal
Physician focus	Overall organ dysfunction	Activity and trajectory of dysfunctional systems
Assessment	Disease classification	Outcome prediction
Treatment	Trial and error	Targeted, optimized
Success measures	Population based	Individual based
Utility of the paradigm	Infectious diseases, Mendelian genetics, single-agent disorders, cancer detection	Inflammatory disease, complex genetics, functional disorders, cancer control, others

NGS, next generation sequencing.
Modified from [2].

Overview of genetics

Two examples of classic genetic disorders that cause CP are hereditary pancreatitis (HP) and cystic fibrosis (CF) (see Chapter 1). HP is caused by mutations in the cationic trypsinogen gene (*PRSS1*) and CF is caused by mutations in the cystic fibrosis transmembrane conductance regulator gene (CFTR). These disorders provide indisputable evidence that genetic variants increase susceptibility to CP. Of the two, HP is most informative because it provides critical insights into more complex gene–environment interactions.

The first observation is that HP is not a congenital disorder. Indeed, some patients with the worst known variant, *PRSS1* R122H, can be asymptomatic into their nineties with absolutely pristine pancreatic histology [3]. In contrast, the average *PRSS1* mutation carrier develops symptoms by the age of 10 years, with a wide variation in the age of onset [4] (Figure 12B.1). This reminds us that a mutation does not equal a disease, but it alters the *risk* for a disease or disease feature. An acquired *disease* occurs when there is an abnormal

response of a biological system linked to an organ when components of the organ are under sufficient stress.

The second observation from HP is that the compilations of CP in affected subjects are not uniform in their age of onset, or in their incidence or prevalence. The major complications in HP are recurrent acute pancreatitis (RAP), which occurs in about 80% of mutation carriers, and pancreatic exocrine insufficiency (PEI) and diabetes mellitus in about 40% of mutation carriers (Figure 12B.1). Since the underlying mutation is the same in all subjects, these complications must involve either additional severity factors or modifying factors, with the consequence that some patients are affected and others are not.

The third observation in HP is that pancreatic ductal adenocarcinoma (PDAC) occurs only late in life, and in some patients but not others. Cancer risk is strongly affected by smoking history, as the incidence of PDAC is doubled, and the age of onset is shifted a decade earlier in smokers [5]. This observation demonstrates that environmental factors can serve as disease modifiers, rather than primary susceptibility factors. We also note, from our HP Registry, that some large kindreds have no cases

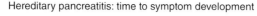

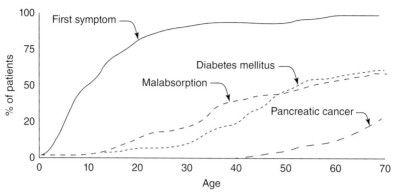

Figure 12B.1 Age of onset of HP-associated symptoms. The cumulative incidence of features and complications of pancreatitis associated with mutations in the *PRSS1* gene. Howes 2004 [3]. Reproduced with permission of Elsevier.

of PDAC, while others suffer from PDAC commonly. This suggests that HP itself provides a high-risk environment for other genetic and environmental factors to manifest. Thus, PDAC in HP is at least a gene × gene × environment condition in most affected patients.

The other informative Mendelian genetic disorder is CF, as reviewed in Chapter 1. Two severe *CFTR* mutations (*CFTR^sev*/*CFTR^sev*) result in classic CF, with pancreatic destruction beginning *in utero*. With mild-variable mutations (*CFTR^m-v*) the onset and severity of pancreatic disease can be delayed and present as RAP and/or CP (Table 12B.2). The first observations with classic CF is that the pancreas develops normally until trypsinogen is expressed, followed by progressive destruction of the developing pancreas. This and other lines of evidence tie duct dysfunction to mishandling of trypsinogen and injury linked to the effects of trypsin activation. Second, disease occurs with milder mutations, illustrating the fact that to cross the threshold required to cause disease is a function of the severity of the genetic variant and the severity of environmental stressor. As the functional effects of pathogenic variants within the gene become weaker, the strength of the environmental stressors must become stronger to overcome the disease-triggering threshold.

Johanson–Blizzard syndrome is a rare but informative disorder with multiple developmental features, as well as CP [6, 7]. The key point of this disorder is that the pathogenesis involves acinar cell stress related to failed clearance of misfolded proteins linked to autosomal

mutational loss of UBR1 function [8]. Thus, it appears that CP can be driven by strong stress signaling from dysfunctional acinar cell biology, eventually linked to the immune–inflammatory systems, and independent of trypsin activation.

Complex genetics

Mutations associated with failed trypsin regulation

Mechanistic insights from HP and CF led to the discovery of multiple genetic factors in HP using a candidate gene approach. Currently, mutations in the coding region of four additional genes linked to the control of trypsin activity in the pancreas have been identified and well defined. Mutations in *CFTR* are among the most important and common risk factors for CP by diminishing the flushing for trypsin from the pancreatic duct, as discussed previously. The expression-altering, loss-of-function genetic variants in the regulatory region of the serine peptidase inhibitor, Kazal type 1 gene (*SPINK1*) represent common and strong-effect risk for CP. Pathogenic variants in both alleles of the gene are commonly seen as major etiologic factors in familial pancreatitis because the threshold for loss of trypsin regulation is presumably very low and requires limited stressors to initiate disease. Smaller risks for CP are seen with mutations in the chymotrypsin C (caldecrin) gene (*CTRC*) and the calcium-sensing receptor gene (*CASR*)

Table 12B.2 Examples of genotype–phenotype correlation and multiorgan syndromes.

Genotype (variants)	Phenotype (syndromes)	Comment
PRSS1 (gain-of-function)	Hereditary pancreatitis (HP)	Genetic counseling recommended
PRSS1/any	HP, worse clinical course	Genetic counseling recommended
PRSS1 (misfolding)	Sporadic, familial (CP)	Pancreatitis only – not well studied
CFTR^{sev}/CFTR^{sev}	Cystic fibrosis (CF)	Manage with a CF center
CFTR^{sev}/CFTR^{m-v}	Atypical CF	Manage with a CF center
SPINK1/SPINK1	Familial pancreatitis	Usually progresses to severe CP
CFTR^{bicarb}/CFTR^{any}	Pancreas/sinus/CBAVD	Newly defined syndrome
CFTR^{any}/SPINK1	RAP/CP	Pancreas only
CFTR^{any}/CTRC^{sev}	RAP/CP	Pancreatitis only
CTRC^{sev}/SPINK1	RAP/CP	Pancreas only – not well studied
CTRC^{G60G}/ETOH/smoke	CP	CP only
CASR+/alcohol	RAP/CP	Pancreas only – not well studied
CASR–/SPINK1	RAP/ CP, familial CP	CP in FHH and sporadic CP
CASR–/CFTR	RAP/CP	Pancreas only – not well studied
PRSS1–PRSS2 locus	Lower RAP/CP risk	Trypsin-linked pathways only
CLDN2 risk allele	CP	Alcoholic, males more common
CEL	MODY 7, CP/DM	Familial, not well studied
CPA1	CP	Mostly children
GGT1	CP, PDAC	Not well studied
MMP1	CP	Not well studied
MTHFR	CP	Not well studied

CFTR: sev, severe mutations (typically functional classes I–III); m-v, mild-variable mutations; (typically *CFTR* functional class IV), bicarb, bicarbonate conductance disrupting variant (e.g., R75Q); any, either severe, mild-variable, or bicarbonate-disrupting variants. *CASR*+, gain-of-function mutations; CASR–, loss-of-function mutations; FHH, familial hypocalciuric hypercalcemia.

(see recent reviews [9–13]), presumably because they require additional susceptibility risk before their effects are relevant. Indeed, these trypsin-controlling gene variants are often seen together in complex, multigenic genotypes [14].

Mutations associated with activation of the unfolded protein response

CEL gene

A different mechanism of CP was discovered in a Norwegian family with maturity-onset diabetes of the young (MODY) type 7 [15]. The majority of the affected family members were found to have steatorrhea, and finally the underlying defect was traced to the carboxyl ester lipase (CEL) gene [16, 17], which is a digestive enzyme [18]. The mutations did not appear to cause premature enzyme activation, such as trypsin, but rather processing and folding defects in the *CEL* gene resulting in failed secretion and, presumably, triggering

the unfolded protein response (UPR) and activation of stress signals resulting in inflammation and CP.

CPA1 gene

Carboxypeptidase A1 is a digestive enzyme that is synthesized in very high amounts, second only to cationic trypsinogen. Using a candidate gene approach, it was found that rare mutations in the carboxypeptidase A1 gene (*CPA1*) were associated with CP, especially in children [19]. Functional analysis determined that the variants associated with CP were not secreted from test cells, but other variants that were not associated with CP were secreted. The interpretation was that this represented another example of CP related to chronic stress signaling from the UPR [19].

PRSS1

Cationic trypsinogen (*PRSS1*) variants that cause gain-of-function changes in the protein are associated with HP (A16V, N29I, and R122H). There are also a number of mutations in *PRSS1* that are associated with specific cases of CP, but do not result in HP. These appear to cause folding defects resulting in failed secretion, and presumably UPR, stress, and CP [20–22].

Alcohol- and smoking-associated risks of CP

Alcohol as long been recognized as a risk factor for CP, but it is also clear that alcohol alone is not sufficient since the majority of heavy drinkers do not have CP, and animals fed high doses of alcohol for years do not develop CP.

Individuals that drink alcohol are also more likely to smoke cigarettes. This fact confounds the analysis of population or cohort data where the effects of alcohol and drinking are being analyzed. Only large studies with well-characterized exposures to alcohol and smoking and variable experiences are needed to tease out the independent and synergistic effects. Compared with Europe, studies in the United States, such as the North American Pancreatitis Study II (NAPS2), are more powerful because of significant numbers of people who smoke but do not drink, who drink but do not smoke, who smoke and drink at different levels, or who neither drink nor smoke.

The year 2009 was a breakthrough year for recognizing the importance of smoking in the etiopathogenesis of CP. Credit for drawing attention to the potential role of smoking in CP must be given to previous investigators [23–27]. However, three large studies with different approaches were published from Denmark [28], Italy [29], and the United States [30], with almost identical findings and convincing evidence for both a limited role for alcohol and a major role for smoking. Among these, the American study from the NAPS2 project [30] had methodological advantages to provide the greatest insight into the question of the role of alcohol and smoking.

The first major finding was that by regression analysis, the risk of CP related to alcohol required very heavy drinking – equal or greater than 5 drinks with 12 g of alcohol per day (>60 gm/day) [30]. Alcohol alone, in patients without smoking, did not have a significant risk of pancreatitis, although there was a trend. Second, in contrast to alcohol, there was a dose-dependent risk of CP with the amount of smoking. Third, the risk of CP in patients *with* both smoking and drinking was quadrupled over either alone, demonstrating a synergist effect.

Complex gene–environment interactions with alcohol and smoking

Further insight into the risk and mechanisms of alcohol- and smoking-related CP were obtained using an unbiased genome-wide association study (GWAS) [31]. Using the deeply phenotyped samples from the NAPS2, we discovered genetic variants in noncoding regions within the *PRSS1–PRSS2* locus and *CLDN2* locus [31]. Rather than classic susceptibility genes, these loci appear to be very important pancreatitis-risk-modifying factors [32].

PRSS1–PRSS2 locus

The *PRSS1–PRSS2* locus is linked to variants in regulatory elements that result in decreased expression of cationic trypsinogen. This results in some protection from CP risk factors associated with control of trypsin activation and activity. The *PRSS1–PRSS2* protective haplotype reduces the likelihood of alcoholic pancreatitis, demonstrating that alcohol is working, in part, through a trypsin-dependent pathway, as predicted by animal studies [33–39].

CLDN2 locus

A surprising locus was *CLDN2* [40]. *CLDN2* codes for the claudin-2 protein, a tight junction protein that is expressed in the pancreas between duct cells along with claudin-4 and other tight junction proteins. Claudin-4 is the common protein that forms a seal between the duct cells to prevent water and solute molecules from crossing the epithelial barrier. Claudin-2 is normally inside the duct cells, but we believe that it is rapidly transferred to the tight junctions in exchange for claudin-4 during active secretion. Claudin-2 differs from claudin-4 because it forms channels that are permeable to water and sodium ions. This is crucial for fluid secretion, as the duct cells secret bicarbonate through CFTR. Together, they produce juice that is high in sodium bicarbonate. This process appears to be normal in patients with the high-risk *CLDN2* haplotype, but claudin-2 may have another biological function related to the immune system. We hypothesize that claudin-2 becomes expressed in acinar cells after acute pancreatitis (AP) as the acinar cells partially dedifferentiate during the regeneration process. Patients with the high-risk *CLDN2* haplotype have overproduction and mislocalization of claudin-2 to interact with macrophages and/or other inflammatory cells to drive further inflammation and the progression from AP to CP. Of note, the *CLDN2* gene is on the X chromosome, and risk in men is directly proportional to the minor allele frequency of the risk allele in the population, ~26%, since men only have one chromosome [40]. In contrast, women have two X chromosomes, with one silenced, such that their risk is only $0.26 \times 0.26 = 0.068$, or ~7% of the population. The risk is also strongly associated with alcohol. Since at-risk drinking in men is ~16% and women is ~10%, the high risk for CP from this mechanism is ~4% of men, and 0.7% of women. This finding may also partly explain the male predominance of CP in many studies.

CTRC G60G

More insight comes from studies of *CTRC* variants in the United States. As noted earlier, rare *CTRC* variants were reported in Europe, India, and China in patients with CP [41–44], but this was not replicated in the NAPS2 study [45]. Instead, we discovered a strong association with the *CTRC* G60G variant, associated with a high-risk haplotype that may affect CTRC expression under some conditions [45]. This was not seen in the European study, but the population was mostly children, who do not smoke or drink. On subset analysis, we found that the risk of CP in *CTRC* G60G carriers was limited to the alcohol-smoking subset, and especially in smokers [45]. Furthermore, the effect was not seen in RAP but only in CP, suggesting that CTRC is not a typical susceptibility factor, but is important in modifying the response of the body to AP in patients who smoke and/or drink.

Other genetic variants associated with CP
GGT1

γ-Glutamyltransferase is an important enzyme used by many cells for detoxifying natural and xenobiotic compounds. We found an association between mutations in γ-glutamyltransferase gene (*GGT1*) and PDAC [46], as well as CP [47]. Further studies on this important pathway are needed.

MMP-1, MTHFR, IL23R

Several genetic factors have been reported that have not been replicated or fully investigated as to functional role in CP. These include mutations in the matrix metalloproteinase-1 gene (*MMP-1*) [48], the 5,10-methylenetetrahydrofolate reductase gene (*MTHFR*) [49], carboxyl ester lipase (CEL) gene – CEL pseudogene (CELP) fusion gene [50].

Framework for understanding genetics of pancreatitis

AP and CP are the most common disorders of the exocrine pancreas. The major risk for the development of these diseases lies with the risk of premature activation of trypsin, followed by zymogen activation, tissue autodigestion, and the generation of a robust immune response with all of its consequences [51]. Of emerging importance is the consequence of protein misfolding and the UPR. Autoimmune pancreatitis (AIP), not discussed here further, is another important entity that is likely a complex disorder.

As noted earlier, the problem with clinicopathologic definitions of disease is that descriptive definitions cannot clearly define very mild or early disease and cannot provide guidance into the design of targeted treatment strategies. Additional challenges for physicians include the variability and unpredictability of disease onset, severity, complications, and managing the clinical course of these disorders. As a result, therapies are primarily symptomatic and supportive rather than targeted at the underlying mechanism and preventing diseases progression. A new conceptual framework is, therefore, needed to better understand and manage patients with pancreatic diseases (reviewed in [2]).

Models of pancreatitis

In simple terms, CP can be viewed as a "two-hit" disorder [52, 53] with the "first hit" being AP, which activates the immune system and starts the process. The magnitude of the triggering event is dependent on the underlying susceptibility factors for trypsin activation and/or injury signaling. As an acquired disorder, the timing of exposure to sufficient stress or injury is random (stochastic) and marks a major change as the patient transfers from disease risk to disease activity and/or outcome. The immune system–activating insult may be recognized clinically as AP. We call this the sentinel acute pancreatitis event (SAPE) model (Figure 12B.2). In our current model, susceptibility to acute pancreatic injury is linked to premature activation of trypsin, either within the acinar cell or in the pancreatic duct. In addition, there are trypsin-independent mechanisms of injury that can activate the inflammatory process such as direct trauma, toxicity, or immune-mediated mechanisms such as AIP.

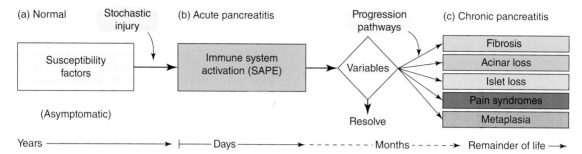

Figure 12B.2 SAPE model of chronic pancreatitis. (a) Patients may spend years with multiple susceptibility risk factors (left) but remain asymptomatic. (b) A stochastic injury to the pancreas is believed to initiate AP, which typically lasts a few days. This is critical to activating the immune system at multiple levels. The resolution phase is affected by multiple variables (yellow diamond) as genetic and environmental risk factors or modifiers that may alter the healing process, leading to progression of pathology depending on the cell type and system. (c) Pathologic variants to the biology of the stellate cell leads to fibrosis, acinar cell loss leads to PEI, islet loss lead to DM, altered neural mechanisms leads to pain syndromes, and altered DNA repair leads to metaplasia and cancer. Modified from Whitcomb [54].

Inflammation is a normal response to injury and, under ideal conditions, should lead to tissue repair and regeneration. A "second hit" that modifies the normal inflammatory response leading to sustained pancreatic stellate cell activation and fibrosis, or other irreversible structural or functional changes, is thought to be needed for development of CP (see reviews [52, 53]). While the first hit centers on factors that cause injury, the second hit centers on factors that drive inflammation and inflammation-associated complications such as fibrosis and sclerosis, failed acinar cell regeneration and atrophy, distorted architecture with morphologic signs of CP, progressive loss of normal parenchyma with exocrine pancreatic insufficiency, metaplasia, dysplasia, cancer, and a variety of pain syndromes. Without the "second hit" (or modifying factors), the pancreas regenerates after mild to moderate injury and resumes normal function. Different genetic variants and environmental factors are relevant to each of these systems as well.

The development of disease models is important for disorders with multiple variables. Modeling allows for the organization of known risk factors and disease-modifying factors into compartments for further study and for providing insight into how multiple risk factors likely interact. In addition, it allows for the organization of sequential events, in which responses are seen to be dependent on initiating conditions thus facilitating the anticipation of potential downstream effects when initial conditions are met. Finally, risk

categories can be constructed based on similarities of therapeutic approaches, linking risk factors with specific therapies.

Susceptibility to AP and RAP

Disorders of the pancreas can be congenital or acquired through trauma, infection, or gallstones, or linked to alcohol, smoking, or genetic factors – or unknown factors (idiopathic disease). The fact that most people do not have pancreatic disease suggests that the system is robust, and that various alternative, adaptive, and protective mechanisms exists.

One of the approaches we have taken to understand the complex genetics is to focus on the specialized cells, which mediate organ function and response to injury. Fortunately, for those who study pancreatitis, the exocrine pancreas is simple, with two major cell types: acinar and duct. Furthermore, each cell has one function, and we know the mechanisms of these functions in detail.

Acinar cells biology and risk of AP

The acinar cells are the primary functional unit of the exocrine pancreas. The primary purpose of the acinar cell is to rapidly produce large amounts of pancreatic digestive proenzymes (zymogens) that are delivered to the duodenum where they are activated and digest ingested nutrients. The key molecule is trypsin, a protease digestive enzyme targeting internal arginine and lysine residues in a peptide chain. Trypsin also serves as the master enzyme in that it is the primary activation mechanism for all of the other zymogens. Pathologically, trypsin can activate the immune system by mimicking the action of the mast cell enzyme tryptase in initiating prolonged immune system signaling through protease-activated receptors [55]. Therefore, maintaining trypsin in its zymogen form as trypsinogen is critical to pancreatic health.

The most important signaling molecule in the acinar cell is calcium [56]. Release of calcium from internal stores is critical for excitation–secretion coupling and expulsion of the zymogen granule content from inside the acinar cell to the duct lumen. Calcium levels are tightly regulated, with ATP required to pump calcium into internal stores and out of the cell [57]. Calcium is also an important modulator of trypsin activity, so danger exists inside the acinar cell when calcium levels are high.

Multiple lines of evidence point to premature activation of trypsin within the acinar cell as a mechanism for initiating acinar cell injury and triggering and inflammatory response recognized clinically as AP (see reviews [57–61]). Trypsinogen is activated to trypsin with the cleavage of trypsinogen activation peptide (TAP) an eight amino acid N-terminus extension that forms a calcium-binding site [62–64]. When the calcium concentration is elevated, the activation site is stabilized allowing trypsin to cleave TAP. Super-physiological calcium concentrations in acinar cells are linked to trypsin activation and the initiation of pancreatitis [58, 65]. Of note, excessive alcohol may disrupt the ability to effectively regulate calcium by damaging mitochondria, which is needed to produce large amounts of ATP to lower intracellular calcium levels [58, 65].

Trypsin activity is also pH dependent [66], with an optimal pH between 7 and 8 [66, 67]. Low pH (e.g., <7.15) as seen in diabetic ketoacidosis or with manipulation of acinar cell pH also promotes activation of trypsin and pancreatitis [68–70] possibly in conjunction with cathepsin B [71].

There are multiple protective mechanisms within the acinar cells that are trypsin specific. The first acinar cell–specific mechanism is trypsin self-destruction (autolysis) in which another trypsin molecule attacks the R122 site. In HP, this site is changed to H122, which is resistant to cleavage. CTRC is another pancreatic

protease activated by trypsin that attacks the trypsin molecule to complete degradation at L81 [72, 73]. However, there is a second calcium-binding site on the trypsin molecule, and calcium binding blocks the R122 and L81 cleavage sites to protect active trypsin [18, 63, 73]. In low calcium concentrations, trypsin is not activated (calcium-binding site 1), but if it is, the molecule is quickly degraded (calcium-binding site 2).

Trypsin activity can be blocked by a second mechanism. In the setting of inflammation, there is marked upregulation of *SPINK1* [2, 74], which codes for the pancreatic secretory trypsin inhibitor (PSTI) that effectively blocks the activity of trypsin. The risks of pancreatitis arising from the acinar cell are linked to trypsin regulation, specifically the molecular structure, the calcium concentration, and the pH. Other key factors for trypsin regulation over time include the upregulation of *CTRC* and *SPINK1*.

Alcohol as a risk for AP

Multiple studies have linked alcohol consumption with an increased risk of developing AP (see reviews [53, 75, 76]). Animal studies suggest that the increased risk is related to lowering the threshold for hyperstimulation-associated pancreatic injury [34, 37]. Other studies suggest that chronic alcohol consumption alters the neurohormonal mechanisms of pancreatic activation with hyperstimulation occurring with alcohol withdrawal (disinhibiting excitatory nerves that adapted to alcohol-associated inhibition) and nutrient feeding (resulting in hyperstimulation) [77], which is consistent with clinical observations [78]. Each of these mechanisms appears to be linked to acinar cell calcium regulation.

Epidemiology studies reveal that less than 3% of heavy alcoholics develop CP [79], and the risk of alcoholic pancreatitis, when adjusted for smoking in regression analysis is low [30]. Furthermore, as noted earlier, a threshold of >5 drinks a day or 35 drinks a week are necessary to detect any risk of pancreatitis [30, 53]. These data indicate that alcohol is a weak susceptibility factor (first hit), but as is discussed later, it is a very strong modifier factor (second hit), especially with smoking [30] and the *CLDN2* risk allele [40].

Duct biology

The primary function of the duct cell is to secrete a bicarbonate-rich fluid to flush the zymogens out of the pancreas and into the duodenum. The most important molecule within the duct is CFTR, an anion channel that is used to transport both chloride and bicarbonate with variable permeability ratios being controlled by duct cell sensors and second messengers [80]. The electrochemical mechanism of pancreatic chloride and bicarbonate secretion has been well defined in animal and mathematical models [81, 82]. The fluid produced in pancreatic ducts is high in calcium (favoring trypsin activation and reducing degradation) but has a high pH (>8), which maintains trypsin in an inactive state.

Risk for pancreatitis is linked with the zymogens within the duct rather than within the duct cell, since risk of CP is diminished in patients with pathogenic *CFTR* variants plus *PRSS1–PRSS2* protective alleles. The duct cells express multiple sensors on the luminal surface that are protective since they sense trypsin activity (e.g., protease activated receptors, PAR 1, PAR2 [83, 84]), while other molecules may sense the calcium concentration and ATP release as an injury signal (e.g., purinoceptors, P2Y2, P2X4, and P2X7 [85]). Activation of these sensors results in the opening of the CFTR channel, secretion of a bicarbonate-rich fluid, and flushing the duct contents into the duodenum [85].

At low intracellular chloride levels, WNL1, an internal sensor, signals CFTR to favor bicarbonate conductance [80, 81]. In addition, there are multiple types of duct cells with different characteristics – with the duct cells nearest to the acinar cells having the highest concentration of CFTR molecules [81]. The duct also contains mucus-secreting cells to further protect the pancreatic duct form zymogens. These sensors and protective mechanisms work in different ways to reduce the risk of injury from active trypsin.

Genetic risk of duct cell dysfunction and AP

Mutations in *CFTR* cause CF, an autosomal recessive disease, which is characterized by the development of CP beginning *in utero*. About 2000 variants in *CFTR* have been identified (http://www.genet.sickkids.on.ca/app), but the functional effect of most of them remains unknown (CFTR2 project – http://www.cftr2.org). The more common variants are classified clinically as severe or mild-variable, based on their effect on the pancreas.

In 1998, two reports noted that there were more *CFTR* variants in patients with idiopathic and some alcoholic CP patients than could be explained by chance

[86, 87]. These findings have been replicated in multiple studies from the United States [88], Europe [14, 89–91], India [92], and China/Taiwan [93, 94]. In most cases, single nucleotide polymorphism (SNP) panels, plus the F508del variant, were tested, and extensive genotyping was not done. In some cases, investigators tested for the *SPINK1* N23S variant. Thus, it could not be determined whether the cases had atypical CF or another *CFTR*-related disorders with underlying complex, pancreas-specific mechanisms [95–98].

Recently, we investigated patients with RAP and CP from the NAPS2 cohort for all *CFTR* variants ever reported more than once in CP cases, plus the more common pathogenic SNPs ($n = 81$) [99]. We discovered nine *CFTR* variants in patients with CP that we previously reported to be benign based on association with normal lung function or sweat chloride levels: *CFTR* R74Q, R75Q, R117H, R170H, L967S, L997F, D1152H, S1235R, and D1270N. In collaboration with Professor Min Goo Lee's group [80, 81], we found that each of these variants, when cloned into wild-type *CFTR* gene and expressed in experimental cells, had normal chloride conductance, but failed to transform into bicarbonate channels when activated with WNK1–SPAK stimulation [99]. These variants were scattered across the coding region of the *CFTR* gene, but when folded into functional conformations, it became apparent that the variants were blocking bicarbonate by four mechanisms.

The findings could be by chance, and the importance of these *CFTR* variants *in vivo* was unclear. We, therefore, looked for organ dysfunction in tissues that use CFTR to secrete bicarbonate, namely the sinuses and the male reproductive system. Comparing pancreatitis patients and controls, the *CFTR* bicarbonate-defective variants significantly increased the risk for rhinosinusitis (OR 2.3, $P < 0.005$) and male infertility (OR 395, $P \ll 0.0001$) [99]. These findings demonstrate that any *CFTR* variant that affects overall function or just bicarbonate conductance without a lung or sweat chloride phenotype are major risk factors for CP.

Progression from RAP to CP

The previous discussion demonstrates that there are multiple etiologies for CP. Modeling CP as a disorder that progresses over years from initial injury to complete gland destruction under the influence of one or more etiologic pathways, however, may be useful for targeting treatments to stop the process, and allow healing and regeneration. We wanted to test the SAPE hypothesis to see whether AP and/or RAP lead to CP. This has recently been tested in a population-based study from Allegheny County (Pittsburgh), PA [100] (Figure 12B.3). These data suggest that following AP, patients progress to CP at different rates based on etiology, with alcohol etiology having the highest risk (Figure 12B.3a) and that the mechanism is linked to RAP (Figure 12B.3b).

SAPE hypothesis – second hit

The SAPE hypothesis model (Figure 12B.2) is built on the observation that individuals go through life for many years with multiple risk factors for CP, then suddenly the process begins and CP develops [52, 53]. The "first hit" is a stochastic event resulting in the activation of the immune system, such as occurs with an episode of AP (SAPE). The outcome of an episode of AP can be either complete recovery, necrosis fibrosis following severe AP, susceptibility to RAP, or the "second hit" with initiation of progressive inflammation and complications of CP over time. Since there is a time period between AP and CP (Figure 12B.2), there is an opportunity to intervene and stop progression. Of note, there are now multiple cell types involved in injury-recovery process that may not respond properly (Figure 12B.2c). Misfunction of the stellate cells results in fibrosis, failed regeneration results in atrophy, susceptibility of islet cells to inflammation results in diabetes mellitus (Type 3c), variant nervous system responses result in chronic pain syndromes, and failed DNA repair results in PDAC.

The approach to preventing RAP and/or progression should therefore be initiated early and be etiology based (such as a cholecystectomy in patients with gallstone pancreatitis but not in patients with alcohol or genetic etiologies), with attention to high-risk of secondary complications such as fibrosis or diabetes. Risk factors for RAP and progression of fibrosis are addressed.

Trypsin activation and progression from RAP to CP

Studies on patients with HP provide an example of how a major susceptibility factor such as *PRSS1* R122H mutations becomes risk factors for AP and CP through RAP [4, 101, 102]. The example of HP provides some evidence that RAP may eventually lead to CP.

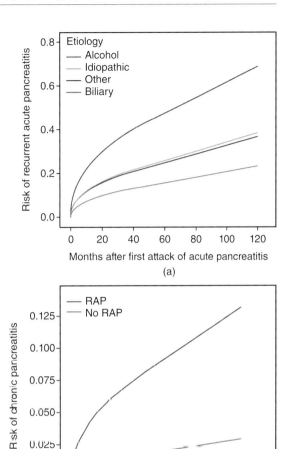

Figure 12B.3 Population-based on 7456 Allegheny County, PA, residents following their first (sentinel) episode of AP. (a) Risk of developing RAP based on etiology. (b) Risk of CP based on the presence or absence of documented RAP. From Yadav, O'Connell and Papachristou [100].

Two genes are important for directly limiting trypsin activity in the pancreas: *SPINK1*, a trypsin inhibitor, and *CTRC*, a trypsin destroyer. The *SPINK1* N34S-haplotype, the most frequent risk variant, likely acts as a disease modifier rather than a susceptibility factor [103, 104]. This is based on the observation that the *SPINK1* N34S high-risk haplotype is common (1–3% of most populations) while CP is uncommon (42/100,000 persons [105]). However, the *SPINK1* N34S variant increases the risk of alcoholic CP (OR 5), idiopathic CP (OR 15), and tropical CP (OR 19) [106]. Furthermore, it is unlikely that *SPINK1* is a susceptibility factor for AP but is closely linked to CP [107, 108]. This suggests that *SPINK1* is normally effective in controlling the effects of *recurrent* intrapancreatic trypsin activation from a variety of etiologies and that mutations in *SPINK1* allow recurrent trypsin-associated injury to drive fibrosis. Furthermore, in genetic studies testing multiple genes, heterozygous *SPINK1* mutations are only seen in patients with RAP or CP when there is also a mutation in a susceptibility gene associated with recurrent trypsin activation such as *PRSS1*, *CFTR*, or *CASR* [14, 88, 92]. Thus, heterozygous *SPINK1* mutations do not cause pancreatitis – they make the clinical outcomes of patients with recurrent pancreatic injury from trypsin activation worse. Of note, *SPINK1* mutations are only slightly more common in alcoholic pancreatitis patients than in the general population [109–112], suggesting that the pathologic pathway from pancreatic injury to CP in patients with alcoholic CP is different [106, 113].

Similarly, the *CTRC* G60G appears to be a disease modifier [45]. The variant is present in about 11% of the general population, making it unlikely that it is an independent susceptibility factor. The frequency of the risk allele is similar in RAP and controls, but significantly increased in CP, and especially CP from alcohol or smoking [45].

Specific therapy for trypsin-related RAP and CP have not been developed and/or tested in adequate human trials. Because of the central role of trypsin in pancreatic exocrine function, it is unclear to our group if targeting trypsin activity directly will be effective in preventing CP.

Alcoholic pancreatitis and progression from RAP to CP

Patients with alcoholic AP are at high risk of RAP [114] and progression from RAP to CP if they continue to drink alcohol and/or smoke [27, 100, 115, 116]. In the NAPS2, the prevalence of *CFTR* variants was equal in RAP and CP, yet only 25% of RAP and 46% of CP subjects had at-risk alcohol drinking [30]. This suggests that alcohol and/or smoking are associated with rapid transition from RAP to CP, decreasing the prevalence in the first category while increasing it in the second.

There are multiple alcohol-associated risks. Alcohol accelerates the rate of fibrosis in animal models beyond what is expected from RAP alone [117, 118]. The mechanism appears to be related to alteration in the immune response to recurrent injury [117]. Alcohol acts synergistically with smoking, and additional pathogenic genetic variants of *CLDN2* and *CLDN2* further increase the risk.

From a therapeutic standpoint, interventions into slowing progression from alcoholic AP to CP are available – namely cessation of alcohol and smoking. In one interesting study, Takeyama et al. [119] found that in patients who continued drinking after developing AP had a 58% chance of RAP and 41% chance of CP. Decreasing drinking but continuing at a lower daily dose resulted in decrease to RAP 37% and CP 23%, while decreasing to occasional or complete cessation decreased recurrence to about 20% for RAP and 13% for CP. These data confirm the premise that alcoholic AP leads to CP and also demonstrate that the risk is reduced with proportional decrease in continued risk exposure.

Relation between developing fibrosis, diabetes, pain, and cancer

In Figure 12B.2c, the complications of CP are listed. As noted earlier, these are all linked to different cell types. The SAPE hypothesis suggests that after the sentinel event, specific secondary risk factors influence the recovery or pathologic complications of failed recovery in the various cell types. While little research has been carried out in this area, a study from the NAPS2 cohort suggests that there is poor correlation between fibrosis (stellate cells) and pain (nerves) [120]. This suggests that the relevant genes and other risk factors differ between these cell types. Similarly, Rebours et al. [121] found that PDAC development in patients with HP did not correlate with severity of inflammation and fibrosis. These findings are very important because it tells us that if we are *only* looking for the morphologic changes in the pancreas to define CP, then we are missing AP followed by pain syndromes, AP followed by diabetes, and so on. In fact, there is no consensus on what to call these disease variants that are clearly part of the CP syndrome in the context of fibrosis – but not in the absence of fibrosis. More work is needed on the new paradigm.

Future directions

Insights gained from the study of genetic variations and/or environmental factors have transformed our understanding of CP. The older approach to making a diagnosis of CP inflammation without infection leading to irreversible damage must be replaced with new disease models that help target therapy. We now understand that CP is a process that begins with immune system activation (first hit), and progression to fibrosis, atrophy, diabetes, pain, and/or cancer if there are additional risk and disease modifiers (second hits). Thus, the future will be one in which patient with early signs of pancreatic disease will receive a structured evaluation that includes genetic testing, and this will provide the data for disease modeling and etiology-targeted treatment. The effectiveness of treatment will be monitored with model-specific biomarkers, leading to therapy adjustments to keep the pancreas close to normal. Such a clinic has already been developed and is operational [2].

References

1 Sarner M, Cotton PB. Classification of pancreatitis. Gut. 1984;25(7):756–759. PMID: 6735257

2 Whitcomb DC. What is personalized medicine and what should it replace? Nature Reviews Gastroenterology & Hepatology. 2012;9(7):418–424. PMID: 22614753

3 Khalid A, Finkelstein S, Thompson B, Kelly L, Hanck C, Godfrey TE, et al. A 93 year old man with the PRSS1 R122H mutation, low SPINK1 expression, and no pancreatitis: insights into phenotypic non-penetrance. Gut. 2006;55(5):728–731. PMID: 16354799

4 Howes N, Lerch MM, Greenhalf W, Stocken DD, Ellis I, Simon P, et al. Clinical and genetic characteristics of hereditary pancreatitis in Europe. Clinical Gastroenterology and Hepatology. 2004;2(3):252–261. PMID: 15017610

5 Lowenfels AB, Maisonneuve P, Whitcomb DC, Lerch MM, DiMagno EP. Cigarette smoking as a risk factor for pancreatic cancer in patients with hereditary pancreatitis. Journal of the American Medical Association. 2001;286(2):169–170. PMID: 11448279

6 Gershoni-Baruch R, Lerner A, Braun J, Katzir Y, Iancu TC, Benderly A. Johanson-Blizzard syndrome: clinical spectrum and further delineation of the syndrome. American Journal of Medical Genetics 1990;35:546–551.

7 Jones NL, Hofley PM, Durie PR. Pathophysiology of the pancreatic defect in Johanson-Blizzard syndrome: a disorder of acinar development. Journal of Pediatrics. 1994;125(3):406–408.

8 Zenker M, Mayerle J, Lerch MM, Tagariello A, Zerres K, Durie PR, et al. Deficiency of UBR1, a ubiquitin ligase of the N-end rule pathway, causes pancreatic dysfunction, malformations and mental retardation (Johanson-Blizzard syndrome). Nature Genetics. 2005; 37(12):1345–1350. PMID: 16311597

9 Witt H, Apte MV, Keim V, Wilson JS. Chronic pancreatitis: challenges and advances in pathogenesis, genetics, diagnosis, and therapy. Gastroenterology. 2007;132(4): 1557–1573. PMID: 17466744

10 Chen JM, Ferec C. Chronic pancreatitis: genetics and pathogenesis. Annual Review of Genomics and Human Genetics 2009;10:63–87. PMID: 19453252

11 Whitcomb DC. Genetic aspects of pancreatitis. Annual Review of Medicine 2010;61:413–424. PMID: 20059346

12 Larusch J, Whitcomb DC. Genetics of pancreatitis. Current Opinion in Gastroenterology. 2011;27(5):467–474. PMID: 21844754

13 Chen JM, Ferec C. Genetics and pathogenesis of chronic pancreatitis: the 2012 update. Clinics and Research in Hepatology and Gastroenterology. 2012;36(4):334–340. PMID: 22749696

14 Rosendahl J, Landt O, Bernadova J, Kovacs P, Teich N, Bodeker H, et al. *CFTR, SPINK1, CTRC* and *PRSS1* variants in chronic pancreatitis: is the role of mutated CFTR overestimated? Gut. 2013;62(4):582–592. PMID: 22427236

15 American Diabetes Association. Diagnosis and classification of diabetes mellitus. Diabetes Care 2014;37 Suppl 1:S81–S90. PMID: 24357215

16 Raeder H, Johansson S, Holm PI, Haldorsen IS, Mas E, Sbarra V, et al. Mutations in the CEL VNTR cause a syndrome of diabetes and pancreatic exocrine dysfunction. Nature Genetics. 2006;38(1):54–62. PMID: 16369531

17 Fjeld K, Weiss FU, Lasher D, Rosendahl J, Chen JM, Johansson BB, et al. A recombinant allele of the lipase gene CEL and its pseudogene CELP confers susceptibility to chronic pancreatitis. Nature Genetics. 2015;47(5):518–522. PMID: 25774637

18 Whitcomb DC, Lowe ME. Human pancreatic digestive enzymes. Digestive Diseases and Sciences. 2007;52(1):1–17. PMID: 17205399

19 Witt H, Beer S, Rosendahl J, Chen JM, Chandak GR, Masamune A, et al. Variants in CPA1 are strongly associated with early onset chronic pancreatitis. Nature Genetics. 2013;45(10):1216–1220. PMID: 23955596

20 Kereszturi E, Szmola R, Kukor Z, Simon P, Weiss FU, Lerch MM, et al. Hereditary pancreatitis caused by mutation-induced misfolding of human cationic trypsinogen: a novel disease mechanism. Human Mutation. 2009;30(4):575–582. PMID: 19191323

21 Nemeth BC, Sahin-Toth M. Human cationic trypsinogen (PRSS1) variants and chronic pancreatitis. American Journal of Physiology: Gastrointestinal and Liver Physiology. 2014;306(6):G466–G473. PMID: 24458023

22 Schnur A, Beer S, Witt H, Hegyi P, Sahin-Toth M. Functional effects of 13 rare PRSS1 variants presumed to cause chronic pancreatitis. Gut. 2014;63(2):337–343. PMID: 23455445

23 Bourliere M, Barthet M, Berthezene P, Durbec JP, Sarles H. Is tobacco a risk factor for chronic pancreatitis and alcoholic cirrhosis? Gut. 1991;32(11):1392–1395.

24 Talamini G, Bassi C, Falconi M, Sartori N, Salvia R, Rigo L, et al. Alcohol and smoking as risk factors in chronic pancreatitis and pancreatic cancer. Digestive Diseases and Sciences. 1999;44(7):1301–1311. PMID: 10489910

25 Lin Y, Tamakoshi A, Hayakawa T, Ogawa M, Ohno Y. Cigarette smoking as a risk factor for chronic pancreatitis: a case–control study in Japan. Research Committee on Intractable Pancreatic Diseases. Pancreas. 2000;21(2): 109–114.

26 Maisonneuve P, Lowenfels AB, Mullhaupt B, Cavallini G, Lankisch PG, Andersen JR, et al. Cigarette smoking accelerates progression of alcoholic chronic pancreatitis. Gut. 2005;54(4):510–514. PMID: 15753536

27 Talamini G, Bassi C, Falconi M, Sartori N, Vaona B, Bovo P, et al. Smoking cessation at the clinical onset of chronic pancreatitis and risk of pancreatic calcifications. Pancreas. 2007;35(4):320–326. PMID: 18090237

28 Tolstrup JS, Kristiansen L, Becker U, Gronbaek M. Smoking and risk of acute and chronic pancreatitis among women and men: a population-based cohort study. Archives of Internal Medicine. 2009;169(6):603–609. PMID: 19307524

29 Frulloni L, Gabbrielli A, Pezzilli R, Zerbi A, Cavestro GM, Marotta F, et al. Chronic pancreatitis: report from a multicenter Italian survey (PanCroInfAISP) on 893 patients. Digestive and Liver Disease. 2009;41(4):311–317. PMID: 19097829

30 Yadav D, Hawes RH, Brand RE, Anderson MA, Money ME, Banks PA, et al. Alcohol consumption, cigarette smoking, and the risk of recurrent acute and chronic pancreatitis. Archives of Internal Medicine. 2009;169(11):1035–1045. PMID: 19506173

31 Whitcomb DC, Yadav D, Adam S, Hawes RH, Brand RE, Anderson MA, et al. Multicenter approach to recurrent acute and chronic pancreatitis in the United States: the North American Pancreatitis Study 2 (NAPS2). Pancreatology. 2008;8(4–5):520–531. PMID: 18765957

32 Whitcomb DC. Genetics of alcoholic and nonalcoholic pancreatitis. Current Opinion in Gastroenterology. 2012;28(5):501–506. PMID: 22885947

33 Thrower EC, Gorelick FS, Husain SZ. Molecular and cellular mechanisms of pancreatic injury. Current Opinion in Gastroenterology. 2010;26(5):484–489. PMID: 20651589

34 Lu Z, Karne S, Kolodecik T, Gorelick FS. Alcohols enhance caerulein-induced zymogen activation in pancreatic acinar cells. American Journal of Physiology: Gastrointestinal and Liver Physiology. 2002;282(3):G501–G507.

35 Gorelick FS. Alcohol and zymogen activation in the pancreatic acinar cell. Pancreas. 2003;24:305–310.

36 Gorelick FS, Thrower E. The acinar cell and early pancreatitis responses. Clinical Gastroenterology and Hepatology. 2009;7(11 Suppl):S10–S14. PMID: 19896090

37 Pandol SJ, Periskic S, Gukovsky I, Zaninovic V, Jung Y, Zong Y, et al. Ethanol diet increases the sensitivity of rats to pancreatitis induced by cholecystokinin octapeptide. Gastroenterology. 1999;117(3):706–716.

38 Gukovskaya AS, Mouria M, Gukovsky I, Reyes CN, Kasho VN, Faller LD, et al. Ethanol metabolism and transcription factor activation in pancreatic acinar cells in rats. Gastroenterology. 2002;122(1):106–118.

39 Pandol SJ, Gukovsky I, Satoh A, Lugea A, Gukovskaya AS. Emerging concepts for the mechanism of alcoholic pancreatitis from experimental models. Journal of Gastroenterology. 2003;38(7):623–628.

40 Whitcomb DC, Larusch J, Krasinskas AM, Klei L, Smith JP, Brand RE, et al. Common genetic variants in the CLDN2 and PRSS1-PRSS2 loci alter risk for alcohol-related and sporadic pancreatitis. Nature Genetics. 2012;44(12): 1349–1354. PMID: 23143602

41 Masson E, Chen JM, Scotet V, Le Marechal C, Ferec C. Association of rare chymotrypsinogen C (CTRC) gene variations in patients with idiopathic chronic pancreatitis. Human Genetics. 2008;123(1):83–91. PMID: 18172691

42 Rosendahl J, Witt H, Szmola R, Bhatia E, Ozsvari B, Landt O, et al. Chymotrypsin C (CTRC) variants that diminish activity or secretion are associated with chronic pancreatitis. Nature Genetics. 2008;40(1):78–82. PMID: 18059268

43 Chang MC, Chang YT, Wei SC, Liang PC, Jan IS, Su YN, et al. Association of novel chymotrypsin C gene variations and haplotypes in patients with chronic pancreatitis in Chinese in Taiwan. Pancreatology. 2009;9(3):287–292. PMID: 19407484

44 Derikx MH, Szmola R, te Morsche RH, Sunderasan S, Chacko A, Drenth JP. Tropical calcific pancreatitis and its association with CTRC and SPINK1 (p.N34S) variants. European Journal of Gastroenterology & Hepatology. 2009;21(8):889–894. PMID: 19404200

45 LaRusch J, Lozano-Leon A, Stello K, Moore A, Muddana V, O'Connell M, et al. The common chymotrypsinogen C (CTRC) variant G60G (C.180T) increases risk of chronic pancreatitis but not recurrent acute pancreatitis in a North American population. Clinical and Translational Gastroenterology. 2015;6:e68. PMID: 25569187

46 Diergaarde B, Brand R, Lamb J, Cheong SY, Stello K, Barmada MM, et al. Pooling-based genome-wide association study implicates gamma-glutamyltransferase 1 (GGT1) gene in pancreatic carcinogenesis. Pancreatology. 2010;10(2–3):194–200. PMID: 20484958

47 Brand H, Diergaarde B, O'Connell MR, Whitcomb DC, Brand RE. Variation in the gamma-glutamyltransferase 1 gene and risk of chronic pancreatitis. Pancreas. 2013; 42(5):836–840. PMID: 23462328

48 Sri Manjari K, Nallari P, Balakrishna N, Vidyasagar A, Prabhakar B, Jyothy A, et al. Influence of matrix metalloproteinase-1 gene −1607 (1G/2G) (rs1799750) promoter polymorphism on circulating levels of MMP-1 in chronic pancreatitis. Biochemical Genetics. 2013;51(7–8): 644–654. PMID: 23644943

49 Singh S, Choudhuri G, Kumar R, Agarwal S. Association of 5,10-methylenetetrahydrofolate reductase C677T polymorphism in susceptibility to tropical chronic pancreatitis in north Indian population. Cellular and Molecular Biology. 2012;58(1):122–127. PMID: 23273201

50 Fjeld K, Weiss FU, Lasher D, Rosendahl J, Chen JM, Johansson BB, et al. A recombined allele of the lipase gene CEL and its pseudogene CELP confers susceptibility to chronic pancreatitis. Nature Genetics. 2015;47(5): 518–522. PMID: 25774637

51 Whitcomb DC. Mechanisms of disease: advances in understanding the mechanisms leading to chronic pancreatitis. Nature Clinical Practice Gastroenterology & Hepatology. 2004;1(1):46–52. PMID: 16265044

52 Whitcomb DC. Hereditary pancreatitis: new insights into acute and chronic pancreatitis. Gut. 1999;45:317–322.

53 Yadav D, Whitcomb DC. The role of alcohol and smoking in pancreatitis. Nature Reviews Gastroenterology & Hepatology. 2010;7(3):131–145. PMID: 20125091

54 Whitcomb DC. Genetic risk factors for pancreatic disorders. Gastroenterology. 2013;144(6):1292–1302. PMID: 23622139

55 Jacob C, Yang PC, Darmoul D, Amadesi S, Saito T, Cottrell GS, et al. Mast cell tryptase controls paracellular permeability of the intestine. Role of protease-activated receptor 2 and beta-arrestins. The Journal of Biological Chemistry. 2005;280(36):31936–31948. PMID: 16027150

56 Mogami H, Nakano K, Tepikin AV, Petersen OH. Ca2+ flow via tunnels in polarized cells: recharging of apical Ca2+ stores by focal Ca2+ entry through basal membrane patch. Cell. 1997;88(1):49–55.

57 Raraty M, Ward J, Erdemli G, Vaillant C, Neoptolemos JP, Sutton R, et al. Calcium-dependent enzyme activation and vacuole formation in the apical granular region of pancreatic acinar cells. Proceedings of the National Academy of Sciences of the United States of America. 2000;97(24):13126–13131.

58 Sutton R, Criddle D, Raraty MG, Tepikin A, Neoptolemos JP, Petersen OH. Signal transduction, calcium and acute pancreatitis. Pancreatology. 2003;3(6):497–505.

59 Lerch MM, Gorelick FS. Early trypsinogen activation in acute pancreatitis. The Medical clinics of North America. 2000;84(3):549–563.

60 Mithofer K, Fernandez-Del Castillo C, Frick TW, Lewandrowski KB, Rattner DW, Warshaw AL. Acute hypercalcemia causes acute pancreatitis and ectopic trypsinogen activation in the rat. Gastroenterology. 1995; 109(1):239–246.

61 Frick TW, Fernandez-del Castillo C, Bimmler D, Warshaw AL. Elevated calcium and activation of trypsinogen in rat pancreatic acini. Gut. 1997;41(3):339–343.

62 Liu JH, Wang ZX. Kinetic analysis of ligand-induced autocatalytic reactions. Biochemical Journal. 2004;379(Pt 3):697–702. PMID: 14705964

63 Colomb E, Figarella C. Comparative studies on the mechanism of activation of the two human trypsinogens. Biochimica et Biophysica Acta. 1979;571(2):343–351. PMID: 508771

64 Guy O, Lombardo D, Bartelt DC, Amic J, Figarella C. Two human trypsinogens. Purification, molecular properties, and N-terminal sequences. Biochemistry. 1978;17(9): 1669–1675. PMID: 656395

65 Criddle DN, Raraty MG, Neoptolemos JP, Tepikin AV, Petersen OH, Sutton R. Ethanol toxicity in pancreatic acinar cells: mediation by nonoxidative fatty acid metabolites. Proceedings of the National Academy of Sciences of the United States of America. 2004;101(29):10738–10743. PMID: 15247419

66 Nemoda Z, Sahin-Toth M. The tetra-aspartate motif in the activation peptide of human cationic trypsinogen is essential for autoactivation control but not for enteropeptidase recognition. The Journal of Biological Chemistry. 2005;280(33):29645–29652. PMID: 15970597

67 Rinderknecht H, Renner IG, Abramson SB, Carmack C. Mesotrypsin: a new inhibitor-resistant protease from a zymogen in human pancreatic tissue and fluid. Gastroenterology. 1984;86(4):681–692. PMID: 6698368

68 Bhoomagoud M, Jung T, Atladottir J, Kolodecik TR, Shugrue C, Chaudhuri A, et al. Reducing extracellular pH sensitizes the acinar cell to secretagogue-induced pancreatitis responses in rats. Gastroenterology. 2009;137(3): 1083–1092. PMID: 19454288

69 Yadav D, Nair S, Norkus EP, Pitchumoni CS. Nonspecific hyperamylasemia and hyperlipasemia in diabetic ketoacidosis: incidence and correlation with biochemical abnormalities. The American Journal of Gastroenterology. 2000;95(11):3123–3128. PMID: 11095328

70 Nair S, Yadav D, Pitchumoni CS. Association of diabetic ketoacidosis and acute pancreatitis: observations in 100 consecutive episodes of DKA. The American Journal of Gastroenterology. 2000;95(10):2795–2800. PMID: 11051350

71 Kukor Z, Mayerle J, Kruger B, Toth M, Steed PM, Halangk W, et al. Presence of cathepsin B in the human pancreatic secretory pathway and its role in trypsinogen activation during hereditary pancreatitis. The Journal of Biological Chemistry. 2002;277(24):21389–21396. PMID: 11932257

72 Beer S, Zhou J, Szabo A, Keiles S, Chandak GR, Witt H, et al. Comprehensive functional analysis of chymotrypsin C (CTRC) variants reveals distinct loss-of-function mechanisms associated with pancreatitis risk. Gut. 2012;62(11): 1616–1624. PMID: 22942235

73 Szabo A, Sahin-Toth M. Increased activation of hereditary pancreatitis-associated human cationic trypsinogen mutants in presence of chymotrypsin C. The Journal of Biological Chemistry. 2012;287(24):20701–20710. PMID: 22539344

74 Ogawa M. Pancreatic secretory trypsin inhibitor as an acute phase reactant. Clinical Biochemistry. 1988; 21:19–25.

75 Sand J, Lankisch PG, Nordback I. Alcohol consumption in patients with acute or chronic pancreatitis. Pancreatology. 2007;7(2–3):147–156. PMID: 17592227

76 Apte M, Pirola R, Wilson J. New insights into alcoholic pancreatitis and pancreatic cancer. Journal of Gastroenterology and Hepatology. 2009;24 Suppl 3:S51–S56. PMID: 19799699

77 Deng X, Wood PG, Eagon PK, Whitcomb DC. Chronic alcohol-induced alterations in the pancreatic secretory control mechanisms. Digestive Diseases and Sciences. 2004;49(5):805–819.

78 Nordback I, Pelli H, Lappalainen-Lehto R, Sand J. Is it long-term continuous drinking or the post-drinking withdrawal period that triggers the first acute alcoholic pancreatitis? Scandinavian Journal of Gastroenterology. 2005;40(10):1235–1239. PMID: 16265780

79 Yadav D, Eigenbrodt ML, Briggs MJ, Williams DK, Wiseman EJ. Pancreatitis: prevalence and risk factors among male veterans in a detoxification program. Pancreas. 2007;34(4):390–398. PMID: 17446836

80 Park HW, Nam JH, Kim JY, Namkung W, Yoon JS, Lee JS, et al. Dynamic regulation of CFTR bicarbonate permeability by [Cl-]i and its role in pancreatic bicarbonate secretion. Gastroenterology. 2010;139(2):620–631. PMID: 20398666

81 Lee MG, Ohana E, Park HW, Yang D, Muallem S. Molecular mechanism of pancreatic and salivary gland fluid and HCO3 secretion. Physiological Reviews. 2012;92(1):39–74. PMID: 22298651

82 Whitcomb DC, Ermentrout GB. A mathematical model of the pancreatic duct cell generating high bicarbonate concentrations in pancreatic juice. Pancreas. 2004;29(2):E30–E40. PMID: 15257112

83 Hansen KK, Sherman PM, Cellars L, Andrade-Gordon P, Pan Z, Baruch A, et al. A major role for proteolytic activity and proteinase-activated receptor-2 in the pathogenesis of infectious colitis. Proceedings of the National Academy of Sciences of the United States of America. 2005;102(23):8363–8368. PMID: 15919826

84 Sharma A, Tao X, Gopal A, Ligon B, Andrade-Gordon P, Steer ML, et al. Protection against acute pancreatitis by activation of protease-activated receptor-2. American Journal of Physiology: Gastrointestinal and Liver Physiology. 2005;288(2):G388–G395. PMID: 15458925

85 Steward MC, Ishiguro H. Molecular and cellular regulation of pancreatic duct cell function. Current Opinion in Gastroenterology. 2009;25(5):447–453. PMID: 19571747

86 Sharer N, Schwarz M, Malone G, Howarth A, Painter J, Super M, et al. Mutations of the cystic fibrosis gene in patients with chronic pancreatitis. New England Journal of Medicine. 1998;339(10):645–652.

87 Cohn JA, Friedman KJ, Noone PG, Knowles MR, Silverman LM, Jowell PS. Relation between mutations of the cystic fibrosis gene and idiopathic pancreatitis. New England Journal of Medicine. 1998;339(10):653–658. PMID: 9725922

88 Schneider A, Larusch J, Sun X, Aloe A, Lamb J, Hawes R, et al. Combined bicarbonate conductance-impairing variants in CFTR and SPINK1 variants are associated with chronic pancreatitis in patients without cystic fibrosis. Gastroenterology. 2011;140(1):162–171. PMID: 20977904

89 Audrezet MP, Chen JM, Le Marechal C, Ruszniewski P, Robaszkiewicz M, Raguenes O, et al. Determination of the relative contribution of three genes-the cystic fibrosis transmembrane conductance regulator gene, the cationic trypsinogen gene, and the pancreatic secretory trypsin inhibitor gene-to the etiology of idiopathic chronic pancreatitis. European Journal of Human Genetics. 2002;10(2):100–106.

90 Sobczynska-Tomaszewska A, Bak D, Oralewska B, Oracz G, Norek A, Czerska K, et al. Analysis of CFTR, SPINK1, PRSS1 and AAT mutations in children with acute or chronic pancreatitis. Journal of Pediatric Gastroenterology and Nutrition. 2006;43(3):299–306. PMID: 16954950

91 de Cid R, Ramos MD, Aparisi L, Garcia C, Mora J, Estivill X, et al. Independent contribution of common CFTR variants to chronic pancreatitis. Pancreas. 2010;39(2):209–215. PMID: 19812525

92 Midha S, Khajuria R, Shastri S, Kabra M, Garg PK. Idiopathic chronic pancreatitis in India: phenotypic characterisation and strong genetic susceptibility due to SPINK1 and CFTR gene mutations. Gut. 2010;59(6):800–807. PMID: 20551465

93 Chang YT, Chang MC, Su TC, Liang PC, Su YN, Kuo CH, et al. Association of cystic fibrosis transmembrane conductance regulator (CFTR) mutation/variant/haplotype and tumor necrosis factor (TNF) promoter polymorphism in hyperlipidemic pancreatitis. Clinical Chemistry. 2008;54(1):131–138. PMID: 17981921

94 Chang MC, Chang YT, Wei SC, Tien YW, Liang PC, Jan IS, et al. Spectrum of mutations and variants/haplotypes of CFTR and genotype-phenotype correlation in idiopathic chronic pancreatitis and controls in Chinese by complete analysis. Clinical Genetics. 2007;71(6):530–539. PMID: 17539902

95 Noone PG, Zhou Z, Silverman LM, Jowell PS, Knowles MR, Cohn JA. Cystic fibrosis gene mutations and pancreatitis risk: relation to epithelial ion transport and trypsin inhibitor gene mutations. Gastroenterology. 2001; 121(6):1310–1319.

96 Bombieri C, Claustres M, De Boeck K, Derichs N, Dodge J, Girodon E, et al. Recommendations for the classification of diseases as CFTR-related disorders. Journal of Cystic Fibrosis. 2011;10 Suppl 2:S86–S102. PMID: 21658649

97 Ooi CY, Dorfman R, Cipolli M, Gonska T, Castellani C, Keenan K, et al. Type of CFTR mutation determines risk of pancreatitis in patients with cystic fibrosis. Gastroenterology. 2011;140(1):153–161. PMID: 20923678

98 Solomon S, Whitcomb DC. Genetics of pancreatitis: an update for clinicians and genetic counselors. Current Gastroenterology Reports. 2012;14(2):112–117. PMID: 22314809

99 LaRusch J, Jung J, General IJ, Lewis MD, Park HW, Brand RE, et al. Mechanisms of CFTR functional variants that impair regulated bicarbonate permeation and increase risk for pancreatitis but not for cystic fibrosis. PLoS Genetics. 2014;10(7):e1004376. PMID: 25033378

100 Yadav D, O'Connell M, Papachristou GI. Natural history following the first attack of acute pancreatitis. The American Journal of Gastroenterology. 2012;107(7):1096–1103. PMID: 22613906

101 Gorry MC, Gabbaizedeh D, Furey W, Gates LK, Jr.,, Preston RA, Aston CE, et al. Mutations in the cationic trypsinogen gene are associated with recurrent acute and chronic pancreatitis. Gastroenterology. 1997;113(4): 1063–1068.

102 Rebours V, Boutron-Ruault MC, Schnee M, Ferec C, Le Marechal C, Hentic O, et al. The natural history of hereditary pancreatitis: a national series. Gut. 2009;58(1):97–103. PMID: 18755888

103 Pfutzer RH, Barmada MM, Brunskill AP, Finch R, Hart PS, Neoptolemos J, et al. SPINK1/PSTI polymorphisms act as disease modifiers in familial and idiopathic chronic pancreatitis. Gastroenterology. 2000;119(3):615–623. PMID: 10982753

104 Threadgold J, Greenhalf W, Ellis I, Howes N, Lerch MM, Simon P, et al. The N34S mutation of SPINK1 (PSTI) is associated with a familial pattern of idiopathic chronic pancreatitis but does not cause the disease. Gut. 2002;50(5):675–681.

105 Yadav D, Timmons L, Benson JT, Dierkhising RA, Chari ST. Incidence, prevalence, and survival of chronic pancreatitis: a population-based study. The American Journal of Gastroenterology. 2011;106(12):2192–2199. PMID: 21946280

106 Aoun E, Chang CC, Greer JB, Papachristou GI, Barmada MM, Whitcomb DC. Pathways to injury in chronic pancreatitis: decoding the role of the high-risk SPINK1 N34S haplotype using meta-analysis. PLoS ONE. 2008;3(4):e2003. PMID: 18414673

107 Aoun E, Muddana V, Papachristou GI, Whitcomb DC. SPINK1 N34S is strongly associated with recurrent acute pancreatitis but is not a risk factor for the first or sentinel acute pancreatitis event. The American Journal of Gastroenterology. 2010;105(2):446–451. PMID: 19888199

108 Masamune A, Ariga H, Kume K, Kakuta Y, Satoh K, Satoh A, et al. Genetic background is different between sentinel and recurrent acute pancreatitis. Journal of Gastroenterology and Hepatology. 2011;26(6):974–978. PMID: 21303407

109 Schneider A, Pfützer RH, Barmada MM, Slivka A, Martin J, Whitcomb DC. Limited contribution of the SPINK1 N34S mutation to the risk and severity of alcoholic chronic pancreatitis – a preliminary report from the United States. Digestive Diseases and Sciences. 2003;48(6):1110–1115.

110 Lee KH, Ryu JK, Yoon WJ, Lee JK, Kim YT, Yoon YB. Mutation analysis of SPINK1 and CFTR gene in Korean patients with alcoholic chronic pancreatitis. Digestive Diseases and Sciences. 2005;50(10):1852–1856. PMID: 16187186

111 Shimosegawa T, Kume K, Masamune A. SPINK1 gene mutations and pancreatitis in Japan. Journal of Gastroenterology and Hepatology 2006;21 Suppl 3:S47–S51. PMID: 16958672

112 Masamune A, Kume K, Shimosegawa T. Differential roles of the SPINK1 gene mutations in alcoholic and nonalcoholic chronic pancreatitis. Journal of Gastroenterology. 2007;42 Suppl 17;135–140. PMID: 17238043

113 Bertin C, Pelletier AL, Vullierme MP, Bienvenu T, Rebours V, Hentic O, et al. Pancreas divisum is not a cause of pancreatitis by itself but acts as a partner of genetic mutations. The American Journal of Gastroenterology. 2012;107(2):311–317. PMID: 22158025

114 Pelli H, Lappalainen-Lehto R, Piironen A, Sand J, Nordback I. Risk factors for recurrent acute alcohol-associated pancreatitis: a prospective analysis. Scandinavian Journal of Gastroenterology. 2008;43(5):614–621. PMID: 18415757

115 Nordback I, Pelli H, Lappalainen-Lehto R, Jarvinen S, Raty S, Sand J. The recurrence of acute alcohol-associated pancreatitis can be reduced: a randomized controlled trial. Gastroenterology. 2009;136(3):848–855. PMID: 19162029

116 Lankisch PG, Breuer N, Bruns A, Weber-Dany B, Lowenfels AB, Maisonneuve P. Natural history of acute pancreatitis: a long-term population-based study. The American Journal of Gastroenterology. 2009;104(11): 2797–2805; quiz 806. PMID: 19603011

117 Deng X, Wang L, Elm MS, Gabazadeh D, Diorio GJ, Eagon PK, et al. Chronic alcohol consumption accelerates fibrosis in response to cerulein-induced pancreatitis in rats. American Journal of Pathology. 2005;166(1):93–106. PMID: 15632003

118 Perides G, Tao X, West N, Sharma A, Steer ML. A mouse model of ethanol dependent pancreatic fibrosis. Gut. 2005;54(10):1461–1467. PMID: 15870229

119 Takeyama Y. Long-term prognosis of acute pancreatitis in Japan. Clinical Gastroenterology and Hepatology. 2009;7(11 Suppl):S15–S17. PMID: 19896091

120 Wilcox CM, Yadav D, Tian Y, Gardner TB, Gelrud A, Sandhu BS, et al. Chronic pancreatitis pain pattern and severity are independent of abdominal imaging findings. Clinical Gastroenterology and Hepatology. 2014; 13(3):552–560. PMID: 25424572

121 Rebours V, Boutron-Ruault MC, Schnee M, Ferec C, Maire F, Hammel P, et al. Risk of pancreatic adenocarcinoma in patients with hereditary pancreatitis: a national exhaustive series. The American Journal of Gastroenterology. 2008;103(1):111–119. PMID: 18184119

PART C: Pancreatic stellate cells: what do they tell us about chronic pancreatitis?

Minoti V. Apte[1,2], Zhihong Xu[1,2], Ron C. Pirola[1,2] & Jeremy S. Wilson[1,2]

[1] Pancreatic Research Group, South Western Sydney Clinical School, Faculty of Medicine, University of New South Wales, Sydney, NSW, Australia
[2] Ingham Institute for Applied Medical Research, Liverpool Hospital, Liverpool, NSW, Australia

Introduction

Chronic pancreatitis, regardless of etiology (alcohol, hereditary, and idiopathic) is characterized by progressive destruction of the pancreas leading to exocrine and endocrine insufficiency [1]. Histologically, the gland exhibits necrotic and atrophied acinar elements surrounded by abundant fibrous tissue [2] (Figure 12C.1). It has now been recognized that the endocrine pancreas (pancreatic islets) also exhibits significant peri- and intra-islet fibrosis in chronic pancreatitis. As recently as two decades ago, the abundant fibrosis of chronic pancreatitis was thought to be a mere end point of chronic inflammation. However, this view changed dramatically in 1998, with the isolation and characterization of the cells responsible for fibrogenesis in the pancreas, namely, pancreatic stellate cells (PSCs). As is discussed in more detail later, evidence that strongly supports the concept of fibrogenesis as an active, dynamic process has now accumulated, suggesting that interventions (at least in the early stages) have the potential to retard/reverse the process.

In contrast to the pancreas, fibrogenesis in the liver has been studied for over a century, ever since the first description of hepatic stellate cells by the renowned pathologist Kupffer [3]. Thus, the hepatic stellate cell biology field has a significant march over the PSC field. PSCs themselves were first described by Watari [4] in 1982 as a result of electron microscopy studies of both rodent and human pancreas. However, it was another 16 years before a method was developed to isolate and culture PSCs from rodent pancreas [5]. The same method was subsequently adapted for the isolation of PSCs from the human pancreas [6]. This isolation method took advantage of the capacity of PSCs to store vitamin A within lipid droplets in their cytoplasm. The cells could, therefore, be separated from other pancreatic cells using a density gradient centrifugation method. The ability to isolate PSCs from the pancreas provided the much-needed impetus to the pancreatic fibrosis field, and characterization of PSCs has moved forward at a rapid pace over the past 17 years.

PSCs are resident cells of the pancreas, located in close proximity to acinar cells (Figure 12C.2), and comprise about 4–7% of all pancreatic parenchymal cells. They have a central cell body and several cytoplasmic extensions that extend around the basolateral aspect of acinar cells. PSCs have also been found around small ducts and blood vessels. In the healthy pancreas, PSCs are in their quiescent state with abundant vitamin A–containing lipid droplets in their cytoplasm (Figure 12C.3). They also stain for the selective markers desmin, glial fibrillary acidic protein (GFAP), nestin, and other neuroectodermal markers; these characteristics help to distinguish PSCs from fibroblasts. During pancreatic injury, PSCs are activated by numerous factors that are known to be upregulated in necroinflammatory states of the gland (listed later), but can also be activated directly by toxic factors such as alcohol and its metabolites (well established causative agents for alcoholic pancreatitis). Upon activation, PSCs invariably lose their vitamin A stores, exhibit a myofibroblast-like phenotype, and express the cytoskeletal protein alpha-smooth muscle actin (αSMA). Activated PSCs have been well identified in fibrotic areas of human chronic pancreatitis sections using immunohistochemistry of serial sections for PSC selective markers such as GFAP and αSMA (Figure 12C.4a) [7] or dual staining of sections

Pancreatitis: Medical and Surgical Management, First Edition.
David B. Adams, Peter B. Cotton, Nicholas J. Zyromski and John Windsor.
© 2017 John Wiley & Sons, Ltd. Published 2017 by John Wiley & Sons, Ltd.

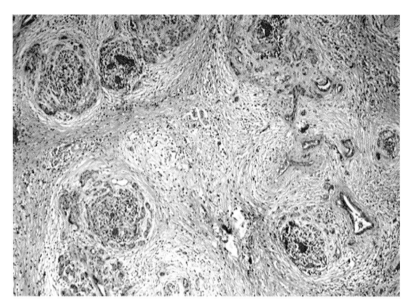

Figure 12C.1   Chronic pancreatitis – a hematoxylin and eosin (H&E) stained section of the pancreas from a patient with chronic pancreatitis showing abundant fibrosis, acinar atrophy, and distorted and dilated ducts. Used with Permission. Copyright, American Gastroenterological Association Institute, Bethesda, MD.

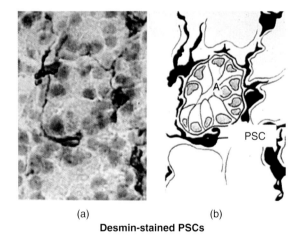

(a)   (b)
Desmin-stained PSCs

Figure 12C.2 Pancreatic stellate cells in rat pancreas stained for the selective marker desmin. (a) A representative photomicrograph of normal rat pancreas immunostained for desmin. (b) The corresponding line diagram. Desmin-positive PSCs with long cytoplasmic projections are located at the basolateral aspect of acinar cells (A). Apte et al., Gut, 1998. Reprinted with permission from BMJ Group.

showing colocalization of αSMA-positive areas with positive staining for ECM proteins such as collagen (Figure 12C.4b). Importantly, using dual staining techniques, it has been unequivocally demonstrated that the αSMA-positive cells in the stroma are the source of the collagen that comprises fibrous tissue in chronic pancreatitis and pancreatic cancer [8, 9].

Over the past decade, the number of factors reported to activate PSCs (based on *in vitro* studies) has increased exponentially, with new activators being identified on a regular basis. A detailed description of the role and postulated mechanism of action of each activating factor is beyond the scope of this article (please refer to the review by Apte et al. [10]). However, it would be pertinent to list the major factors identified to date. As noted earlier, the commonest association of chronic pancreatitis in the western world is alcohol abuse. It is well established that the pancreas has the capacity to metabolize alcohol to its toxic metabolites, which exert injurious effects on the gland. In this regard, it is of interest that both rat and human PSCs have the capacity to metabolize alcohol via the oxidative pathway, due to the activity of the ethanol-metabolizing enzyme alcohol dehydrogenase 1 (ADH1), within the cells [11, 12]. These *in vitro* observations are supported by an *in vivo* study, demonstrating increased expression of ADH1C (an ADH1 isozyme), namely in activated PSCs in histological sections of the pancreas from patients with chronic pancreatitis and pancreatic cancer [12].

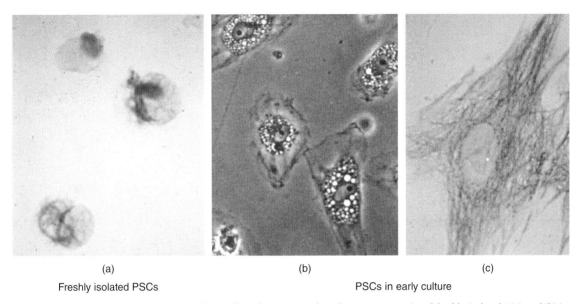

(a)   (b)   (c)

Freshly isolated PSCs   PSCs in early culture

Figure 12C.3 Freshly isolated pancreatic stellate cells and PSCs in early culture. (a) Cytospin of freshly isolated PSCs exhibiting desmin staining (brown) in the cytoplasm adjacent to the nucleus (blue). (b) PSCs in early culture exhibiting a flattened polygonal shape with abundant lipid droplets (containing vitamin A) in the cytoplasm, surrounding the central nucleus. (c) PSC in early culture showing positive desmin staining characteristic of a cytoskeletal protein. Apte et al., Gut, 1998. Reprinted with permission from BMJ Group.

Other known PSC-activating factors closely relevant to the setting of pancreatic injury include oxidant stress, inflammatory mediators (cytokines, chemokines), cyclooxygenase 2, hypoxia, hyperglycemia, and angiotensin. One of the intriguing features with regard to PSC activation is the fact that upon activation by the exogenous factors noted earlier, PSCs are themselves able to secrete cytokines, which can act on the cells in an autocrine manner. This ability to produce endogenous cytokines confers on the cells a capacity to remain in a perpetually activated state (even when the original activating factors are no longer present) (Figure 12C.5). This can lead to uncontrolled production of ECM proteins eventually leading to pathological fibrosis.

In parallel with studies identifying the exogenous factors responsible for activating PSCs during pancreatic injury, researchers have been assessing the signaling pathways that may mediate the responses of PSCs to such activating factors. It is now well established that PSC functions such as proliferation, αSMA expression, migration, and ECM expression are regulated by the MAP kinase, PI3 kinase, and PKC pathways [13–15]. More recently, the Hedgehog pathway has also been implicated in PSC migration [16], while downstream signaling molecules such as JAK-STAT and Smads regulate cell proliferation and ECM synthesis, respectively [17, 18]. Rho kinases are thought to regulate cytoskeletal stress protein expression in PSCs [19], while transcription factors such as AP-1, NF-κB, and Gli-I act as downstream regulators of several PSC functions. While the pathways noted earlier generally regulate the induction of the activating process in PSCs, there is one pathway that is unique because it mediates the *inhibition* of PSC activation – thus, binding of glita-zone ligands to their receptor, peroxisome proliferator activator receptor-gamma (PPARγ), has been shown to prevent/retard the activation process in PSCs [20].

Although initial interest in PSC biology revolved around their possible role in pathological fibrosis, recent studies indicate a wider functional scope for these cells, such as protecting the pancreas against initial pancreatic injury via their role in innate immunity [21]. In this regard, PSCs have been shown to express the receptors that recognize pathogen-associated molecular patterns (PAMPs), namely toll-like receptors 2, 3, 4, 5, and 9 [22]. Moreover, they have been shown to

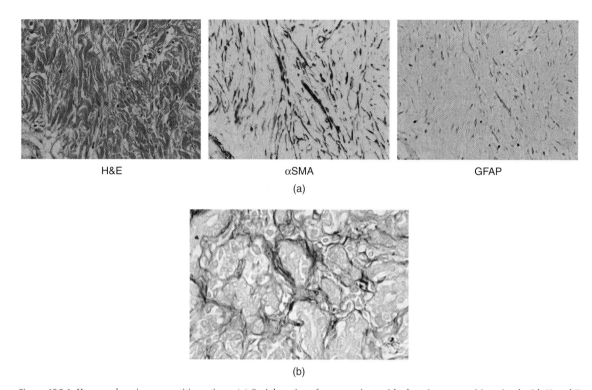

H&E   αSMA   GFAP

(a)

(b)

Figure 12C.4 Human chronic pancreatitis sections. (a) Serial sections from a patient with chronic pancreatitis stained with H and E and immunostained for α-smooth muscle actin (αSMA) and glial fibrillary acidic protein (GFAP), demonstrating positive staining for the PSC activation marker αSMA and the PSC selective marker GFAP in fibrotic areas. Tahara et al., Laboratory Investigation, 2013. Reprinted with permission from Nature Publishing Group. (b) Dual staining of a human chronic pancreatitis section immunostained for the PSC activation marker αSMA and for collagen using Sirius Red. The brown staining for αSMA is colocalized with the red staining for collagen indicating the presence of activated PSCs in fibrotic areas of the pancreas. Haber 1999. Reproduced with permission of Elsevier.

have a capacity for endocytosis and phagocytosis of necrotic cells. However, in contrast to hepatic stellate cells, PSCs appear to be unlikely to play a role in acquired immunity since they do not appear to function as antigen-presenting cells as evidenced by lack of expression of antigen-presenting cell markers such as MHC class II molecules or HLA-DR molecules [23]. This difference between HSCs and PSCs may reflect the fact that HSCs are routinely exposed to antigens via the portal circulation, whereas PSCs are located in a relatively sheltered microenvironment.

PSCs and chronic pancreatitis

In order to elucidate the specific role of PSCs in chronic pancreatitis, researchers have assessed pancreatic sections from patients with chronic pancreatitis (these are necessarily cross-sectional studies) and in experimental models of pancreatic injury, which allow the examination of chronological changes during disease development.

Human chronic pancreatitis sections have been stained for ECM deposition (using trichrome stains), collagen (using Sirius Red), and also immunostained for ECM proteins, PSC selective markers, fibrogenic cytokines such as TGFβ and other indices of injury such as oxidant stress. It has now been consistently demonstrated that fibrotic areas in chronic pancreatitis exhibit the presence of increased numbers of activated PSCs [9]. Moreover, using dual staining techniques for αSMA and procollagen mRNA, it has been shown that activated PSCs are the predominant source of collagen in pancreatic fibrosis [9].

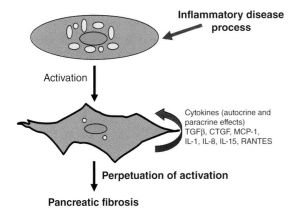

Figure 12C.5 Perpetuation of PSC activation. A diagrammatic representation of the postulated pathway for a perpetually activated state for PSCs. Pancreatic stellate cells are activated via paracrine pathways by exogenous factors during pancreatic necroinflammation. Activated PSCs synthesize and secrete endogenous cytokines, which influence PSC function via autocrine pathways. It is possible that this autocrine loop in activated PSCs perpetuates the activated state of the cell, even in the absence of the initial trigger factors, leading to excessive ECM production and eventually causing pancreatic fibrosis.

As noted earlier, a number of PSC-activating factors have been identified through *in vitro* studies including cytokines, growth factors, and oxidant stress. Supportive evidence for a role of these factors during the development of pancreatic fibrosis comes from the following observations : (i) significantly increased expression of the profibrogenic cytokine transforming growth factor beta (TGFβ) in acinar cells in the vicinity of fibrotic areas and in spindle-shaped cells within fibrotic bands, suggesting a paracrine effect of the growth factor on PSC activation [9]; (ii) increased expression of the receptor for platelet-derived growth factor (PDGF, a well-known mitogenic factor for PSCs) in areas of fibrosis, suggesting that PDGF-induced proliferation is responsible for the increased numbers of PSCs in chronic pancreatitis [9]; (iii) increased expression of nerve growth factor (NGF, a PSC selective marker) in chronic pancreatitis [24], indicating that apart from neuronal cells, PSCs may also contribute to the observed increase in NGF expression in chronic pancreatitis; and (iv) increased evidence of oxidant stress (as assessed by the staining for 4-hydroxynonenal, a lipid peroxidation product) in fibrotic areas of chronic pancreatitis [25].

Animal models

Researchers turned to experimental models of pancreatic fibrosis to overcome the limitation of "point-in-time" studies using human chronic pancreatitis sections. Several animal models (mostly rodent models) have been described in the literature, the majority of which have used relatively nonphysiological interventions to cause pancreatic fibrosis (see review Apte et al. [10]). A detailed description of each of these models is not within the scope of this chapter, but the approaches used to produce pancreatic fibrosis in rats have included retrograde infusions of toxins into the pancreatic duct [9], duct ligation with simultaneous secretory stimulation (hypertension obstruction model) [26], repeated injections of a superoxide dismutase inhibitor (thus causing increased oxidant stress within the gland) [27], chronic alcohol administration with repeated cyclosporine and caerulein injections [28], and chronic alcohol administration followed by endotoxin (LPS) challenge [29]. A model of spontaneous chronic pancreatitis in Wbn/Kob rats has also been studied [30]. Mouse models of pancreatic fibrosis have involved the use of transgenic animals overexpressing TGF or the EGF receptor ligand heparin epidermal growth factor-like growth factor (HB-EGF) [31] or IL-1β [32] and chronic pancreatitis produced by repeated injections of supraphysiological caerulein [33].

Each of the models noted earlier has provided useful experimental evidence in support of a role for PSCs in progressive pancreatic fibrosis, but only one of the models could be said to closely represent the clinical situation, that is, the rat model of alcoholic chronic pancreatitis produced by repeatedly challenging alcohol-fed rats with endotoxin (LPS) [29]. This model is based on the well-recognized clinical observation of endotoxemia in heavy drinkers (secondary to alcohol-mediated increase in gut mucosal permeability) [34]. In this model, a synergistic effect of alcohol and LPS was observed whereby pancreatic injury was significantly more severe (as evidenced by acinar atrophy and fibrosis) in rats treated with alcohol and LPS, compared with animals treated with either factor alone (Figure 12C.6).

Regardless of the model used however, in general, the aforementioned studies have demonstrated that PSCs are activated early during pancreatic injury. Once activated they not only produce significantly increased

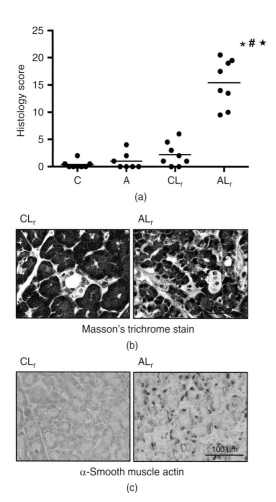

Figure 12C.6 Rat model of alcoholic chronic pancreatitis involving chronic ethanol administration and repeated endotoxin (LPS) challenge. (a) Graphical representation of histological injury in four groups of rats as assessed by scoring for vacuolization, necrosis, inflammatory infiltrate, hemorrhage, and edema: (i) control diet–fed rat, no alcohol (C); (ii) alcohol-fed rat (A); (iii) control diet–fed rat challenged with repeated LPS injections (CL_r) ; (iv) alcohol-fed rat challenged with repeated LPS injections (AL_r). Alcohol and LPS alone caused minimal histological damage to the pancreas. AL_r animal exhibited the highest histological injury scores compared with the other three groups. 25 HPF/section, three sections per rat were examined (*$P < 0.001$ AL_r vs. CL_r, A and C; $n = 7$ rats/group). (b) Masson's trichrome staining for pancreatic connective tissue: representative micrographs from CL_r and AL_r animals showing increased fibrosis (blue Masson's staining) in the latter group. (c) αSMA staining for activated PSCs: representative micrographs from CL_r and AL_r animals showing significantly increased αSMA in the latter group. Vonlaufen 2007. Reproduced with permission of Elsevier.

amounts of ECM proteins but also modulate the proportion of matrix-degrading enzymes and their inhibitors, such that deposition of excess ECM is facilitated.

One of the well-recognized complications of chronic pancreatitis is diabetes, postulated to occur due to islet cell destruction secondary to progressive fibrosis. Interestingly, recent evidence using Goto-Kakizaki rats (a model of type 2 diabetes) indicates that activated PSCs (as identified by positive immunostaining for αSMA and the PSC selective marker GFAP) are present in fibrotic areas around and within pancreatic islets [35]. *In vitro* studies by Kikuta et al. [36] have examined the interaction between PSCs and β-cells and have reported increased apoptosis and decreased insulin production by β-cells upon co-incubation with PSCs. In turn, β-cells (specifically the beta cell line INS-1) have been shown to increase proliferation, while at the same time, inhibiting ECM synthesis and cytokine production by PSCs [37]. The authors hypothesize that the inhibitory effects of beta cells on PSCs may represent a mechanism by which β-cells protect themselves from PSC-induced injury. Although further studies will be required to clarify the observed differential responses of PSCs to islet cells, the aforementioned work suggests a role for PSCs in chronic pancreatitis–related islet dysfunction.

While it is agreed that a major proportion of the increased numbers of activated PSCs in experimental chronic pancreatitis reflect increased proliferation of resident PSCs, it is possible that a small fraction of activated PSCs in the diseased pancreas come from circulating bone marrow cells. Using a chimeric approach, where bone marrow from male, GFP-enhanced transgenic mice was infused into irradiated female mice that were then subjected to repeated caerulein injections to produce chronic pancreatitis, Watanabe et al. [38] demonstrated that at least 20% of αSMA-positive (activated) PSCs were sourced from the bone marrow. These findings support the concept that during pancreatic injury, bone marrow–derived PSCs home to areas of injury, thereby contributing to the fibrotic process in the injured gland.

Reversal of pancreatic fibrosis in chronic pancreatitis

In view of the central role of activated PSCs in the fibrosis of chronic pancreatitis, any steps to retard/reverse the process would necessarily entail removal of excess ECM from the pancreas and restitution of the activated and proliferating PSC population to its normal quiescent phenotype. Loss of activated PSCs could occur through a reversion to quiescence, apoptosis, or senescence. *In vitro* studies have shown that culture of cells on Matrigel (a basement membrane-like matrix) [39] or exposure of cells to albumin [40] or retinol metabolites such as all *trans*-retinoic acid (ATRA) [13] can induce a partial reversion to quiescence. ATRA treatment *in vivo*, albeit in a model of pancreatic cancer, has been shown to inhibit PSC activation [41]. However, there are no *in vivo* studies yet pertaining to ATRA treatment in chronic pancreatitis. Apoptosis of PSCs has been better studied, with both *in vitro* and *in vivo* evidence demonstrating that withdrawal of alcohol from culture medium, or from the diet in rats, promoted PSC apoptosis and a reversal of fibrosis [42]. Interestingly, Li and colleagues [43] have reported that an acute phase reactant protein (pancreatic stone protein, PSP, known to be upregulated in pancreatitis) can induce apoptosis of PSCs and also decreases TIMP production by the cells, effectively facilitating MMP activity, which eventually leads to fibrinolysis.

Based on accumulating knowledge regarding the mechanisms mediating PSC activation and quiescence, several potentially useful antifibrotic strategies have now been trialed *in vivo* although these have been limited mainly to experimental models. Significant reductions in fibrosis have been reported using the following approaches: (i) inhibition of cytokines such as TGFβ or TNFα by decreasing production (e.g., pentoxifylline for TNFα) [44], by using neutralizing antibodies to prevent cytokine activity [45, 46], or via inhibition of relevant signaling pathways (e.g., halofuginone to suppress downstream Smad3 phosphorylation in the case of TGFβ) [47]; (ii) inhibition/prevention of oxidant stress, using antioxidants such as vitamin E, xanthine oxidase inhibitors, and free radical scavengers [44, 48–51]; (iii) inhibition of inflammation using protease inhibitors or the synthetic carboxamide derivative IS-741, which reduces macrophage infiltration of the injured pancreas [52, 53]; (iv) stimulation of the PPARγ pathway using its ligand troglitazone [20]; (v) inhibition of the renin–angiotensin system using the antiangiotensin drug losartan [54]; (vi) decreasing collagen synthesis via silencing of collagen mRNA in PSCs, using vitamin A–coupled liposomes containing siRNA for a collagen-specific chaperone [55] and (vii) calcipotriol, a vitamin D receptor ligand recently shown to induce PSC quiescence [56]. As regards alcohol-induced pancreatic fibrosis, it has now been shown by Vonlaufen and colleagues [42] that withdrawal of dietary alcohol from rats with established alcoholic pancreatitis can reverse parenchymal injury as well as fibrosis in the pancreas. Notably, these findings provide the first experimental evidence to support the clinical advice of abstinence that is routinely offered to heavy drinkers by their treating doctors.

In conclusion, cellular and molecular mechanisms regulating fibrogenesis in the pancreas in health as well as in disease have become increasingly clarified over the past 15 years. Through *in vitro* and *in vivo* studies, researchers have unraveled some of the complex interactions between PSCs and other cells as well as between PSCs and the extracellular matrix in the pancreatic parenchyma. Furthermore, using the information gained, novel therapeutic options have been tested and these have proved reasonably successful in reducing/preventing fibrosis in the experimental setting. Transferring these new insights into the clinical situation is the next logical step in this field. Our improved understanding of PSC biology in animal models as well as in humans provides a firm foundation for the genesis of new approaches in the near future, which can successfully interrupt pathological fibrosis in the clinical setting, thereby improving patient outcome in diseases such as chronic pancreatitis.

References

1 Forsmark CE. Management of chronic pancreatitis. Gastroenterology 2013; 144:1282–1291; e3.

2 Kloppel G. Pathology of chronic pancreatitis and pancreatic pain. Acta Chirurgica Scandinavica 1990; 156:261–265.

3 Friedman SD. The cellular basis of hepatic fibrosis. New England Journal of Medicine 1993; 328:1828–1835.

4 Watari N, Hotta Y, Mabuchi Y. Morphological studies on a vitamin A-storing cell and its complex with macrophage observed in mouse pancreatic tissues following excess vitamin A administration. Okajimas Folia Anatomica Japonica 1982; 58:837–858.

5 Apte MV, Haber PS, Applegate TL, et al. Periacinar stellate shaped cells in rat pancreas - identification, isolation, and culture. Gut 1998; 43:128–133.

6 Vonlaufen A, Phillips PA, Xu ZH, et al. Isolation of quiescent human pancreatic stellate cells; a useful in vitro tool to study hPSC biology. Pancreatology 2010; 10:434–443.

7 Tahara H, Sato K, Yamazaki Y, et al. Transforming growth factor-alpha activates pancreatic stellate cells and may be involved in matrix metalloproteinase-1 upregulation. Laboratory Investigation 2013; 93:720–732.

8 Apte MV, Wilson JS, Lugea A, Pandol SJ. A starring role for stellate cells in the pancreatic cancer microenvironment. Gastroenterology 2013; 144:1210–1219.

9 Haber P, Keogh G, Apte M, et al. Activation of pancreatic stellate cells in human and experimental pancreatic fibrosis. American Journal of Pathology 1999; 155:1087–1095.

10 Apte MV, Pirola RC, Wilson JS. Pancreatic stellate cells: a starring role in normal and diseased pancreas. Frontiers in Physiology 2012; 3:344.

11 Apte MV, Phillips PA, Fahmy RG, et al. Does alcohol directly stimulate pancreatic fibrogenesis? Studies with rat pancreatic stellate cells. Gastroenterology 2000; 118:780–794.

12 Chiang CP, Wu CW, Lee SP, et al. Expression pattern, ethanol-metabolizing activities, and cellular localization of alcohol and aldehyde dehydrogenases in human pancreas: implications for pathogenesis of alcohol-induced pancreatic injury. Alcoholism: Clinical and Experimental Research 2009; 33:1059–1068.

13 McCarroll JA, Phillips PA, Santucci N, Pirola RC, Wilson JS, Apte MV. Vitamin A inhibits pancreatic stellate cell activation: implications for treatment of pancreatic fibrosis. Gut 2006; 55 1:79–89.

14 McCarroll JA, Phillips PA, Kumar RK, et al. Pancreatic stellate cell migration: role of the phosphatidylinositol 3-kinase(PI3-kinase) pathway. Biochemical Pharmacology 2004; 67:1215–1225.

15 McCarroll JA, Phillips PA, Park S, et al. Pancreatic stellate cell activation by ethanol and acetaldehyde: is it mediated by the mitogen-activated protein kinase signaling pathway? Pancreas 2003; 27:150–160.

16 Shinozaki S, Ohnishi H, Hama K, et al. Indian hedgehog promotes the migration of rat activated pancreatic stellate cells by increasing membrane type-1 matrix metalloproteinase on the plasma membrane. Journal of Cellular Physiology 2008; 216:38–46.

17 Masamune A, Satoh M, Kikuta K, Suzuki N, Shimosegawa T. Activation of JAK-STAT pathway is required for platelet-derived growth factor-induced proliferation of pancreatic stellate cells. World Journal of Gastroenterology 2005; 11:3385–3391.

18 Ohnishi H, Miyata T, Yasuda H, et al. Distinct roles of Smad2-, Smad3-, and ERK-dependent pathways in transforming growth factor-beta1 regulation of pancreatic stellate cellular functions. Journal of Biological Chemistry 2004; 279:8873–8878 ; Epub 2003 Dec 18.

19 Masamune A, Shimosegawa T. Signal transduction in pancreatic stellate cells. Journal of Gastroenterology 2009; 44:249–260.

20 Shimizu K, Shiratori K, Kobayashi M, Kawamata H. Troglitazone inhibits the progression of chronic pancreatitis and the profibrogenic activity of pancreatic stellate cells via a PPARgamma-independent mechanism. Pancreas 2004; 29:67–74.

21 Shimizu K, Kobayashi M, Tahara J, Shiratori K. Cytokines and peroxisome proliferator-activated receptor gamma ligand regulate phagocytosis by pancreatic stellate cells. Gastroenterology 2005; 128:2105–2118.

22 Masamune A, Kikuta K, Watanabe T, Satoh K, Satoh A, Shimosegawa T. Pancreatic stellate cells express Toll-like receptors. Journal of Gastroenterology 2008; 43:352–362.

23 Shimizu K, Hashimoto K, Tahara J, Imaeda H, Andoh A, Shiratori K. Pancreatic stellate cells do not exhibit features of antigen-presenting cells. Pancreas 2012; 41:422–427.

24 Friess H, Zhu ZW, di Mola FF, et al. Nerve growth factor and its high-affinity receptor in chronic pancreatitis. Annals of Surgery 1999; 230:615–624.

25 Casini A, Galli A, Pignalosa P, et al. Collagen type I synthesized by pancreatic periacinar stellate cells (PSC) co-localizes with lipid peroxidation-derived aldehydes in chronic alcoholic pancreatitis. Journal of Pathology 2000; 192:81–89.

26 Murayama KM, Barent BL, Gruber M, et al. Characterization of a novel model of pancreatic fibrosis and acinar atrophy. Journal of Gastrointestinal Surgery 1999; 3:418–425.

27 Matsumura N, Ochi K, Ichimura M, Mizushima T, Harada H, Harada M. Study on free radicals and pancreatic fibrosis–pancreatic fibrosis induced by repeated injections of superoxide dismutase inhibitor. Pancreas 2001; 22:53–57.

28 Gukovsky I, Lugea A, Shahsahebi M, et al. A rat model reproducing key pathological responses of alcoholic chronic pancreatitis. American Journal of Physiology: Gastrointestinal and Liver Physiology 2008; 294:G68-G79.

29 Vonlaufen A, Xu ZH, Joshi S, et al. Bacterial endotoxin – a trigger factor for alcoholic pancreatitis? Findings of a novel physiologically relevant model. Gastroenterology 2007; 133:1293–1303.

30 Ohashi K, Kim JH, Hara H, Aso R, Akimoto T, Nakama K. WBN/Kob rats. A new spontaneously occurring model of chronic pancreatitis. International Journal of Pancreatology 1990; 6:231–247.

31 Blaine SA, Ray KC, Branch KM, Robinson PS, Whitehead RH, Means AL. Epidermal growth factor receptor regulates pancreatic fibrosis. American Journal of Physiology: Gastrointestinal and Liver Physiology 2009; 297:G434-G441.

32 Marrache F, Tu SP, Bhagat G, et al. Overexpression of interleukin-1beta in the murine pancreas results in chronic pancreatitis. Gastroenterology 2008; 135:1277–1287.

33 Neuschwander-Tetri BA, Burton FR, Presti ME, et al. Repetitive self-limited acute pancreatitis induces pancreatic fibrogenesis in the mouse. Digestive Diseases and Sciences 2000; 45:665–674.

34 Bode C, Fukui H, Bode JC. Hidden endotoxin in plasma of patients with alcoholic liver disease. European Journal of Gastroenterology and Hepatology 1993; 5:257–262.

35 Saito R, Yamada S, Yamamoto Y, et al. Conophylline suppresses pancreatic stellate cells and improves islet fibrosis in Goto-Kakizaki rats. Endocrinology 2011; 153: 621–630.

36 Kikuta K, Masamune A, Hamada S, Takikawa T, Nakano E, Shimosegawa T. Pancreatic stellate cells reduce insulin expression and induce apoptosis in pancreatic beta-cells. Biochemical and Biophysical Research Communications 2013; 433:292–297.

37 Li F, Chen B, Li L, et al. INS-1 cells inhibit the production of extracellular matrix from pancreatic stellate cells. Journal of Molecular Histology 2013; 45:321–327.

38 Watanabe T, Masamune A, Kikuta K, et al. Bone marrow contributes to the population of pancreatic stellate cells in mice. American Journal of Physiology: Gastrointestinal and Liver Physiology 2009; 297:G1138–G1146.

39 Apte MV, Yang L, Phillips PA, et al. Extracellular matrix composition significantly influences pancreatic stellate cell gene expression pattern: role of transgelin in PSC function. American Journal of Physiology: Gastrointestinal and Liver Physiology 2013; 305:G408–G417.

40 Kim N, Choi S, Lim C, Lee H, Oh J. Albumin mediates PPAR-gamma or C/EBP-alpha-induced phenotypic changes in pancreatic stellate cells. Biochemical and Biophysical Research Communications 2010; 391:640–644.

41 Froeling FE, Feig C, Chelala C, et al. Retinoic acid induced pancreatic stellate cell quiescence reduces paracrine Wnt-beta-catenin signaling to slow tumor progression. Gastroenterology 2011; 141:1486–1497; 1497.e1–e14.

42 Vonlaufen A, Phillips P, Xu ZH, et al. Alcohol withdrawal promotes regression of pancreatic fibrosis via induction of pancreatic stellate cell (PSC apoptosis). Gut 2011; 60:238–246.

43 Li L, Bachem MG, Zhou S, et al. Pancreatitis-associated protein inhibits human pancreatic stellate cell MMP-1 and -2, TIMP-1 and -2 secretion and RECK expression. Pancreatology 2009; 9:99–110.

44 Pereda J, Sabater L, Cassinello N, et al. Effect of simultaneous inhibition of TNF-alpha production and xanthine oxidase in experimental acute pancreatitis: the role of mitogen activated protein kinases. Annals of Surgery 2004; 240:108–116.

45 Hughes CB, Gaber LW, Mohey el-Din AB, et al. Inhibition of TNF alpha improves survival in an experimental model of acute pancreatitis. American Surgeon 1996; 62:8–13.

46 Menke A, Yamaguchi H, Gress TM, Adler G. Extracellular matrix is reduced by inhibition of transforming growth factor beta1 in pancreatitis in the rat. Gastroenterology 1997; 113:295–303.

47 Zion O, Genin O, Kawada N, et al. Inhibition of transforming growth factor beta signaling by halofuginone as a modality for pancreas fibrosis prevention. Pancreas 2009; 38:427–435.

48 Gomez JA, Molero X, Vaquero E, Alonso A, Salas A, Malagelada JR. Vitamin E attenuates biochemical and morphological features associated with development of chronic pancreatitis. American Journal of Physiology: Gastrointestinal and Liver Physiology 2004; 287:G162–G169; Epub 2004 Mar 4.

49 Lu XL, Dong XY, Fu YB, et al. Protective effect of salvianolic acid B on chronic pancreatitis induced by trinitrobenzene sulfonic acid solution in rats. Pancreas 2009; 38:71–77.

50 Suzuki N, Masamune A, Kikuta K, Watanabe T, Satoh K, Shimosegawa T. Ellagic acid inhibits pancreatic fibrosis in male Wistar Bonn/Kobori rats. Digestive Diseases and Sciences 2009; 54:802–810.

51 Tasci I, Deveci S, Isik AT, et al. Allopurinol in rat chronic pancreatitis: effects on pancreatic stellate cell activation. Pancreas 2007; 35:366–371.

52 Gibo J, Ito T, Kawabe K, et al. Camostat mesilate attenuates pancreatic fibrosis via inhibition of monocytes and pancreatic stellate cells activity. Laboratory Investigation 2005; 85:75–89.

53 Kaku T, Oono T, Zhao H, et al. IS-741 attenuates local migration of monocytes and subsequent pancreatic fibrosis in experimental chronic pancreatitis induced by dibutyltin dichloride in rats. Pancreas 2007; 34:299–309.

54 Madro A, Korolczuk A, Czechowska G, et al. RAS inhibitors decrease apoptosis of acinar cells and increase elimination of pancreatic stellate cells after in the course of experimental chronic pancreatitis induced by dibutyltin dichloride. Journal of Physiology and Pharmacology 2008; 59 Suppl 2:239–249.

55 Ishiwatari H, Sato Y, Murase K, et al. Treatment of pancreatic fibrosis with siRNA against a collagen-specific chaperone in vitamin A-coupled liposomes. Gut 2012; 62:1328–1339.

56 Sherman MH, Yu RT, Engle JE, et al. Vitamin D Receptor-Mediated Stromal Reprogramming Suppresses Pancreatitis and Enhances Pancreatic Cancer Therapy. Cell 2014; 159(1):80–93.

PART D: Autoimmune pancreatitis: an update

Thiruvengadam Muniraj[1], Raghuwansh P. Sah[2], & Suresh T. Chari[2],

[1] Section of Digestive Diseases, Yale University School of Medicine, New Haven, CT, USA
[2] Division of Gastroenterology and Hepatology, Mayo Clinic College of Medicine, Rochester, MN, USA

Introduction

Autoimmune pancreatitis (AIP) is rare but distinct form of chronic pancreatitis that mimics pancreatic cancer in presentation and is characteristically responsive to steroids. Initially reported from Japan in 1995, AIP is now increasingly recognized worldwide [1]. High serum IgG4, first described in AIP patients in 2001 [2], was thought to be a characteristic feature of the disease; now it has become clear that a subset of AIP patients do not have elevated serum IgG4. With increasing recognition of this disease, several other distinct features have now been recognized. Over the last decade, these features have resulted in the formulation of diagnostic criteria such as the Japan Pancreas Society, Mayo Clinic (HISORt), Korean, Asian, and European criteria. Recently, international consensus diagnostic criteria (ICDC) have been formulated for a consistent platform for the diagnosis of AIP across the world. The process of recognition of this disease, description of various features, and development of the diagnostic criteria and treatment strategies over the last 20 years has yielded in several key lessons for the pancreas community in general. In this review, we provide a concise update on AIP and discuss various lessons learnt from the developments in AIP.

Consensus definition and subtypes

AIP is a distinct form of pancreatitis characterized clinically by frequent presentation with obstructive jaundice with or without a pancreatic mass, histologically by a lymphoplasmacytic infiltrate and fibrosis, and therapeutically by a dramatic response to steroids [3].

Two distinct subtypes of AIP, namely Types 1 and 2 AIP, are now recognized [3, 4].

Type 1 AIP

Type 1 AIP is characterized by lymphoplasmacytic inflammatory infiltration of the pancreas with abundant IgG4-positive plasma cells. Serum IgG4 elevation is seen in up to 80% patients [5]. A multifocal disease beyond the pancreas, with histopathologic features in other involved organs paralleling that in the pancreas, is seen in a large proportion of Type 1 AIP patients. In fact, this observation was critical in the recognition of a novel disease entity called IgG4-related disease (IgG4-RD) associated with IgG4-positive plasma cell infiltration in the affected organs. Now, it is clear that Type 1 AIP is the pancreatic manifestation of IgG4-RD (Figure 12D.1). The list of affected extrapancreatic organs continues to expand. The well-characterized and frequently affected organs include extrapancreatic bile duct, salivary and lacrimal glands, lymph nodes, retroperitoneum, kidneys, lungs, prostate, and so on.

Type 2 AIP

Type 2 AIP is characterized by the presence of granulocyte epithelial lesions (GEL) in the pancreas along with lymphoplasmacytic inflammatory infiltrate. Type 2 AIP appears to be a pancreas-specific disorder that is not associated with serum IgG4 elevation or tissue infiltration with IgG4+ cells. Type 2 AIP differs from Type 1 AIP not only in clinical presentation but also in relapse rate. The recurrences are infrequent, if not rare, in Type 2 AIP [5].

Pancreatitis: Medical and Surgical Management, First Edition.
David B. Adams, Peter B. Cotton, Nicholas J. Zyromski and John Windsor.
© 2017 John Wiley & Sons, Ltd. Published 2017 by John Wiley & Sons, Ltd.

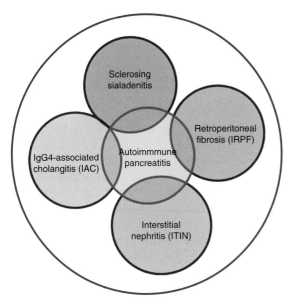

Figure 12D.1 AIP and other organ involvement in IgG4 related disease [6]. Adapted from Chari et al. Gastroenterology 2008; 134:625–8.

Epidemiology

Based on the experience over the last few decades, it is clear that AIP is an uncommon disease. However, no population-based studies have evaluated the incidence or prevalence of AIP. Based on the nationwide hospital-based survey conducted in Japan in 2002 in which a total of 900 AIP patients were found, the prevalence of AIP was estimated to be 0.82 per 100,000 individuals [7]. This study also estimated the male:female ratio of 3:1 and the mean age at onset over 45 years. Another similar hospital-based survey in 2009 noted an increase in prevalence with a total of 2709 patients with AIP seen in that year and an additional 5190 patients with IgG4-RD without pancreatic involvement [8]. The mean age at presentation in our cohort at Mayo Clinic is 63 and 37 years, respectively, with a male:female ratio of 4:1 and 1.5:1, respectively, for Type 1 AIP and for Type 2 AIP (Table 12D.1).

Table 12D.1 Summary of the clinical profile of Types 1 and 2 autoimmune pancreatitis (AIP).

	Type 1 AIP (*n* = 116)	Type 2 AIP (*n* = 44)	*P* value
Age at diagnosis, mean (SD)	63.4 (13.3)	37.0 (19.2)	<0.01
Male gender, *n* (%)	93 (80.2)	26 (59.1)	<0.01
Presenting symptoms			
Jaundice	75 (64.7)	18 (40.9)	<0.01
Pancreatic mass	48 (41.4)	14 (31.8)	0.27
Pancreatitis	13 (11.2)	24 (54.5)	<0.01
Other	8 (6.9)	2 (4.5)	0.72
Serum IgG4 status			
>ULN, *n* (%)	71/99 (71.7)	2/33 (6.1)	<0.01
>2 × ULN, *n* (%)	41/99 (41.4)	0/33	<0.01
Parenchymal imaging at presentation			
Diffuse enlargement	49 (30.6)	11 (25.0)	0.04
Focal enlargement	20 (17.2)	6 (13.6)	0.64**
Indeterminate (includes atypical)	27 (23.3)	23 (52.3)	<0.01
N/A	20 (17.2)	4 (9.1)	
Biliary involvement at presentation			
Distal only	54 (46.7)	20 (45.4)	0.90
Proximal ± distal	30 (25.9)	-	<0.01
None	32	24	<0.01
Other organ involvement (excluding IBD)	58 (50.4)	0	<0.01
Relapses (at least one relapse)	50 (44.2)	4 (9)	<0.01

Data reported based on the Mayo Clinic Cohort. Percentages are reported in parentheses.

Pathogenesis

An autoimmune mechanism is generally thought to be the most probable pathogenic mechanism responsible for the development of AIP based on multiple lines of evidence including lymphoplasmacytic inflammatory infiltration, association with serum autoantibodies including IgG4 and others, improvement with steroids, recent studies linking HLA haplotypes with IgG4-RD, and lack of other obvious inciting factors. However, a pathogenic antibody has not been recognized so far in Types 1 or 2 AIP. In 2010, the Italian group described a novel antibody that showed homology with plasminogen-binding protein of *Helicobater pylori* [9]. This and other prior reports led to the hypothesis that *H. pylori* infection through antigen mimicry resulted in AIP in "genetically" susceptible individuals. An alternate hypothesis proposed based on the association of eosinophilia and allergic diseases with AIP is that an allergic IgE-mediated pathogenesis might be involved in AIP [10]. However, so far no further evidence has emerged for these hypotheses that remain speculations at best.

HLA haplotype DRB1*0405-DQB1*0401 was found to be associated with Japanese patients [11]. This was not confirmed in Korean patients, but instead this population seemed to have association with substitution of aspartic acid at DQβ1 57, which was identified as a genetic factor predisposing to relapses in AIP [12].

T-cell-mediated responses have been recognized in AIP and IgG4-RD with contradicting observations of Th1 responses predominating in peripheral blood [13], whereas Th2 responses predominating in the affected organs in Type 1 AIP [14] lead to the hypothesis that Th1 cytokines may be important in disease induction and Th2 cytokines in disease progression [15]. Th2-mediated responses and increased expression of a specific subset of Tregs leading to IL-10 production, which induces class switching to IgG4 subtype, and TGFβ production, which leads to fibrosis, has been suggested in IgG4-RD including Type 1 AIP [14, 16]. It is still unclear if the increased IgG4 levels constitute pathogenic phenomenon causing AIP or they just represent an epiphenomenon. No IgG4 antibodies are found against any specific antigens. The increase in IgG4 responses are known to be controlled by Type 2 helper T-cells [17, 18]. Mislocalization of CFTR in pancreatic ducts was demonstrated in AIP

that was corrected with steroid treatment suggesting possible CFTR-mediated duct dysfunction as a potential pathogenic mechanism. However, duct dysfunction and CFTR mislocalization have now been demonstrated in other forms of chronic pancreatitis as well. A recent study induced AIP-like changes in a mouse model by acinar-specific overexpression of lymphotoxin α and β [19]. Recently, based on flow cytometry on AIP patient blood samples compared with other pancreatic diseases, a specific subset (CD19+ CD24high CD27+) were demonstrated to be deregulated in AIP [20]. While the ultimate question of pathogenesis of AIP is still not resolved, treatment directed toward the ablation of B-cells (plasma cells are mature form of B-cells that secrete IgG antibodies) with sole agent CD20 antibody, rituximab, has shown a dramatic response even in hard-to-treat patients such as relapsing patients after steroids, and steroid-intolerant and immunomodulator-resistant patients [21].

Clinical profile of AIP

The common clinical presentation of AIP (both subtypes) is obstructive jaundice and pancreatic enlargement on imaging, which can be diffuse or focal. The presentation closely mimics pancreatic cancer [3, 22, 23]. Abdominal pain can be seen during acute presentation but chronic pain is uncommon. Acute pancreatitis is a common at presentation in Type 2 AIP (50% cases), while only 10% of Type 1 AIP patients present with acute pancreatitis [22]. While features of chronic pancreatitis including steatorrhea and pancreatic atrophy generally develop in the course of AIP, these can occasionally be the only presenting features (late presentation). In addition, patients with Type 1 AIP can have symptoms related to involvement of other organs such as biliary strictures, cholangitis, interstitial nephritis, and retroperitoneal fibrosis with complications [24]. Type 2 AIP is frequently associated with inflammatory bowel disease. The differences between the clinical profile of Types 1 and 2 AIP have been summarized in Table 12D.2. Type 2 patients are clearly distinct with younger age of presentation, lack of other organ involvement (OOI), frequent presentation with acute pancreatitis, lack of association with IgG4, higher incidence of IBD, and infrequent relapses [5].

Table 12D.2 Summary of diagnostic features in the International consensus diagnostic criteria (ICDC) for autoimmune pancreatitis (AIP).

Features	Level 1 (strong)	Level 2 (supportive)
International consensus diagnostic criteria (ICDC) for AIP diagnosis		
Histology (see text)	At least 3/4 histological features	Two histological features
Imaging (see text)	Typical	Supportive/atypical/indeterminate
IgG4 serology	IgG4 >2 × ULN	IgG4 >1 but <2 × ULN
Other organ involvement (OOI) (any one of the listed features)	1 Proximal BD 2 RPF 3 At least 3/4 histological features on biopsy	1 Renal 2 Salivary/lacrimal gland 3 IgG4+ lymphoplasmacytic infiltration on biopsy
Response to steroids (dramatic radiologic improvement at 2 weeks)		

For other organ involvement, evidence may be radiologic for bile duct, RPF, and renal involvement and clinical for salivary/lacrimal gland enlargement. See text for details.
ULN, upper limit of normal; BD, bile duct; RPF, retroperitoneal fibrosis.

Diagnosis of AIP

The diagnosis of AIP can be a challenge, particularly as AIP can mimic pancreatic cancer. In the past, many diagnostic criteria have been published from different countries, focusing more on Type 1 AIP [23, 25–28]. The ICDC for AIP have been proposed understanding the differences in subtypes of AIP and geographical variations [3]. ICDC incorporated the five cardinal components of AIP as proposed by HISORt criteria [23, 27], Histology (H), Imaging (I), Serology (S), OOI, and Response to steroid treatment (Rt), which are described later and in Table 12D.2.

Histology

The four histologic features of Type 1 AIP (in the pancreas) and IgG4-related disease (in the affected organs) are

1 periductal lymphoplasmacytic infiltrate without granulocyte infiltration
2 obliterative phlebitis
3 storiform fibrosis
4 abundant (>10 cells/HPF) IgG4-positive cells.

Type 2 AIP may demonstrate lymphoplasmacytic infiltrate with storiform fibrosis on histology but it is considered diagnostic in the presence of both

1 granulocytic infiltration of duct wall (GEL) with or without granulocytic acinar inflammation,
2 absent or scant (0–10 cells/HPF) IgG4-positive cells.

Parenchymal imaging

The following features, which are similar in both AIP subtypes, may be seen on pancreatic parenchymal imaging with a CT/MRI scan

1 Diffuse enlargement of the pancreas (also called "sausage-shaped" pancreas) with delayed enhancement (considered *typical imaging*). A capsule-like rim surrounding the diffusely enlarged gland can sometimes be seen.
2 Focal/segmental enlargement with delayed enhancement (considered *supportive imaging*).
3 *Atypical* features (low density mass, upstream duct dilatation, pancreatic duct cut-off, and distal atrophy), which are strongly suggestive of pancreatic cancer. Normal looking pancreas (*indeterminate imaging*) can be seen occasionally.

Ductal imaging

ERP features of long (>1/3 length of the main pancreatic duct) or multiple strictures without marked upstream dilatation (duct size <5 mm) are strongly suggestive of Type 1 AIP while segmental/focal narrowing without marked upstream dilatation are supportive.

Diagnostic strategy

We recommend review of parenchymal imaging and collateral evidence (OOI or IgG4 serology) in suspected patients for diagnosis of AIP and differentiating them from pancreatic cancer. In the absence of typical imaging features, next steps in diagnosis should only be considered after a negative work-up for pancreatic cancer.

Type 1 AIP can be diagnosed if one of the following is fulfilled:

1 Level 1 histologic features in the pancreas.
2 Level 1 parenchymal imaging features with any (Level 1 or 2) collateral evidence.
3 Positive response to steroid trial in patients without typical (Level 1) parenchymal imaging and one strong (Level 1) collateral evidence or (Level 2)

supportive collateral evidence + consistent ERP features (ductal imaging).

A definitive diagnosis of Type 2 AIP can be made in the presence of characteristic histology.

Though histology from tissue obtained through EUS-core biopsy provides definitive diagnosis, this requires high level of expertise and may not be readily available [29, 30]. We also wish to highlight here that the elevation in IgG4 alone is not sufficient to make a diagnosis of AIP. In addition, steroid trial should only be considered in a select patient group as noted in point 2 earlier after a negative work-up for pancreatic cancer.

Management and long-term outcomes

AIP (both subtypes) dramatically responds to corticosteroids. Use of steroids have shown to have significantly higher remission rates (98%) and lower relapse rates, and rapid symptom alleviation when compared with not using steroids [31–33]. Therefore, the administration of oral steroid is the standard treatment for inducing remission in active AIP [32, 34]. At Mayo Clinic, we use prednisone 40 mg daily for 4 weeks followed by a taper of 5 mg per week (total 11-week course). By then, most patients have had their biliary stents removed, are clinically asymptomatic, and are not placed on maintenance treatment [34]. In Japan, slower taper over 3–6 months followed by low-dose maintenance steroid for up to 3 years is routinely used [32]. The response is assessed based on radiological improvement and improvement of liver function tests (LFTs). Symptoms alone or serological monitoring is not useful for monitoring of responses. The advantages of long-term steroid maintenance have not been established.

Disease relapse is common in Type 1 AIP, while relapses in patients with Type 2 AIP are very infrequent [5, 35]. During a median clinical follow-up period of 42 and 29 months, respectively, 47% of patients with Type 1 AIP and none of those with Type 2 AIP experienced a relapse [5]. Relapses seem to occur most frequently in the proximal bile duct (in 60% of patients with relapses), presenting as biliary stricture, jaundice, and cholangitis. Relapses can also affect the pancreas (in 25% of patients in relapses) and other extrapancreatic organs with lesser frequency [5, 36]. Patients with proximal bile duct involvement or diffuse enlargement of the pancreas at presentation are more likely to experience

relapses [5]. These patients should be monitored closely for relapses. The treatment of relapses is also variable among different centers. We typically use short course of steroids for the induction of remission combined with 12–18 months of azathioprine for the maintenance of remission [21]. In steroid-intolerant patients or those who relapse while on azathioprine, we use rituximab [21].

The long-term survival in both Types 1 and 2 AIP patients are found to be similar [5]. Despite long-term complications such as pancreatic insufficiency, diabetes, extrapancreatic involvement, and complication related to therapy, both Types 1 and 2 AIP do not alter the long-term survival of the patients [5]. However, a recent UK study showed that the risk of death in Type 1 AIP and IgG4- related sclerosing cholangitis was increased compared with matched population [37]. Reports on the risk of malignancy in AIP are conflicting. Kamisawa et al. have noted significant frequency of KRAS mutation occurring in the pancreatobiliary region of AIP patients, rendering them at high risk of pancreatobiliary cancers [38]. Huggett et al. recently noted 11% malignancy shortly before or after the diagnosis of AIP/IgG4-RD [37]. Our own data did show any increased risk in AIP compared with matched cohort of controls.

Lessons learnt from AIP experience

Recognition of an uncommon disease

AIP is an increasingly diagnosed clinical entity in recent years; however, for a long time this disease went unrecognized. There were clues on AIP described as early as in 1961 when Sarles et al. noticed chronic inflammatory sclerosis of the pancreas and proposed the idea of autoimmune pancreatic disease [39]. In 1963, two case reports of steroid-responsive pancreatic mass with biliary obstruction were reported from Mayo Clinic, though they could not derive a clear etiopathogenesis at that time [16]. Similarly, in 1965, Wenger et al. reported a patient who presented as obstructive jaundice, serum gamma-globulin elevation with nonmalignant diffuse thickening of bile duct walls, responding well to steroids [40]. It is fascinating that many important features that we discuss currently in AIP were described so many years ago but remained undiagnosed for all this period. Cumulative knowledge over the decades led to the recognition of unusual subsets of pancreatic inflammation that had been given various names including lymphoplasmacytic sclerosing pancreatitis (LPSP), nonalcoholic duct destructive pancreatitis (NADDP), idiopathic duct centric pancreatitis (IDCP), "sausage" pancreatitis, and so on. Increasing experience of this steroid-responsive pancreatitis or pancreatic mass over the decades resulted in the recognition of AIP as a distinct entity in 2003.

An example of controversies and collaboration

Even though both Types 1 and 2 are called "autoimmune" pancreatitis, it took many years to reach this unifying diagnosis. Historically, what is now called as Type 1 AIP was proposed mainly in Japan focusing mainly on clinical phenotype [1, 4, 5, 26, 41, 42]. Later, the concept of what was termed later as Type 2 AIP was first proposed in Europe, based on histopathologic features [43]. The American contribution and further collaboration paved the way for incorporating these two diseases as subtypes of a single disease AIP [4, 5].

In 2011, a multinational collaborative group formed a consensus diagnostic criteria unifying the different diagnostic criteria around the world and incorporating both subtypes of AIP [3]. The diversity of diagnostic criteria for AIP from individual countries reflected differences in practice patterns, for example, Asian diagnostic criteria have focused on Type 1 AIP, and American and Italian diagnostic criteria may pertain to both subtypes. Though the individual items of these criteria are very similar, the approach for analyzing each feature varies depending on the country. For example, Japanese criteria mandate endoscopic retrograde pancreatography (ERP) but are usually precluded in the United States to avoid causing or worsening pancreatitis [44]. According to the ICDC, the performance of diagnostic ERP is not mandatory and reserved only for a subset of patients without typical parenchymal imaging features and only supportive (level 2) collateral evidence (see Table 12D.2) under consideration of a steroid trial [3, 45].

Is neuritis the cause of chronic pain in CP?

Despite the presence of intense inflammation, AIP is relatively painless. Even when patient presents with pain, this is often mild and resolves with treatment. Chronic pain, which is common in chronic pancreatitis, is almost unheard of in AIP patients. It is currently believed that pancreatic neuritis and sensitization of visceral nerves in chronic pancreatitis is responsible for chronic pain. Recent studies have even suggested that nerve growth factors and receptors such as TRPV1 may be an exciting new target for treating the pain of chronic pancreatitis [46]. However, the fact that AIP has intense inflammation and fibrosis but lacks pain raises the question whether inflammation in CP (along with accompanying neuritis) is indeed responsible for pain. Furthermore, if this were true, how can the lack of pain in AIP be explained? Another possibility is something unique about chronic inflammation in AIP that renders it painless despite the intense inflammation. These issues need to be explored in future studies and exemplify how characterization of an uncommon form of chronic pancreatitis (AIP) is affecting our understanding about chronic pancreatitis, chronic pain, and pancreatic neuroinflammation in a broader sense.

Do other forms of CP have distinct histologies?

Recognition of distinct histopathologic features in AIP brought up an interesting question whether histology can be used to distinguish other etiologies of CP. To answer this, a blinded two-phase study was conducted at Mayo Clinic involving 13 pathologists to study a mixed group of resected specimens of AIP, and other forms of CP. Pathologists were able to distinguish AIP from other causes of CP and Type 1 AIP from Type 2 AIP. But they were not able to differentiate alcoholic CP from other forms of obstructive CP [47].

Recognition of IgG4-related disease

In 2003, Kamisawa et al. found that IgG4-positive plasma cells had extensively infiltrated the organs and tissues of patients with AIP, and this led to the novel proposal that AIP is not simply pancreatitis but that it is a pancreatic lesion involved in IgG4-related systemic disease [4, 41]. This concept was similar to that proposed by Comings et al. on multifocal fibrosclerosis [48]. The steroid responses and the prognoses of AIP patients with sclerosing cholangitis differ from patients with primary sclerosing cholangitis (PSC), which suggests that they are different pathological conditions. These findings led to the concept of "IgG4-related disease" and suggestion that AIP is a pancreatic lesion reflecting this systemic disease [49, 50].

The OOI seen in patients with Ig4-RD associated with AIP include chronic sclerosing sialadenitis (CSS), IgG4-associated retroperitoneal fibrosis (IRPF), IgG4-associated nephritis (ITIN), and IgG4-associated cholangitis (IAC)) (see Figure 12D.1) [6]. The frequency of OOI varies depending on which organ is the focus of study as the primary manifestation. Whether AIP is necessarily "the center of the universe" of ISD is not clear [6]. A nephrologist might see ITIN as a more common manifestation as opposed to a pancreatologist noticing AIP as the commonest presentation of IgG4-RD. Though it is still unclear, it is likely that the indication for treatment, response to treatment, and natural history of disease may vary with the organ affected.

Is serum IgG4 a good marker for AIP?

Elevated serum IgG4 levels are characteristic of Type 1 AIP, first recognized in 2001. A diagnostic test for AIP appeared to have been found, and IgG4 in some sense got popularized as a success story in medical diagnosis understanding that a single diagnostic test is uncommon for many diseases. However, it is now clear that IgG4 level alone has poor diagnostic accuracy for Type 1 AIP [51]. Despite this, measurement of serum IgG4 is popularly perceived as the diagnostic test for AIP. Recently, in a study of 4366 unique patients who had IgG4 levels measured, we have found that the positive predictive value of elevated IgG4 is low for Type 1 AIP and IgG4-related diseases. We now understand that IgG4 measurement is useful for AIP diagnosis when used in combination with other diagnostic features and IgG4 elevations in patients with low pretest probability of having AIP are likely to represent false positives.

Is response to steroids diagnostic of AIP?

AIP closely mimics relatively more common pancreatic cancer and, therefore, any false diagnosis of AIP could be disastrous. However, differentiating AIP and cancer based on a steroid trial has been proposed sometimes to be useful in the diagnosis of AIP based on a study of 22 patients who received a 2 week steroid trial [52]. This brings up the danger of indiscriminate use of this strategy and delaying cancer diagnosis. Diagnosis of AIP can be challenging without biopsy, and steroid trial is useful in a select situation (as discussed earlier in this chapter) for a noninvasive diagnosis after a thorough negative work for excluding pancreatic cancer. Steroid trial can

be tempting but it is important to emphasize here that the strategy "If it responds, it must be AIP," is dangerous.

Summary

AIP is a chronic fibro-inflammatory disease of the pancreas, only recently recognized. Two distinct subtypes are now characterized. Steroids are the mainstay of treatment of both subtypes of AIP. Recognition of extra-pancreatic organ involvement in AIP has led now to the recognition of systemic disease – IgG4-related disease, with Type 1 AIP being the pancreatic manifestation. With increasing recognition of AIP, our experience with this novel disease is increasing.

References

1 Yoshida K, Toki F, Takeuchi T, Watanabe S, Shiratori K, Hayashi N. Chronic pancreatitis caused by an autoimmune abnormality. Proposal of the concept of autoimmune pancreatitis. Digestive diseases and sciences 1995;40:1561–1568.

2 Hamano H, Kawa S, Horiuchi A, et al. High serum IgG4 concentrations in patients with sclerosing pancreatitis. The New England Journal of Medicine 2001;344:732–738.

3 Shimosegawa T, Chari ST, Frulloni L, et al. International consensus diagnostic criteria for autoimmune pancreatitis: guidelines of the International Association of Pancreatology. Pancreas 2011;40:352–358.

4 Chari ST, Kloeppel G, Zhang L, Notohara K, Lerch MM, Shimosegawa T. Histopathologic and clinical subtypes of autoimmune pancreatitis: the Honolulu consensus document. Pancreas 2010;39:549–554.

5 Sah RP, Chari ST, Pannala R, et al. Differences in clinical profile and relapse rate of type 1 versus type 2 autoimmune pancreatitis. Gastroenterology 2010;139:140–148; quiz e12–e13.

6 Chari ST, Murray JA. Autoimmune pancreatitis, Part II: the relapse. Gastroenterology 2008;134:625–628.

7 Nishimori I, Tamakoshi A, Otsuki M. Prevalence of autoimmune pancreatitis in Japan from a nationwide survey in 2002. Journal of Gastroenterology 2007;42 Suppl 18:6–8.

8 Uchida K, Masamune A, Shimosegawa T, Okazaki K. Prevalence of IgG4-Related Disease in Japan Based on Nationwide Survey in 2009. International Journal of Rheumatology 2012;2012:358371.

9 Frulloni L, Lunardi C, Simone R, et al. Identification of a novel antibody associated with autoimmune pancreatitis. The New England Journal of Medicine 2009;361:2135–2142.

10 Kamisawa T, Anjiki H, Egawa N, Kubota N. Allergic manifestations in autoimmune pancreatitis. European Journal of Gastroenterology & Hepatology 2009;21:1136–1139.

11 Kawa S, Ota M, Yoshizawa K, et al. HLA DRB10405-DQB10401 haplotype is associated with autoimmune pancreatitis in the Japanese population. Gastroenterology 2002;122:1264–1269.

12 Park do H, Kim MH, Oh HB, et al. Substitution of aspartic acid at position 57 of the DQbeta1 affects relapse of autoimmune pancreatitis. Gastroenterology 2008;134:440–446.

13 Okazaki K, Uchida K, Ohana M, et al. Autoimmune-related pancreatitis is associated with autoantibodies and a Th1/Th2-type cellular immune response. Gastroenterology 2000;118:573–581.

14 Zen Y, Fujii T, Harada K, et al. Th2 and regulatory immune reactions are increased in immunoglobulin G4-related sclerosing pancreatitis and cholangitis. Hepatology (Baltimore, MD) 2007;45:1538 1546.

15 Okazaki K, Uchida K, Fukui T. Recent advances in autoimmune pancreatitis: concept, diagnosis, and pathogenesis. Journal of Gastroenterology 2008;43:409–418.

16 Bartholomew LG, Cain JC, Woolner LB, Utz DC, Ferris DO. Sclerosing cholangitis: its possible association with Riedel's struma and fibrous retroperitonitis. Report of two cases. The New England Journal of Medicine 1963;269:8–12.

17 Stone JH, Zen Y, Deshpande V. IgG4-related disease. The New England Journal of Medicine 2012;366:539–551.

18 Kamisawa T, Chari ST, Lerch MM, Kim MH, Gress TM, Shimosegawa T. Republished: recent advances in autoimmune pancreatitis: type 1 and type 2. Postgraduate Medical Journal 2014;90:18–25.

19 Seleznik GM, Reding T, Romrig F, et al. Lymphotoxin beta receptor signaling promotes development of autoimmune pancreatitis. Gastroenterology 2012;143:1361–1374.

20 Sumimoto K, Uchida K, Kusuda T, et al. The role of $CD19^+$ $CD24^{high}$ $CD38^{high}$ and $CD19^+$ $CD24^{high}$ $CD27^+$ regulatory B cells in patients with type 1 autoimmune pancreatitis. Pancreatology 2014;14:193–200.

21 Hart PA, Topazian MD, Witzig TE, et al. Treatment of relapsing autoimmune pancreatitis with immunomodulators and rituximab: the Mayo Clinic experience. Gut 2013;62:1607–1615.

22 Kamisawa T, Chari ST, Lerch MM, Kim MH, Gress TM, Shimosegawa T. Recent advances in autoimmune pancreatitis: type 1 and type 2. Gut 2013;62:1373–1380.

23 Chari ST, Smyrk TC, Levy MJ, et al. Diagnosis of autoimmune pancreatitis: the Mayo Clinic experience. Clinical Gastroenterology and Hepatology 2006;4:1010–1016; quiz 934.

24 Park DH, Kim MH, Chari ST. Recent advances in autoimmune pancreatitis. Gut 2009;58:1680–1689.

25 Otsuki M, Chung JB, Okazaki K, et al. Asian diagnostic criteria for autoimmune pancreatitis: consensus of the Japan-Korea Symposium on Autoimmune Pancreatitis. Journal of Gastroenterology 2008;43:403–408.

26 Kim KP, Kim MH, Kim JC, Lee SS, Seo DW, Lee SK. Diagnostic criteria for autoimmune chronic pancreatitis revisited. World Journal of Gastroenterology 2006;12:2487–2496.

27 Chari ST, Takahashi N, Levy MJ, et al. A diagnostic strategy to distinguish autoimmune pancreatitis from pancreatic cancer. Clinical Gastroenterology and Hepatology 2009;7:1097–1103.

28 Shimosegawa T. The amendment of the Clinical Diagnostic Criteria in Japan (JPS2011) in response to the proposal of the International Consensus of Diagnostic Criteria (ICDC) for autoimmune pancreatitis. Pancreas 2012;41:1341–1342.

29 Kamisawa T, Shimosegawa T. Pancreas: histological diagnostic criteria for autoimmune pancreatitis. Nature Reviews Gastroenterology & Hepatology 2012;9:8–10.

30 Detlefsen S, Mohr Drewes A, Vyberg M, Kloppel G. Diagnosis of autoimmune pancreatitis by core needle biopsy: application of six microscopic criteria. Virchows Archiv 2009;454:531–539.

31 Ghazale A, Chari ST. Optimising corticosteroid treatment for autoimmune pancreatitis. Gut 2007;56:1650–1652.

32 Kamisawa T, Shimosegawa T, Okazaki K, et al. Standard steroid treatment for autoimmune pancreatitis. Gut 2009;58:1504–1507.

33 Kamisawa T, Okamoto A, Wakabayashi T, Watanabe H, Sawabu N. Appropriate steroid therapy for autoimmune pancreatitis based on long-term outcome. Scandinavian Journal of Gastroenterology 2008;43:609 613.

34 Pannala R, Chari ST. Corticosteroid treatment for autoimmune pancreatitis. Gut 2009;58:1438–1439.

35 Detlefsen S, Zamboni G, Frulloni L, et al. Clinical features and relapse rates after surgery in type 1 autoimmune pancreatitis differ from type 2: a study of 114 surgically treated European patients. Pancreatology 2012;12:276–283.

36 Naitoh I, Nakazawa T, Ohara H, et al. Clinical significance of extrapancreatic lesions in autoimmune pancreatitis. Pancreas 2010;39:e1–e5.

37 Huggett MT, Culver EL, Kumar M, et al. Type 1 autoimmune pancreatitis and IgG4-related sclerosing cholangitis is associated with extrapancreatic organ failure, malignancy, and mortality in a prospective UK cohort. The American Journal of Gastroenterology 2014;109:1675–1683.

38 Kamisawa T, Tsuruta K, Okamoto A, et al. Frequent and significant K-ras mutation in the pancreas, the bile duct, and the gallbladder in autoimmune pancreatitis. Pancreas 2009;38:890–895.

39 Sarles H, Sarles JC, Muratore R, Guien C. Chronic inflammatory sclerosis of the pancreas--an autonomous pancreatic disease? The American Journal of Digestive Diseases 1961;6:688–698.

40 Wenger J, Gingrich GW, Mendeloff J. Sclerosing cholangitis--a manifestation of systemic disease. Increased serum gamma-globulin, follicular lymph node hyperplasia,

and orbital pseudotumor. Archives of Internal Medicine 1965;116:509–514.

41 Kamisawa T, Funata N, Hayashi Y, et al. A new clinico-pathological entity of IgG4-related autoimmune disease. Journal of Gastroenterology 2003;38:982–984.

42 Kamisawa T, Egawa N, Nakajima H, Tsuruta K, Okamoto A. Morphological changes after steroid therapy in autoimmune pancreatitis. Scandinavian Journal of Gastroenterology 2004;39:1154–1158.

43 Ectors N, Maillet B, Aerts R, et al. Non-alcoholic duct destructive chronic pancreatitis. Gut 1997;41:263–268.

44 Okazaki K, Kawa S, Kamisawa T, et al. Amendment of the Japanese Consensus Guidelines for Autoimmune Pancreatitis, 2013 I. Concept and diagnosis of autoimmune pancreatitis. Journal of Gastroenterology 2014;49:567–588.

45 Kim JH, Kim MH, Byun JH, et al. Diagnostic strategy for differentiating autoimmune pancreatitis from pancreatic cancer: is an endoscopic retrograde pancreatography essential? Pancreas 2012;41(4):636–638.

46 Schwartz ES, Christianson JA, Chen X, et al. Synergistic role of TRPV1 and TRPA1 in pancreatic pain and inflammation. Gastroenterology 2011;140:1283–1291; e1–e2.

47 Zhang L, Chari S, Smyrk TC, et al. Autoimmune pancreatitis (AIP) type 1 and type 2: an international consensus study on histopathologic diagnostic criteria. Pancreas 2011;40:1172–1179.

48 Comings DE, Skubi KB, Van Eyes J, Motulsky AG. Familial multifocal fibrosclerosis. Findings suggesting that retroperitoneal fibrosis, mediastinal fibrosis, sclerosing cholangitis, Riedel's thyroiditis, and pseudotumor of the orbit may be different manifestations of a single disease. Annals of Internal Medicine 1967;66:884–892.

49 Kamisawa T, Okamoto A. Autoimmune pancreatitis: proposal of IgG4-related sclerosing disease. Journal of Gastroenterology 2006;41:613–625.

50 Okazaki K, Kawa S, Kamisawa T, et al. Clinical diagnostic criteria of autoimmune pancreatitis: revised proposal. Journal of Gastroenterology 2006;41:626–631.

51 Ghazale A, Chari ST, Smyrk TC, et al. Value of serum IgG4 in the diagnosis of autoimmune pancreatitis and in distinguishing it from pancreatic cancer. The American Journal of Gastroenterology 2007;102:1646–1653.

52 Moon SH, Kim MH, Park DH, et al. Is a 2-week steroid trial after initial negative investigation for malignancy useful in differentiating autoimmune pancreatitis from pancreatic cancer? A prospective outcome study. Gut 2008;57:1704–1712.

PART E: Etiology and pathophysiology: tropical pancreatitis

Rajesh Gupta[1], Sunil D. Shenvi[2], Ritambhra Nada[3], Surinder S. Rana[4] & Deepak Bhasin[4]

[1] Division of Surgical Gastroenterology, Department of General Surgery, PGIMER, Chandigarh, India
[2] Department of Surgery, Division of Transplant Surgery, MUSC, Charleston, SC, USA
[3] Department of Histopathology, PGIMER, Chandigarh, India
[4] Department of Gastroenterology, PGIMER, Chandigarh, India

Alcoholic chronic pancreatitis (ACP) is the commonest type of chronic pancreatitis seen in the Western world, while in the tropics there is a distinct nonalcoholic type of chronic pancreatitis of uncertain etiology, which is far more common. It is seen almost exclusively in developing countries of the tropical world (23.5° to either side of equator), which include parts of Asia, Africa, and Central America.

First report about tropical pancreatitis (TP) came from Zuidema in 1959 from Indonesia who reported a series of 45 patients with pancreatic calcification with diabetes mellitus who were poor and consumed a protein- and calorie-deficient diet, and also had striking clinical features of malnutrition [1]. The largest series was reported by Geevarghese, a pioneer in this field from Kerala, India, who immortalized the uniqueness of this entity by the aphorism "pain in childhood, diabetes in adolescence and death during prime of life" [2]. This was followed by a series of reports of similar patients from various tropical countries following which **TP** came to be recognized as a distinct entity with unique clinical and epidemiological features different from that of ACP [2–7].

Highest prevalence of chronic pancreatitis has been reported from Kerala state of South India, that is, 125/100,000 population, which is much higher than chronic pancreatitis reported from Japan – 45/100,000, and West where prevalence is 10–15/100,000 population [6].

Definition

TP is a juvenile form of chronic calcific, nonalcoholic pancreatitis. Some of its distinctive features are younger onset, presence of large intraductal calculi, accelerated course of the disease, and high susceptibility to pancreatic cancer.

The classical triad of clinical presentation includes abdominal pain, maldigestion leading to steatorrhea, and diabetes (fibrocalculous pancreatic diabetes (FCPD)). Diabetes is inevitable and occurs a decade or two after first episode of abdominal pain and is related to the duration of pain and calcification but unrelated to exocrine deficiency. Diabetes tends to be severe, and up to 90% of patients require insulin, often in high doses. Episodes of hypoglycemia are common, whereas ketosis is uncommon. Demonstration of high blood sugar level and pancreatic calculi on plain abdominal X-ray clinches the diagnosis. Microvascular complications are as frequent as Type 2 diabetes, while macrovascular complications are uncommon [8, 9].

Etiology

Although the etiology of TCP is not clearly determined, epidemiologic, clinical, and experimental data strongly suggest a certain pattern, which include role of malnutrition, dietary toxins, oxidant stress, trace element deficiency, familial clustering, and genetic factors.

Malnutrition

TP is reported primarily in poorer population of developing world where the diet is poor in proteins and rich in carbohydrates. Moreover, earlier reports on TP emanated from southern India and most patients with TP were undernourished, implicating malnutrition as a cause [2, 10, 11].

Hair and skin changes, cyanotic lips, bilateral parotid gland enlargement, and pancreatic fibrosis were seen in both TP and classic kwashiorkor. Structural and functional changes in the pancreas in primary protein deficiency also supported malnutrition as a possible etiological candidate [1].

However, recent observations question this hypothesis. The large pockets of malnutrition in many parts of the world present with relative low frequency of TP, for example, Ethiopia [12], which suggests that malnutrition by itself is unlikely to have an etiological role. Furthermore, kwashiorkor seldom leads to permanent pancreatic damage, and pancreatic stones are absent even in advanced stages of kwashiorkor [8, 13].

In an experiment on monkeys, Sandhyamani et al. [14] studied the effect of high-carbohydrate and low-protein diet and observed that monkeys developed inflammatory and vascular changes in the pancreas. These lesions were different from that seen in chronic pancreatitis. The heart and vessels were predominantly involved.

Ironically Kerala, a state in southern India with the highest literacy and lowest infant mortality rates, has the highest prevalence of TP. Malnutrition may be the effect rather than the cause of the disease because attendant malabsorption could itself lead to malnutrition. This is borne out by two recent studies as well. In the recent study by Regunath and coworkers [15], it was found that malnutrition occurred equally commonly in TP and ACP, and this appears to develop after the onset of illness. In the study by Sathiaraj et al. [16], it was also noticed that malnutrition was not a cause of TP (idiopathic CP) as only 15% patients were malnourished before the onset of disease and 52% lost weight subsequently.

The consensus, therefore, is that protein calorie malnutrition cannot be considered as the main etiological factor of TCP.

Cassava toxicity (cyanogen toxicity)

Cassava (tapioca, *Manihot esculenta*) is a tuber consumed as a staple food by poor people in some parts of the world including Kerala. A potential toxic effect of Cassava through its content of cyanogenic glycosides (linamarin and linamarase) is cited as a possible etiologic factor based on epidemiologic data [17, 18]. It is seen that TCP is prevalent in those areas, where people eat Cassava as their staple diet such as Kerala, Nigeria, Indonesia, Uganda, Malawi, and Thailand.

Cassava root contains 65 mg of toxic glycosides/l00 g. Hydrocyanic acid is liberated when the glycosides react with HCL in the stomach, which is alleged to cause pancreatic injury. The enzyme rhodanase acts on hydrocyanic acid to produce thiocyanate in the presence of adequate amounts of methionine and cystine, which are deficient in protein malnutrition [17, 18].

Experimental evidence in support of Cassava as a cause of TCP was obtained from rats fed with a diet containing 22.8 g of cassava for 18 months. The pancreatic changes noticed were dilated ductules, papillary infoldings, eosinophilic materials in ductular lumina, and round cell infiltration, as seen in TP [19].

However, none of the rats developed permanent diabetes or chronic pancreatitis. A recent study on rats fed cassava diets for up to 1 year did not produce either pancreatitis or diabetes [20]. Thus, the cassava hypothesis lacks experimental support.

Epidemiologic studies also have shown conflicting data. In the study by Chari et al. [21], none of their patients consumed cassava as a staple diet. Also, TP is prevalent in many parts of India and Africa where cassava is not consumed, and TP is also not seen in a rural West African population consuming a high cassava diet [22].

At the same time, these findings do not rule out these factors completely, as in any chronic diseases the suggested etiologic factor cannot be demonstrated in 100% of cases. Cyanogens impair a number of enzymes including superoxide dismutase, an important scavenger of free radicals, which can cause cell injury. On the other hand, malnutrition such as deficiencies of methionine, zinc, copper, and selenium interferes with cyanogen detoxification. Cassava containing cyanogen along with malnutrition creates an ideal setting for free radical injury by promoting the generation of free radicals and by decreasing the ability to scavenge them.

From these discussions, it may be presumed that TCP is a multifactorial disease. Malnutrition and cyanogen toxicity may lead to free radical injury but there might be other etiologic factors such as genetic, familial, and immunological.

Xenobiotics and micronutrients

The role of xenobiotic on pathogenesis of chronic pancreatitis has been highlighted by Braganza et al. [23]. Inhaled xenobiotics that survive the pulmonary circulation could pose the biggest threat by striking this *xenobiotic-metabolizing organ* directly via its rich arterial supply. The authors found increased exposure to xenobiotics, especially polycyclic aromatic hydrocarbons (cigarette and firewood smoke and vehicular fumes) in patients of TP compared with controls. This was associated with rapid theophylline clearance (a marker for heightened cytochrome P450-I activity) in TP subjects compared with controls, suggesting a role of oxidant stress in causation of TP [24, 25].

Studies on the antioxidant status of TP patients showed low levels of vitamin C and β-carotene, and this may well tilt the balance in favor of oxidant stress [26]. Malnutrition induces a state of defective ability to scavenge free radicals, which could enhance the susceptibility for organ damage [23]. In a randomized controlled trial [27], cocktail of antioxidant supplementation was associated with relief in abdominal pain and decrease in oxidative stress, thus supporting the oxidative stress hypothesis.

These interesting observations need to be substantiated before an etiological role to these factors can be assigned.

Familial aggregation

TP sometimes affects many members of the same family [28, 29]. In one study [28], familial aggregation was seen in 8% of TP patients. In some families, there was evidence of vertical transmission of TP from the parents to the offspring, while in others there was horizontal distribution of the disease among siblings. Familial aggregation suggests, but does not necessarily prove, a hereditary etiology for TP, since several family members could be exposed to the common toxic or other environmental factors.

Genetic factors

The description and characterization of genetic factors in TP has added a new dimension to the understanding of pathogenesis of the disease.

Mutations in a gene that regulates inactivation of excess trypsin produced by pancreatic acinar cells by autolysis, the *SPINK1* (serine protease inhibitor, Kazal type 1), was the first gene associated with TP. Since the inhibitory molecule provides the first line of defense against premature activation of trypsinogen inside the pancreas, it has attracted a lot of attention as a possible cause of chronic pancreatitis. The association between the *SPINK1* gene and TP has now been reported by a number of groups [30–32].

Since all the aforementioned studies on TP and on other forms of chronic pancreatitis have shown a strong association with this gene, it is likely that this could be at least one of the genes predisposing to chronic pancreatitis in general and TCP in particular and present consensus is that this plays a "modifier role" rather than disease inducer [33–35].

Loss-of-function alterations in chymotrypsin C (*CTRC*) could predispose to pancreatitis by diminishing its protective trypsin-degrading activity [36]. A large study from India [37] examined role for chymotrypsin C variants in the pathogenesis of TP. Authors investigated its interaction with p.N34S SPINK1, which is the strongest predictor of risk for TP, and also with cathepsin B. Cathepsin B can activate trypsinogen, while CTRC is capable of inactivating trypsinogen, the probable gain-of-function mutation in *CTSB* and loss-of-function mutations in *CTRC* could increase susceptibility to pancreatitis in Indians. However, the findings of the study suggest a role for chymotrypsin C variants in exons 3 and 7 in the pathogenesis of TP independent of *SPINK1* and *CTSB* mutations.

The molecular basis for hereditary pancreatitis has been attributed to mutations in exons 2 and 3 of the trypsinogen gene [38]. Hassan et al. did not find the link between CP/FCPD and common mutations in the trypsinogen gene [39].

Mutations in the *CFTR* (cystic fibrosis transmembrane conductance regulator) gene could be important in TCP [40]. Cathepsin B, anionic trypsinogen, and *CASR* genes are few other genes studied [41].

Despite these recent advances, we still find that many patients do not carry mutations in any of the known pancreatitis susceptibility genes, suggesting the involvement of other yet unidentified genes.

In a recent review, a two-hit model for the pathogenesis of tropical calcific pancreatitis was proposed. The first hit may be loss of balance between activation and degradation of trypsin leading to the presence of persistent "super-trypsin" within the acinar cell, due to mutations in one or more genes such as *SPINK1, CTSB, CTRC*, and other yet unidentified genes, resulting in inflammation. Presence of additional genetic and/or environmental factors, which constitute the second hit, may lead to one or more phenotypes such as stone formation, fibrosis, and/or diabetes mellitus [9].

Pathology of tropical pancreatitis

There is marked heterogeneity from one area to another resulting in soft to firm hard areas along with ductal calculi in the main ducts. Microscopically, these are seen as areas of normal pancreas to areas of fibrosis and fat replacement, with other areas showing ductal dilatation with concretions and periductal fibrosis (Figure 12E.1).

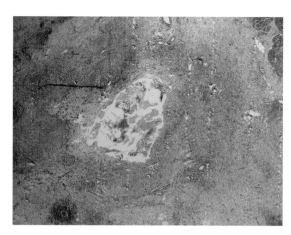

Figure 12E.2 Photomicrographs show dilated duct with denuded epithelium contains concretions with extensive periductal fibrosis. (H&E, ×20 original magnification.)

Ducts show dilatation and contain calcified stone/concretions resulting in surface denudation at the site of impaction (Figure 12E.2). It results in periductal fibrosis, which extends as interlobular fibrosis.

Acinar tissue show infiltration by lymphomononuclear cells along with eosinophils. This results in acinar loss and lipoid metaplasia of acinar cells (Figure 12E.3). Acinar tissue is replaced by fibrosis and later lipoid metaplasia replaces fibrosis with mature adipose tissue. Neural hyperplasia and perineural inflammation can be seen (Figure 12E.4).

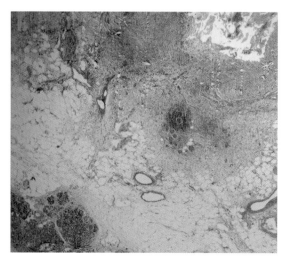

Figure 12E.1 Photomicrographs show marked heterogeneity of pathology ranging from normal acini to ductal concretions with periductal fibrosis and lymphoid follicles indicating chronic changes. (H&E, ×10 original magnification.)

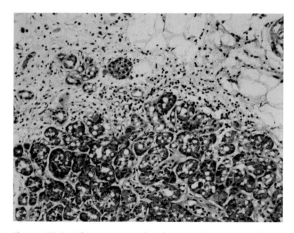

Figure 12E.3 Photomicrographs show mild peripheral lymphomononuclear infiltration with lipoid metaplasia of acinar cells, which is seen in early phase. (H&E, ×40 original magnification.)

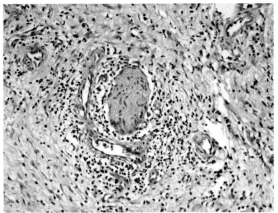

Figure 12E.4 Photomicrographs show neural hyperplasia with perineural inflammation. (H&E, ×40 original magnification.)

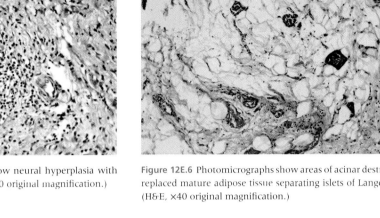

Figure 12E.6 Photomicrographs show areas of acinar destruction replaced mature adipose tissue separating islets of Langerhans. (H&E, ×40 original magnification.)

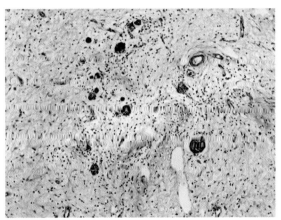

Figure 12E.5 Photomicrographs show areas of acinar destruction replaced by young fibroblasts accompanied by edema separating islets of Langerhans. (H&E, ×20 original magnification.)

Islets are entrapped in fibrous tissue and later seen floating in adipose tissue (Figures 12E.5 and 12E.6). Loss of islets and hyperplasia along with nesidioblastosis has been documented.

Pathophysiology

Pancreatic calculi

In over 90% of patients with TP, pancreatic calculi may be detected especially in the later stages. Stones vary from small sand particles to large stones weighing up to 20 g. The calculi may be smooth, rounded, or stag-horn-like in shape and are usually incarcerated in the main pancreatic duct or its branches [12].

Maldigestion/steatorrhea

Overt steatorrhea is only present in about 20% of patients. The low frequency of steatorrhea is attributed to the low fat intake in the diet. When the fat intake of the diet was experimentally increased to 100 g/day from the average intake of 27 g/day, 76% of TCP patients developed steatorrhea [43].

Pancreatic diabetes

Diabetes in TCP is called FCPD, which is now classified under the broad category of other specific types both in the American Diabetes Association and the WHO consultation classifications of diabetes [44].

One of the characteristic clinical features of FCPD is that despite requiring insulin for control, patients rarely become ketotic on withdrawal of insulin. Ketosis resistance may be attributed to the following factors [45]:

1 residual β-cell function, adequate to prevent ketosis;
2 concomitant destruction of α-cells and thus loss of glucagon, a major ketogenic hormone;
3 subcutaneous fat loss and, therefore, reduced supply of NEFA – the fuel for ketogenesis;

4 resistance to subcutaneous adipose tissue lipolysis by adrenalin;

5 carnitine deficiency affecting transfer of NEFA across mitochondrial membrane.

Complications related to diabetes

It was earlier believed that patients with FCPD do not develop long-term complications of diabetes. This belief was based mainly on the assumption that being a secondary form of diabetes, patients with FCPD do not live long enough to develop specific diabetes-related complications, which normally set in only after 10–15 years of diabetes. However, it has been shown that both microvascular and macrovascular complications do occur in patients with FCPD [46]. Macrovascular complications, though, are rare in FCPD. This is believed to be due to three reasons: the patients are young, lean, and have low lipid levels [8].

Changing scenario

The presentation of the disease has become more heterogeneous, though about 10–15% of patients still present with the classical picture of TP. In the patients without a classical clinical picture, no definite clinical or biochemical markers are available to confidently diagnose TP, as distinct from idiopathic CP [9]. Compared with the very young age in the earlier reports, the mean age of patients with CP is reported to be late twenties and early thirties. Now, the patients are not dying in their second or third decade of life probably due to earlier detection, improvement in hospital care, and overall improved facilities. However, overall disease frequency is not decreasing simultaneously. Moreover, it is also detected even in obese and business executives. Unchanged are its geographical segregation, occurrence in strict nonalcoholics, and early onset of the disease [9, 47, 48]. Most patients still present with pain, though milder and often controlled with drugs. The diabetes is milder, and can often be controlled using dietary measure and oral hypoglycemic agents; about one-third of the patients require insulin. Many patients initially have diabetes and develop pain a few years later [9]. These recent studies describing the change in phenotype of idiopathic chronic pancreatitis in India

make us ponder why this change has happened in last two decades. It probably appears that this change has been brought about by changes in diet and environment caused by economic development in India. We feel that genetic studies will probably throw more light on the pathogenesis of this intriguing disease and answer some important questions like whether TP of south India and Idiopathic pancreatitis of North seen now are same or different diseases. However, despite this change in phenotype, patients with classical features of TP are still seen occasionally in north India also. Till the time we are able to better understand the pathogenesis of idiopathic chronic pancreatitis, we will continue to designate this disease by geographical locations [49]. Quite intriguingly, TP has recently been reported from northern India, Bangladesh, and even China, regions that fall outside the "tropics" [48, 50, 51].

References

1 Zuidema PJ. Cirrhosis and disseminated calcification of the pancreas in patients with malnutrition. Tropical and Geographical Medicine 1959;11:70–74.

2 Geevarghese PJ. Pancreatic Diabetes. Bombay, Popular Prakashan. 1968, 110–115.

3 Illangovekara V. Malnutrition related diabetes in Sri Lanka fact or fiction? Journal of the Ceylon College of Physicians 1995;28:16–25.

4 Mngola EN. Diabetes mellitus in the African environment—the dilemma. In: Mngola EN (Ed). Diabetes 1982. Proceedings of the II Congress of the IDF. Amsterdam, Excerpta Medica. 1983, 309–313.

5 Dani R, Penna FJ, Nogueira CED. Etiology of chronic pancreatitis in Brazil: a report of 329 consecutive cases. International Journal of Pancreatology 1986(5–6):399–406.

6 Tandon RK, Sato N, Garg PK. Chronic pancreatitis: Asia-Pacific consensus report. Journal of Gastroenterology and Hepatology 2002;17: 508–518.

7 Pitchumoni CS. Special problems of tropical pancreatitis. Journal of Clinical Gastroenterology 1985; 13: 941–959.

8 Barman KK, Premalatha G, Mohan V. Tropical chronic pancreatitis. Postgraduate Medical Journal 2003; 79: 606–615.

9 Balakrishnan V, Nair P, Radhakrishnan L, Narayanan V A. Tropical pancreatitis – a distinct entity, or merely a type of chronic pancreatitis? Indian Journal of Gastroenterology 2006;25:74–81.

10 GeeVarghese PJ, Pitchumoni CS, Nair SR. Is protein malnutrition a initiating cause of pancreatic calcification? Journal of the Association of Physicians of India 1969;14:417–419.

11 Shaper AG. Aetiology of chronic pancreatic fibrosis with calcification seen in Uganda. British Medical Journal 1964;1:1607–1609.

12 Lester FT. A search for malnutrition related diabetes mellitus in an Ethiopian diabetes clinic. Bulletin of the International Diabetes Federation 1984;29:14.

13 Davies JNP. The essential pathology of kwashiorkor. Lancet 1948; 251: 317–320.

14 Sandhyamani S. Vasculopathic and cardiomyopathic changes induced by low-protein high carbohydrate tapioca based diet in bonnet monkey. Vasculopathic and cardiomyopathic changes in induced malnutrition. The American Journal of Cardiovascular Pathology 1992;4:41–50.

15 Regunath H, Shivakumar BM, Kurien A, Satyamoorthy K, Pai GC. Anthropometric measurements of nutritional status in chronic pancreatitis in India: Comparison of tropical and alcoholic pancreatitis. Indian Journal of Gastroenterology 2011: 30; 78–83.

16 Sathiaraj E, Gupta S, Chutke M, et al. Malnutrition is not an etiological factor in the development of tropical pancreatitis—a case-control study of southern Indian patients. Tropical Gastroenterology 2010;31:169–174.

17 Narendranathan M. Chronic calcific pancreatitis in the tropics. Tropical Gastroenterology 1981; 2: 40–45.

18 Pitchumoni CS Special problem of tropical pancreatitis. Clinical Gastroenterology 1984; 13: 941–959.

19 McMillan DE, Geevarghese PJ. Dietary cyanide and tropical malnutrition diabetes. Diabetes Care 1979;2:202–208.

20 Mathangi DC, Deepa R, Mohan V, et al. Long term ingestion of cassava (tapioca) does not produce diabetes or pancreatitis in the rat model. International Journal of Pancreatology 2000; 27: 203–208.

21 Chari ST, Mohan V, Jayanthi V, et al. Comparative study of the clinical profiles of alcoholic chronic pancreatitis and tropical chronic pancreatitis in Tamil Nadu, south India. Pancreas 1992; 7: 52–58

22 Tuescher T, Rosman JB, Baillod R, et al. Absence of diabetes in rural west African population with a high carbohydrate/cassava diet. Lancet 1987;1:765–768.

23 Braganza JM, Lee SH, McCloy RF, McMahon MJ. Chronic pancreatitis. Lancet 2011; 377: 1184–1197.

24 Braganza JM, John S, Padmayalam I, et al. Xenobiotics and tropical pancreatitis. International Journal of Pancreatology 1990; 7: 231–245.

25 Chaloner C, Sandle LN, Mohan V, et al. Evidence for induction of cytochrome p-4501 in patients with tropical chronic pancreatitis. International Journal of Clinical Pharmacology, Therapy, and Toxicology 1990;28: 235–240.

26 Braganza JM, Schofield D, Snehalatha C, et al. Micronutrient antioxidant status in tropical compared with temperate zone chronic pancreatitis. Scandinavian Journal of Gastroenterology 1993;28:1098–1104.

27 Bhardwaj P, Garg PK, Maulik SK, Saraya A, Tandon RK, Acharya SK. A randomized controlled trial of antioxidant supplementation for pain relief in patients with chronic pancreatitis. Gastroenterology 2009;136:149–159.

28 Mohan V, Chari S, Hitman GA, et al. Familial aggregation in tropical fibrocalculous pancreatic diabetes. Pancreas 1989; 4: 690–693.

29 Kambo PK, Hitman GA, Mohan V, et al. The genetic predisposition to fibrocalculous pancreatic diabetes. Diabetologia 1989;32:45–51.

30 Hassan Z, Mohan V, Ali L, et al. SPINK1 is a major gene for susceptibility to fibrocalculous pancreatic diabetes in subjects from southern Indian subcontinent. The American Journal of Human Genetics 2002;71:964–968.

31 Chandak GR, Idris MM, Reddy DN, et al. Mutations in the pancreatic secretory trypsin inhibitor gene (*PSTI/SPINK1*) rather than the cationic trypsinogen gene (*PRSS1*) are significantly associated with tropical calcific pancreatitis. Journal of Medical Genetics 2002;39:347–351.

32 Schneider A, Suman A, Rossi L, et al. SPINK 1/PSTI 1 mutation are associated with tropical pancreatitis and type 2 diabetes in Bangladesh. Gastroenterology 2002;123:1026–1030.

33 Pfutzer RH, Barmada MM, Brunskill AP, et al. SPINK/PSTI polymorphisms act as disease modifiers in familial and idiopathic chronic pancreatitis. Gastroenterology 2000;119: 615–623.

34 Mahurkar S, Reddy DN, Rao GV, Chandak GR. Genetic mechanisms underlying the pathogenesis of tropical calcific pancreatitis. World Journal of Gastroenterology 2009;15:264–269.

35 Singh S, Choudhuri G, Agarwal S. Frequency of CFTR, SPINK1, and cathepsin B gene mutation in north Indian population: connections between genetics and clinical data. ScientificWorldJournal 2014; 2014: 763195 ; Published online 2014 January 27. doi: 10.1155/2014/763195

36 Derikx MH, Szmola R, te Morschea RH, et al. Tropical calcific pancreatitis and its association with CTRC and SPINK1 (p.N34S) variants. European Journal of Gastroenterology & Hepatology 2009;21:889–894.

37 Paliwal S, Bhaskar S, Mani KR, et al. Comprehensive screening of chymotrypsin C (CTRC) gene in tropical calcific pancreatitis identifies novel variants. Gut 2013; 62: 1602–1606.

38 Whitcomb DC. Hereditary pancreatitis: new insights into acute and chronic pancreatitis. Gut 1999; 45:317–322.

39 Hassan Z, Mohan V, McDermott MF, et al. Pancreatitis in fibrocalculous pancreatic diabetes mellitus is not associated with common mutations in the trypsinogen gene. Diabetes/Metabolism Reviews 2000;16:454–457.

40 Rajesh G, Elango EM, Vidya V, Balakrishnan V. Genotype phenotype correlations in 9 patients with tropical pancreatitis and identified gene mutations. Indian Journal of Gastroenterology 2009;28:68–71.

41 Murugaian EE, Premkumar RM, Radhakrishnan L, Vallath B. Novel mutations in the calcium sensing receptor gene in tropical chronic pancreatitis in India. Scandinavian Journal of Gastroenterology 2008;43:117.

42 Chari ST, Jayanthi V, Mohan V, et al. Radiological appearance of pancreatic calculi in tropical and alcoholic chronic pancreatitis. Journal of Gastroenterology and Hepatology 1992;7:42–44.

43 Balakrishnan V, Sauniere JH, Hariharan M, et al. Diet, pancreatic function and chronic pancreatitis in South India and France. Pancreas 1988;3:30–35.

44 Alberti KGMM, Zimmet PZ. Definition, diagnosis and classification of diabetes mellitus and its complications. Part 1: diagnosis and classification of diabetes mellitus: provisional report of a WHO consultation. Diabetic Medicine 1998;78:539–553.

45 Mohan V, Nagalotimath SJ, Yajnik CS, et al. Fibrocalculous pancreatic diabetes. Diabetes/Metabolism Reviews 1998;14:153–170.

46 Shelgikar KM, Yajnik CS, Mohan V. Complications in fibrocalculous pancreatic diabetes—the Pune and Madras experience. International Journal of Diabetes in Developing Countries 1995;15:70–75.

47 Bhasin DK, Singh G, Rana SS, Chowdry S, Shafiq N, Malhotra S, Sinha SK, Nagi B. Clinical profile of idiopathic chronic pancreatitis in North India. Clinical Gastroenterology and Hepatology 2009;7:594–599.

48 Garg PK. Chronic pancreatitis in India and Asia. Current Gastroenterology Reports 2012; 14:118–124.

49 Bhasin DK, Rana SS, Singh K. Idiopathic chronic pancreatitis in India: looking for a name! Futile or fruitful exercise?. Gut. 2011;60:1164.

50 Bhasin DK, Rana SS, Chandail VS, Singh G, Gupta R, Kang M, Sinha SK, Singh K. Clinical profile of calcific and noncalcific chronic pancreatitis in north India. Journal of Clinical Gastroenterology 2011;45:546–550.

51 Balakrishnan V, Unnikrishnan AG, Thomas V et al. Chronic pancreatitis. A prospective nationwide study of 1,086 subjects from India. Journal of the Pancreas (Online) 2008; 9(5):593–600.

Dana A. Dominguez & Kimberly S. Kirkwood

Department of Surgery, University of California, San Francisco, San Francisco, CA, USA

Introduction

Severe, disabling abdominal pain is the hallmark of chronic pancreatitis. Currently available treatments for pancreatitis pain are inadequate and expensive, both in health-care dollars and in lost productivity. Pain is the most common reason for hospitalization among chronic pancreatitis patients, and as many as 40% require three or more admissions during their lifetime for pain management [1]. Improved treatments depend on a better understanding of the mechanisms of chronic visceral pain, a subject that has gained attention recently with the development of suitable animal models and reproducible experimental measures of sustained pancreatic pain.

Manifestations and treatment of pancreatic pain

Chronic pain syndrome: a downward spiral

Among the many clinical sequelae of chronic pancreatitis, pain has been shown to be the most important factor affecting quality of life [2]. The pain often becomes the focal point around which work, leisure activities, and relationships must revolve. In a study of 265 patients, Wehler et al. showed that as abdominal pain index scores increased across subgroups, there was a significant and profound decrease in all quality-of-life indices. Since eating can trigger pain exacerbations, patients typically respond by decreasing food intake. Many patients also suffer nutrient malabsorption due to pancreatic exocrine insufficiency, and this combination leads to progressive weight loss and malnutrition. Decreased BMI has been correlated with impairment in quality-of-life measurements [3].

Pain theories

Traditional theories of the origin of pancreatic pain in chronic pancreatitis focused on structural abnormalities causing ductal hypertension [4]. Such abnormalities ranged from stones and strictures to fibrosis due to toxic effects and ischemia [5]. While this ductal obstruction theory is logical, studies in patients with chronic pancreatitis have failed to show a correlation between ductal pressure and pain levels; moreover, ductal pressures do not accurately predict the success of ductal decompression procedures [6–9]. In fact, Bornman et al. demonstrated that there was no significant difference in either the anatomy or the morphological changes between groups of patients with either painful or painless pancreatitis [10]. Rather than a single mechanism of pain, recent research has favored a more complex relationship between these structural and morphological components, and their interaction with neurobiological mechanisms [11]. Nociceptive pathways, inflammatory mediators, and sensitization of both central and peripheral pathways have been shown to play important roles in pancreatic pain [12].

Models

Pancreatic atrophy and fibrosis can be induced experimentally in a variety of ways; however, measures of visceral pain have proven more difficult. Studies in rats evaluated spontaneous activity qualitatively by video tracking and sensitivity of the abdomen to mechanical

Pancreatitis: Medical and Surgical Management, First Edition.
David B. Adams, Peter B. Cotton, Nicholas J. Zyromski and John Windsor.
© 2017 John Wiley & Sons, Ltd. Published 2017 by John Wiley & Sons, Ltd.

and electrical stimulation [13]. The most widely used of these rat models was developed in 1996 by Puig et al. who injected trinitrobenzene sulfonic acid (TNBS) directly into the pancreatic duct of rats to induce early severe acute pancreatitis that evolved over weeks into painful chronic pancreatitis [14]. This model was further characterized and modified to provide better face validity and generalization to human disease by Winston et al. in 2005. This model has proved invaluable in providing insight into the complex nature of pain from chronic pancreatitis. Further progress in identifying specific pathways that might be therapeutic targets, however, was hampered by the lack of a murine model in which putative mediators could be genetically deleted.

Adaptation of the TNBS model to mice was fraught with early experimental failure related to the high mortality of severe acute pancreatitis in the physiologically fragile mice. Our laboratory adapted the model to mice by dramatically reducing the dose of TNBS and by providing perioperative fluid resuscitation during the first 24 hours [15]. The resultant chronic pancreatitis is apparent after 1–2 weeks with severe fibrosis, monocyte infiltration, atrophy, and fatty replacement of the gland. We used Von Frey filament probing of the abdomen to demonstrate referred mechanical hyperalgesia, in which heightened withdrawal responses were measured to a mildly painful stimulus, as well as allodynia, in which probes that do not cause pain in control mice evoke withdrawal responses. TNBS-injected mice also showed reduced spontaneous activity (distance and time) on a running wheel and longer periods of immobility during open field testing. This model can be used to examine both peripheral and central mechanisms of sustained pain and for comparison with models of somatic pain, such as peripheral or spinal nerve ligation, so that both shared and unique pathways can be identified.

Components of pancreatic pain

Nociceptive neurons

In addition to parasympathetic cholinergic innervation from the vagus nerve and sympathetic innervation mainly derived from the celiac ganglia, the pancreas is also innervated by nociceptive sensory neurons. These afferent neurons have their cell bodies in the dorsal root ganglia (DRG), and they give off projections that map to the dorsal horn of the spinal cord [12]

(Figure 12F.1). They are responsible for transmission of noxious visceral stimuli from the pancreas and the relay of this information to the central nervous system.

Uncontrolled proteolysis

The pancreas is rich in cysteine and serine proteases that can be released following a variety of insults and are known to activate, either directly or indirectly, nociceptive neurons. Using a near infrared-labeled activity-based probe that covalently modifies active cathepsins, our laboratory found significant accumulation of cathepsins B, L, and S in both the inflamed rodent pancreas and in human juice from patients with painful chronic pancreatitis [16]. Cathepsins, in turn, cleave and activate trypsinogens, yielding active trypsins, some of which are resistant to endogenous degradation by ubiquitous inhibitors, and are thereby free to bind and activate receptors on peptidergic neurons [17]. Following activation, peptidergic neurons release neuropeptides and inflammatory mediators including calcitonin gene–related peptide (CGRP), substance P (SP), vasoactive intestinal polypeptide (VIP), and bradykinin, that act both peripherally where they promote vasodilation, plasma extravasation, and neutrophil infiltration (so-called neurogenic inflammation) and centrally where they activate central pain pathways [18].

Sensory neuron receptors

Vanilloid receptors

One of the best characterized pain receptors is transient receptor potential vanilloid 1 (TRPV1). A member of the family of vanilloid nociceptive receptors found on sensory neurons, it functions as a nonselective cation channel, permitting flow of sodium and calcium into cells, leading to depolarization of the cell membrane and release of neurotransmitters such as SP and CGRP [12]. Originally known as the capsaicin receptor, it is activated by heat and local acidification, as well as multiple endogenous chemical mediators including leukotrienes and arachidonic acid metabolites [19]. Caterina et al. used TRPV1 knockout mice to clearly demonstrate the role of TRPV1 in nociception and tissue-injury-induced hyperalgesia [20]. We showed that TRPV1 plays an important role in nociceptive mediation in acute pancreatitis through the induction of SP and CGRP release by pancreatic sensory nerves, increasing *c-fos*

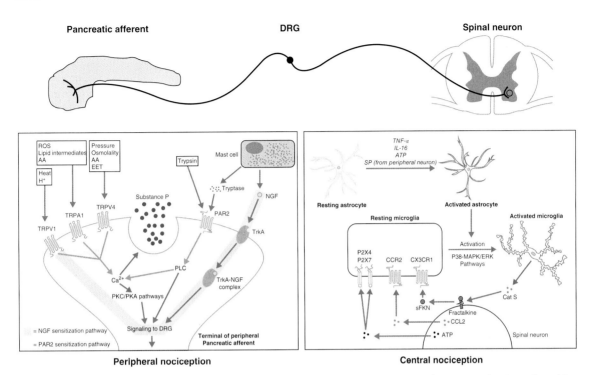

Figure 12F.1 Pathways of pancreatic pain signal transmission in chronic pancreatitis with emphasis on mechanisms of sensitization. Peripherally, extracellular inflammatory agents including NGF, trypsin, and tryptase sensitize and activate pancreatic afferent nociceptive neurons through integrative calcium signaling pathways. Centrally, sensitization is mediated through positive feedback loops among dorsal horn neurons and the activated neuronal supporting cells, microglia and astrocytes, via Cat S-mediated cleavage and release of soluble FKN. Abbreviations: ROS, reactive oxygen species; AA, arachidonic acid metabolites; TRPV, transient receptor potential vanilloids; NGF, nerve growth factor; PAR2, protease-activated receptor 2; PLC, phospholipase C; PKC, protein kinase C; PKA, protein kinase A; DRG, dorsal root ganglia; EET, epoxyeicosatrienoic acids; TrkA, trypomyosin-related kinase A; SP, substance P; FKN, fractalkine; sFKN, soluble fractalkine; Cat S, cathepsin S; CCR2, chemokine receptor 2; CCL2, chemokine ligand 2; MAPK, map kinase pathway; ERK, extracellular signal–regulated kinase pathway.

expression in the spinal cords of rats. Administration of a TRPV1 antagonist attenuated this effect [21]. TRPV1 is upregulated in chronic pancreatitis and has been demonstrated as a mediator of hyperalgesia and inflammation in this condition [22]. In addition, it has been implicated to have interactions with other TRP receptors as well as protease-activated receptor 2 (PAR2), a G-protein-coupled receptor with unique roles in inflammation and pain sensitization [12], described later.

TRPV1 can work alone or in concert with other TRP receptors, such as TRP Ankyrin 1 (TRPA1), to amplify nociceptive signaling. Required for sensory neuron excitation, TRPA1 functions as a "gatekeeper" of chronic inflammation by serving two major roles: controlling peripheral release of inflammatory neuropeptides and facilitating neuronal activation by inflammatory mediators released through local tissue injury [23]. Though

it had been previously shown to mediate inflammation and visceral pain in acute pancreatitis [24], the first evidence of TRPA1's direct role in pain from chronic pancreatitis came in 2013 with the establishment of a TNBS murine model of chronic pancreatitis. In this model of painful chronic pancreatitis following severe acute pancreatitis, we found that TRPA1 knockout mice had less inflammation and fibrosis and markedly reduced pain indices, including referred mechanical hyperalgesia, spontaneous running activity, and mobility in open field testing, as compared with wild-type controls [15].

Over the past decade, it has been demonstrated using knockout mice [20, 25, 26], TRPA1 knockdowns [27], and the use of antagonists [28] that TRPA1 works in concert with TRPV1 to mediate inflammation-induced stimulus transmission in sensory neurons. Evidence for a direct interaction between the two channels was shown by Staruschenko et al. using FRET constructs of the respective channels [29]. Recently, TRPA1 and TRPV1 were implicated in the transition from acute to chronic inflammation in the pancreas. Schwartz et al., using a cerulein model of acute pancreatitis, demonstrated that morphologic acute to chronic changes were mitigated by the administration of TRP antagonists [30].

Increasing evidence also supports a role for TRPV4 in pancreatic pain. TRPV4 is directly activated by shear stress, osmotic stimuli, and lipid mediators, as well as indirectly via G-protein-coupled receptors that regulate TRP channels [31, 32]. TRPV4 knockout mice [33] and TRPV4 knockdowns [34] have demonstrated abnormal osmotic regulation and decreased responses to changes in pressure and tonicity. Alessandri-Haber et al. proposed the attractive notion that the "soup" of inflammatory mediators that surround local tissue injury, including bradykinin, SP, prostaglandin E2 (PGE_2), serotonin, and histamine, among others, may induce mechanical hyperalgesia through activation of TRPV4, sensitizing it for a triggering event. They demonstrated that activation of TRPV4 by hypotonic saline was enhanced in the presence of PGE2, and increased nociceptive behavior in rats. These effects were absent in their TRPV4 knockout rats [34]. They also demonstrated the involvement of protein kinase A and C intracellular second messenger pathways in the activation of TRPV4 [35]. This activation in turn mediates pain transmission through subsequent activation of nociceptive spinal neurons in the superficial laminae of the spinal cord. In the pancreas, we showed that injection of a TRPV4 agonist into the pancreatic duct increased c-Fos-LI expression in the spinal cord in the input regions of pancreatic sensory neurons located by retrograde tracing, suggesting that TRPV4 could play a role in pain signaling in the inflamed pancreas [24]. Further experiments are needed to clarify the importance of TRPV4 in acute and chronic pancreatic inflammatory pain.

Protease-activated receptor 2 (PAR2)

Protease-activated receptor 2 (PAR2) is one of the four GPCRs that is activated by serine proteases such as trypsin and thrombin. These proteases cleave an N-terminal fragment, revealing a tethered receptor agonist (ligand), which can then bind and activate signaling pathways [36]. Steinhoff et al. provided initial

evidence of a neurogenic inflammatory role for PAR2 by demonstrating its coexpression with neuropeptides CGRP and substance P in DRG neurons. Activation of PAR2 leads to release of neuropeptides in peripheral tissues as well as the spinal cord, increasing local inflammation and edema [37].

In addition to causing the direct release of inflammatory neuropeptides from sensory neurons, activated PAR2 leads to increased intracellular calcium, which lowers the threshold for activation of TRP channels by other inflammatory mediators and products of tissue injury, so-called "sensitization." Thus, the addition of trypsin or PAR2-activating peptide (AcPep) in dorsal root ganglion cell culture led to significantly increased capsaicin-evoked CGRP release, an indication of PAR2 sensitization of TRPV1. *In vivo*, preinjection of AcPep into the pancreatic duct increased capsaicin-induced FOS expression in pancreatic spinal cord segments compared with the control peptide, suggesting that PAR2 sensitizes TRPV1 in the pancreas [38]. Under normal physiologic conditions, concentrations of active trypsin in the pancreas are low due to its release in a zymogen form as trypsinogen. However, following pancreatic inflammation, early activation of trypsins by cysteine proteases, as well as the recruitment of mast cells that release tryptase, can, in turn, activate PAR2 [39]. Indirect evidence of the importance of mast cell products in chronic pancreatitis pain derives from the observation that mast cells were present in significantly higher numbers in patients with painful chronic pancreatitis than in patients with nonpainful pancreatitis (33.8 vs. 9.4 average mast cell/10 high power field; $P < 0.01$) or with healthy controls (33.8 vs. 6.1 average mast cell/10 high-power field; $P < 0.01$) [40]. Intraductal injection of trypsin into the pancreatic duct of mice in subinflammatory concentrations causes increased FOS expression in pancreas-specific spinal cord DRG. This effect was mitigated by pretreatment with AcPep, indicating that PAR2 and trypsin may share this pain pathway [41]. PAR2 activation in these neurons leads to sustained hyperalgesia [42]. Thus, serine proteases contribute to pancreatic pain via multiple pathways mediated by PAR2 activation [17].

PAR2 has also been shown to sensitize both TRPV4 and TRPA1, and thereby lower the threshold for activation of pancreatic sensory neurons [43, 44]. PAR2-mediated sensitization of these TRP channels has been associated with neuropathic pain induced by the chemotherapy agent paclitaxel, which indicates that these pathways have clinical importance [45]. Peripheral sensitization represents an important pathway by which the painful effects of inflammatory mediators that result from tissue injury are amplified and sustained.

Nerve growth factor (NGF) and receptor tyrosine kinase A (TrkA)

Nerve growth factor (NGF), a protein that contributes to the development and survival of neurons, also plays an important role in the peripheral sensitization of sensory neurons [46]. It acts mainly through its high-affinity tyrosine kinase receptor, TrkA, which is found in highest concentration within the pancreas in the perineurium. Coexpression of TrkA with NGF is increased in the pancreas from patients with chronic pancreatitis [47]. NGF exerts its effects through multiple mechanisms including a direct effect on ion channels, posttranslational modifications by second messengers, as well as by translocation of the NGF/trkA complex to the nucleus where it regulates transcriptional modifications to certain genes [48]. Early evidence for its role in mediating visceral pain came from expression studies by McMahon et al. in 1994, which demonstrated that almost all afferent neurons innervating visceral targets expressed trkA, while its expression in those innervating skeletal muscle was very low [49]. Immunodepletion studies using a trkA–IgG on cultured neurons, showed a sustained hypoalgesia and a downregulation of CGRP [50]. This was further supported by studies using animals lacking the *trkA* gene, which also experienced a significant hypoalgesic state [51]. This same hypoalgesic effect was noted after administration of a blocking antibody for NGF to rats with chronic pancreatitis, which significantly increased A-type potassium currents, thereby decreasing the likelihood of depolarization [52]. Conversely, both neonatal and adult rats that were injected with excess exogenous NGF showed a profound behavioral hyperalgesia [53]. Recent reports suggest that NGF/trkA can sensitize neurons via interaction with the vanilloid receptor TRPV1, and NGF can regulate TRPV1 expression through both transcriptional and posttranslational mechanisms (Figure 12F.1) [48].

Neurokinin receptor 1 (NK-1R)

Substance P, neurokinin A (NKA), and neurokinin B (NKB) are the main tachykinins involved in sensory neural transmission and nociception. Substance P and NKA share a receptor, neurokinin receptor 1 (NK-1R), and NKB binds preferentially to neurokinin receptor 2 (NK-2R) [54]. Through a study of human pancreatic tissue, Di Sebastiano et al. found that although there was an increase in substance P surrounding pancreatic nerve fibers, there was not a concomitant increase in the gene encoding substance P. This observation led to the early understanding that substance P was being synthesized in extrapancreatic ganglia and transported to the pancreas [55]. Thus, activation of peripheral sensory nerve endings leads to the release of substance P and CGRP peripherally within the pancreas, where they promote neurogenic inflammation in a positive feedback loop that leads to amplification of inflammatory pain, and centrally, where substance P binds to NK-1R in the dorsal horn of the spinal cord and activates central pain pathways [56, 57] Shrikhande et al. was the first to examine NK-1R expression in pancreata from patients with painful chronic pancreatitis. They established a definitive relationship between mRNA levels and intensity, frequency, and duration of pain in these patients [58].

Central sensitization

Nervous system support cells
Microglia

Microglia are immune cells in the central nervous system that respond to tissue injury by switching from a quiescent to an active state, in which they secrete inflammatory mediators to recruit other immune cells and promote cellular hypertrophy and proliferation [59, 60]. Their function in the CNS is similar to that of macrophages in peripheral tissues.

How are microglia activated? The initial activation of microglia likely occurs through multiple pathways. Excitation of nociceptive neurons leads to release of the chemokine CCL2 that binds to its receptor CCR2 on microglia, a critical signaling event in microglial activation [61] that promotes pain signal amplification (Figure 12F.1). Another potential pathway is through the receptors P2X4 and P2X7, which are upregulated in microglia after nerve injury and activated in response to injury by ATP released by primary sensory and dorsal horn neurons as well as dorsal horn astrocytes [62]. P38, a mitogen-activated protein kinase (MAPK) has been implicated as a major participant in the activation of spinal microglia (Figure 12F.1). Originally demonstrated in a neuropathic pain model using sciatic nerve ligation, Jin et al. showed early p38 activation in spinal microglia (12–24 hours after injury), with subsequent activation in DRG neurons [63]. Inhibition of this activation with a p38-inhibitor also inhibited the development of pain hypersensitivity [59]. P38 activation has also been reported in the rat model of chronic pancreatitis pain by Liu et al., suggesting that this pathway is important in sustained visceral pain [64]. Once activated, these loops can function without further external stimulus. Thus, excitation of nociceptive spinal neurons leads to activation of spinal microglia via multiple parallel pathways that provide an efficient means to amplify inflammatory nociceptive signals.

How does microglial activation cause sustained pain? It has been well established that support cells of the nervous system participate in maintaining neuropathic pain pathways in somatic pain models [59, 65, 66]. Activation of spinal microglia leads to the release of the soluble chemokine fractalkine (FKN), which is expressed in CNS sensory neurons as a transmembrane protein that can be cleaved to a soluble form (Figure 12F.1). This cleavage was originally shown to occur after excitotoxic stimuli, suggesting that fractalkine cleavage represented an early event in the neurogenic inflammatory process [67]. It is now known that membrane-bound FKN is cleaved by the cysteine protease cathepsin S (Cat S), which is secreted peripherally by macrophages [68] and centrally by activated microglia. Cat S cleaves FKN on dorsal horn neurons, releasing its soluble form, which then binds its own receptor CX3CR1 [69]. This receptor is only expressed in microglia that is in the activated state [70] and binding further activates the p38 pathway in a positive feedback loop. Using the rat model of peripheral nerve ligation, Clark et al. showed that using a Cat S inhibitor reduced pain behavior 7- and 14-days after sciatic nerve ligation in rats, whereas it did not prevent the initial development of pain. This suggests that Cat S is important in the maintenance of neuropathic pain, rather than the development of hyperalgesia [69]. The release of Cat S and subsequent binding and activation of the p38 pathway is dependent on microglial activation.

Recent evidence supports the importance of activated microglia in the development and maintenance of sustained visceral pain. In a rat model of TNBS-induced chronic pancreatitis, Liu et al. found that the microglial activation inhibitor, minocycline, significantly decreased nociceptive behavior, and that withdrawal of minocycline caused a return to baseline. Also, pretreatment with minocycline, prior to injection of TNBS, prevented chronic visceral hyperalgesia for as long as 3 weeks [64]. We found similar results in the TNBS-induced chronic pancreatitis mouse treated with minocycline, with normalization of the expected heightened responses to Von Frey filament probing (unpublished results). These data suggest that microglial activation may play an important role in sustained pancreatic pain.

Astrocytes

Astrocytes demonstrate activated morphology in neuropathic pain models [71], and drugs used to treat pain in these experimental conditions attenuate activation [66, 72]. Activation of astrocytes by mediators, such as ATP, SP, prostaglandins, and glutamate, released by sensory nerves in response to injury stimulates release of proinflammatory mediators. These mediators include cytokines such as IL-1B, IL-6, and TNFα, as well as the molecules that activate them, including ATP and prostaglandins [66]. Multiple intracellular signaling pathways have been implicated in the regulation of astrocyte activation, including p38, c-Jun-N-terminal kinase (JNK) and, perhaps most importantly, the extracellular signal–regulated kinase (ERK) pathway [73]. Zhuang et al. demonstrated increased expression of phosphorylated ERK in both microglia and dorsal horn astrocytes 10 days after spinal nerve ligation. In this study, intrathecal injection of an ERK inhibitor significantly reduced mechanical allodynia [74]. In the rat model of TNBS-induced chronic pancreatitis pain, Feng et al. reported an increase in glial fibrillary acidic protein (GFAP), an astrocyte marker that is upregulated in somatic models of neuropathic pain. This study also importantly demonstrated that attenuation of neuropathic pain in this model was possible using l-α-aminoadipate (LAA), a specific inhibitor of astrocyte activation, [75] suggesting a potential therapeutic target.

Reorganization

Observational studies in humans with chronic visceral pain have led to the notion that changes in inhibitory and amplification processes in the CNS contribute to reorganization of referred pain signal mapping. Mertz et al. meticulously mapped pain patterns in patients with inflammatory bowel syndrome (IBS). In response to rectal distension, IBS patients had increased hypersensitivity in areas remote from the stimulus, as well as larger overall pain areas, as compared with healthy controls. These changes were associated with increased thalamic activation in the brain. They suggested that increased afferent signaling from the gut may lead to perceptual reorganization of pain signals [76]. Interestingly, in contrast to these results, Dimcevski and colleagues reported that chronic pancreatitis patients had hypoalgesia in response to balloon distension of viscera surrounding the pancreas compared with healthy controls [77]. It is worth noting that duodenal distension is less well established as a marker of referred visceral hyperalgesia than rectal distension, which could contribute to these results. In other studies by this group, electrical visceral pain stimulation in chronic pancreatitis patients was associated with reduced evoked potential latency in the brain, thereby suggesting that central modulation of pain pathways contributes to visceral hypersensitivity. Similar to prior findings in IBS patients, chronic pancreatitis patients also demonstrated an increase in the mean size of areas of referred pain following electrical visceral stimulation, suggesting reorganization of pain perception [78].

Opioid-induced hyperalgesia

Opioids are the mainstay of treatment for patients with severe chronic pancreatitis pain. As early as the nineteenth century, it was recognized that chronic opioid use leads not only to tolerance and physical and psychological dependence but, ironically, also to increased sensitivity to painful stimuli or opioid-induced hyperalgesia (OIH). Unlike opioid tolerance, OIH cannot be mitigated by increased dosage regimens [79]. Multiple studies in animal models have shown a reduction in mechanical and thermal thresholds to nociceptive stimuli with opioid treatment [80–82]. Similarly, there have been multiple clinical studies in humans describing varying levels of hyperalgesic states among both patients and healthy controls treated with chronic opioids [83–86]. Much remains to be defined about the mechanisms of this hyperalgesia, but they are thought to be closely intertwined with the pathways of opioid tolerance. Pathways involving the N-methyl-d-aspartate receptor (NMDAR), spinal glutamate activity, protein kinase C activity, and spinal dynorphin have all been

implicated as vital to both tolerance and hyperalgesia [87]. It is likely that this phenomenon contributes, in part, to the exasperation experienced by both patients and physicians at the progressive worsening of chronic pancreatitis pain experienced by some patients on escalating opioid dosages.

Conclusion

Research into the mechanisms of chronic pancreatitis pain has been accelerated by the recent availability of validated rat and mouse models, which provide interested investigators with a wider array of reproducible measures of experimental visceral pain. Emerging models illustrate the complexity, redundancy, interconnectedness, and plasticity of chronic visceral pain pathways. Current treatments do not address the underlying mechanisms of sensitization and amplification of both peripheral and central pain signals, which may, in part, explain the high level of medical and surgical treatment failure. In the periphery, integrative channels offer potentially high-leverage targets, as do positive feedback loops in the spinal cord, where selective inhibition could have profound beneficial results. The development of clinically useful inhibitors of these potential targets is expected to improve both treatment effectiveness and quality of life for patients with debilitating chronic pancreatitis pain.

Acknowledgment

Parts of images from motifolio.com were used to construct figure.

References

1 Mullady DK et al. Type of pain, pain-associated complications, quality of life, disability and resource utilisation in chronic pancreatitis: a prospective cohort study. Gut 2011;60:77–84.

2 Pezzilli R et al. Quality of life in patients with chronic pancreatitis. Digestive and Liver Disease 2005;37:181–189.

3 Wehler M et al. Factors associated with health-related quality of life in chronic pancreatitis. The American Journal of Gastroenterology 2004;99:138–146.

4 Bradley EL III. Pancreatic duct pressure in chronic pancreatitis. American Journal of Surgery 1982;144:313–316.

5 Demir IE, Tieftrunk E, Maak M, Friess H, Ceyhan GO. Pain mechanisms in chronic pancreatitis: of a master and his fire. Langenbeck's Archives of Surgery/Deutsche Gesellschaft fur Chirurgie 2011;396:151–160.

6 Ebbehoj N. Pancreatic tissue fluid pressure and pain in chronic pancreatitis. Danish Medical Bulletin 1992;39:128–133.

7 Ebbehoj N et al. Evaluation of pancreatic tissue fluid pressure measurements intraoperatively and by sonographically guided fine-needle puncture. Scandinavian Journal of Gastroenterology 1990;25:1097–1102.

8 Ebbehoj N, Borly L, Madsen P, Matzen, P. Pancreatic tissue fluid pressure during drainage operations for chronic pancreatitis. Scandinavian Journal of Gastroenterology 1990;25:1041–1045.

9 Ebbehoj N, Borly L, Madsen P, Matzen P. Comparison of regional pancreatic tissue fluid pressure and endoscopic retrograde pancreatographic morphology in chronic pancreatitis. Scandinavian Journal of Gastroenterology 1990;25:756–760.

10 Bornman PC et al. Pathogenesis of pain in chronic pancreatitis: ongoing enigma. World Journal of Surgery 2003;27:1175–1182.

11 Drewes AM et al. Pain in chronic pancreatitis: the role of neuropathic pain mechanisms. Gut 2008;57:1616–1627.

12 Pasricha PJ. Unraveling the mystery of pain in chronic pancreatitis. Nature Reviews. Gastroenterology & Hepatology 2012;9:140–151.

13 Winston JH, He ZJ, Shenoy M, Xiao SY, Pasricha PJ. Molecular and behavioral changes in nociception in a novel rat model of chronic pancreatitis for the study of pain. Pain 2005;117:214–222.

14 Puig-Divi V et al. Induction of chronic pancreatic disease by trinitrobenzene sulfonic acid infusion into rat pancreatic ducts. Pancreas 1996;13:417–424.

15 Cattaruzza F et al. Transient receptor potential ankyrin 1 mediates chronic pancreatitis pain in mice. American Journal of Physiology: Gastrointestinal and Liver Physiology 2013;304:G1002–G1012.

16 Lyo V et al. Active cathepsins B, L, and S in murine and human pancreatitis. American Journal of Physiology: Gastrointestinal and Liver Physiology 2012;303:G894–G903.

17 Cattaruzza F et al. Serine proteases and protease-activated receptor 2 mediate the proinflammatory and algesic actions of diverse stimulants. British Journal of Pharmacology 2014;171:3814–3826.

18 Larsson LI. Innervation of the pancreas by substance P, enkephalin, vasoactive intestinal polypeptide and gastrin/CCK immunoractive nerves. The Journal of Histochemistry and Cytochemistry 1979;27:1283–1284.

19 Hwang SW et al. Direct activation of capsaicin receptors by products of lipoxygenases: endogenous capsaicin-like substances. Proceedings of the National Academy of Sciences of the United States of America 2000;97:6155–6160.

20 Caterina MJ et al. Impaired nociception and pain sensation in mice lacking the capsaicin receptor. Science 2000;288:306–313.

21 Wick EC et al. Transient receptor potential vanilloid 1, calcitonin gene-related peptide, and substance P mediate nociception in acute pancreatitis. American Journal of Physiology: Gastrointestinal and Liver Physiology 2006;290:G959–G969.

22 Liddle RA. The role of transient receptor potential vanilloid 1 (TRPV1) channels in pancreatitis. Biochimica et Biophysica Acta 2007;1772:869–878.

23 Bautista DM, Pellegrino M, Tsunozaki M. TRPA1: a gatekeeper for inflammation. Annual Review of Physiology 2013;75:181–200.

24 Ceppa E et al. Transient receptor potential ion channels V4 and A1 contribute to pancreatitis pain in mice. American Journal of Physiology: Gastrointestinal and Liver Physiology 2010;299:G556–G571.

25 Bautista DM et al. TRPA1 mediates the inflammatory actions of environmental irritants and proalgesic agents. Cell 2006;124:1269–1282.

26 Kwan KY et al. TRPA1 contributes to cold, mechanical, and chemical nociception but is not essential for hair-cell transduction. Neuron 2006;50:277–289.

27 Obata K et al. TRPA1 induced in sensory neurons contributes to cold hyperalgesia after inflammation and nerve injury. The Journal of Clinical Investigation 2005;115:2393–2401.

28 Petrus M et al. A role of TRPA1 in mechanical hyperalgesia is revealed by pharmacological inhibition. Molecular Pain 2007;3:40.

29 Staruschenko A, Jeske NA, Akopian AN. Contribution of TRPV1-TRPA1 interaction to the single channel properties of the TRPA1 channel. The Journal of Biological Chemistry 2010;285:15167–15177.

30 Schwartz ES et al. TRPV1 and TRPA1 antagonists prevent the transition of acute to chronic inflammation and pain in chronic pancreatitis. The Journal of Neuroscience 2013;33:5603–5611.

31 Nilius B. TRP channels in disease. Biochimica et Biophysica Acta 2007;1772:805–812.

32 Poole DP et al. Protease-activated receptor 2 (PAR2) protein and transient receptor potential vanilloid 4 (TRPV4) protein coupling is required for sustained inflammatory signaling. The Journal of Biological Chemistry 2013;288:5790–5802.

33 Liedtke W, Friedman JM. Abnormal osmotic regulation in trpv4$^{-/-}$ mice. Proceedings of the National Academy of Sciences of the United States of America 2003;100:13698–13703.

34 Alessandri-Haber N, Joseph E, Dina OA, Liedtke W, Levine JD. TRPV4 mediates pain-related behavior induced by mild hypertonic stimuli in the presence of inflammatory mediator. Pain 2005;118:70–79.

35 Alessandri-Haber N, Dina OA, Joseph EK, Reichling D, Levine JD. A transient receptor potential vanilloid

4-dependent mechanism of hyperalgesia is engaged by concerted action of inflammatory mediators. The Journal of Neuroscience 2006;26:3864–3874.

36 Vu TK, Hung DT, Wheaton VI, Coughlin SR. Molecular cloning of a functional thrombin receptor reveals a novel proteolytic mechanism of receptor activation. Cell 1991;64:1057–1068.

37 Steinhoff M et al. Agonists of proteinase-activated receptor 2 induce inflammation by a neurogenic mechanism. Nature Medicine 2000;6:151–158.

38 Hoogerwerf WA et al. The proteinase-activated receptor 2 is involved in nociception. The Journal of Neuroscience 2001;21:9036–9042.

39 Dery O, Corvera CU, Steinhoff M, Bunnett NW. Proteinase-activated receptors: novel mechanisms of signaling by serine proteases. The American Journal of Physiology 1998;274:C1429–C1452.

40 Hoogerwerf WA et al. The role of mast cells in the pathogenesis of pain in chronic pancreatitis. BMC Gastroenterology 2005;5:8.

41 Hoogerwerf WA et al. Trypsin mediates nociception via the proteinase-activated receptor 2: a potentially novel role in pancreatic pain. Gastroenterology 2004;127:883–891.

42 Vergnolle N et al. Proteinase-activated receptor-2 and hyperalgesia: A novel pain pathway. Nature Medicine 2001;7:821–826.

43 Dai Y et al. Sensitization of TRPA1 by PAR2 contributes to the sensation of inflammatory pain. The Journal of Clinical Investigation 2007;117:1979–1987.

44 Grant AD et al. Protease-activated receptor 2 sensitizes the transient receptor potential vanilloid 4 ion channel to cause mechanical hyperalgesia in mice. The Journal of Physiology 2007;578:715–733.

45 Chen Y, Yang C, Wang, ZJ. Proteinase-activated receptor 2 sensitizes transient receptor potential vanilloid 1, transient receptor potential vanilloid 4, and transient receptor potential ankyrin 1 in paclitaxel-induced neuropathic pain. Neuroscience 2011;193:440–451.

46 Woolf CJ, Safieh-Garabedian B, Ma QP, Crilly P, Winter J Nerve growth factor contributes to the generation of inflammatory sensory hypersensitivity. Neuroscience 1994;62:327–331.

47 Friess H et al. Nerve growth factor and its high-affinity receptor in chronic pancreatitis. Annals of Surgery 1999;230:615–624.

48 Zhu Y et al. Nerve growth factor modulates TRPV1 expression and function and mediates pain in chronic pancreatitis. Gastroenterology 2011;141:370–377.

49 McMahon SB, Armanini MP, Ling LH, Phillips HS. Expression and coexpression of Trk receptors in subpopulations of adult primary sensory neurons projecting to identified peripheral targets. Neuron 1994;12:1161–1171.

50 McMahon SB, Bennett DL, Priestley JV, Shelton DL. The biological effects of endogenous nerve growth factor on adult sensory neurons revealed by a trkA-IgG fusion molecule. Nature Medicine 1995;1:774–780.

51 Barbacid M. The Trk family of neurotrophin receptors. Journal of Neurobiology 1994;25:1386–1403.

52 Zhu Y et al. Systemic administration of anti-NGF increases A-type potassium currents and decreases pancreatic nociceptor excitability in a rat model of chronic pancreatitis. American Journal of Physiology: Gastrointestinal and Liver Physiology 2012;302:G176–G181.

53 Lewin GR, Ritter AM, Mendell LM. Nerve growth factor-induced hyperalgesia in the neonatal and adult rat. The Journal of Neuroscience 1993;13:2136–2148.

54 Mantyh PW, Mantyh CR, Gates T, Vigna SR, Maggio JE. Receptor binding sites for substance P and substance K in the canine gastrointestinal tract and their possible role in inflammatory bowel disease. Neuroscience 1988;25:817–837.

55 Di Sebastiano P et al. Expression of interleukin 8 (IL-8) and substance P in human chronic pancreatitis. Gut 2000;47:423–428.

56 Grady EF et al. Substance P mediates inflammatory oedema in acute pancreatitis via activation of the neurokinin-1 receptor in rats and mice. British Journal of Pharmacology 2000;130:505–512.

57 Hutter MM et al. Transient receptor potential vanilloid (TRPV-1) promotes neurogenic inflammation in the pancreas via activation of the neurokinin-1 receptor (NK-1R). Pancreas 2005;30:260–265.

58 Shrikhande SV et al. NK-1 receptor gene expression is related to pain in chronic pancreatitis. Pain 2001;91:209–217.

59 Tsuda M, Inoue K, Salter MW. Neuropathic pain and spinal microglia: a big problem from molecules in "small" glia. Trends in Neurosciences 2005;28:101–107.

60 Wen YR, Tan PH, Cheng JK, Liu YC, Ji RR. Microglia: a promising target for treating neuropathic and postoperative pain, and morphine tolerance. Journal of the Formosan Medical Association 2011;110:487–494.

61 Thacker MA et al. CCL2 is a key mediator of microglia activation in neuropathic pain states. European Journal of Pain 2009;13:263–272.

62 Tsuda M et al. P2X4 receptors induced in spinal microglia gate tactile allodynia after nerve injury. Nature 2003;424:778–783.

63 Jin SX, Zhuang ZY, Woolf CJ, Ji RR. p38 mitogen-activated protein kinase is activated after a spinal nerve ligation in spinal cord microglia and dorsal root ganglion neurons and contributes to the generation of neuropathic pain. The Journal of Neuroscience 2003;23:4017–4022.

64 Liu PY et al. Spinal microglia initiate and maintain hyperalgesia in a rat model of chronic pancreatitis. Gastroenterology 2012;142:165–173; e162.

65 Smith HS. Activated microglia in nociception. Pain Physician 2010;13:295–304.

66 Watkins LR, Milligan ED, Maier SF. Spinal cord glia: new players in pain. Pain 2001;93:201–205.

67 Chapman GA et al. Fractalkine cleavage from neuronal membranes represents an acute event in the inflammatory response to excitotoxic brain damage. The Journal of Neuroscience 2000;20:RC87.

68 Barclay J et al. Role of the cysteine protease cathepsin S in neuropathic hyperalgesia. Pain2007; 130:225–234.

69 Clark AK et al. Inhibition of spinal microglial cathepsin S for the reversal of neuropathic pain. Proceedings of the National Academy of Sciences of the United States of America 2007;104:10655–10660.

70 Clark AK, Yip PK, Malcangio M. The liberation of fractalkine in the dorsal horn requires microglial cathepsin S. The Journal of Neuroscience 2009;29:6945–6954.

71 Garrison CJ, Dougherty PM, Kajander KC, Carlton SM. Staining of glial fibrillary acidic protein (GFAP) in lumbar spinal cord increases following a sciatic nerve constriction injury. Brain Research 1991;565:1–7.

72 Garrison CJ, Dougherty PM, Carlton SM. GFAP expression in lumbar spinal cord of naive and neuropathic rats treated with MK-801. Experimental Neurology 1994;129:237–243.

73 Ji RR, Kawasaki Y, Zhuang ZY, Wen YR, Decosterd I. Possible role of spinal astrocytes in maintaining chronic pain sensitization: review of current evidence with focus on bFGF/JNK pathway. Neuron Glia Biology 2006;2:259–269.

74 Zhuang ZY, Gerner P, Woolf CJ, Ji RR. ERK is sequentially activated in neurons, microglia, and astrocytes by spinal nerve ligation and contributes to mechanical allodynia in this neuropathic pain model. Pain2005; 114:149–159.

75 Feng QX et al. Astrocytic activation in thoracic spinal cord contributes to persistent pain in rat model of chronic pancreatitis. Neuroscience 2010;167:501–509.

76 Mertz H. Role of the brain and sensory pathways in gastrointestinal sensory disorders in humans. Gut 2002;51 Suppl 1:i29–i33.

77 Dimcevski G et al. Hypoalgesia to experimental visceral and somatic stimulation in painful chronic pancreatitis. European Journal of Gastroenterology & Hepatology 2006;18:755–764.

78 Dimcevski G et al. Pain in chronic pancreatitis: the role of reorganization in the central nervous system. Gastroenterology 2007;132:1546–1556.

79 Lee M, Silverman SM, Hansen H, Patel VB, Manchikanti L. A comprehensive review of opioid-induced hyperalgesia. Pain Physician 2011;14:145–161.

80 Celerier E, Laulin J, Larcher A, Le Moal M, Simonnet G. Evidence for opiate-activated NMDA processes masking opiate analgesia in rats. Brain Research 1999;847:18–25.

81 Mao J, Sung B, Ji RR, Lim G. Chronic morphine induces downregulation of spinal glutamate transporters: implications in morphine tolerance and abnormal pain sensitivity. The Journal of Neuroscience 2002;22: 8312–8323.

82 Vanderah TW, Ossipov MH, Lai J, Malan TP, Jr., Porreca F. Mechanisms of opioid-induced pain and antinociceptive tolerance: descending facilitation and spinal dynorphin. Pain 2001;92:5–9.

83 Chu LF, Clark DJ, Angst MS. Opioid tolerance and hyperalgesia in chronic pain patients after one month of oral morphine therapy: a preliminary prospective study. The Journal of Pain 2006;7:43–48.

84 Compton P, Charuvastra VC, Ling W. Pain intolerance in opioid-maintained former opiate addicts: effect of long-acting maintenance agent. Drug and Alcohol Dependence 2001;63:139–146.

85 Hay JL et al. Hyperalgesia in opioid-managed chronic pain and opioid-dependent patients. The Journal of Pain 2009;10:316–322.

86 Reznikov I, Pud D, Eisenberg E. Oral opioid administration and hyperalgesia in patients with cancer or chronic nonmalignant pain. British Journal of Clinical Pharmacology 2005; 60:311–318.

87 Mao J. Opioid-induced abnormal pain sensitivity: implications in clinical opioid therapy. Pain 2002;100:213–217.

CHAPTER 13

PART A: Imaging of chronic pancreatitis

Ferenc Czeyda-Pommersheim, Bobby Kalb & Diego Martin

Department of Medical Imaging, University of Arizona, College of Medicine, Tucson, AZ, USA

Introduction

Chronic pancreatitis (CP) is a common cause of chronic abdominal pain, with a significant health burden in the United States, associated with approximately 86,000 admissions annually [1]. CP is a progressive disease in which the normal pancreatic acinar tissue and islet cells are destroyed and replaced by fibrosis. Although the exact etiology remains to be clearly defined, it is thought that the histological events leading to CP are initiated by clinical or subclinical episodes of acute pancreatitis in genetically susceptible individuals [2]. Regardless of the etiology, affected patients present with chronic abdominal pain and varying levels of exocrine and endocrine insufficiency. However, many patients with early CP and parenchymal fibrosis demonstrate no biochemical abnormalities and present a diagnostic challenge for accurate diagnosis.

Various imaging modalities have been used in the evaluation of CP. When patients present with advanced disease, the morphological changes of pancreatic atrophy, pancreatic duct dilatation, and parenchymal calcifications are straightforward and easily evaluated with noninvasive imaging methods. However, a large number of patients with early or minimal change CP demonstrate symptoms with no identifiable changes in the morphology of the pancreas. Laboratory analyses, including directed pancreatic function testing of cholecystokinin and other biochemical markers, are also not reliable in early-stage disease. There is a continued need for reliable methods of disease detection that can provide a noninvasive analysis of pancreatic tissue composition in the absence of morphologic changes. Ultrasound (US) and computed tomography (CT) have been the most highly utilized imaging methods for evaluation of the pancreas; however, they have been unable to reliably differentiate normal from early fibrotic disease. Magnetic resonance imaging (MRI) is a noninvasive imaging method that has excellent soft tissue contrast compared with US and CT. For this reason, MRI has potential with regard to development of noninvasive imaging biomarkers for the diagnosis of early CP, where accurate diagnosis relies upon the differentiation of different tissue types (such as fibrosis and normal pancreatic tissue) rather than morphologic changes of parenchymal atrophy and duct dilatation. In this chapter, we discuss the imaging methods commonly employed for the diagnosis of CP, with special emphasis on MRI as the optimum imaging technique for early disease detection through a combination of established methods and novel MRI techniques that hold promise for more reliable detection of minimal change disease.

Imaging modalities

Ultrasound

Transabdominal US has been widely used to image the pancreas due to its availability, speed, and relatively low cost. However, transabdominal US may be limited by gas in the stomach or large bowel, patient body habitus, operator skill, and the difficulty to obtain an adequate scan window to image the distal body and tail, all of which decrease the utility for assessing pancreatic pathology. The diagnostic criteria for CP on US depend exclusively on gross morphologic changes. When these changes are detected, they often indicate CP that is highly advanced. Many of the typical sonographic findings such as gland atrophy, heterogeneous parenchymal echotexture, calcification, and irregular central duct may be absent even in moderate disease. Punctate parenchymal calcifications, for example, are identified in only 40% of patients [3]. In early or moderate disease, the pancreas often is sonographically normal [4]. As an additional confounder, focal CP may present as a focal hypoechoic lesion, which is rarely possible to confidently distinguish from ductal adenocarcinoma on sonography alone.

Compared with transabdominal imaging, endoscopic ultrasound (EUS) is more reliable in identifying CP [5, 6]. However, similar to transabdominal US, diagnostic criteria again depend on morphologic changes. When using the diagnostic criteria of hyperechoic foci, parenchymal strands, lobulations, hyperechoic duct wall, irregular duct, visible side branches, ductal dilation, calcification, and cysts, EUS has a positive predictive value of 85% to diagnose CP when two or more of the criteria are present [7, 8]. However, the utility of EUS is limited by its invasive nature – a disadvantage compared with both transabdominal scanning and other cross-sectional imaging modalities.

Computed tomography

The use of CT has increased exponentially over the past two decades. Due to its ready availability and ease of use, CT is currently the most commonly used modality to image inflammatory and neoplastic diseases of the pancreas. Compared with US, CT is less operator dependent, less affected by patient body habitus, and in the majority of cases allows visualization of the entire gland. Comprehensive evaluation by CT requires the administration of iodinated intravenous contrast. Since iodinated contrast is nephrotoxic, its use is often contraindicated in patients with borderline (Stage 3 and below) kidney function who are not on dialysis. In addition, CT imaging protocols for dedicated pancreatic evaluation often require thin collimation scanning and multiple scan phases with and without contrast, which results in a relative increase in radiation exposure when compared with routine, single-phase abdominal CT protocols.

Similar to US, diagnostic criteria for CP with CT depends entirely on morphologic changes in the gland, which are frequently absent in early or moderate cases. Intraductal calcifications, representing calcium carbonate within inspissated protein plugs in the main duct, and punctate parenchymal calcifications are the most sensitive finding of CP on CT [4]. Other findings include atrophy or enlargement of the gland, ectasia, and irregularity of the main pancreatic duct and/or side branches and parenchymal calcifications.

Compared with US, CT provides a more comprehensive evaluation of the peripancreatic soft tissues and retroperitoneum. CT provides a more detailed evaluation of complications related to acute pancreatitis, such as pseudocysts, splenic vein thrombosis, and splenic artery pseudoaneurysm, and is also more sensitive for the detection of pancreatic neoplasms. Similar to US, it may be difficult to distinguish focal pancreatitis from pancreatic ductal adenocarcinoma on CT [9]. The sensitivity of CT for CP is 65–95%, though the gland often appears normal in early or mild disease [10].

MRI

MRI provides excellent soft tissue resolution of the abdominopelvic visceral tissues, which aids in the detection of parenchymal changes of CP, even in the absence of morphologic changes [11]. MRI does not employ ionizing radiation, and the gadolinium-chelate-based intravenous contrast does not have the nephrotoxicity associated with iodine-based CT contrast agents. MRI may be contraindicated in some patients with implanted metallic hardware; however, many devices – including most implanted cardiac devices – can safely be scanned with proper institutional safety protocols.

Advanced morphological changes of CP are easily demonstrated on MRI, including abnormalities of the main pancreatic duct and side branches, parenchymal atrophy, duct strictures, and intraductal stones. Parenchymal calcifications are not well seen by MRI, and CT is the most sensitive exam for the detection of CP-associated pancreatic calcifications. However, calcifications remain a late-stage finding of CP, and MRI may detect parenchymal signal changes of diseased and fibrotic tissue in early-stage disease, well before the development of parenchymal calcifications. The subtle signal alterations due to histological changes of fibrosis is more easily identified with MRI due to its superior soft tissue contrast, with new techniques that allow for the assessment of active inflammation, lipid content, and parenchymal perfusion on dynamic contrast-enhanced imaging [12]. This allows earlier detection of disease, serial follow-up of disease severity in the same patient over time, and comparison of disease severity among different patients. MRI may also more confidently differentiate pancreatic adenocarcinoma from its mimics of focal pancreatic fat infiltration or focal pancreatitis [13].

MRI features of chronic pancreatitis

While MR imaging protocols have the potential to be complex and widely varied, we have advocated a simplified, uniform protocol that may be applied to multiple indications, including pancreatic assessment. This protocol consists of dynamic contrast-enhanced T1-weighted (T1W) multiphase imaging, which allows for the assessment of parenchymal perfusion patterns that may be indicative of fibrosis. Arterial phase images are acquired at an 8–10 second delay from the bolus trigger point; venous phase imaging is initiated at 70 seconds and delayed phase imaging at 180 seconds after the trigger point. Motion-insensitive T2-weighted (T2W) sequences are the second major component of this simplified imaging protocol, providing an alternate method of tissue interrogation, which helps increase the specificity of diagnosis, especially to more reliably differentiate acute from chronic pancreatitis (Figures 13A.2d, 13A.4d). Magnetic resonance cholangiopancreatography (MRCP) techniques are T2W sequences that provide excellent visibility of the pancreatic duct morphology and are helpful in tumor diagnosis and presurgical planning. Finally, diffusion-weighted imaging (DWI) is an additional noncontrast technique that has the potential to improve sensitivity for small malignant lesions in certain pancreatic tumor subtypes, especially related to neuroendocrine tumors.

Normal pancreas
Normal pancreatic parenchyma is filled with zymogens and other proteinaceous material. The pancreas is also well vascularized by an extensive peripancreatic vascular plexus. These features of the normal pancreatic parenchyma have a direct influence on the appearance of the gland on MRI. On precontrast, fat-saturated T1W sequences, the pancreas shows uniformly high signal, typically demonstrating the highest signal

intensity of all solid visceral organs in the abdomen and pelvis (Figure 13A.1a). The extensive arterial vascular network supplying the pancreas causes the peak parenchymal enhancement to occur in the arterial phase, with relatively less enhancement in venous and interstitial delayed phase images (Figure 13A.1b,c).

On T2W images, the pancreatic signal is isointense to normal hepatic and adrenal tissues (Figure 13A.1d). The pancreatic duct is thin and uniform, measuring no more than 1–2 mm in diameter. Pancreatic duct side branches are not typically seen on MRI unless diseased.

Chronic pancreatitis
A variety of insults to the pancreas may result in increased pressure within the duct and side branches, leading to periductal inflammation and progressive cycles of parenchymal necrosis and hemorrhage, resulting in parenchymal fibrosis and glandular atrophy [14]. The proteinaceous fluid content of the pancreas is diminished due to the process of chronic inflammation and fibrosis, causing a decrease in the intrinsic T1 signal of the pancreas on precontrast fat-suppressed T1W images (Figures 13A.2a, 13A.3a, 13A.4a and 13A.6a) [12, 15]. A resultant decrease in parenchymal vascularity causes a decrease in early arterial enhancement of the pancreatic parenchyma; the fibrotic tissue replacing the pancreatic parenchyma shows delayed uptake of the intravenous gadolinium chelate. For these reasons, patients with CP have a shift in peak enhancement of the parenchyma to the late venous phase, instead of the normal early arterial peak (Figures 13A.2b, 13A.2c, 13A.3b, 13A.3c, 13A.4b, 13A.4c, 13A.5b, 13A.6b and 13A.6c) [16, 17]. Note that (unlike CT and US), these MR features do not rely on late-stage morphologic changes of the pancreas, such as parenchymal atrophy and duct obstruction. While these findings are also well-depicted with MRI, the early findings of fibrosis result in alterations of the intrinsic signal features of the pancreas on MRI, allowing for earlier detection of disease before morphologic changes become evident.

T2W images are the mainstay for imaging of the pancreatic duct in the setting of CP. Tortuosity, stricture, calcification, and side branch dilation of the pancreatic duct often develop due to strictures in the main pancreatic duct and are features of moderate to severe CP (Figure 13A.3d). Due to an imbalance of the components of pancreatic fluid, protein plugs consisting of precipitated pancreatic enzymes and other proteins

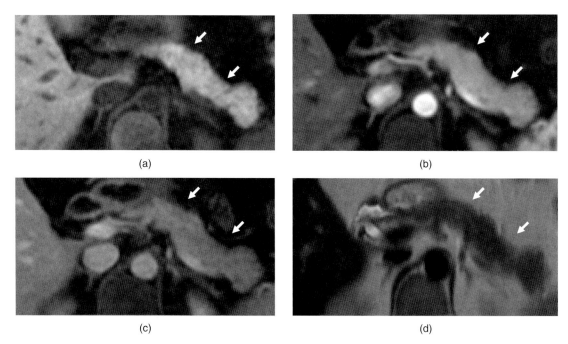

(a)　　　　　　　　　　　(b)

(c)　　　　　　　　　　　(d)

Figure 13A.1 Normal pancreas. Axial precontrast T1W 3D gradient echo with fat saturation (3D GRE FS) (a) shows that T1 signal in the normal pancreas (arrows) is more intense than that of the liver and spleen. Axial postcontrast T1W 3D GRE FS in the arterial (b) and delayed (c) phase shows the normal peak enhancement of the pancreas, in the arterial phase, with relative decreased enhancement in the delayed phase. Axial T2W image (d) demonstrates the normal T2 signal is similar in the pancreas compared with the liver.

form and serve as a nidus for the deposition of calcium carbonate seen as intraductal calcification. In severe cases due to multiple plugs and strictures, the duct assumes the classic "chain of lakes" configuration of strictured segments alternating with dilated duct segments and several cystic-appearing dilated side branches [14]. The anatomic depiction of the pancreatic duct is well seen on heavily T2W MRCP sequences, which provide the most sensitive noninvasive imaging method for the detection of pancreatic duct abnormalities.

Novel MRI techniques

T1 mapping

Since the intrinsic T1 signal of the normal pancreas is diminished in CP due to a decrease in the proteinaceous fluid content of the gland, mapping of T1 values allows both for qualitative global assessment and also more quantitative assessment through calculation of T1 relaxation times at various locations in the gland. By measuring T1 values for each voxel, the degree

of parenchymal changes may be directly measured to provide improved reproducibility, instead of relying on subjective comparison of signal intensities of normal versus diseased gland parenchyma. T1 mapping techniques have been in routine clinical use in cardiac MRI to quantify postinfarction myocardial scar and are easily adapted to the abdomen [18]; newer techniques have recently been developed with significant gains in scan time and further improved by automated postprocessing [19] that would allow for application to abdominal viscera, including the pancreas.

Perfusion

In addition to changing the intrinsic T1 signal of the pancreas, CP also alters the perfusion dynamics of the gland, shifting the peak enhancement to the venous/delayed phase in a dynamic contrast-enhanced study. Objective quantification of gland perfusion may be performed by MRI perfusion mapping. This technique uses a high temporal resolution T1-weighed spoiled gradient echo sequence to follow contrast agent uptake and washout in the pancreas during a dynamic

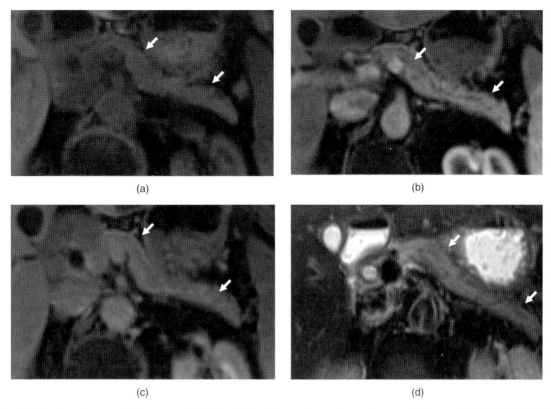

(a)   (b)

(c)   (d)

Figure 13A.2 Chronic pancreatitis, presumed due to radiation therapy for esophageal cancer. Axial precontrast T1W 3D GRE FS image (a) shows relative decreased T1 signal intensity of the pancreas (arrows) compared with the liver. Postcontrast arterial (b) and delayed phase (c) T1W images demonstrate that peak enhancement has shifted to the delayed phase. On the axial T2W fat-saturated image (d), there is uniform increased T2 signal throughout the pancreas.

contrast-enhanced examination. The entire gland can usually be imaged with adequate spatial resolution, allowing for comparison of the relative severity of involvement in various anatomic locations through the gland. To quantify enhancement at a specific anatomic location, specific regions of interest may be drawn and signal intensity versus time curves may be obtained [20]. The spoiled gradient echo method is heavily influenced by multiple factors including intrinsic T1 tissue properties and scan parameters such as TR, TE, and the flip angle. As an alternative, T1 mapping–based perfusion analysis can avoid many of these pitfalls. Techniques recently developed for rapid combined T1/B1 mapping are relatively independent of scan parameters, tissue variables, and extrinsic factors [21].

T2 mapping

Active inflammation causes an increase of the intrinsic T2 signal of the pancreas. Characterization of the pancreatic T2 signal can be performed qualitatively or quantitatively. The pancreas normally has relatively hypointense T2 signal and may be visually compared with another visceral organs (typically isointense to normal hepatic parenchyma) for qualitative assessment of its intrinsic signal.

T2 mapping provides an objective technique for quantitative assessment of pancreatic T2 signal. Radial acquisition-based fast spin-echo methods allow for rapid measurement of T2 values and are relatively unaffected by the challenges in signal-to-noise ratio or motion artifacts encountered in HASTE or 2D-FSE imaging [22].

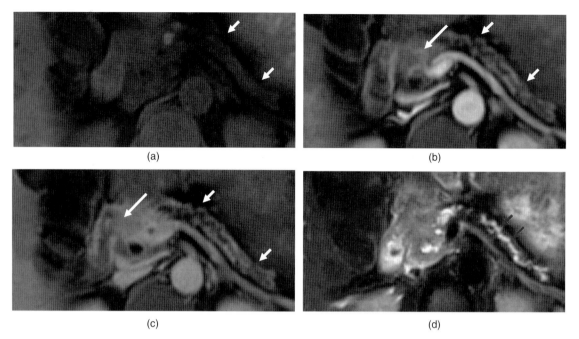

Figure 13A.3 Chronic pancreatitis due to pancreatic ductal adenocarcinoma. Axial precontrast T1W 3D GRE FS image (a) shows decreased T1 signal throughout the pancreas (short white arrows) with peak enhancement shifted to the delayed postcontrast phase (c) compared with the arterial phase (b). The T2W fat-saturated image (d) demonstrates dilation of the pancreatic duct (red arrows). A mass in the head of the pancreas (long white arrow in b and c) was biopsied, showing ductal adenocarcinoma.

Dixon method

The Dixon acquisition using a rapid gradient echo sequence allows quantitation of microscopic lipid in a single breath-hold [23]. This technique exploits the difference in precessional frequency of protons in water and fat in an external magnetic field. The difference in precessional frequency produces a phase shift, which brings the magnetization vector of water and fat protons in and out of alignment at periodic intervals. When water and fat protons are present in the same voxel and process in phase, their signal is additive, and when they are out of phase, their combined signal is decreased (Figure 13A.5). The data acquired during an "in phase" and "opposed phase" scan may be postprocessed to display a "fat only" and a "water only" image and quantify the degree of fat deposition.

MR spectroscopy

High-speed T2 corrected multiecho proton MR spectroscopy (HISTO-MRS) allows for the rapid acquisition of multiple echoes to simultaneously assess tissue lipid and water content. This sequence may be collected in a single breath-hold (approximately 15 seconds) with highly reproducible results both *in vivo* and *in vitro*. This technique allows for reproducible, quantitative assessment of hepatic lipid and iron content, helpful for presurgical planning especially for potential total pancreatectomy with auto-islet cell transfusion (Figure 13A.6d). Postprocessing is automated, making this technique a robust tool even for sites with limited experience in advanced MRI techniques [24].

Elastography

MR elastography provides quantitative assessment of the mechanical properties of tissues based on the propagation of shear waves and has been successfully used in abdominal imaging for tissue characterization [25]. The MR elastography system consists of an acoustic driver for the generation of shear waves in the tissue of interest. The tissues are then imaged with a conventional MR pulse sequence with the inclusion of motion encoding gradients, which allow the propagating shear waves to be imaged. These images are postprocessed to generate quantitative images that depict tissue stiffness (elastograms).

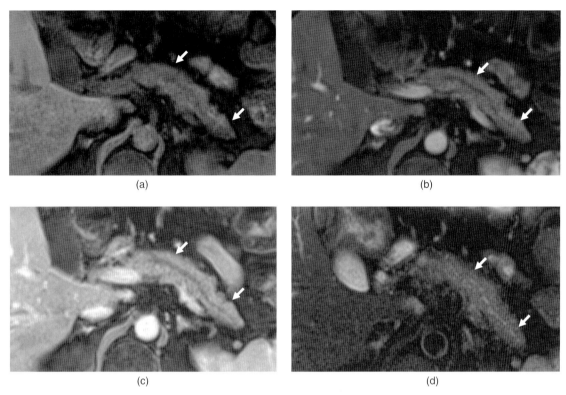

(a)   (b)

(c)   (d)

Figure 13A.4 Chronic pancreatitis. Axial precontrast T1W 3D GRE FS image (a) shows relative decreased T1 signal intensity of the pancreas (arrows) compared with the liver. Postcontrast arterial (b) and delayed phase (c) T1W images demonstrate that peak enhancement has shifted to the delayed phase. On the axial T2W fat-saturated image (d), there is uniform mildly increased T2 signal throughout the pancreas.

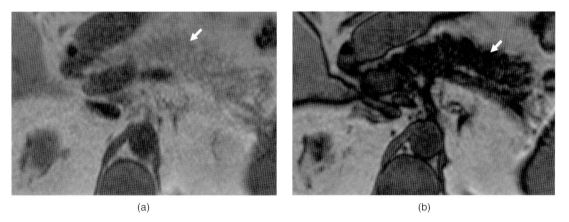

(a)   (b)

Figure 13A.5 Fatty infiltration of the pancreas in chronic pancreatitis. In-phase (a) and opposed-phase (b) T1W images show marked signal dropout on the opposed-phase image due to microscopic lipid throughout the pancreas (arrow).

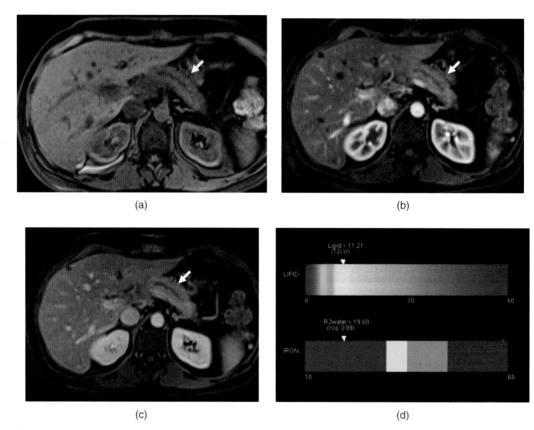

(a)　　　　　　　　　　　　　(b)

(c)　　　　　　　　　　　　　(d)

Figure 13A.6 Chronic pancreatitis in a patient status post-Whipple procedure. Axial precontrast T1W 3D GRE FS image (a) shows relative decreased T1 signal intensity of the pancreas (arrow) compared with the liver. Postcontrast arterial (b) and delayed phase (c) T1W images demonstrate that peak enhancement has shifted to the delayed phase. (d) Spectroscopic analysis demonstrates hepatic lipid correlating to 11%; quantitative evaluation of hepatic lipid and iron may be routinely obtained with MRI.

The use of elastography has been well documented in the quantification primarily of hepatic fibrosis and has been found to be technically feasible in other organs including the pancreas [26, 27]. While this technique continues to undergo research, some preliminary studies using US elastography have shown success in distinguishing focal pancreatitis from pancreatic adenocarcinoma [28].

Conclusion

Multiple imaging modalities are available for evaluation of the pancreas, aiding the diagnosis of CP, identifying its complications, and following disease progression. MRI, well validated as a potent diagnostic tool in pancreatic diseases, is the subject of ongoing research that in recent years has shown its reliability for quantitative and qualitative assessments of the gland. With increasing awareness of the risks of ionizing radiation and the ongoing development of novel sequences that allow rapid, tissue-level characterization of the gland, MRI holds advantages with respect to noninvasive imaging of CP, especially for early or minimal change disease in the absence of typical morphologic changes to the gland.

References

1 Yadav D, et al. Incidence, prevalence, and survival of chronic pancreatitis: a population-based study. The American Journal of Gastroenterology 2011;106(12): 2192–2199.

2 Ketwaroo GA, Freedman SD, Sheth SG. Approach to patients with suspected chronic pancreatitis: a comprehensive review. Pancreas 2015;44(2):173–180.

3 Alpern M, et al. Chronic pancreatitis: ultrasonic features. Radiology 1985;155(1):215–219.

4 Siddiqi AJ, Miller F. Chronic pancreatitis: ultrasound, computed tomography, and magnetic resonance imaging features. In: Seminars in Ultrasound, CT and MRI, Vol. 28. No. 5. WB Saunders. 2007

5 Pungpapong S, et al. Accuracy of endoscopic ultrasonography and magnetic resonance cholangiopancreatography for the diagnosis of chronic pancreatitis: a prospective comparison study. Journal of Clinical Gastroenterology 2007;41(1):88–93.

6 Raimondo M, Wallace MB. Diagnosis of early chronic pancreatitis by endoscopic ultrasound. Are we there yet. Journal of the Pancreas 2004;5(1):1–7.

7 Sahai AV, et al. Prospective assessment of the ability of endoscopic ultrasound to diagnose, exclude, or establish the severity of chronic pancreatitis found by endoscopic retrograde cholangiopancreatography. Gastrointestinal Endoscopy 1998;48(1):18–25.

8 Kahl S, et al. EUS in the diagnosis of early chronic pancreatitis: a prospective follow-up study. Gastrointestinal Endoscopy 2002;55(4):507–511.

9 Kim T, et al. Pancreatic mass due to chronic pancreatitis: correlation of CT and MR imaging features with pathologic findings. American Journal of Roentgenology 2001;177(2):367–371.

10 Choueiri NE, et al. Advanced imaging of chronic pancreatitis. Current Gastroenterology Reports 2010;12(2):114–120.

11 Balcı C. MRI assessment of chronic pancreatitis. Diagnostic and Interventional Radiology 2011;17(3):249–254.

12 Miller, F.H., et al., MRI of pancreatitis and its complications: part 2, chronic pancreatitis. American Journal of Roentgenology, 2004. 183(6):1645–1652.

13 Kim JK, et al. Focal pancreatic mass: distinction of pancreatic cancer from chronic pancreatitis using gadolinium-enhanced 3D-gradient-echo MRI. Journal of Magnetic Resonance Imaging 2007;26(2):313–322.

14 Strate T, et al. Chronic pancreatitis: etiology, pathogenesis, diagnosis, and treatment. International Journal of Colorectal Disease 2003;18(2):97–106.

15 Semelka RC, et al. Chronic pancreatitis: MR imaging features before and after administration of gadopentetate dimeglumine. Journal of Magnetic Resonance Imaging 1993;3(1):79–82.

16 Coenegrachts K, et al. Dynamic contrast-enhanced MRI of the pancreas: initial results in healthy volunteers and patients with chronic pancreatitis. Journal of Magnetic Resonance Imaging 2004;20(6):990–997.

17 Zhang XM, et al. Suspected early or mild chronic pancreatitis: enhancement patterns on gadolinium chelate dynamic MRI. Magnetic resonance imaging. Journal of Magnetic Resonance Imaging 2003;17(1):86–94.

18 Messroghli DR, et al. Myocardial T1 mapping: application to patients with acute and chronic myocardial infarction. Magnetic Resonance in Medicine 2007;58(1):34–40.

19 Piechnik SK, et al. Shortened Modified Look-Locker Inversion recovery (ShMOLLI) for clinical myocardial T1-mapping at 1.5 and 3 T within a 9 heartbeat breathhold. Journal of Cardiovascular Magnetic Resonance 2010;12:69.

20 Taouli B, Ehman RL, Reeder SB. Advanced MRI methods for assessment of chronic liver disease. American Journal of Roentgenology 2009;193(1):14.

21 Treier R. et al. Optimized and combined T1 and B1 mapping technique for fast and accurate T1 quantification in contrast-enhanced abdominal MRI. Magnetic Resonance in Medicine 2007;57(3):568–576.

22 Altbach MI, et al. Radial fast spin-echo method for T2-weighted imaging and T2 mapping of the liver. Journal of Magnetic Resonance Imaging 2002;16(2):179–189.

23 Fishbein MH. Stevens WR. Rapid MRI using a modified Dixon technique: a non-invasive and effective method for detection and monitoring of fatty metamorphosis of the liver. Pediatric Radiology 2001;31(11):806–809.

24 Pineda N, et al. Measurement of hepatic lipid: high-speed T2-corrected multiecho acquisition at 1H MR spectroscopy—a rapid and accurate technique 1. Radiology 2009;252(2):568–576.

25 Yin M, et al. Abdominal MR elastography. Topics in Magnetic Resonance Imaging 2009;20(2):79.

26 Yin M, et al. Assessment of the pancreas with MR elastography. Paper presented at: Proceedings of the International Society for Magnetic Resonance in Medicine. 2008.

27 Shi Y, et al. Feasibility of using 3D MR elastography to determine pancreatic stiffness in healthy volunteers. Journal of Magnetic Resonance Imaging 2014;41:369–375.

28 Itokawa F, et al. EUS elastography combined with the strain ratio of tissue elasticity for diagnosis of solid pancreatic masses. Journal of Gastroenterology 2011;46(6):843–853.

Brenda Hoffman & Nathaniel Ranney

Division of Hepatology and Gastroenterology, Medical University of South Carolina, Charleston, SC, USA

Introduction

Chronic pancreatitis (CP) is characterized by inflammation and irreversible changes in the pancreatic parenchyma. Those changes may lead to chronic abdominal pain and both exocrine and endocrine insufficiency. The diagnosis of CP is often suggested by the clinical manifestations of the disease (i.e., abdominal pain, steatorrhea); however, a diagnosis should be confirmed by imaging the pancreas. Despite recent advances in high-resolution cross-sectional imaging, the diagnosis may be elusive. Endoscopic ultrasound (EUS) has a theoretic advantage over other modalities in that the probe in placed in the gastrointestinal tract in close proximity to the pancreas, allowing improved visualization. The role of EUS in patients with CP can be categorized as follows:

- Establishing the diagnosis through established criteria.
- Expanding the differential diagnosis: exclusion of other causes of recurrent pancreatitis or chronic pain.
- Excluding malignancy: detection of small neuroendocrine tumors or evaluation of pancreatic masses.
- Providing therapy: neurolysis, cyst drainage, accessing obstructed bile duct, or pancreatic ducts.

Endoscopic ultrasound features of the normal pancreas

With EUS, the normal pancreas appears as a homogenous structure with a fine, diffusely speckled pattern ("salt-and-pepper" appearance). The pancreatic duct is seen as a smooth anechoic tubular structure that can be traced from the head to the tail of the pancreas. The normal pancreas measures 10–15 mm in thickness

(anterior–posterior). A thickness of <10 mm would qualify as "atrophy," although the clinical significance of this finding is unclear. The normal pancreatic duct measures 3 mm in the head and should taper to 2 mm in the body and 1mm in the tail of the pancreas. Of importance, it is common to see a distinct transition between the ventral and dorsal anlage, as the ventral anlage appears less echogenic and overall darker as compared with the brighter dorsal anlage, and this should not be confused as an abnormal finding. When assessing for CP, it should be noted that the head of the pancreas is generally more heterogeneous in appearance than the body or tail. Therefore, when assessing the pancreatic parenchyma for criteria of CP, only the appearance of the body and tail should be taken into account.

Endoscopic ultrasound features of chronic pancreatitis

EUS was first developed in the early 1980s as a means to better examine the pancreas. As endosonographers gained experience, the sonographic criteria for diagnosing CP were identified and expanded upon. William Lees can be credited as the first to recognize many of the features still used in modern EUS classifications for CP [1]. The characteristics he described and examples of normal and abnormal scans are shown in Figures 13B.1–13B.3. Many of these features were adapted from the parenchymal changes seen on transabdominal ultrasound and the Cambridge classification (Table 13B.1) of ductal changes noted on endoscopic retrograde cholangiopancreatography (ERCP) [2]. These features were initially studied in symptomatic patients only; Wiersema and his colleagues later studied these criteria in normal, asymptomatic subjects in

Pancreatitis: Medical and Surgical Management, First Edition.
David B. Adams, Peter B. Cotton, Nicholas J. Zyromski and John Windsor.
© 2017 John Wiley & Sons, Ltd. Published 2017 by John Wiley & Sons, Ltd.

Reported EUS features of chronic pancreatitis

- Ductal
  - Dilatation
  - Echogenic walls
  - Irregular contour
  - Side branch dilation
  - Calcifications

- Parenchymal
  - Echogenic foci
  - Small cysts
  - Lobular outer contour
  - Echogenic strands
  - Inhomogeneity

Lees WR, Scandinavian Journal of Gastroenterology 1986; 21:123–129

Figure 13B.1 EUS features of chronic pancreatitis.

Histologic correlates

- Echogenic walls
- Irregular duct wall
- Intraductal foci
- Echogenic foci
- Cysts
- Lobularity
- Echogenic strands

- Periductal fibrosis
- Obstruction
- Stones
- Fibrosis
- Duct leaks
- Acute inflammation
- Fibrosis

Lees WR, Scandinavian Journal of Gastroenterology, 1986

Figure 13B.2 Histologic correlates of EUS features of chronic pancreatitis.

addition to patients with chronic abdominal pain [3]. Using logistic regression analysis, the EUS features most indicative of CP were identified. These criteria have become the accepted standard, or "conventional" EUS criteria (synonymous with Wiersema criteria), as shown in Table 13B.2. Furthermore, the investigators of this study developed a receiver operating characteristic (ROC) curve to define the number of criteria needed to achieve maximum sensitivity and specificity in making a diagnosis of CP. Of the nine accepted criteria, four (hyperechoic foci, hyperechoic strands, hypoechoic lobules, and cysts) describe features of the pancreatic parenchyma. The remaining criteria (irregular duct, visible side branches, hyperechoic duct margins, dilated main duct, and intraductal stones) describe the features of the pancreatic duct.

In the standard, or "conventional," classification system, equal weight is given to each of the nine criteria, and the absolute score is used. The presence of 0–2 criteria represents a normal pancreas, or low probability of CP. The presence of three or four criteria represents indeterminate or intermediate probability. The presence

of five or greater criteria is determinate, or high probability, for CP.

Most gastroenterologists would agree that certain criteria are more important than others, with the finding of parenchymal calcifications and lobules being the most meaningful. In an attempt to rank the criteria in order of importance, a group of experienced endosonographers under the auspices of the American Society of Gastrointestinal Endoscopy met in Rosemont, Illinois, to develop a consensus [4]. The result of their efforts was the Rosemont criteria (RC), which is summarized in Table 13B.3. The differences between the conventional and RC and classification systems are illustrated in Tables 13B.4 and 13B.5.

Inter- and intraobserver variability in chronic pancreatitis

In order for EUS to be considered a reliable diagnostic test for CP, it is important to establish that the criteria are reproducible for the observer and for other endosonographers. Wallace and colleagues [5] performed the first intraobserver study utilizing video clips. Eleven experienced endosonographers were blinded to clinical information and independently evaluated videotaped examinations for the presence of CP based on conventional criteria (CC). There was moderately good agreement on the diagnosis of CP, with kappa of 0.45. Although this was a modest result, it did compare favorably with other gastrointestinal studies, including a study on intraobserver agreement of hemorrhage stigmata in bleeding peptic ulcers [6]. A later study by Lieb and colleagues [7] used 30 EUS images from patients with suspected CP, and showed them twice in random order to five different blinded endosonographers. The intraobserver agreement was good among all five endosonographers. It was found to be better than the previously published interobserver agreement for EUS features and was better than published intraobserver agreement for ERCP imaging for CP. Another study by Gardner et al. [8] evaluated back-to-back EUS examinations performed on the same day by two different endosonographers, which showed good Kappa scores for the presence of hyperechoic strands and parenchymal cysts only – but not for other features.

After the RC were published, Kalmin et al. [9] performed a study to determine and compare the

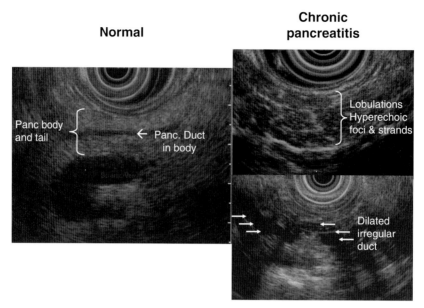

Normal

Chronic pancreatitis

Figure 13B.3 EUS images demonstrating normal pancreatic parenchymal and ductal anatomy in comparison to EUS features in chronic pancreatitis.

Table 13B.1 Cambridge classification.

Classification	Main duct	Abnormal side branches	Additional features
0: Normal	Normal	None	
1: Equivocal	Normal	<3	
2: Mild changes of chronic pancreatitis	Normal	≥3	
3: Moderate changes of chronic pancreatitis	Abnormal	>3	Presence of small cysts (<10 mm)
4: Marked/severe changes of chronic pancreatitis	Abnormal	>3	Presence of any of the following: large cysts (>10 mm), gross irregularity of the main duct, intraductal calculus, stricture, obstruction with severe dilation of main duct

interobserver reliability and intertest agreement of the CC versus the RC in diagnosing CP. Images from 36 consecutive patients who underwent EUS for suspected CP were reviewed separately by three sonographic experts who were asked to record the presence of both CC and RC features. The kappa for interobserver agreement for CC was higher than that for RC for both agreement on the classification of CP and for agreement on a positive diagnosis. This was further studied by Del Pozo et al. [10] who had 69 patients undergo same day back-to-back EUS procedures by different endosonographers. Data were collected in regard to findings of both CC and RC, and interobserver agreement was calculated. The kappa was slightly higher for conventional as compared with Rosemont, and the authors drew the conclusion that the RC did not provide an advantage in diagnosing CP as compared with the CC. Given the lack of evidence to support benefit with using the RC, it has not been widely adopted.

Table 13B.2 Wiersema (conventional) criteria.

Endoscopic ultrasound criteria	Classification
Parenchymal criteria	
Hyperechoic foci	**Normal (or low probability)**
Hyperechoic strands	0–2 criteria
Hypoechoic lobules, foci, or areas	
Cyst	**Indeterminate or intermediate probability** 3–4 criteria
Duct criteria	
Irregular duct contour	
Visible side branches	**High probability**
Hyperechoic duct margin	5–9 criteria
Dilated main duct	Presence of calcifications/stones
Intraductal stone	

Table 13B.3 Rosemont criteria

Endoscopic ultrasound criteria	Classification
Major criteria A	**Consistent with CP:**
Hyperechoic foci with shadowing	2 major A criteria
Major duct calculi	1 major A + 1 major B criteria
	1 major A + ≥3 minor criteria
Major criteria B	**Suggestive of CP:**
Lobularity with "honeycombing"	1 major A + <3 minor criteria
Minor criteria	1 major B + ≥3 minor criteria
Cyst	≥5 minor, no major criteria
Dilated main duct	
Irregular duct contour	**Indeterminate for CP:**
Dilated side branch	1 major B + <3 minor criteria
Hyperechoic duct wall	
Hyperechoic strands	**Normal:**
Hyperechoic foci without shadowing	<3 minor, no major criteria
Lobularity without "honeycombing"	

Table 13B.4 Conventional and Rosemont EUS criteria for diagnosis of chronic pancreatitis.

Conventional	Rosemont
Parenchymal criteria	**Major criteria A**
Hyperechoic foci	Hyperechoic foci (>2 mm in length/width) with shadowing
	Major duct calculi
Hyperechoic strands	
Hypoechoic lobules, foci, or areas	
Cyst	**Major criteria B** Lobularity with "honeycombing" (≥3 contiguous lobules)
Duct criteria	**Minor criteria**
Irregular duct contour	Cyst
Visible side branches	Dilated main duct (≥3.5 mm in body or >1.5 mm in tail)
Hyperechoic duct margin	Irregular duct contour
Dilated main duct	Dilated side branch (>3 each measuring ≥1 mm in width)
Intraductal stone	Hyperechoic duct wall
	Hyperechoic strands (≥3 mm in at least 2 dimensions)
	Hyperechoic foci without shadowing (>2 mm in length/width)
	Lobularity without "honeycombing" (>5 mm, noncontiguous lobules)

EUS in comparison with ERCP

ERCP is limited as a diagnostic tool in that it can only assess for ductal changes and/or the presence of cysts that communicate with the pancreatic ducts. It is unable to assess for parenchymal changes outside of the ducts, except in cases where there are large radiopaque stones that can be seen on fluoroscopy. On the other hand, EUS is able to assess both for parenchymal changes and ductal changes to help make a diagnosis of CP. This allows for the detection of more subtle changes not easily detected with ERCP. However, the primary advantage of EUS over ERCP is that EUS is an inherently safer test and carries no risk of causing acute pancreatitis (except when performing EUS-FNA, which carries 1–2% risk). As summarized in Table 13B.6, studies have shown

Table 13B.5 Classification of patients based on conventional and Rosemont EUS criteria.

Conventional	Rosemont
Normal (or low probability)	**Consistent with CP:**
0–2 criteria	2 major A criteria
	1 major A + 1 major B criteria
Indeterminate or intermediate probability	1 major A + ≥3 minor criteria
3–4 criteria	**Suggestive of CP:** 1 major A + <3 minor criteria
High probability	1 major B + ≥3 minor criteria
5–9 criteria	≥5 minor, no major criteria
Presence of calcifications/stones	
	Indeterminate for CP:
	1 major B + <3 minor criteria
	Normal:
	<3 minor, no major criteria

that higher number of EUS criteria (≥3) has strong correlation to higher Cambridge classification by ERCP. It is not clear whether those patients who meet criteria for CP by EUS but have normal diagnostic ERCP have early disease or are overdiagnosed. There have been few studies that have included clinical follow-up of patients as it relates to the diagnostic performance of EUS. Chen et al. (abstract) [16] performed a retrospective study of 19 patients with suspected CP who underwent EUS and ERCP that were then repeated >12 months later. They found that 5/6 patients (83%) who had normal initial ERCP but abnormal EUS were found to have abnormalities consistent with CP on the repeat ERCP, suggesting that the early changes of CP seen on EUS progressed to more advanced disease that was later detectable by ERCP.

EUS versus pancreatic function testing

There are multiple forms of pancreatic function testing available, and they can be neatly divided into two groups: noninvasive (indirect) and invasive (direct) testing. Noninvasive testing includes fecal fat analysis, measurement of fecal chymotrypsin, the measurement of fecal elastase, the ^{13}C-mixed triglyceride breath test, and the plasma pancreatic polypeptide test. Invasive testing includes the secretin-stimulated bicarbonate testing on duodenal aspirates or pure pancreatic juice. Despite the multitude of options, pancreatic function testing remains of limited value. None of the available tests are able to accurately and reliably detect mild or moderate pancreatic insufficiency [17]. On the other hand, EUS is very sensitive but not specific for late CP. It is unclear whether it is more or less sensitive than pancreatic function testing for early CP. Of the multiple studies performed, the data still seem mixed. In a study by Dominguez-Munoz et al. [18], 128 consecutive patients with CP were evaluated to see whether EUS could serve as an indirect measure of exocrine insufficiency. All patients underwent ^{13}C-mixed triglyceride breath testing as a means to diagnose pancreatic insufficiency. EUS was then performed and the EUS criteria for CP was evaluated and recorded by two separate endosonographers who were blinded to the results of the breath test. The investigators found a direct correlation between the number of EUS criteria present and the probability of the patient having pancreatic insufficiency. In addition, the presence of pancreatic ductal calcifications, main duct dilation, and hyperechoic foci with shadowing were all independently associated with the presence of pancreatic insufficiency.

EUS in comparison to other imaging modalities

Computed tomography (CT) and magnetic resonance imaging (MRI) are commonly used imaging modalities that are often utilized in making a diagnosis of CP. In fact, the first studies of CT scan for CP date as far back as the 1970s. Imaging quality has clearly improved over the years, particularly for pancreatic protocol CT and for secretin-stimulated MRCP. However, the sensitivity for diagnosing CP with cross-sectional imaging still remains poor, especially in the early stages of the disease. The diagnosis of CP with MRI relies on findings of pancreatic duct dilation and the presence of cysts calcifications – all findings that are included in the ERCP Cambridge criteria as markers of severe disease.

Table 13B.6 Diagnostic performance of EUS versus ERCP and PFTs in diagnosis of chronic pancreatitis (CP).

Study	Number of patients	Design	Results
Wiersema et al. [3]	89	Prospective. 20 asymptomatic patients underwent EUS only, and 69 patients with abdominal pain underwent EUS followed by ERCP. 16/69 patients also underwent secretin-stimulated PPJ collection	30/69 patients found to have CP based on clinical, ERCP, and/or PPJ data. EUS was abnormal in 24/30 patients with CP. 22/30 patients with CP had "early disease" (none or minimal changes per ERCP). Sensitivity, specificity, and accuracy of EUS in diagnosing CP were 80%, 86%, and 84% respectively. Versus ERCP, SN was 100% and SP was 79% for EUS.
Catalano et al. [11]	80	Prospective. 80 patients with recurrent pancreatitis underwent ERCP, EUS, and secretin test.	Abnormal studies were EUS = 63, ERCP = 36, secretin test = 25. SN 86% and SP 95% for EUS versus ERCP. EUS criteria of 0 had 100% NPV, 1–2 had 17% +ERCP and 13% +secretin, 3–5 criteria 92% +ERCP and 50% +secretin, ≥6 criteria had 100% PPV.
Sahai et al. [12]	126	Prospective. 126 patients undergoing ERCP for suspected CP underwent EUS by blinded endosonographers.	For EUS, NPV <85% when <3 criteria present. PPV >85% when ≥ 6 criteria present. SN and SP not specified.
Hollerbach et al. [13]	37	Prospective. 37 patients with suspected CP underwent ERCP, EUS, and indirect pancreatic function testing. EUS-FNA was performed in 27 of the patients.	For EUS without FNA, SN was 97% with SP 60% versus ERCP. With FNA, SP increased to 67% but caused acute pancreatitis in 2/27 (7%) patients. SN was 52% with SP 75% vs. indirect PFT.
Chowdhury et al. [14]	21	Prospective. 21 patients with suspected CP that underwent secretin testing also underwent EUS.	For EUS, ≥4 criteria yielded SN 57% and SP 64% as compared with direct PFT. SP increased to 92% with ≥6 criteria.
Stevens et al. [15]	83	Retrospective. 83 patients with suspected CP who underwent EUS, ERCP, and secretin PFT. Secretin PFT used as "gold standard" for diagnosis.	EUS and ERCP had similar SN (68% vs. 72%) and SP (79% vs. 76%). Associations were similar for both mild and moderate–severe disease.

EUS, endoscopic ultrasound; ERCP, endoscopic retrograde cholangiopancreatography; CP, chronic pancreatitis; PPJ, pure pancreatic juice; SN, sensitivity; SP, specificity; PPV, positive predictive value; NPV, negative predictive value; PFT, pancreatic function tests.

Therapeutic EUS

To date, the main therapeutic applications of EUS have been in the management of pseudocysts and providing pain relief by celiac plexus neurolysis. These techniques are covered in separate chapters.

References

1 Lees WR. Endoscopic ultrasonography of chronic pancreatitis and pancreatic pseudocysts. Scandinavian Journal of Gastroenterology, Supplement 1986;123:123–129.

2 Axon AT, Classen M, Cotton PB, Cremer M, Freeny PC, Lees WR. Pancreatography in chronic pancreatitis: international definitions. Gut. 1984;25(10):1107–1112.

3 Wiersema MJ, Hawes RH, Lehman GA, Kochman ML, Sherman S, Kopecky KK. Prospective evaluation of endoscopic ultrasonography and endoscopic retrograde cholangiopancreatography in patients with chronic abdominal pain of suspected pancreatic origin. Endoscopy. 1993;25(9):555–564.

4 Catalano MF, Sahai A, Levy M, Romagnuolo J, Wiersema M, Brugge W, et al. EUS-based criteria for the diagnosis of chronic pancreatitis: the Rosemont classification. Gastrointestinal Endoscopy. 2009;69(7):1251–1261.

5 Wallace MB, Hawes RH, Durkalski V, Chak A, Mallery S, Catalano MF, et al. The reliability of EUS for the diagnosis of chronic pancreatitis: interobserver agreement among experienced endosonographers. Gastrointestinal Endoscopy. 2001;53(3):294–299.

6 Lau JY, Sung JJ, Chan AC, Lai GW, Lau JT, Ng EK, et al. Stigmata of hemorrhage in bleeding peptic ulcers: an interobserver agreement study among international experts. Gastrointestinal Endoscopy. 1997;46(1):33–36.

7 Lieb JG, 2nd, Palma DT, Garvan CW, Leblanc JK, Romagnuolo J, Farrell JJ, et al. Intraobserver agreement among endosonographers for endoscopic ultrasound features of chronic pancreatitis: a blinded multicenter study. Pancreas. 2011;40(2):177–180.

8 Gardner TB, Gordon SR. Interobserver agreement for pancreatic endoscopic ultrasonography determined by same day back-to-back examinations. Journal of Clinical Gastroenterology. 2011;45(6):542–545.

9 Kalmin B, Hoffman B, Hawes R, Romagnuolo J. Conventional versus Rosemont endoscopic ultrasound criteria for chronic pancreatitis: comparing interobserver reliability and intertest agreement. Canadian Journal of Gastroenterology. 2011;25(5):261–264.

10 Del Pozo D, Poves E, Tabernero S, Beceiro I, Moral I, Villafruela M, et al. Conventional versus Rosemont endoscopic ultrasound criteria for chronic pancreatitis: interobserver agreement in same day back-to-back procedures. Pancreatology. 2012;12(3):284–287.

11 Catalano MF, Lahoti S, Geenen JE, Hogan WJ. Prospective evaluation of endoscopic ultrasonography, endoscopic retrograde pancreatography, and secretin test in the diagnosis of chronic pancreatitis. Gastrointestinal Endoscopy. 1998;48(1):11–17.

12 Sahai AV, Zimmerman M, Aabakken L, Tarnasky PR, Cunningham JT, van Velse A, et al. Prospective assessment of the ability of endoscopic ultrasound to diagnose, exclude, or establish the severity of chronic pancreatitis found by endoscopic retrograde cholangiopancreatography. Gastrointestinal Endoscopy. 1998;48(1):18–25.

13 Hollerbach S, Klamann A, Topalidis T, Schmiegel WH. Endoscopic ultrasonography (EUS) and fine-needle aspiration (FNA) cytology for diagnosis of chronic pancreatitis. Endoscopy. 2001;33(10):824–831.

14 Chowdhury R, Bhutani MS, Mishra G, Toskes PP, Forsmark CE. Comparative analysis of direct pancreatic function testing versus morphological assessment by endoscopic ultrasonography for the evaluation of chronic unexplained abdominal pain of presumed pancreatic origin. Pancreas. 2005;31(1):63–68.

15 Stevens T, Conwell DL, Zuccaro G, Jr., Vargo JJ, Dumot JA, Lopez R. Comparison of endoscopic ultrasound and endoscopic retrograde pancreatography for the prediction of pancreatic exocrine insufficiency. Digestive Diseases and Sciences. 2008;53(4):1146–1151.

16 Chen RYM, Hino S, Aithal GP, et al. Endoscopic ultrasound (EUS) features of chronic pancreatitis predate subsequent development of abnormal endoscopic retrograde pancreatogram (ERP) (abstract). Gastrointestinal Endoscopy 55:AB242 2002

17 Boeck WG, Adler G, Gress TM. Pancreatic function tests: when to choose, what to use. Current Gastroenterology Reports. 2001;3(2):95–100.

18 Dominguez-Munoz JE, Alvarez-Castro A, Larino-Noia J, Nieto L, Iglesias-Garcia J. Endoscopic ultrasonography of the pancreas as an indirect method to predict pancreatic exocrine insufficiency in patients with chronic pancreatitis. Pancreas. 2012;41(5):724–728.

CHAPTER 14

PART A: Pancreatic enzyme replacement therapy (PERT)

Ravi K. Prakash, Alexander Schlachterman & Chris E. Forsmark

Division of Gastroenterology, Hepatology, and Nutrition, University of Florida, Gainesville, FL, USA

Pancreatic enzyme replacement therapy

Oral pancreatic enzymes have been utilized for more than a century to treat maldigestion associated with pancreatic exocrine insufficiency [1]. The main goal of the use of pancreatic enzymes is to restore near-normal digestion and, in doing so, improve nutritional status, symptoms, and quality of life. Although the general principle of delivering the right amount of pancreatic enzymes to the duodenum and proximal jejunum at the right time and in the right milieu (an alkaline environment) seems achievable, this is often not the case in practice. This chapter briefly reviews the basic physiology of pancreatic secretion and digestion, outlines the most effective approaches to diagnosis and monitoring of exocrine insufficiency, and discusses the currently available enzyme formulations with a focus on appropriate patient selection and dosage needed to achieve reasonable digestion of fats, carbohydrates, and protein.

The pancreas produces about 500–1000 mL of digestive juices per day [2]. This process is tightly controlled and hormonally mediated. Entry of food from the stomach into the small intestine is the most potent stimulator. This effect is mediated mainly through two hormones: notably, secretin, which acts on the pancreatic and biliary ducts to stimulate bicarbonate secretion, and cholecystokinin (CCK), which acts on acinar cells to stimulate enzyme secretion [3]. The normal pancreas secretes approximately 900,000 USP units of lipase with each meal. While lipase and amylase are secreted in an active form, the proteolytic enzymes (trypsinogen, chymotrypsin A and B, procarboxypeptidase A and B) are stored and secreted as inactive zymogens. Trypsinogen is activated to trypsin in the duodenum by the brush border enzyme enterokinase, and trypsin then activates the other proteases in the duodenum. In the basal state, the pancreas secretes protein-rich and mildly alkaline fluid. Pancreatic enzymes are secreted rapidly after food ingestion and reach their peak effect in about an hour. This is followed by a continuous sustained release of enzyme secretion for about 3–4 hours following meal ingestion [4].

The majority of digestion occurs in the duodenum and most absorption occurs in the duodenum and jejunum. As exocrine pancreatic insufficiency develops, fat maldigestion occurs first and is more severe than protein or carbohydrate maldigestion. There are a number of reasons for this, including increased opportunities for compensatory mechanisms for carbohydrates (salivary amylase) and proteins (brush border enteropeptidases and pepsin) than for lipase (only a small increase in gastric lipase). In addition, lipase is a rather fragile enzyme and is rapidly denatured. Normal fat and fat-soluble vitamin absorption is a closely coordinated and complex process, which begins with nutrient delivery to the intestines. Subsequent bicarbonate secretion by the pancreatic and biliary ducts neutralizes gastric acid. This is an essential step, as both

Pancreatitis: Medical and Surgical Management, First Edition.
David B. Adams, Peter B. Cotton, Nicholas J. Zyromski and John Windsor.
© 2017 John Wiley & Sons, Ltd. Published 2017 by John Wiley & Sons, Ltd.

lipase and bile acids may be irreversibly denatured in the presence of acid. Appropriate control of luminal pH, coupled with the presence of sufficient concentrations of both digestive enzymes and bile acids, is necessary for fat digestion. The human pancreas has a substantial reserve capacity for secretion, and pancreatic exocrine insufficiency does not appear until lipase secretion is reduced by 90% or more [5]. This would suggest that delivering approximately 10% of normal pancreatic enzyme output of enzyme replacement therapy with each meal would be sufficient to eliminate maldigestion and exocrine insufficiency.

A number of disorders may result in disruption of the normal process of pancreatic enzyme secretion. These conditions include loss of acinar cell mass (chronic pancreatitis, necrotizing acute pancreatitis, or pancreatic surgery), obstruction of the pancreatic duct (benign, premalignant, and malignant causes), rare genetic syndromes (Shwachman–Diamond and Johanson–Blizzard syndromes), previous upper gut surgery leading to asynchronous delivery of enzymes and food to the intestine, and reduced pH in the duodenum leading to inactivation of enzymes and bile acids.

Chronic pancreatitis is associated with slowly progressive fibrosis and destruction of the gland. In addition to destruction of parenchyma, a number of ductal changes including strictures and stones may result in duct blockage, which augments exocrine insufficiency. Steatorrhea and other signs of maldigestion generally do not occur until late in the course of chronic pancreatitis [6], often years or even decades after disease onset. Exocrine insufficiency is seen most commonly in those with chronic pancreatitis due to alcohol or smoking, and in certain genetic causes (e.g., hereditary pancreatitis or cystic fibrosis). In addition, these patients often undergo pancreatic surgery, which may further reduce enzyme secretory capacity. A majority of patients continue to require pancreatic enzyme supplementation after surgical treatment [7].

Patients with severe acute pancreatitis with complications such as pancreatic necrosis are at a high risk of developing pancreatic insufficiency. The risk of pancreatic exocrine (and endocrine) insufficiency is highest in patients who have undergone necrosectomy due to the resulting loss of pancreatic parenchyma, but exocrine insufficiency may occur after less severe episodes of acute pancreatitis [8]. Pancreatic cancer patients are also at risk of pancreatic insufficiency depending on the location and degree of pancreatic ductal obstruction. These can include patients with ductal adenocarcinoma of the pancreatic head, which prevents enzyme access to the duodenum. Exocrine insufficiency may also be seen due to intraductal papillary mucinous neoplasms (IPMN) involving the main pancreatic duct, in which the gelatinous mucin obstructs the pancreatic duct. Most patients with tumors in the pancreas requiring pancreatic resection either had exocrine insufficiency at diagnosis or became exocrine insufficient soon after surgical resection [9].

Patients who undergo upper gastrointestinal surgery are at risk of asynchrony of pancreatic secretions in response to nutrient entry into the lumen, thereby causing inadequate mixing of enzymes with food resulting in malabsorption [10]. This occurs most frequently in patients who have a Roux limb from surgery. In these patients, the enzymes have to travel through the Roux limb before entering the efferent limb where nutrients are entering the digestive tract. Malabsorption can ensue, as simultaneous mixing following nutrient intake does not happen [11]. This contributes to the maldigestion and malabsorption associated with Roux-en-Y gastric bypass.

Low intraluminal pH in the duodenum results in inactivation of lipase and bile acids, which can result in maldigestion. This is seen in gastric hypersecretory states such as Zollinger–Ellison syndrome, which is a result of autologous gastrin secretion by gastrinoma. The duodenal bicarbonate concentration may be insufficient to neutralize the acid, thereby resulting in malabsorption [12]. Another mechanism for low duodenal pH is dumping of gastric contents too quickly into the duodenum, thereby giving inadequate time for bicarbonate action. This can result in denaturation of pancreatic enzymes [13]. It is noteworthy that patients with chronic pancreatitis often have a lower duodenal pH than normal controls, and this may also contribute to the maldigestion seen in these patients.

Diagnosis of pancreatic exocrine insufficiency

Two diagnostic challenges exist in these patients. The first is establishing accurately the diagnosis of chronic pancreatitis or alternative diagnosis that may cause exocrine insufficiency. That topic is covered in other sections. The second challenge is establishing the presence of exocrine insufficiency. Patients with pancreatic exocrine insufficiency do not present clinically until the majority of glandular production of enzymes has been compromised. In careful analyses, fat maldigestion does not occur until pancreatic lipase falls below 10% of normal secretion [5]. However, patients who have pancreatic cancer may present with maldigestion after removal of as little as 30% of the parenchyma. This is probably the result of diminished functional capacity of the remnant parenchyma, coupled with asynchrony after surgery. Patients may present with oily clay colored stools, abdominal bloating and gas, loose stools or diarrhea, and an inability to maintain weight despite adequate oral intake. It is important to note that diarrhea is probably present in only about 50–60% of patients with confirmed maldigestion [14]. Many patients can have dramatic steatorrhea, despite having only one formed bowel movement a day. The lack of diarrhea is often attributed to better preserved carbohydrate and protein digestion, compared with diseases of the small bowel producing malabsorption of all dietary components.

Clinical symptoms are insufficient for diagnosis. The most accurate diagnosis of steatorrhea requires measurement of the coefficient of fat absorption (CFA – % of dietary fat digested and absorbed). Measuring unabsorbed carbohydrates or protein is also possible, but more complex than fat. The 72-hour fecal fat test was designed to quantify fat malabsorption, which remains the gold standard for quantification of steatorrhea. Patients are required to go off of pancreatic enzymes for at least a week and should be consuming at least 100 g/day of fat for 3 days preceding the test as well as the 3 days during the test. The fat in the diet needs to be high and needs to be precisely quantified. It is noteworthy that unlike when the test was originally developed, an intake of 100 g/day of fat is significant but is still less than the average daily fat intake in the United States (>160 g daily per capita) and many other developed countries. The need to know rather precisely the fat content of the diet during the test makes it difficult to perform accurately in an outpatient setting and often requires the services of a dietician or a metabolic kitchen. In the setting of normal fat digestion and absorption, the CFA should be at least 93% (i.e., presence of greater than 7 g/day of fecal fat on a 100 g fat/day intake is diagnostic of steatorrhea). The levels

of steatorrhea are often much higher (>20 g/day) in patients with confirmed pancreatic disease [15]. This test proves the presence of steatorrhea, but does not determine the cause. The test is not widely used in clinical practice, due to the number of practical and logistical issues mentioned earlier. Spot fecal fat testing involves Sudan staining of random stool samples. The test is simpler than a 72-hour fecal fat analysis but must also be performed on a high-fat diet. The finding of >100 fat globules/HPF or the presence of larger fat globules >6 μm is abnormal. This is a relatively insensitive test with positive results mainly in patients who have greater than 25 g of fecal fat per day [16]. A similar test, which is not available, is the acid steatocrit in which stool is acidified and centrifuged, with the height of the fat layer compared with the total height of the sample being used to quantify fat in stool (>31% fat layer of total sample height in a test tube is abnormal).

Several noninvasive tests have also been developed over time to diagnose pancreatic insufficiency in the outpatient and inpatient setting. Measuring the presence of pancreatic enzymes in stool is one such test. Chymotrypsin is one of the relatively stable enzymes secreted by the pancreas. Chymotrypsin avoids degradation in the small bowel by binding to insoluble debris in the stool and remains detectable for several days. Fecal chymotrypsin below 3 U/g of stool is suggestive of pancreatic insufficiency [17]. Pancreas elastase −1 is a pancreas-specific elastase that evades digestion and degradation in the small bowel and can be reliably detected in stool. Similar to fecal chymotrypsin, the levels correlate well with the functionality of the pancreas. Typically, values less than 100 mcg/g of stool is diagnostic of pancreatic insufficiency [18]. The accuracy of fecal elastase exceeds that of fecal chymotrypsin, and it is preferred as it is more stable during intestinal passage [19, 20]. A number of conditions other than exocrine insufficiency can produce a falsely low fecal elastase. Chief among these is watery diarrhea, in which the enzyme is diluted. Similarly, the test may be abnormal in diabetics. Fecal elastase (human) may be measured while the patient is taking exogenous porcine enzymes as the assay is not affected. Serum measurements are also available to estimate pancreatic function. Serum trypsin is abnormally low in patients with advanced chronic pancreatitis and steatorrhea, but may be normal in other conditions associated with pancreatic exocrine insufficiency and in those with less-advanced chronic pancreatitis. Low levels below 20 mg/mL are consistent with advanced chronic pancreatitis [21].

A number of breath tests have also been developed to identify exocrine insufficiency, using triglycerides radiolabeled with ^{13}C or ^{14}C. In the presence of sufficient lipase, the radiolabeled carbon is liberated during lipolysis, and the excreted CO_2 can be measured. Mass spectrometry or infrared analysis is required to measure ^{13}C. These tests are available at a few research centers but are not available for patients in the United States [20].

Direct measurement of pancreatic secretion is also possible. The conventional secretin stimulation test (SST), involves placing a 26-Fr oroduodenal tube with both gastric and duodenal ports. The tube is introduced fluoroscopically with the weighted tip positioned close to the ligament of Treitz and the tapered radiopaque portion of the tube is kept close to the pylorus [22]. Basal duodenal and gastric pH along with the volume secreted is then measured over 15 minutes. This is followed by the injection of a supraphysiologic dose of synthetic human secretin at a dose of 0.2 mg/kg [23]. Secretin stimulates the ducts in the pancreas to secrete bicarbonate [24]. SST has mainly been used as a test to diagnose chronic pancreatitis, rather than to determine the presence or absence of exocrine insufficiency. It does appear to be reasonably sensitive and specific as a diagnostic tool, with sensitivities of over 90% for late stages of chronic pancreatitis, and about 75% in early-stage chronic pancreatitis [25]. After secretin infusion, the duodenal fluid is then collected every 15 minutes for 60 minutes, and this fluid is measured for volume, pH, and bicarbonate concentration in mEq/L. The normal range for peak bicarbonate secretion is about 80–130 mEq/L. The secretin test measures maximal stimulated secretory capacity of ductal cells and is not a direct measurement of enzyme secretion. Maximum stimulated secretory capacity drops prior to the later development of exocrine insufficiency, but there is not a specific bicarbonate concentration cutoff below which exocrine insufficiency invariably occurs. In general, however, peak bicarbonate concentrations less than 50 mEq/L are associated with exocrine insufficiency while levels of 50–80 are often not.

CCK can also be used to test the functional capacity of the pancreas with the CCK stimulation test and, in the past, has also been combined with secretin. The CCK stimulation test is a better test for pancreatic insufficiency than the SST, as it measures actual enzyme output. As a diagnostic tool for chronic pancreatitis, it parallels the overall accuracy of the SST [26]. In the CCK stimulation test, a tube with gastric and duodenal ports (Dreiling tube) is placed, followed by the collection and measurement of basal secretion. Subsequently, CCK is injected and collection of duodenal contents is performed at 20-minute intervals for a total of 80 minutes. During the first 20–40 minutes, CCK stimulates the contraction of the gallbladder followed by the secretion of bile, which affects the measurement of pancreatic output. The fluid is analyzed for lipase secretion, which has shown to be sensitive for diagnosis of early- and late-stage chronic pancreatitis [27].

The CCK stimulation test is no longer performed, owing to a variety of reasons. Even the secretin test is rarely performed except at a few research centers, and even there it was not possible for several years due to an unavailability of secretin. Both tests require unsedated placement of a relatively large caliber oroduodenal tube, which also limits their acceptability by patients. One alternative to conventional pancreatic function testing is to utilize endoscopy to collect fluid in the duodenum after secretin injection. This test is called endoscopic SST or eSST [28]. Endoscopic SST has shown results that are similar to conventional SST, although with less specificity as the collection time is often shortened to 30–45 minutes. This test is likely better tolerated than the Dreiling tube insertion under fluoroscopy as the patient is well sedated for the procedure. There are, however, cost and time constraints in using an endoscopy room for 60 minutes for the procedure. Similar to the standard secretin test, the eSST is mainly used for the diagnosis of less-advanced chronic pancreatitis, rather than the documentation of exocrine insufficiency.

In addition to testing of pancreatic function to determine the presence of pancreatic exocrine insufficiency, the presence of exocrine insufficiency may be suspected based on imaging tests of the pancreas documenting features consistent with advanced chronic pancreatitis. In the case of chronic pancreatitis, the development of a dilated pancreatic duct, pancreatic gland atrophy, or diffuse pancreatic calcification often signal disease, which is advanced enough to be likely associated with exocrine insufficiency. These features may be visible on

EUS, CT, or MRI with MRCP. A quasi-function test uti-lizing MRCP examination of the pancreas coupled with secretin stimulation can estimate pancreatic function (ductal fluid secretion rather than enzyme secretion) and is used in some centers. This secretin-enhanced MRCP (S-MRCP) assesses the volume of fluid in the duodenum after secretin injection. One of the main drawbacks with this system is that it measures volume rather than bicarbonate concentration. In addition, obstructive lesions of the ampulla can also give false-positive results [29].

Pancreatic function tests, whether invasive or non-invasive, do very well in detecting advanced disease, the setting in which exocrine insufficiency is most commonly encountered. However, the diagnosis of early chronic pancreatitis or even the diagnosis of pancreatic exocrine insufficiency is more challenging. In many patients, the diagnosis of exocrine insuf-ficiency is empiric, considered in the right clinical setting and with the right constellation of symptoms and supported by tests such as fecal elastase or serum trypsin.

Consequences of pancreatic exocrine insufficiency

In addition to diagnosis, additional testing of nutritional status is often useful to gauge the degree and severity of nutritional complications of exocrine insufficiency as enzyme therapy is begun. This testing may include anthropometric measurements (BMI or change in BMI over time), serum measures of general malnutrition (albumin, prealbumin, cholesterol, RBP, CBC with lymphocyte count), and measures of fat-soluble vitamin deficiency (INR, vitamins D, A, and E levels). Those with exocrine insufficiency may develop frank malnutrition, although this is unusual unless p.o. intake is signifi-cantly restricted as well. In those without malnutrition, deficiencies of fat-soluble vitamins may develop even in the presence of rather mild steatorrhea. Deficiency of vitamin D is particularly important, and numerous studies have documented high rates of osteopenia and osteoporosis in patients with chronic pancreatitis. Thus, it is important to not only measure vitamin D levels at the onset of therapy but to monitor this over time and to also assess bone density.

Pancreatic enzymes

Pancreatic enzyme products (PEPs) contain a mixture of digestive enzymes including amylase, lipase, and vari-ous proteases. For many years, these products were mar-keted in the United States as unapproved products. As a result, the PEPs contained variable amounts of enzyme concentrations, and a concern was raised as to quality of manufacture and resulting under- or overdosing caus-ing patient intolerance or side effects. In July 1991, the US Food and Drug Administration (US FDA) intervened and announced that all PEPs should be approved, and any new product should submit a New Drug Application (NDA) before marketing it. The drug companies were instructed to demonstrate that they were able to man-ufacture their products with sufficient consistency and quality to ensure that patients did not experience dose variation. The goal was to assure safety, effectiveness, and product quality for all the PEPs. In 2004, the US FDA notified manufacturers of its intent to permit mar-keting of the unapproved products while the companies were working on their applications. In 2006, the US FDA issued guidance documentation about the requirements manufacturers had to meet for the US FDA approval. In 2007, the US FDA extended the deadline of approval to April 28, 2010 due to the difficulties encountered in manufacturing these products. The guidelines for effi-cacy were based on CFA, and the minimum change on enzyme therapy was defined as an increase of 10% or more. In addition, in those with a CFA <40% at baseline an increase of at least 30% was considered a clinically meaningful change. Approval was based on these cri-teria in at least 200 patients studied over 6 months (or 100 patients over 1 year). Approval was granted for both cystic fibrosis and chronic pancreatitis, even if the sup-porting clinical studies only analyzed those with cystic fibrosis. Currently, there are six products that are US FDA approved (Table 14A.1). The approved list includes the following:

- Creon and Zenpep – approved 2009
- Pancreaze – approved April 2010
- Ultresa and Viokace – approved March 2012
- Pertzye – approved May 2012.

Five of these products are capsules containing enteric-coated microspheres, including one (Pertzye) that includes bicarbonate. One product (Viokace) is a not enteric coated and is supplied as a tablet. Pancreatic

Table 14A.1 Current food and drug administration approved pancreatic enzyme replacement therapy.

Product	Formulation	Manufacturer	Lipase content/capsule or pill
Zenpep®	Enteric-coated porcine	Aptalis	3,000; 5,000; 10,000; 15,000; 20,000; 25,000
Creon®	Enteric-coated porcine	AbbVie	3,000; 6,000; 12,000; 24,000; 36,000
Pancreaze®	Enteric-coated porcine	Janssen	4,200; 10,500; 16,800; 21,000
Viokace®	Tablet non-enteric-coated porcine	Aptalis	10,440; 20,880
Ultresa®	Enteric-coated porcine	Aptalis	13,800; 20,700; 23,000
Pertzye®	Enteric-coated porcine with bicarbonate	Digestive care	8,000; 16,000

enzymes (particularly lipase) become irreversibly denatured in the acidic gastric environment, hence the fact that most preparations are available in an enteric-coated formulation. The microspheres in these enteric-coated agents have a polyacrylic acid layer that dissolves only in an environment with pH >5.5 [30]. This prevents the granules from being released in the stomach where the pH is normally less than 4. Once in the intestinal lumen, the contents are released for digestion, but this may occur significantly downstream in the small bowel. In the normal state, these enzymes are most active in the duodenum, whereas in patients on pancreatic enzyme replacement therapy the release may be in the distal jejunum or even the ileum. This creates some limitation on effectiveness. These capsules are designed to be taken orally as whole capsules without being chewed [31]. Viokace is the only non-enteric-coated pancreatic enzyme preparation. Since it will be deactivated in an acidic environment, it is necessary to coadminister proton pump inhibitors (PPIs) or H2-receptor antagonists to increase the pH of the gastric environment and prevent deactivation.

There is some evidence to suggest that the addition of a PPI even in patients on enteric-coated PEPs may enhance efficacy [32], although the data on this point are mixed. There are several potential explanations. In addition to enzyme secretion, the pancreas secretes a significant quantity of bicarbonate, which is responsible for maintaining an alkaline milieu in the small intestine. This also facilitates interaction between fatty acids and bile. In an acidic environment, even bile acids are precipitated. Studies have demonstrated that bicarbonate secretion may not drop proportionately to the degree of enzyme secretion drop in pancreatic insufficiency. Therefore, not all patients require PPI therapy in order for PEPs to function optimally [14].

There is no evidence to suggest that enteric-coated PEPs are superior to non-enteric-coated PEPs and vice versa in terms of absolute capacity to reduce steatorrhea. It is, however, definitely worth considering a trial of PPI in patients who are not responding to high doses of enteric-coated PEPs.

The goal of enzyme supplementation is the elimination of steatorrhea with normal absorption of fat and fat-soluble vitamins, protein, and carbohydrates. Completely normal absorption is difficult to achieve. In clinical practice, a goal of improved absorption, maintenance or gain of weight and muscle mass, and avoidance of complications (e.g., vitamin D deficiency and osteoporosis) is reasonable. For proper digestion, the enzymes need to adequately combine with nutrients and interact within the digestive lumen. The timing is crucial. Normally, the enteric-coated capsule covering disintegrates once they enter the stomach. At this point, the microspheres are released and can mix with the food ingested. The microspheres remain inactive until they reach the intestine where the alkaline milieu releases the enzymes. Peak activity is reached about 30 minutes after ingestion, and the enzymes remain active for about 2 hours. Studies have demonstrated that pancreatic enzymes taken with food report superior absorption compared with those taken after meals [33]. It is crucial for physicians to stress the importance of dosing and timing of the enzymes. More often than not, patients are left with minimal instructions, and studies have shown a large percentage of patients still symptomatic while on therapy [34].

In patients with surgically altered anatomy, such as partial gastrectomy, duodenectomy, or Roux-en-Y anatomy, it may be difficult to achieve adequate mixing of enzymes and food. Delayed gastric emptying or rapid intestinal transit can create a delay in activation of these enzymes [35]. Due to delayed activation, the enzymes do not have adequate time to mix with the food, thereby decreasing their efficacy. Endogenous lipase achieves highest concentrations in the duodenum and progressively reduces to nearly undetectable levels in the ileum. One study demonstrated that exogenous lipase supplementation of about 40,000 U with meals increased the duodenal concentrations only minimally, but enormously increased the ileal concentrations due to limited proximal release of enzymes. Therefore, the enteric-coated enzymes abolished the normal postcibal lipase gradient between the duodenum and ileum. In this situation, the majority of ingested enzyme is wasted as fat hydrolysis does not occur before the ileum where surface area for digestion and absorption is minimal. Even though enzyme supplementation managed to reduce steatorrhea in patients with severe pancreatic insufficiency, the small bowel digestive and absorptive capabilities were only partially utilized [36].

The goal of enzyme supplementation is to abolish steatorrhea and ensure adequate absorption of nutrients but especially fat, fat-soluble vitamins, and essential fatty acids. While all enzyme products contain proteases, lipase, and amylase, it is the lipase content that is most clinically important. Endogenous or exogenous lipase activity can be measured in International Units (IU) or United States Pharmacopeia (USP) units. Commercial products in the United States are rated in USP units (1 IU = 3 USP units). In a single normal meal, more than 900,000 USP units of lipase are delivered into the duodenum from the pancreas. Clinical studies have demonstrated that when this falls to about 10% of that normal amount, steatorrhea develops. This has led to a minimum target for enzyme replacement therapy of around 90,000 USP units of lipase with each meal. Not all patients require this amount, some require more. Fat digestion is aided by gastric lipase, which is increased in a compensatory manner in those with advanced chronic pancreatitis. In addition, even in patients with advanced chronic pancreatitis, there may remain some residual enzyme secretion.

Some studies have documented that lower doses of enzymes may be effective in certain situations. In one study, around 30,000 USP units of unprotected lipase given with meals abolished steatorrhea as long as the enzymes were able to mix with meals and were not destroyed by gastric acidity [37]. Studies have shown that the effect of therapy on steatorrhea is greater in individuals where the gastric and duodenal pH remained greater than 4 for longer periods [38]. Reliable enzyme therapy is more achievable in achlorhydria patients where the pH barrier is absent. Graham et al demonstrated that administration of a smaller dose (about 18,000 USP units) in microsphere formulation that is enterically coated is also effective in abolishing steatorrhea [39]. Nonetheless, the effectiveness of exogenous enzyme supplementation is often substantially less than this, and higher dosages are required in the vast majority of patients.

In the clinical studies of recently approved enzyme products [40–44], the overall change in CFA ranged from 26% to 41% (Table 14A.2). In those with a baseline CFA <40%, improvements of 52–60% were demonstrated, while in those with better CFAs the improvement is more modest (20–30%). It should be noted that these registration trials were largely in patients with CF, not chronic pancreatitis. These studies generally treated patients with 6000–11,000 USP units of lipase/kg/day. These are substantially greater than the 10% of normal range mentioned earlier. For an average 70 kg patient with chronic pancreatitis, this could be 140,000–250,000 USP units of lipase with each of three daily meals, which is approximately 3–5 times the typical dosage.

Recent reviews suggest a starting dose of 40,000–50,000 USP units of lipase with each meal, which assumes some gastric lipase activity remains and some residual pancreatic secretion remains. The dose is increased based on clinical response. Underdosing is very common. Two surveys from the Netherlands [34, 45] noted that significant underdosing was common in patients with chronic pancreatitis, pancreatic surgery, and pancreatic cancer. In these surveys, nearly three-fourths of the patients continued to experience steatorrhea despite enzymes, and more than 40% had ongoing weight loss. Another impediment to effective prescribing is the cost of medications. As no generic enzymes remain, the cost per prescription tripled over the last 5 years, reaching a level of nearly $600/month.

A reasonable approach is to make sure the diagnosis is accurate and to identify patients with possible exocrine insufficiency based on the appropriate clinical situation (e.g., evidence of chronic pancreatitis, previous pancreatic surgery, pancreatic cancer, or IPMN) and/or suspicious clinical features (steatorrhea, weight loss, vitamin D deficiency, etc.). The diagnostic suspicion

Table 14A.2 Some randomized controlled trials on PERT, study design and outcome.

Drug	Study	Patients, N	Study design	Change in CFA or CFA
Creon	Safdi [15]	CP, N = 27	DBRPC	Δ 37% vs. 12%
	Whitcomb [40]	CP or pancreatic surgery, N = 54	DBRPC	Δ 32% vs. 9%
		CF, N = 36	DBRPC	Δ 35% vs. 3%
		CF, N = 16	DBRPC	83% vs. 47%
		Pancreatic surgery, N = 58	DBRPC	Δ 21% vs. 4.2%
	Ramesh [43]	CP, N = 62	DBRPC	Δ 18% vs. 4.1%
Zenpep	Toskes [42]	CP, N = 72	DBR crossover	90% vs. 80%
		CF, N = 33	DBRPC	88% vs. 63%
Pancreaze		CF, N = 40	DBRPC	Δ 34% vs. 1.5%

Δ = change in fat absorption with drug versus placebo. Percentages without Δ imply absolute values of CFA in drug versus placebo.
CP, chronic pancreatitis; CF, cystic fibrosis; DBRPC, double-blind randomized placebo-controlled study; CFA, coefficient of fat absorption.

may be able to be confirmed by fecal elastase, serum trypsin, or fecal fat. Baseline assessment can include anthropometrics, albumin, prealbumin, cholesterol, retinal binding protein, CBC with lymphocyte count, and fat-soluble vitamin levels (A, D, E, and K). Therapy should begin with at least 40,000 USP units of lipase with each meal (taken during the meal). There is no need to restrict fat in the diet. In some patients, a higher initial dose may be considered (significant pancreatic resection, pancreatic cancer, or IPMN blocking the main pancreatic duct). The response to therapy can be measured by clinical features (weight gain, less steatorrhea), fecal fat tests, or laboratory tests of fat-soluble vitamin levels. When enzyme therapy does not seem to be effective, the most likely explanation is an inadequate dose (either prescribed or unable to afford drug). The wrong timing of ingestion is also a common reason for inadequate response. If neither of these is responsible, consider adding acid suppression therapy. If still not effective, consider alternative diagnoses and especially small intestinal bacterial overgrowth, gastroparesis, or secondary pancreatic cancer.

References

1 Layer P, Keller J, Lankisch PG. Pancreatic enzyme replacement therapy. Current Gastroenterology Reports 2001;3(2):101–108.

2 Parrish CR, Quatrara B. The art of reinfusing intestinal secretions. Journal of Supportive Oncology 2010; 8(2):92–96.

3 Berry AJ. Pancreatic enzyme replacement therapy during pancreatic insufficiency. Nutrition in Clinical Practice 2014;29(3):312–321.

4 Go VL, Hofmann AF, Summerskill WH. Pancreozymin bioassay in man based on pancreatic enzyme secretion: potency of specific amino acids and other digestive products. Journal of Clinical Investigation 1970;49(8):1558–1564.

5 DiMagno EP, Go VL, Summerskill WH. Relations between pancreatic enzyme outputs and malabsorption in severe pancreatic insufficiency. New England Journal of Medicine 1973;288(16):813–815.

6 Layer P, et al. The different courses of early- and late-onset idiopathic and alcoholic chronic pancreatitis. Gastroenterology 1994;107(5):1481–1487.

7 Riediger H, et al. Long-term outcome after resection for chronic pancreatitis in 224 patients. Journal of Gastrointestinal Surgery 2007;11(8):949–959; discussion 959–960.

8 Das SL, et al. Relationship between the exocrine and endocrine pancreas after acute pancreatitis. World Journal of Gastroenterology 2014;20(45):17196–17205.

9 Matsumoto J, Traverso LW. Exocrine function following the Whipple operation as assessed by stool elastase. Journal of Gastrointestinal Surgery 2006;10(9):1225–1229.

10 Mossner J, Keim V. Pancreatic enzyme therapy. Deutsches Ärzteblatt International 2010;108(34–35):578–582.

11 Rogers C. Postgastrectomy nutrition. Nutrition in Clinical Practice 2011;26(2):126–136.

12 Fabian E, Kump P, Krejs GJ. Diarrhea caused by circulating agents. Gastroenterology Clinics of North America 2012;41(3):603–610.

13 Long WB, Weiss JB. Rapid gastric emptying of fatty meals in pancreatic insufficiency. Gastroenterology 1974;67(5):920–925.

14 Lankisch PG, et al. Functional reserve capacity of the exocrine pancreas. Digestion 1986;35(3):175–181.

15 Safdi M, et al. The effects of oral pancreatic enzymes (Creon 10 capsule) on steatorrhea: a multicenter, placebo-controlled, parallel group trial in subjects with chronic pancreatitis. Pancreas 2006;33(2):156–162.

16 Drummey GD, Benson Jr., JA, Jones CM. Microscopical examination of the stool for steatorrhea. New England Journal of Medicine 1961;264:85–87.

17 Adham NF, et al. Stool chymotrypsin and trypsin determinations. American Journal of Digestive Diseases 1967;12(12):1272–1276.

18 Sziegoleit A, Linder D. Studies on the sterol-binding capacity of human pancreatic elastase 1. Gastroenterology 1991;100(3):768–774.

19 Leeds JS, Oppong K, Sanders DS. The role of fecal elastase-1 in detecting exocrine pancreatic disease. Nature Reviews Gastroenterology & Hepatology 2011;8(7):405–415.

20 Lohr JM, Oliver MR, Frulloni L. Synopsis of recent guidelines on pancreatic exocrine insufficiency. United European Gastroenterology Journal 2013;1(2):79–83.

21 Jacobson DG, et al. Trypsin-like immunoreactivity as a test for pancreatic insufficiency. New England Journal of Medicine 1984;310(20):1307–1309.

22 Go VL, Hofmann AF, Summerskill WH. Simultaneous measurements of total pancreatic, biliary, and gastric outputs in man using a perfusion technique. Gastroenterology 1970;58(3):321–328.

23 Somogyi L, et al. Comparison of biologic porcine secretin, synthetic porcine secretin, and synthetic human secretin in pancreatic function testing. Pancreas 2003;27(3):230–234.

24 Heij HA, et al. Relationship between functional and histological changes in chronic pancreatitis. Digestive Diseases and Sciences 1986;31(10):1009–1013.

25 Steer ML, Waxman I, Freedman S. Chronic pancreatitis. New England Journal of Medicine 1995;332(22): 1482–1490.

26 Hansky J, et al. Relationship between maximal secretory output and weight of the pancreas in the dog. Proceedings of the Society for Experimental Biology and Medicine 1963;114:654–656.

27 Bank S, et al. The pancreatic-function test--method and normal values. South African Medical Journal 1963;37:1061–1066.

28 Conwell DL, et al. An endoscopic pancreatic function test with synthetic porcine secretin for the evaluation of chronic abdominal pain and suspected chronic pancreatitis. Gastrointestinal Endoscopy 2003;57(1):37–40.

29 Schneider AR, et al. Does secretin-stimulated MRCP predict exocrine pancreatic insufficiency? A comparison with noninvasive exocrine pancreatic function tests. Journal of Clinical Gastroenterology 2006;40(9):851–855.

30 Tran TC, et al. Functional changes after pancreatoduodenectomy: diagnosis and treatment. Pancreatology 2009;9(6):729–737.

31 Kuhn RJ, et al. CREON (pancrelipase delayed-release capsules) for the treatment of exocrine pancreatic insufficiency. Advances in Therapy 2010;27(12):895–916.

32 Regan PT, et al. Reduced intraluminal bile acid concentrations and fat maldigestion in pancreatic insufficiency: correction by treatment. Gastroenterology 1979;77(2):285–289.

33 Dominguez-Munoz JE, et al. Effect of the administration schedule on the therapeutic efficacy of oral pancreatic enzyme supplements in patients with exocrine pancreatic insufficiency: a randomized, three-way crossover study. Alimentary Pharmacology and Therapeutics 2005;21(8):993–1000.

34 Sikkens EC, et al. The daily practice of pancreatic enzyme replacement therapy after pancreatic surgery: a northern European survey: enzyme replacement after surgery. Journal of Gastrointestinal Surgery 2012;16(8):1487–1492.

35 Paik CN, et al. The role of small intestinal bacterial overgrowth in postgastrectomy patients. Neurogastroenterology and Motility 2011;23(5):e191–e196.

36 Guarner L, et al. Fate of oral enzymes in pancreatic insufficiency. Gut 1993;34(5):708–712.

37 Keller J, et al. Duodenal and ileal nutrient deliveries regulate human intestinal motor and pancreatic responses to a meal. American Journal of Physiology 1997;272(3 Pt 1):G632–G637.

38 Graham DY. Enzyme replacement therapy of exocrine pancreatic insufficiency in man. Relations between in vitro enzyme activities and in vivo potency in commercial pancreatic extracts. New England Journal of Medicine 1977;296(23):1314–1317.

39 Graham DY. An enteric-coated pancreatic enzyme preparation that works. Digestive Diseases and Sciences 1979;24(12):906–909.

40 Whitcomb DC, et al. Pancrelipase delayed-release capsules (CREON) for exocrine pancreatic insufficiency due to chronic pancreatitis or pancreatic surgery: a double-blind randomized trial. American Journal of Gastroenterology 2010;105(10):2276–2286.

41 Gubergrits N, et al. A 6-month, open-label clinical trial of pancrelipase delayed-release capsules (Creon) in patients with exocrine pancreatic insufficiency due to chronic pancreatitis or pancreatic surgery. Alimentary Pharmacology and Therapeutics 2011;33(10):1152–1161.

42 Toskes PP, et al. Efficacy of a novel pancreatic enzyme product, EUR-1008 (Zenpep), in patients with exocrine pancreatic insufficiency due to chronic pancreatitis. Pancreas 2011;40(3):376–382.

43 Ramesh H, et al. A 51-week, open-label clinical trial in India to assess the efficacy and safety of pancreatin 40000 enteric-coated minimicrospheres in patients with pancreatic exocrine insufficiency due to chronic pancreatitis. Pancreatology 2013;13(2):133–139.

44 Trang T, Chan J, Graham DY. Pancreatic enzyme replacement therapy for pancreatic exocrine insufficiency in the 21(st) century. World Journal of Gastroenterology 2014;20(33):11467–11485.

45 Sikkens EC, et al. Patients with exocrine insufficiency due to chronic pancreatitis are undertreated: a Dutch national survey. Pancreatology 2012;12(1):71–73.

PART B: Nutritional treatment: antioxidant treatment

Ajith K. Siriwardena[1,2]

[1] Department of Hepatobiliary Surgery, University of Manchester, Manchester, UK
[2] Regional Hepato-Pancreato-Biliary Surgery Unit, Manchester Royal Infirmary, Manchester, UK

Introduction

Chronic pancreatitis (CP) is defined as an inflammatory disorder of the pancreas characterized clinically by recurrent abdominal pain associated with the eventual development of pancreatic exocrine and endocrine insufficiency [1]. These changes are matched histologically by loss of normal parenchymal architecture with replacement by fibrotic scar tissue, parenchymal and ductal calcification together with distortion and abnormalities of the main pancreatic duct.

Abdominal pain is the dominant symptom and has a complex basis of origin [2]. Current concepts of pain in CP suggest that there is a pancreatic glandular component, probably related to parenchymal inflammation and ductal obstruction or hypertension and that in addition there is an extra-pancreatic component related to changes in visceral afferent pain nerves and also to alterations in central nervous system perception and processing of pain [3, 4].

As neither endoscopic nor surgical intervention provide reliable pain relief in all patients, the search for alternative treatments led Braganza and colleagues to propose the oxidative stress paradigm of cellular injury in CP [5]. This theory proposed that CP arose as a result of pathologic exposure of pancreatic acinar cells to short-lived oxygen-derived free radicals produced as a result of an imbalance between their production and quenching [5]. Essential cellular oxygen reduction (redox) pathways were overcome in CP leading to the clinical syndrome. Micronutrient antioxidant therapy was developed as a tablet-based medication to restore components of these deficient pathways and was introduced into clinical practice in Manchester, England, in the 1980s, setting up a controversy in pancreatology that to some extent continues to this day. In its favor, the oxidative stress hypothesis is elegant and scientifically plausible with micronutrient antioxidant therapy having the attraction of treating all disease variants of CP and of avoiding surgical intervention. Against the hypothesis questions are raised as to the validity of the evidence base underlying both the hypothesis and the clinical effectiveness of antioxidant therapy.

This chapter provides a concise review of the hypothesis (and the evidence base for this) and undertakes a reappraisal of current evidence for antioxidant therapy as a treatment for CP.

Basis of the "oxidative stress–micronutrient antioxidant" hypothesis

There were four key components of the micronutrient antioxidant hypothesis [5]. The first premise of the hypothesis was that exposure to toxic xenobiotic substances (such as inhaled volatile hydrocarbons) caused pancreatic injury. The second premise was that the mechanism of injury was by pathological induction of the cytochrome P450 system within the pancreatic acinar cell. The third was that hepatic cytochrome P450 induction led to the exposure of pancreatic acinar cells to oxidative stress by-products by reflux of liver-originated toxic compounds into the pancreatic duct via passage in the bile duct, and the final pillar of this concept was that micronutrient antioxidant therapy given in tablet form would restore intra-acinar pharmacological balance, reduce inflammation, and thus be a treatment for pain in CP.

Modern re-appraisal of the "oxidative stress–micronutrient antioxidant" hypothesis

Much of the evidence for the first component of the hypothesis comes from an occupational health study carried out in Manchester, UK, in the 1980s [6]. McNamee and colleagues matched 102 cases of CP with 204 age and sex-matched referents from the same geographic areas of the Manchester conurbation obtaining information about their occupational histories, alcohol intake, cigarette smoking, and diet. Exposure to hydrocarbons was inferred from interview responses by four assessors who were blind to disease state and these data were then summarized by a cumulative hydrocarbon exposure (CHE) score. The key finding of the study was that high hydrocarbon exposure was present in 24 (24%) of patients with CP compared with 21 (10%) of controls. The authors concluded "These results support the original hypothesis."

A modern reappraisal of this evidence immediately highlights two important deficiencies. First, high hydrocarbon exposure was present in only 24 of 102 patients with CP; thus, high hydrocarbon exposure is not a necessary prerequisite for the development of CP.

Second, this study does not adequately control for the confounding effect of alcohol with almost half of patients in the CP group consuming over 50 units of alcohol per week.

A computerized literature search reveals that only one other study examines the role of xenobiotic exposure as an etiological agent for CP and this South African study takes the form of an interview with a case series of 112 patients with CP [7]. Although 86 (77%) described exposure to burning firewood and coal, 104 (93%) consumed alcohol, with 44 (39%) of these patients consuming alcohol on a daily basis.

In summary, occupational exposure to hydrocarbons is not a necessary etiological agent for the development of CP.

The second component of the hypothesis is that xenobiotic exposure leads to induction of cytochrome P450 within pancreatic acinar cells [5]. The pancreas is recognized as one of the extrahepatic sites of production of cytochrome P450. Chronic exposure to xenobiotics, either in the form of ingested toxins such as alcohol or inhaled volatile chemicals was hypothesized as leading to cytochrome induction. In turn, cytochrome metabolism led to the intra-acinar generation of toxic free radicals.

The past three decades have witnessed a substantial increase in the understanding of cytochrome biology both in terms of function, role in drug detoxification, and in terms of patterns of differential expression and function [8, 9].

However, in relation to the pancreas, modern knowledge suggests that intra-acinar functional expression of cytochromes is a small fraction of hepatocyte expression of these proteins and a further consistent finding is that much pancreatic expression is within islets [10]. Thus, although intra-acinar expression of cytochromes in response to toxins is likely to occur, it is a small component of a pathophysiological response to injury and not the key or unique step it was once thought to be.

The third component of the hypothesis was that hepatocyte-derived oxidant by-products may contribute to pancreatic injury by passage along the bile duct and reflux into the pancreatic duct. This theory led to the highly idiosyncratic operation of bile duct ligation to divert bile in patients with CP [11]. These patients continued to experience recurrent pancreatitis after biliary diversion, and it is clear that bile duct ligation has no helpful effect on the clinical course of CP.

Taken together, the evidence base for these three components of the hypothesis is not strong. Setting this evidence in the context of current knowledge of the pathophysiology of CP would suggest that free-radical-mediated cellular injury is one of a host of cell damage mechanisms rather than an isolated causal factor. Importantly, in terms of practical clinical advice to patients, there is no strong evidence linking xenobiotic exposure to subsequent CP.

However, a nonsustainable hypothesis does not necessarily preclude antioxidant therapy from being effective and thus the clinical evidence for this treatment should be assessed separately.

Clinical trials of antioxidant therapy in chronic pancreatitis

Assessment of the clinical efficacy of antioxidant therapy for pain relief in CP is affected by the lack of consistency in the use of the term antioxidant. Furthermore, antioxidant therapy has been evaluated in a range of pancreatic inflammatory diseases including acute pancreatitis with a broad range of therapeutic interventions in a range of clinical disease with a variety of endpoints. Thus, conventional systematic review is not applicable. These limitations notwithstanding, Cai and colleagues undertook a systematic review of nine randomized controlled trials (RCTs) of antioxidant therapy in CP [12]. It is noteworthy that the nine trials contained in their systematic review include a total of 390 patients highlighting the relatively small size of the majority of these trials. Their key finding was that overall, antioxidant therapy was not associated with a reduction in pain in patients with CP while there was evidence that antioxidant therapy increased adverse effects [12]. The broad range of interventions for which the label "antioxidant therapy" is attached is seen as the systematic review included trials of compound selenium-methionine-based antioxidant therapy, curcumin, allopurinol, and selenomethionine. Also, the duration of therapy, patient populations, and assessment of interventions and endpoints differ with only one study undertaking a formal assessment of the effect of intervention on quality of life. Broadly similar findings were reported in a recent Cochrane systematic review [13].

To provide a more in-depth assessment of the potential clinical role of antioxidant therapy in CP, the randomized trials of compound selenium/methionine/vitamin C-based antioxidant therapy can be dichotomized into the older small trials and two more recent larger and well-conducted trials from the twenty-first century.

In the former category, the index Manchester study was a randomized, placebo-controlled trial in 20 patients with recurrent acute pancreatitis, which used a cross-over design comparing 10 weeks of antioxidant therapy with placebo [14]. The principal clinical outcome was the assessment of frequency of episodes of pancreatitis, and there were six episodes of pancreatitis on placebo versus none on treatment ($P = 0.032$). A more recent randomized, placebo-controlled trial in 19 patients with well-characterized CP from Belfast used compound antioxidant therapy (antox; Pharmanord, UK) as an intervention and compared 10 weeks of treatment with 10 weeks of placebo in a cross-over design [15]. The primary endpoint was completion of the Short Form-36 (SF-36) questionnaire. The principal clinical outcome was that 17 patients reported improvement in quality of life on antox compared with 7 on

placebo. Eight patients reported improvement in social functioning on antox compared with seven on placebo. These results highlight the importance of the placebo response in assessing interventions in patients with CP.

For their time, these were pathfinding studies. However, they were trials of small sample size assessing an intervention of unknown efficacy in a disease with an unknown responsiveness to this intervention. The probability of type I error is high, and no modern treatment strategy can any longer be based on this evidence.

Modern randomized controlled clinical trials of antioxidant therapy in chronic pancreatitis

The modern era features two larger and well-conducted RCTs of antioxidant therapy in CP. Bhardwaj and colleagues from Delhi undertook a double-blind, placebo-controlled randomized trial of antioxidant therapy in CP [16]. Patients were selected for inclusion on the basis of magnetic resonance (MR) scan, endoscopic retrograde pancreatography (ERP), or computed tomography (CT). There was no prior pancreatic intervention of any form and those who were narcotic addicts were excluded. The study intervention was compound antioxidant therapy in the form of 600 μg selenium, ascorbic acid, β-carotene, α-tocopherol, and methionine manufactured commercially as Betamore (G Osper, India). Pain was assessed as the number of "painful days." The patient profiles show that the majority had idiopathic CP and that the median body mass index in the treatment group was 20.2 ± 3.1 (compared with 19.7 ± 3.5 in placebo). Strikingly, 18 (32%) patients in the treatment group were malnourished with a BMI of <18.5 (with a comparable number in placebo). The principal outcome was a reduction in days in pain in the treatment arm from 9.1 ± 7.6 at baseline to 1.6 ± 2.8 at 6 months. This reduction was significant when compared with the placebo group at 6 months. However, the striking finding in this assessment is the dramatic placebo response (at 6 months: 3.3 ± 4.3 days in pain from a baseline level of 7.2 ± 5.3 days in pain).

Almost in parallel to this trial, the ANTICIPATE study in Manchester set out to evaluate the effect of antox (a compound antioxidant therapy) in patients with established painful CP [17]. Patients with a clinical diagnosis of CP were identified by a combination of

CT scan and assessment of pancreatic elastase. Patients maintained pain diaries in a 1-month run-in period to establish that their symptoms were stable and that self-scored pain was at least 5 on at least 7 in 30 days on a numerical rating scale (NRS) of 11 points from 0 to 10. Patients were randomized to receive either compound antioxidant therapy (Antox, Morpeth, UK) with each tablet of antox comprising 480 mg methionine, 38.5 mg of selenium, and 126.3 mg of ascorbic acid (vitamin C) or a matched placebo. The primary endpoint was pain scores assessed in the outpatient clinic at 2, 4, and 6 months. Secondary endpoints included pain diary pain scores maintained by patients (as a correlate to the scores assessed in clinic) and quality of life assessed by a variety of measures including the EORTC QLQ-Pan28 score validated for use in CP. Patients were stratified by prior pancreatic intervention.

A total of 356 patients were screened and 92 randomized with 70 completing 6 months of either intervention or placebo (37 in placebo and 33 in antioxidant arm). The demographic profile revealed a median (range) age of 49.8 ± 12.7 years in the antioxidant group. This was not significantly different from the 50 ± 9 years in the control group but this represents a much older age group than that seen in the Delhi trial. Further the demographic profile of ANTICIPATE comprised mainly male patients with a disease duration of 4.2 ± 2.4 years, with clinic pain scores of 5.2 ± 1.6 (on a 0–10 scale) at baseline and a predominantly alcohol-related etiology (72% in the antioxidant arm and 73% in the placebo arm).

A further important difference between the Delhi and Manchester trials is in the morphology of CP, as in the Manchester study only 45% of patients in the treatment arm had pancreatic duct dilatation with the majority having the European normal disease variant of a pancreatic head mass.

The final results of ANTICIPATE showed that there was no difference in the primary endpoint with clinic pain scores Similarly, there was no difference in any of the secondary endpoints of patient-recorded diary pain scores or quality-of-life measures. Antioxidant therapy was associated with a significant elevation in antioxidant levels (change from baseline for selenium values in the placebo group was 0.92 (12.39) mg/mL compared with an increase in the treatment arm: change from baseline to 6 months in the treatment arm: 42.73 (32.27) mg/mL with this difference being significant ($P < 0.001$).

Thus, ANTICIPATE concluded that "in patients with painful chronic pancreatitis of predominantly alcoholic origin, antioxidant therapy does not reduce pain or improve quality of life, despite increasing blood levels of antioxidants."

Comparing and contrasting the Delhi and Manchester clinical trials

Whenever two similar trials reach contrasting conclusions, there is an apparent discord. Both studies are credible and can be believed so how can the apparent difference be reconciled? Although both studies used antioxidant therapy, the specific intervention was different and thus potentially of different efficacy. It is also possible that the differences arise simply from chance. However, the likely explanation lies in the different demographic profiles with the Delhi study including predominantly young patients with idiopathic CP and significant malnutrition.

The benefits seen in the Delhi study may be related to the treatment of malnutrition in a cohort of patients where up to a third had a BMI of <18.5. At the least, the confounding effect of treatment of malnutrition cannot be excluded.

Interestingly in the Delhi study, there was no benefit of antioxidant therapy in the subgroup with CP of alcohol etiology.

Risks associated with high-dose selenium therapy

It could be argued that a pragmatic approach to antioxidant therapy could be adopted with the reasoning being that if treatment may benefit some patients it could continue to be evaluated as a first-line treatment. The risk with this approach is that there is an increasing body of evidence suggesting that selenium therapy may be harmful. For example, SELECT an RCT of selenium + vitamin E (alone or combined) for the reduction of prostate cancer risk in 35,333 participants reported that while neither selenium nor vitamin E supplementation reduced risk, selenium was associated with a 91% increase in the risk of prostate cancer ($P < 0.007$) with vitamin E also increasing the risk of prostate cancer

[18]. Thus, casual use of antioxidant therapy should be discouraged.

Current recommendation for antioxidant therapy in chronic pancreatitis

In its time, the micronutrient antioxidant theory provided a genuine stimulus to research and clinical practice in pancreatology. Free-radical-induced cellular damage is accepted as one of the mechanisms of acinar injury in CP. However, the passage of time makes it clear that the assumption that biochemical pathways were compromised as a result of cytochrome P450 induction due to environmental xenobiotic exposure is not sustainable on reappraisal of evidence applying modern assessment criteria.

Although the hypothesis does not stand the test of time, is it still possible that micronutrient antioxidant therapy could be beneficial in CP? The two large contemporary trials from Delhi and Manchester were both conducted and reported to acceptable standards but reached different conclusions. Reaching a sustainable consensus view from both trials, it appears that antioxidant therapy is ineffective in patients in their fourth or fifth decades of life with disease of alcohol etiology. The apparent benefit in patients in their twenties with idiopathic CP may relate to the benefits of treatment of malnutrition.

Casual prescription of antioxidant therapy cannot be sustained in view of the well-demonstrated risks associated with the use of selenium and vitamin E therapy.

The EUROPAC 2 study evaluating antox is ongoing (having opened to recruitment in 2005) and, although this study evaluates antioxidant therapy only in hereditary pancreatitis and idiopathic CP, it is still to report and no final conclusion has been reached until this time [19].

However, the current recommendation, pending the reporting of this final study is that antioxidant therapy should no longer be prescribed for patients with painful CP.

Declaration

The ANTICIPATE study was supported by an unrestricted educational grant from Pharmanord, Morpeth,

UK. The author has no other disclosures or conflicts of interest.

References

1 Singer MV, Gyr K, Sarles H. nclassification of pancreatitis. Report of the second international symposium on the classification of pancreatitis in Marseille, France March 28–30 1984. Gastroenterology 1985; 89:683–685.
2 Mullady DK, Yadav D, Amann ST, et al. Type of pain, pain-associated complications, quality of life, disability and resource utilisation in chronic pancreatitis: a prospective cohort study. Gut 2011; 60:77–84.
3 Ceyhan GO, Bergmann F, Kadihasanoglu M, et al. Pancreatic neuropathy and neuropathic pain-a comprehensive pathomorphological study of 546 cases. Gastroenterology 2009; 136: 177–186.
4 Drewes AM, Krarup AL, Detlefsen S, et al. Pain in chronic pancreatitis: the role of neuropathic pain mechanisms. Gut 2008; 57:1616–1627.
5 Braganza JM, Dormandy TL. Micronutrient therapy for chronic pancreatitis: rationale and impact. Journal of the Pancreas 2010; 11:99–112.
6 Mcnamee R, Braganza JM, Hogg J, et al. Occupational exposure to hydrocarbons and chronic pancreatitis: a case-referent study. Occupational and Environmental Medicine 1994; 51:631 637.
7 Jeppe CV, Smith MD. Transversal descriptive study of xenobiotic exposures in patients with chronic pancreatitis and pancreatic cancer. Journal of the Pancreas 2008;9:235–239.
8 Nelson DR. The cytochrome P450 homepage. Human Genomics 2009; 4:59–65.
9 Zordoky BN, El-Kadi BO. Role of NF-kappaB in the regulation of cytochrome P450 enzymes. Current Drug Metabolism 2009; 10:164–178.
10 Standop J, Schneider M, Ulrich A, et al. Differences in immunohistochemical expression of xenobiotic-metabolizing enzymes between normal pancreas, chronic pancreatitis and pancreatic cancer. Toxicologic Pathology 2003; 31:506–513.
11 Sandilands D, Jeffrey IJM, Haboubi NY, et al. Abnormal drug metabolism in chronic pancreatitis. Gastroenterology 1990; 98:766–772.
12 Cai G-H, Huang J, Zhao Y, et al. Antioxidant therapy for pain relief in patients with chronic pancreatitis: systematic review and meta-analysis. Pain Physician 2013; 16:521–532
13 Ahmed AU, Jens S, Busch OR, et al. Antioxidants for pain in chronic pancreatitis. Cochrane Database Systematic Reviews 2014;21(8):CD008945.
14 Uden S, Bilton D, Nathan L, et al. Antioxidant therapy for recurrent pancreatitis: placebo-controlled trial. Alimentary Pharmacology and Therapeutics 1990;4:357–371.
15 Kirk GR, White JS, McKie L, et al. Combined antioxidant therapy reduces pain and improves quality of life in chronic

pancreatitis. Journal of Gastrointestinal Surgery 2006; 10:499–503.

16 Bhardwaj P, Garg PK, Maulik SK, et al. A randomized controlled trial of antioxidant supplementation for pain relief in patients with chronic pancreatitis. Gastroenterology 2009;136:149–159.

17 Siriwardena AK, Mason JM, Sheen AJ et al. Antioxidant therapy does not reduce pain in patients with chronic pancreatitis: the ANTICIPATE study. Gastroenterology 2012; 43:655–663.

18 Kristal A, Darke AK, Morris JS, et al. Baseline selenium status and effects of selenium and vitamin e supplementation on prostate cancer risk. Journal of the National Cancer Institute 2014; 106:1–8.

19 www.clinicaltrials.gov>home>find studies>EUROPAC 2. Accessed December 7, 2014.

PART C: Pancreatogenic diabetes: etiology, implications, and management

Dana K. Andersen

Division of Digestive Diseases and Nutrition, National Institute of Diabetes and Digestive and Kidney Diseases, National Institutes of Health, Bethesda, MD, USA

Introduction

Pancreatogenic diabetes, also referred to as pancreatic diabetes or apancreatic diabetes, is a form of secondary diabetes classified as type 3c diabetes (T3cD) by the American Diabetes Association (ADA) [1]. Although known as a form of diabetes from the time of Von Mering and Minkowski's demonstration in 1889 of the diabetogenic effects of pancreatectomy [2], the clinical incidence and prevalence of T3cD are incompletely understood, and it is frequently misdiagnosed as either type 1 diabetes (T1D) or type 2 diabetes (T2D) [3].

The purposes of this review are threefold: (i) to review the known causative illnesses, prevalence, and mechanism(s) associated with T3cD, (ii) to describe the practical importance of distinguishing T3cD from other types of diabetes and the evidence that identifies T3cD as a high-risk group for the subsequent development of pancreatic ductal adenocarcinoma (PDAC), and (iii) to provide a rationale for the approach to management of T3cD.

Etiology of T3cD

Classification of T3cD by ADA

The ADA characterizes the types of diabetes that are caused by underlying diseases or conditions as secondary, or type 3, diabetes [1] (see Table 14C.1). Included within the category of T3cD are those congenital or acquired diseases of the exocrine pancreas, including (acute or chronic) pancreatitis, pancreatic resection or trauma, pancreatic neoplasia, cystic fibrosis, hemochromatosis, and pancreatic agenesis. This classification system has been adopted by the Centers for Disease Control and Prevention [4], The European Association for the Study of Diabetes [5], and the World Health Organization [6].

Despite the widespread recognition of T3cD, there are no guidelines for the treatment of T3cD by these organizations, and no universally accepted procedure or system for the identification of T3cD separately from other forms of diabetes. A consensus conference on T3cD secondary to chronic pancreatitis (CP) was organized by the annual PancreasFest meeting in 2012, and consensus recommendations from that conference regarding the diagnosis and treatment of T3cD were published by Rickels et al. [7].

Clinical characteristics and prevalence of T3cD

T3cD has a variable clinical presentation, which ranges from mild glucose intolerance to severe periods of hyperglycemia alternating with profound hypoglycemia. The most extreme pattern is also referred to as "brittle diabetes," which implies ongoing insulin dependency despite exaggerated sensitivity to insulin [8]. Several clinical and laboratory findings distinguish T3cD from T1D and T2D, and help to explain the mechanisms for the "brittleness" (see Table 14C.2). Because T3cD is usually accompanied by exocrine insufficiency, metabolic abnormalities include nutritional abnormalities, vitamin deficiencies, and malnutrition in addition to diabetes. Moreover, exocrine insufficiency results in

Table **14C.1** American Diabetes Association etiologic classification of diabetes mellitus.

I. **Type 1 diabetes** (β-cell destruction, usually leading to absolute insulin deficiency)
   a) **Immune mediated**
   b) **Idiopathic**
II. **Type 2 diabetes** (insulin resistance with relative or severe insulin secretory deficiency)
III. **Other specific types** (secondary diabetes)
   a) **Genetic defects of β-cell function** (such as chromosomal defects causing maturity-onset diabetes of the young, or MODY, syndromes)
   b) **Genetic defects in insulin action** (such as type A insulin resistance, leprechaunism, and lipoatrophic diabetes)
   c) **Diseases of the Exocrine Pancreas**
     i. Acute and chronic pancreatitis
     ii. Trauma/pancreatectomy
     iii. Neoplasia
     iv. Cystic fibrosis
     v. Hemochromatosis
     vi. Fibrocalculous pancreatopathy
     vii. Pancreatic agenesis
     viii. Others
   d) **Endocrinopathies** (such as acromegaly, Cushing syndrome, glucagonoma, somatostatinoma, pheochromocytoma)
   e) **Drug or chemical induced** (such as glucocorticoids, diazoxide, thiazide diuretics, cyclosporine, dilantin, β-adrenergic agonists)
   f) **Infections** (such as congenital rubella, cytomegalovirus)
   g) **Uncommon forms of immune-mediated diabetes** (such as Stiff-man syndrome)
   h) **Other genetic syndromes sometimes associated with diabetes** (such as Down syndrome, porphyria, Prader–Willi syndrome, myotonic dystrophy)
IV. **Gestational diabetes mellitus**

Adapted from: American Diabetes Association [1] with permission.

Table **14C.2** Clinical and laboratory findings in types of diabetes.

Parameter	T1D	T2D	T3cD
Ketoacidosis	Common	Rare	Rare
Hyperglycemia	Severe	Usually mild	Mild
Hypoglycemia	Common	Rare	Common
Peripheral insulin sensitivity	Normal or increased	Decreased	Increased
Hepatic insulin sensitivity	Normal	Normal or decreased	Decreased
Insulin levels	Low	High	Low
Glucagon levels	Normal or high	Normal or high	Low
PP levels	High (early), low (late)	High	Low
GIP levels	Normal or low	Normal or high	Low
GLP-1 levels	Normal	Normal or high	Normal or high
Typical age of onset	Childhood or adolescence	Adulthood	Any

Adapted from: Cui and Andersen [9] with permission.

fat malabsorption, which results in an impaired incretin response to nutrients [10]. Therefore, the mechanisms of disordered glucose metabolism in T3cD are complex and incompletely understood.

There are no published data on the prevalence of T3cD in North America. In the most definitive study available, Hardt and Ewald studied over 1900 diabetic patients referred to an academic medical center in

Germany and carefully examined the records, clinical findings, and laboratory studies of this population. They found that 8% of their entire diabetic population were properly characterized as T3cD and that half of this cohort had been previously misdiagnosed as T1D (6%) or T2D (45%) [3]. CP was found to be the etiology in 78% of patients with T3cD (see Figure 14C.1).

Diabetes caused by CP is an important contributor to the T3cD population. The prevalence of diabetes in CP varies from 20% to 70% in various studies [11–13] and is dependent of the duration of the CP. A study of 500 patients with mostly alcoholic CP revealed that 85% of patients eventually developed diabetes when followed for over 25 years [14]. Progressive fibrosis with loss of vascularity and ischemic atrophy of the pancreas results in eventual loss of islet tissue and is assumed to be the cause of T3cD secondary to CP.

Recently, a study by Das et al. revealed that diabetes and/or "prediabetes" was seen in 37% of people after an initial episode of acute pancreatitis (AP) [15]. In this meta-analysis of over 1100 patients described in 24 clinical studies, newly diagnosed diabetes developed in 15% of patients within 12 months after a single episode of AP. Furthermore, the prevalence of this otherwise uncharacterized diabetes increased progressively over the following 5 years. Surprisingly, there was no association with the severity (i.e., extent of pancreatic necrosis) of AP and the subsequent development of diabetes, nor any correlation with the age of the patient at the time of AP. It is not known whether these patients progressed to CP, although patients with a known diagnosis of CP were excluded from the analysis. Furthermore, the incidence of diabetes exceeded the known rate for the development of CP after an episode of AP. As AP is now the leading hospital discharge diagnosis of gastrointestinal disease in the United States, representing over 270,000 patients annually [16], the implication of these findings is that a single prior episode of AP alone may be an important etiologic event in the subsequent development of T3cD.

Pathophysiology of T3cD

Pancreatogenic diabetes was known to be associated with low levels of circulating insulin and a compensatory increased sensitivity to insulin by the early 1980s [17], but the alterations in insulin action in T3cD were poorly understood until the glucose clamp technique of Andres [18] was used with isotopic glucose infusion in dogs with CP. Sun et al. showed that although levels of circulating insulin were low, hepatic sensitivity to insulin was greatly reduced despite normal or increased peripheral insulin sensitivity [19]. This dichotomy in insulin sensitivity explained the hyperglycemia of the condition, due to unsuppressed hepatic glucose production, despite increased glucose uptake by peripheral tissues when insulin was administered. Subsequently, such paradoxical hepatic insulin resistance was documented in T3cD secondary to pancreatic resection [20], CP [21], pancreatic carcinoma [22], and cystic fibrosis [23].

The cause of persistent hepatic glucose production and isolated hepatic insulin resistance in T3cD appears to be multifactorial. Insulin-regulated hepatic glucose

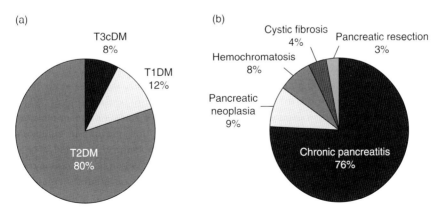

Figure 14C.1 Prevalence of types of diabetes. (a) Distribution of types of diabetes and (b) causes of type 3c (pancreatogenic) diabetes based on studies of 1922 diabetic patients reported by Hardt et al. [3]. From Cui and Andersen [9] with permission.

production is dependent upon the availability and function of insulin receptors as well as the availability and function of glucose transporter type 2 (GLUT2) proteins on the hepatocyte plasma membrane [24]. Seymour et al. showed that in T3cD, due to CP, the number of available hepatic insulin receptors was significantly decreased [25], and Nathan et al. showed that the internalization (endocytosis) of hepatocyte plasma membrane GLUT2 is impaired in CP [26]. Further studies by this group suggested that insulin receptors and GLUT2 transporters are physically linked on the hepatocyte plasma membrane and that impaired clathrin-mediated endocytosis of an insulin receptor–glucose transporter complex may explain the dual abnormality, which results in persistent hepatic glucose production [27].

In addition to altered insulin receptor availability, altered hepatic insulin function in CP has also been linked to inflammation-based activation of hepatocyte I-kappa beta kinase (IKK)-beta (IKK-β) and nuclear factor-κB (NF-κB) [28]. Blockade of NF-κB activation results in improved hepatic insulin sensitivity, possibly due to suppressed expression of proinflammatory cytokines [29]. This effect can be achieved by the activation of peroxisome proliferator-activated receptor-gamma (PPAR-γ), which is the mechanism of action of the thiozolidinedione (TZD) class of antidiabetic drugs; the TZD rosiglitazone has been shown to reverse hepatic insulin resistance in rats with CP [30].

Diagnosis of T3cD

A prior history of pancreatic disease, such as acute or CP, is an important factor in making the diagnosis of T3cD, but this alone does not rule out the possibility that the diabetes was antecedent to the development of pancreatitis. Therefore, Ewald and Hardt screened patients with anti-β-cell antibodies to rule out autoimmune disease. In addition, they performed screening studies of exocrine function (fecal elastase levels) and selected pancreatic imaging to detect those patients with undiagnosed but clinically detectable pancreatic disease [3].

In their consensus conference report on the diabetes associated with CP, Rickels et al. stressed that patients with CP should be screened annually with fasting glucose levels and hemoglobin A_{1c} levels [7]. If either of these values becomes abnormal, formal glucose tolerance testing should be performed to confirm a diagnosis of diabetes. In addition to the historical and laboratory

Table 14C.3 Criteria for the diagnosis of pancreatogenic (type 3c) diabetes.

1 Absence of anti-islet antibodies
2 Documented history or radiographic evidence of pancreatic disease
3 Pancreatic exocrine insufficiency
4 Deficient pancreatic polypeptide response to ingested nutrients

From: Rickels et al. [7] with permission.

criteria used by Ewald and Hardt, however, Rickels and colleagues recommended testing for a failure of nutrient-induced release of pancreatic polypeptide (PP) as a specific indicator to differentiate T3cD from the 10-fold more prevalent T2D (see Table 14C.3).

Pancreatic polypeptide (PP) – a marker for T3cD?

PP physiology and pathophysiology

PP was discovered by Kimmel et al. as a by-product during the purification of avian insulin [31]. Simultaneously, it was found by Chance and coworkers to be an islet hormone in several species [32]. It is a highly conserved 36 amino acid peptide, which is secreted almost exclusively from the F-cells, or PP-cells, of the pancreatic islet (see Figure 14C.2). PP-cells are found predominantly in islets located in the uncinate process or posterior pancreatic head. In these islets, the PP-cells form a mantle around the periphery of the islet and are second only to β-cells in their concentration. A small number (~5%) of PP-cells are scattered throughout the dorsal pancreas [34]. The uncinate process of the pancreas originates as the ventral pancreatic bud, which eventually fuses with the dorsal pancreatic bud in gestational week 5. The dorsal pancreas (the origin of the body and tail of the pancreas) is relatively rich in α-cells or glucagon-containing cells, which are nearly absent from the ventral pancreas. Therefore, the contrasting presence of PP- or α-cells is the only histologic feature that differentiates the ventral and dorsal portions, respectively, of the pancreas [35] (see Figure 14C.3).

PP is one of three members of the "PP family" of regulatory peptides. Neuropeptide Y (NPY) and peptide YY (PYY) comprise the other members of the family and share considerable amino acid sequence homology

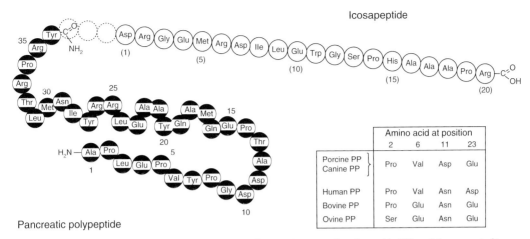

Figure 14C.2 Pancreatic polypeptide. The amino acid structure of (canine) pancreatic polypeptide (PP) and the connected icosapeptide that is synthesized as a precursor molecule in PP- or F-cells of the pancreatic islets. The amino acids that differ in mammalian PPs are shown in the box. The "hairpin fold" of the peptide is conserved among all members of the PP family of peptides. From Schwartz [33] with permission.

[36]. Despite their similar chemical structure, the PP family members have distinct regulatory roles. PYY is released from small intestinal "L" cells where it is colocalized with the incretin glucagon-like peptide-1 (GLP-1) and serves as a regulator of pancreatic growth and function. NPY is a neuropeptide that regulates food intake, among other functions, and is found within the central nervous system. A class of six G-protein-coupled receptors named "Y" receptors binds the PP family members with variable affinity [37]. The Y4 receptor subtype has the highest affinity for PP and is located throughout the gastroenterohepatic system as well as in the central nervous system [38].

Soon after its discovery, PP was found to be released promptly after ingestion of nutrients, with a four- to fivefold increase in plasma levels that lasted for up to 3 hours after a meal [39]. This response was initially found to be stimulated by cholecystokinin (CCK) [40], and has been shown to be linked to the secretion of glucose-dependent insulinotropic polypeptide (GIP) [41, 42]. The PP response to nutrients is exquisitely cholinergically dependent, however, and is obliterated by truncal vagotomy or atropine [33, 43]. The prolonged release and vigorous response of PP after feeding suggested that it had a regulatory role in digestion or metabolism, but studies of purified PP administration in normal human volunteers failed to demonstrate any changes in glucose, insulin, glucagon, or other nutrients

or hormones [44]. Laboratory studies suggested that PP had an inhibitory effect on choleresis [44] and pancreatic exocrine secretion [45, 46], but the physiologic role of PP remained obscure until studies were performed in states of PP deficiency.

Early clinical studies demonstrated that PP levels were elevated in obesity, in normal aging, in T2D, and in early T1D [47–49]. In addition, PP levels were seen to be markedly elevated in pancreatic neuroendocrine tumors [50, 51] although no symptoms were associated with PP hypersecretion *per se*. Decreased PP levels after nutrient ingestion were observed in severe CP [52, 53], after proximal pancreatectomy [54], in cystic fibrosis [55], and in diabetic autonomic neuropathy [56]. The observations of increased PP levels in glucose intolerant states associated with T2D suggested a role of PP in the regulation of glucose metabolism, and laboratory studies of congenitally obese rodents suggested an insulin-sparing effect of PP [57, 58]. However, the early studies of PP administration to normal volunteers were unrevealing, so the role of PP and its relationship to glucoregulation remained unclear.

Clinical studies of PP deficiency and PP replacement

As PP deficiency was known to be a feature of CP [52, 53], the effect of PP replacement was examined in a canine model of T3cD due to CP. Although acute

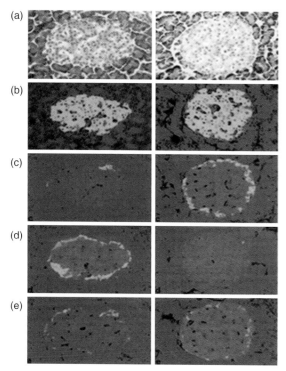

Figure 14C.3 Endocrine anatomy of pancreatic islets. Serial sections of a representative islet found in the head or ventral (left panel) and tail or dorsal (right panel) portions of the pancreas. (a) Tissue stained with hematoxylin and eosin. (b) β-Cells immunohistochemically stained with anti-insulin antibody. (c) α-Cells stained with antiglucagon antibody. (d) Pancreatic polypeptide (PP) cells stained with anti-PP antibody. (e) δ-Cells stained with antisomatostatin antibody. Note the differential presence of α-cells and PP-cells in the dorsal and ventral portions of the pancreas, respectively. Adapted from: Orci [35] with permission.

treatment with PP resulted in no apparent effect [59], prolonged PP administration was found to reverse the hepatic resistance to insulin and to reverse the glucose intolerance in animals with CP [19]. To determine whether this effect was a direct result of hepatic dysfunction, Seymour et al. applied a rodent model of CP and found that *in vitro* perfusion of livers harvested from rats with CP also demonstrated hepatic insulin resistance [60] and that this resistance was reversed by PP administration [61]. The hepatic defect was found to be due to a loss of hepatic insulin receptor availability in PP-deficient animals, and PP was subsequently shown

to increase hepatic insulin receptor availability and hepatic insulin receptor gene expression [62].

PP deficiency had been documented in patients who had undergone proximal pancreatectomy [54], and in a study of patients who had recovered from pancreatic resections performed for trauma Seymour et al. showed that PP-deficient patients demonstrated hepatic insulin resistance during isotopic glucose clamp studies, whereas subjects with normal PP levels after distal pancreatectomy did not [20]. After an 8-hour intravenous infusion of PP, the hepatic insulin resistance was reversed in PP-deficient subjects, whereas PP administration had no effect on the normal hepatic insulin sensitivity of subjects with normal levels of PP. Subsequently, Brunicardi et al. performed the same studies in patients with documented CP and showed that a similar period of PP administration reversed the hepatic insulin resistance of PP-deficient subjects [21]. Furthermore, the PP infusion resulted in lowered glycemic levels in CP patients with hyperglycemia after oral glucose challenge (see Figure 14C.4). The association of impaired hepatic insulin sensitivity was subsequently shown in patients with pancreatic cancer [22] and in patients with cystic fibrosis [23]. Finally, in a randomized, blinded, placebo-controlled study, a 72-hour subcutaneous infusion of PP was found to improve overall insulin sensitivity in PP-deficient type 1 and type 3c diabetic patients who were on chronic insulin pump therapy [63].

So PP is a glucoregulatory hormone that regulates hepatic insulin sensitivity, and PP deficiency is a ubiquitous finding in all of the forms of T3cD studied thus far. Preliminary clinical studies suggest that PP replacement may have a therapeutic role in this form of diabetes, but native PP is rapidly metabolized in the circulation with a half-life of about 7 minutes. Therefore, recent efforts have focused on methods to protect PP from rapid degradation by lipid encapsulation [64] or other methods [65] to facilitate further studies of a possible therapeutic role on PP in T3cD.

Role of PP measurement in differentiating T3cD from T2D

The loss of PP responsiveness to ingested nutrients in T3cD contrasts dramatically with the elevated levels of PP seen in T2D and in normal aging (see Figure 14C.5), and this difference forms the basis for differentiating the less common T3cD from the larger population of T2D. In addition to a deficiency in the PP response to ingested

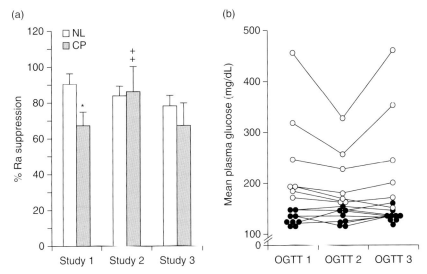

Figure 14C.4 Hepatic insulin sensitivity and glucose tolerance in patients with chronic pancreatitis before, during, and after PP administration. (a) Percent suppression of hepatic glucose production (Ra) during 2.0 mU/kg/min insulin infusion in six normal subjects (NL) and five patients with chronic pancreatitis accompanied by PP deficiency (CP), before (Study 1), during (Study 2), and 1 month after (Study 3) an 8-hour infusion of 2.0 pmol/kg/min of bovine PP. *$P < 0.05$ versus NL, ‡$P < 0.05$ versus Study 1. (b) Mean plasma glucose concentration during 180-minute oral glucose tolerance test in 6 normal subjects and 10 patients with chronic pancreatitis before (OGTT 1), 18 hours after (OGTT2), and 1 month after (OGTT3) an 8-hour infusion of 2.0 pmol/kg/min of bovine PP. Closed circles indicate normal glucose tolerance status on initial testing; open circles indicate impaired glucose tolerance or diabetes on initial glucose tolerance testing. After PP infusion, every patient with abnormal glucose tolerance demonstrated a lower mean glucose value. From Cui and Andersen [9] with permission.

nutrients, the absence of circulating anti-islet antibodies, a history or imaging evidence of pancreatic disease, and the demonstration of pancreatic exocrine insufficiency (PEI) have been proposed as the criteria for the diagnosis of T3cD [7, 67]. Further validation studies are needed, however, to determine whether these criteria are appropriate for all forms of T3cD.

PP deficiency cannot be determined from basal levels of the hormone; basal levels are similar in normal and PP-deficient subjects. PP secretion in response to oral nutrients varies with the type of nutrient; glucose is a relatively weak stimulant for PP release, whereas a mixed meal or a combined protein–fat–carbohydrate supplement is a strong stimulus for PP release. An 8 ounce volume of a commercial dietary supplement such as Boost® or Ensure® serves as a convenient standard test meal (STM) for the stimulated release of PP (and other enteric hormones) [7, 9]. Peak PP levels are seen 30–60 minutes after STM ingestion; a loss of PP responsiveness in the setting of fasting glucose levels greater than 126 mg/dL (7 mmol/L) or a hemoglobin

A_{1c} level greater than 7% is consistent with a diagnosis of T3cD.

Implications for risk for other diseases in T3cD

Metabolic disorders associated with exocrine insufficiency

In T3cD due to CP, the loss of exocrine function usually precedes the loss of endocrine function, as the islets remain relatively conserved despite progressive replacement of acinar tissue with fibrosis [24]. Therefore, patients with T3cD uniformly demonstrate PEI when it is quantified. As a result of a deficiency in lipase secretion, fat digestion is impaired, as is the absorption of the fat-soluble vitamins A, D, E, and K [9, 68].

The most prevalent adverse effect of the loss of fat soluble vitamins is the development of metabolic bone disease due to vitamin D deficiency. Osteopenia, osteoporosis, and an increased incidence of bone

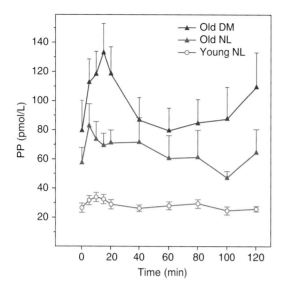

Figure 14C.5 PP responses to oral glucose in young normal, old normal, and old diabetic subjects. Serum PP responses to 75 g glucose ingested at time 0 in 10 healthy subjects aged less than 40 years with normal glucose tolerance (Young NL), 19 healthy subjects aged greater than 65 years with normal glucose tolerance (Old NL), and 21 elderly subjects with T2D (Old DM). Data are shown as mean ± SE. From Magruder et al. [66] with permission.

fractures have been documented in patients with CP, both without and with pancreatic enzyme replacement therapy (PERT) [68, 69].

Fat malabsorption is manifested by steatorrhea in some patients, but is not uniformly reported by patients with PEI. Some patients spontaneously adhere to a low-fat diet when they discover that "rich foods" result in multiple bowel movements and "indigestion." Other patients report that they can eat "whatever I want" but never gain weight. These symptoms of malabsorption should prompt assessment of exocrine function with fecal elastase levels or serum trypsin measurement [70]. When PEI is confirmed, restoration of adequate fat absorption helps to correct the consequences of vitamin deficiency and also helps to restore normal function of the incretin-based augmentation of insulin release [9, 71].

In addition to metabolic bone disease, nonalcoholic fatty liver disease (NAFLD) and nonalcoholic steatohepatitis (NASH) have been found to be associated with PEI in patients undergoing pancreatic resection [72, 73]. Treatment with PERT has been shown to improve the

findings of NAFLD on serial imaging. NAFLD and NASH are known to be associated with diabetes, and it is likely that T3cD is an important predisposing condition.

Association of T3cD with pancreatic ductal adenocarcinoma (PDAC)

Epidemiologic studies have repeatedly demonstrated an increased risk of PDAC in patients with both diabetes [74] and CP [75], and patients with PDAC are known to have coexisting diabetes in at least half of all cases [76, 77]. In most cohort studies, however, the type of diabetes has not been well characterized, or characterized at all, and the risk related to T3cD, *per se*, has remained unclear [66]. Two recent studies have appeared in which the risk of PDAC was examined in large populations of patients in which a history of CP was accompanied by (presumably type 3c) diabetes. In an examination of 200,000 patients enrolled in the Taiwan National Health System database, Liao and colleagues found that the risk of PDAC was increased 33-fold in patients in whom CP was accompanied by diabetes [78]. In a similar study of 9 million British National Health System patients, Brodovicz et al. found that the risk of PDAC was increased more than 12-fold in patients with a history of CP accompanied by diabetes [79].

In CP, the development of T3cD is a late manifestation of pancreatic exocrine destruction, and therefore the increase in PDAC risk associated with the presence of T3cD may merely reflect the advanced degree of the inflammatory processes, which contribute to the development of the malignancy. However, in patients with PDAC in whom no history of CP is present, new onset diabetes occurs in 25–50% of patients [74, 80]. This new-onset diabetes typically occurs anywhere from 6 months to 3 years before the PDAC is diagnosed and is believed to be caused by the PDAC due to an as yet unknown mechanism; roughly half of the patients with new-onset diabetes show improvement or resolution of their diabetes after resection of the malignancy [77, 81, 82]. Because PDAC is typically diagnosed at an advanced stage of disease, the presence of new-onset diabetes has been examined as a possible harbinger of the presence of otherwise asymptomatic PDAC. Unfortunately, due to the relatively low incidence of PDAC and the high incidence of diabetes in the aging population, new-onset but otherwise uncharacterized diabetes is not a sufficiently strong risk factor to justify imaging studies for PDAC [83–85]. In a study of over

2000 new-onset adult diabetic subjects in Ohmsted County, Minnesota, fewer than 1% developed PDAC within 3 years of the diagnosis [86].

It is, therefore, important to identify the T3cD that is caused by PDAC, as differentiated from the T2D that is the cause of new-onset diabetes in 99% of adults. One indicator of the presence of T3cD due to PDAC in a new-onset diabetic is the absence of a family history of diabetes and the presence of weight loss (or the absence of obesity). A history of prior pancreatitis or symptoms of exocrine insufficiency are additional historical clues. A family history of PDAC in two or more relatives increases the risk further and is taken as an indication for imaging studies of the pancreas [87]. Historical and clinical features do not clearly differentiate patients with PDAC-induced T3cD from patients with new-onset T2D, however, and hormonal markers have been evaluated as indicators of T3cD due to PDAC.

An elevated glucagon-to-insulin ratio in oral glucose tolerance test samples has been reported to correlate significantly with PDAC-induced diabetes as opposed to T2D [88], but it is unclear whether this can identify PDAC-associated diabetes with specificity. To distinguish T3cD caused by PDAC from T2D, Hart et al. have reported a pilot study in which the PP response to a mixed meal was significantly blunted in patients with PDAC with new-onset diabetes compared with T2D controls [89]. Not surprisingly, the effect was more pronounced in patients with tumors located in the pancreatic head, but the results suggest that larger studies are indicated to assess the value of surveying the PP response to nutrients.

Several investigators have searched for a biomarker of PDAC-induced T3cD. Pfeffer et al. described connexin-26, a gap junction protein, as being highly overexpressed in diabetic patients with PDAC [90], and a PDAC-derived S-100A8 N-terminal peptide has been described as a diabetogenic agent by Basso et al. [91]. Huang et al. described two upregulated genes in 27 patients with PDAC associated with new-onset diabetes, vanin-1 and matrix metalloproteinase 9, that showed high correlation [92] and a variety of micro-RNA fragments have been suggested as possibly having predictive usefulness [93]. Chari's group at the Mayo Clinic has suggested adrenomedullin as a peptide mediator of the impaired insulin sensitivity and secretion seen in PDAC-associated T3cD [94]. Adrenomedullin is a multifunctional vasoactive peptide, which has been

implicated in inflammation and sepsis [95]. Together with vanin-1, which is also expressed in response to inflammation, these finding suggest that mediators of inflammation may play a role in altered islet function and insulin action in PDAC. Further studies are currently underway to determine the usefulness of these and other markers of PDAC-associated T3cD.

The implications of validating T3cD as a harbinger of PDAC is an important goal, but there are several steps that remain to be delineated in order to progress from the identification of new-onset T3cD to the identification of early, potentially curable PDAC. The discrimination of T3cD from the larger population of new-onset T2D is a first step. Then, the etiology of T3cD needs to be established, to separate the minority of patients with T3cD who actually harbor PDAC from the majority who do not. Finally, if an early, curable, but probably radiographically invisible tumor is present, it remains to be determined what additional information or findings are needed in order to proceed with a therapeutic intervention.

Management of T3cD

The overriding principle in the care of patients with T3cD is that both exocrine and endocrine deficiencies exist, and both require treatment. Because exocrine insufficiency precedes endocrine dysfunction, essentially all patients with T3cD require treatment with PERT. If no symptoms of maldigestion are present, it is recommended that fecal elastase or serum trypsin levels be obtained and documented as normal before PERT is declined, as failure to correct indolent lipase deficiency greatly increases the risk of metabolic bone disease and fractures [96]. It has been estimated that 90,000 USP units of lipase are needed for adequate digestion after a meal, so it is reasonable to begin PERT with 70,000–80,000 USP units of enzyme (1000 USP units per kg) administered in divided doses during and after a meal [70, 96]. Enteric-coated products are more resistant to breakdown by gastric acid, and uncoated preparations usually require combination with an antacid medication [70]. Dose modifications are based on the resolution of symptoms and the measurements of vitamin levels.

Exocrine insufficiency also contributes to glucose abnormalities due to an impaired secretion of the incretin hormones, GIP and GLP-1. Therefore, exocrine replacement improves glucose homeostasis and should be the first line of drug therapy after the patient has been counseled on weight loss, smoking cessation, and abstention from alcohol, if needed (see Figure 14C.6). Although no clinical guidelines for the treatment of T3cD have been published, initial therapy with an antidiabetic drug should follow the recommendations of the ADA-EASD consensus group, which advises a trial of metformin as first-line oral therapy for T2D [97]. When hyperglycemia is mild and (hepatic) insulin resistance is suspected, therapy with metformin should be considered in the absence of contraindications

and provided it is well tolerated [7]. Side effects of metformin include nausea, abdominal discomfort, and diarrhea, with which the patient with T3cD may have particular difficulty, but a trial of gradually increasing doses beginning with 500 mg once or twice a day escalating up to 2000 or 2500 mg per day as tolerated can usually result in a substantial improvement in $HgbA_{1c}$ levels (see Table 14C.4). The choice of what to do if metformin fails to control $HgbA_{1c}$, or if metformin is not tolerated, is unclear. Sulfonylureas are commonly prescribed, but their associated side effects of hypoglycemia are of particular concern in patients with T3cD. In addition, insulin secretagogues are a concern in patients

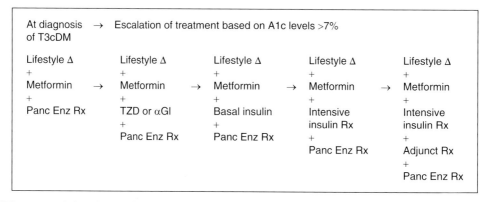

Figure 14C.6 Suggested algorithm for the treatment of patients with T3cD. Recommend and reinforce lifestyle changes (weight loss if obese, exercise, diet, abstention from alcohol, and smoking cessation) at every visit. Begin metformin and advance to maximum dose based on blood glucose and hemoglobin A_{1c} ($HgbA_{1c}$) levels. Add pancreatic enzyme replacement therapy (Panc Enz Rx) if fecal elastase C1 is less than 100 ug/g or patient has signs or symptoms of pancreatic exocrine insufficiency. If $HgbA_{1c}$ levels persist above 7%, add an additional oral agent such as a thiazolidinedione (TZD), an α-glucosidase inhibitor (αGI), or a sodium glucose cotransporter-2 inhibitor. If $HgbA_{1c}$ > 7% persists, add basal intermediate- or long-acting insulin. Convert to intensive (multidose) insulin treatment but continue metformin if $HgbA_{1c}$ persists > 7%. Consider adjunct treatment (Adjunct Rx) such as pramlintide before escalating insulin dose if $HgbA_{1C}$ > 7% persists. From Cui and Andersen [9] with permission.

Table 14C.4 Titration of metformin.

1 Begin with low dose (500 mg) of metformin taken once or twice a day (before breakfast and/or dinner) or 850 mg once a day before breakfast.

2 After 5–7 days, if gastrointestinal side effects have not occurred, advance dose to 850–1000 mg twice a day.

3 If gastrointestinal side effects appear as dose is increased, drop back to previous dose and wait 2–4 weeks before increasing the dose again.

4 Maximum effective dose is 1000 mg twice a day, although increasing the dose to 2500 mg per day may have additional benefit if gastrointestinal side effects do not intervene.

5 Generic metformin is preferred based on cost considerations but a longer acting formulation that may allow once-a-day dosing is available in some countries. Metformin is contraindicated in patients with renal failure or in whom glomerular filtration rate is less than 30 mL/min.

Adapted from Nathan et al. [97] with permission.

at increased risk for recrudescence of pancreatitis and pancreatic cancer. For this reason, the incretin-based therapies of GLP-1 receptor agonists and dipeptidyl peptidase-4 inhibitors are discouraged in T3cD until clinical studies confirm their safety in patients with T3cD [7]. Although no clinical trials have been published, thiazolidinediones, α-glucosidase inhibitors, and sodium-glucose cotransporter-2 inhibitors all seem to be reasonable choices in patients with T3cD as second-line drugs. Rosiglitazone has been shown to improve hepatic insulin resistance in an animal model of CP [30], and similar to the TZD compounds, both α-glucosidase inhibitors and sodium glucose cotransporter-2 inhibitors avoid the hyperinsulinema and hypoglycemia risks of sulfonylureas and incretin-based therapies [98, 99].

In patients with elevated $HgbA_{1c}$ levels refractory to these agents, baseline insulin therapy with low doses of insulin with intermediate length of action is often a necessary next step. If this fails to control the hyperglycemia, multiple-dose insulin schedules are reasonable, but it is advisable to continue metformin therapy if side effects can be avoided, as metformin may have preventative effects on the risk of pancreatic cancer [100]. The important goal is to reduce $HgbA_{1c}$ levels to less than 7%, as the retinal and renal risks of persistent hyperglycemia are the same in T3cD as they are in T1D and T2D [101].

Summary

Pancreatogenic or T3cD probably accounts for 5% or more of the diabetic patient population in western countries. More than 75% of T3cD is due to CP, but it is also caused by pancreatic cancer, pancreatic resection, and cystic fibrosis. The spectrum of severity of the diabetic state in T3cD ranges from mild to severe. The most difficult pattern to treat is referred to as "brittle diabetes," due to enhanced peripheral sensitivity to insulin combined with hepatic insulin resistance, caused by the combined deficiencies of insulin and PP secretion. The combination of CP and T3cD carries an especially high risk for the development of metabolic bone disease and pancreatic cancer. Insulin secretagogues have been associated with the risk of pancreatic cancer, so metformin should be the first-line therapy of T3cD, with avoidance of newer secretagogue therapy until studies confirm safety. Aggressive replacement of pancreatic enzymes can reduce the risk of disease due to a loss of fat-soluble vitamin absorption. New onset T3cD is an indication to consider screening for pancreatic cancer.

References

1 American Diabetes Association. Diagnosis and classification of diabetes. Diabetes Care 2014; 37(suppl 1):S81–S90.

2 Von Mering J, Minkowski O. Diabetes mellitus nach pankreasexstirpation. Archives of Experimental Pathology and Pharmacology 1889; 26:371–387.

3 Hardt PD, Kloer HU, Brendel HG, Bretzel RG. Is pancreatic (type 3c) diabetes underdiagnosed and misdiagnosed? Diabetes Care 2008; 31(suppl 2):S165–S169.

4 Centers for Disease Control and Prevention. National Diabetes Fact Sheet. 2014. http://www.cdc.gov/diabetes/data/statistics2014S.pdf. Accessed December 11, 2014.

5 Task force on diabetes, pre-diabetes and cardiovascular diseases of the European Society of Cardiology (ESC) and the European Association for the Study of Diabetes (EASD). ESC guidelines on diabetes, pre-diabetes and cardiovascular diseases developed in collaboration with the EASD. European Heart Journal 2013; ePub ahead of print August 2013. Doi: 10.1093/eurheartj/eht108.

6 World Health Organization (WHO) Consultation. Definition and diagnosis of diabetes and hyperglycemia. 2006. http://www.who.int/diabetes/publications/Definitions%20and%20diagnosis%20of%20diabetes_new.pdf. Accessed July 26, 2016

7 Rickels MR, Bellin M, Toledo FGS, et al. Detection, evaluation and treatment of diabetes mellitus in chronic pancreatitis. Recommendations from PancreasFest 2012. Pancreatology 2013; 13:336–342.

8 Alberti KGM. Diabetes secondary to pancreatopathy: an example of brittle diabetes. In: Tiengo A, Alberti KGM, DelPrato S, Vranic M (Eds). Diabetes Secondary to Pancreatopathy. Proceedings of the Post-EASD International Symposium on Diabetes Secondary to Pancreatopathy. Padova September 21–22, 1987. International Congress Series 762. Amsterdam, Excerpta Medica, 1988, 35–50.

9 Cui YF, Andersen DK. Pancreatogenic diabetes: special considerations for management. Pancreatology 2011; 11:279–294.

10 Ebert R, Creutzfeldt WO. Reversal of impaired GIP and insulin secretion in patients with pancreatogenic steatorrhea following enzyme substitution. Diabetologia 1980; 19:198–204.

11 Nyboe Andersen B, Krarup T, Thorsgaard Petersen NT, et al. B cell function in patients with chronic pancreatitis and its relation to exocrine pancreatic function. Diabetologia 1982; 23(2):86–89.

12 Howes N, Lerch MM, Greenhalf W, et al. Clinical and genetic characteristics of hereditary pancreatitis in

Europe. Clinical Gastroenterology and Hepatology 2004; 2(3):252–261.

13 Wang W, Guo Y, Liao Z, et al. Occurrence of and risk factors for diabetes mellitus in Chinese patients with chronic pancreatitis. Pancreas 2011; 40(2):206–212.

14 Malka D, Hammel P, Sauvanet A, et al. Risk factors for diabetes mellitus in chronic pancreatitis. Gastroenterology 2000; 119(5):1324–1332.

15 Das SLM, Singh PP, Phillips ARJ, et al. Newly diagnosed diabetes mellitus after acute pancreatitis: a systematic review and meta-analysis. Gut 2014; 63:818–831.

16 Peery AF, Dellon ES, Lund J, et al. Burden of gastrointestinal disease in the United States: 2012 update. Gastroenterology 2012; 143:1179–1187.

17 Nosadini R, del Prato S, Tiengo A, et al. Insulin sensitivity, binding, and kinetics in pancreatogenic and type 1 diabetes. Diabetes 1982; 31:346–355.

18 Andres R, Swerdloff R, Pozefsky T, et al. Manual feedback technique for control of glucose concentration. In: Skeggs L Jr, (Ed) Automation in Analytic Chemistry. New York, Mediad, Inc. 1966. 486–501.

19 Sun YS, Brunicardi FC, Druck P, et al. Reversal of abnormal glucose metabolism in chronic pancreatitis by administration of pancreatic polypeptide. American Journal of Surgery 1986; 151:130–140.

20 Seymour NE, Brunicardi FC, Chaiken RL et al. Reversal of abnormal glucose production after pancreatic resection by pancreatic polypeptide in man. Surgery 1988; 104:119–129.

21 Brunicardi FC, Chaiken RL, Ryan AS, et al. Pancreatic polypeptide administration improves abnormal glucose metabolism in patients with chronic pancreatitis. Journal of Clinical Endocrinology and Metabolism 1996; 81:3566–3572.

22 Cerosimo E, Pisters PW, Pescola G, et al. Insulin secretion and action in patients with pancreatic cancer. Cancer 1991; 67:486–493.

23 Kien CL, Horswill CA, Zipf SB, et al. Elevated hepatic glucose production in children with cystic fibrosis. Pediatric Research 1995; 37:600–605.

24 Andersen DK. Mechanisms and emerging treatments of the metabolic complications of chronic pancreatitis. Pancreas 2007; 35:1–15.

25 Seymour NE, Volpert AR, Lee EL, et al. Alterations in hepatocyte insulin binding in chronic pancreatitis: effects of pancreatic polypeptide. American Journal of Surgery 1995; 169:105–110.

26 Nathan JD, Zdankiewicz PD, Wang JP, et al. Impaired hepatocyte glucose transport protein (GLUT2) internalization in chronic pancreatitis. Pancreas 2001; 22:172–178.

27 Eisenberg ML, Maker AV, Slezak LA, et al. Insulin receptor and glucose transporter 2 proteins form a complex on the rat hepatocyte membrane. Cellular Physiology and Biochemistry 2005; 15:51–58.

28 Cai D, Yuan M, Frantz DF, et al. Local and systemic insulin resistance resulting from hepatic activation of IKK-beta and NF-kappaBeta. Nature Medicine 2005; 11:183–190.

29 Kiechl S, Wittmann J, Giaccari A, et al. Blockade of receptor activator of nuclear factor-K-B (RANKL) signaling improves hepatic insulin resistance and prevents development of diabetes mellitus. Nature Medicine 2013; 19:358–363.

30 Zhou X, You S. Rosiglitazone inhibits hepatic insulin resistance induced by chronic pancreatitis and IKK-β/NF-kB expression in liver. Pancreas 2014; 43:1291–1298.

31 Kimmel JR, Hayden LJ, Pollock HG. Isolation and characterization of a new pancreatic polypeptide hormone. Journal of Biological Chemistry 1975; 250:9369–9376.

32 Lin TM, Chance RE. Gastrointestinal actions of a new bovine pancreatic polypeptide (BPP). In: Chey WY, Brooks FP (Eds). Endocrinology of the Gut. Thorofare, NJ, Charles B. Slack Inc. 1974, 143–145.

33 Schwartz TW. Pancreatic polypeptide: a hormone under vagal control. Gastroenterology 1983; 85:1411–1425.

34 Orci L, Baetens D, Ravazzola M, et al. PP and glucagon: non-random distribution in pancreatic islets. Life Sciences 1976; 19:1811–1816.

35 Orci L. Macro- and micro-domains in the endocrine pancreas. Diabetes 1982; 31:538–565.

36 Hazelwood RL. The pancreatic polypeptide (PP-fold) family: gastrointestinal, vascular, and feeding behavioral implications. Proceedings of the Society for Experimental Biology and Medicine 1993; 202:44–63.

37 Gehlert DR. Multiple receptors for the pancreatic polypeptide (PP fold) family: physiological implications. Proceedings of the Society for Experimental Biology and Medicine 1998; 218:7–22.

38 Berglund MM, Hipskind PA, Gehlert DR. Recent developments in our understanding of the physiological role of PP-fold peptide receptor subtypes. Experimental Biology and Medicine 2003; 228:217–244.

39 Hazelwood RL. Synthesis, storage, secretion, and significance of pancreatic polypeptide in vertebrates. In: Cooperstein SJ, Watkins SD (Eds). The islets of Langerhans: Biochemistry, Physiology, and Pathology. New York, Academic Press. 1981, 275–318.

40 Lonovics J, Guzman S, Devitt P, et al. Release of pancreatic polypeptide in humans by infusion of cholecystokinin. Gastroenterology 1980; 79:817–822.

41 Amland PF, Jorde R, Aanderud S, et al. Effects of intravenously infused porcine GIP on serum insulin, plasma C-peptide, and pancreatic polypeptide in non-insulin dependent diabetes in the fasting state. Scandinavian Journal of Gastroenterology 1985; 20:315–320.

42 Chia CW, Odetunde JO, Kim W, et al. GIP contributes to islet trihormonal abnormalities in type 2 diabetes. Journal of Clinical Endocrinology and Metabolism 2014; 99:2477–2485.

43 Glaser B, Vinik AI, Sive AA, Floyd JC. Plasma human pancreatic polypeptide responses to administered secretin: effects of surgical vagotomy, cholinergic blockade, and chronic pancreatitis. Journal of Clinical Endocrinology and Metabolism 1980; 50:1094–1099.

44 Adrian TE, Greenberg GR, Bloom SR. Actions of pancreatic polypeptide in man. In: Bloom SR, Polak M (Eds). Gut Hormones. Edinburgh, Churchill-Livingstone. 1981. 206–212.

45 Chance RE, Cieszkowski M, Jaworek J, et al. Effect of pancreatic polypeptide and its C-terminal hexapeptide on meal and secretion-induced pancreatic secretion in dogs. Journal of Physiology (London) 1981; 314:1–9.

46 Putnam WS, Liddle RA, Williams JA. Inhibitory regulation of rat exocrine pancreas by peptide YY and pancreatic polypeptide. American Journal of Physiology 1989; 256:G698–G703.

47 Floyd JC, Fajans SS, Pek S, Chance RE. A newly recognized pancreatic polypeptide: plasma levels in health and disease. Recent Progress in Hormone Research 1977; 33:519–570.

48 Berger D, Crowther R, Floyd JC, et al. Effect of age on fasting levels of pancreatic hormones in man. Journal of Clinical Endocrinology and Metabolism 1978; 47:1183–1189.

49 Glaser B, Zoghlin G, Pienta K, Vinik AI. PP response to secretin in obesity: effects of glucose intolerance. Hormone and Metabolic Research 1988; 20:288–292.

50 Schwartz TW. Pancreatic polypeptide and endocrine tumors of the pancreas. Scandinavian Journal of Gastroenterology 1979; 14 (suppl 53):93–100.

51 Friesen SR, Kimmel JR, Tomita T. Pancreatic polypeptide as screening marker for pancreatic polypeptide apudomas in multiple endocrinopathies. American Journal of Surgery 1980; 139:61–72.

52 Sive AS, Vinik AI, Van Tonder S, Lund A. Impaired pancreatic polypeptide secretion in chronic pancreatitis. Journal of Clinical Endocrinology and Metabolism 1978; 47:556–559.

53 Valenzuela JE, Taylor IL, Walsh JH. Pancreatic polypeptide (PP) response to a meal in chronic pancreatitis. Gastroenterology 1978; 74:1149–1152.

54 Inoue K, Tobe T, Suzuki T, et al. Plasma cholecystokinin and pancreatic polypeptide response after radical pancreaticoduodenectomy with Billroth I and Billroth II type of reconstruction. Annals of Surgery 1987; 206:148–154.

55 Adrian TE, McKiernan J, Johnstone DI, et al. Hormonal abnormalities of the pancreas and gut in cystic fibrosis. Gastroenterology 1980; 79:460–465.

56 Krarup T, Schwartz TW, Hilsted J, et al. Impaired response of pancreatic polypeptide to hypoglycemia: an early sign of autonomic neuropathy in diabetics. British Medical Journal 1979; 15:1544–1546.

57 Gates RJ, Lazarus NR. The ability of pancreatic polypeptide (APP and BPP) to return to normal the hyperglycemia,

58 hyperinsulinemia, and weight gain of New Zealand obese mice. Hormone Research 1977; 8:189–202.

58 Gettys TW, Garcia R, Savage K, et al. Insulin-sparing effects of pancreatic polypeptide in congenitally obese rodents. Pancreas 1991; 6:46–53.

59 Bastidas JA, Couse NF, Yeo CJ, et al. The effects of pancreatic polypeptide infusion on glucose tolerance and insulin response in longitudinal-studied pancreatitis-induced diabetes. Surgery 1990; 107:661–668.

60 Seymour NE, Turk JB, Lasker MK, et al. In vitro hepatic insulin resistance in chronic pancreatitis in the rat. Journal of Surgical Research 1989; 46:450–456.

61 Goldstein JA, Kirwin JD, Seymour NE, et al. Reversal of hepatic insulin resistance in chronic pancreatitis by pancreatic polypeptide in the rat. Surgery 1989; 106:1128–1132.

62 Seymour NE, Andersen DK. Pancreatic polypeptide and glucose metabolism. In: Greeley GH (Ed) Gastrointestinal Endocrinology. Totowa, NJ, Humana Press. 1999. 321–334.

63 Rabiee A, Galiatsatos P, Salas-Carrillo R, et al. Pancreatic polypeptide enhances insulin sensitivity and reduces the insulin requirement of patients on insulin pump therapy. Journal of Diabetes Science and Technology 2011; 5:1521–1528.

64 Banerjee A, Onyuksel H. A novel treatment nanomedicine for treatment of pancreatogenic diabetes. Nanomedicine: Nanotechnology, Biology and Medicine 2013; 9:722–720.

65 Bellmann-Sickert K, Elling CE, Madsen AN, et al. A long acting lipidated analog of human pancreatic polypeptide is slowly released into circulation. Journal of Medicinal Chemistry 2011; 54:2658–2667.

66 Magruder JT, Elahi D, Andersen DK. Diabetes and pancreatic cancer: chicken or egg? Pancreas 2011; 40:339–351.

67 Ewald N, Hardt PD. Pancreatogenic (type 3c) diabetes. World Journal of Gastroenterology 2013; 19:7276–7281.

68 Sikkens ECM, Cahen DL, Koch AD, et al. The prevalence of fat-soluble vitamin deficiencies and a decreased bone mass in patients with chronic pancreatitis. Pancreatology 2013; 13(3):238–242.

69 Van Staa TP, Dennison EM, Leufkens HG, Cooper C. Epidemiology of fractures in England and Wales. Bone 2001; 29:517–522.

70 Berry AJ. Pancreatic enzyme replacement therapy during pancreatic insufficiency. Nutrition in Clinical Practice 2014; 29:312–321.

71 Knop FK, Visboll T, Larsen S, et al. Increased post-prandial responses of GLP-1 and GIP in patients with chronic pancreatitis and steatorrhea following pancreatic enzyme substitution. American Journal of Physiology, Endocrinology and Metabolism 2007; 292:E324–E330.

72 Yu H-H, Yan Y-S, Lin P-W. Effect of pancreaticoduodenectomy on the course of hepatic steatosis. World Journal of Surgery 2010; 34:2122–2127.

73 Song SC, Choi SH, Choi DW, et al. Potential risk factors for non-alcoholic steatohepatitis related to pancreatic secretions following pancreaticoduodenectomy. World Journal of Gastroenterology 2011; 17(32):3716–3723.

74 Cui YF, Andersen DK. Diabetes and pancreatic cancer. Endocrine-Related Cancer 2012; 19:F9–F26.

75 Maisonneuve P, Lowenfels AB, Bueno-de-Mesquita HB, et al. Past medical history and pancreatic cancer risk: results from a multi-center case–control study. Annals of Epidemiology 2010; 20:92–98.

76 Green RC Jr, Baggenstoss AH, Sprague RG. Diabetes mellitus in association with primary carcinoma of the pancreas. Diabetes 1958; 7:308–311.

77 Pannala R, Leirness JB, Bamlet WR, et al. Prevalence and clinical profile of pancreatic cancer-associated diabetes mellitus. Gastroenterology 2008; 134:981–987.

78 Liao KF, Lai SW, Li CI, Chen WC. Diabetes mellitus correlates with increased risk of pancreatic cancer: a population-based cohort study in Taiwan. Journal of Gastroenterology and Hepatology 2012; 27; 709–713.

79 Brodovicz KG, Kou TD, Alexander CM, et al. Impact of diabetes duration and chronic pancreatitis on the association between type 2 diabetes and pancreatic cancer risk. Diabetes, Obesity & Metabolism 2012; 14; 1123–1128.

80 Pannala R, Basu A, Petersen GM, Chari ST. New-onset diabetes: a potential clue to the early diagnosis of pancreatic cancer. Lancet Oncology 2009; 10:88–95.

81 Permert J, Ihse I, Jorfeldt L, et al. Improved glucose metabolism after subtotal pancreatectomy for pancreatic cancer. British Journal of Surgery 1993; 80:1047–1050.

82 Fogar P, Pasquali C, Basso D, et al. Diabetes mellitus in pancreatic cancer follow up. Anticancer Research 1994; 14:2827–2830.

83 Ogawa Y, Tanaka M, Inoue K, et al. A prospective pancreatographic study of the prevalence of pancreatic carcinoma in patients with diabetes mellitus. Cancer 2002; 94:2344–2349.

84 Damiano J, Bordier L, Le Berre JP, et al. Should pancreas imaging be recommended in patients over 50 years when diabetes is discovered because of acute symptoms? Diabetes & Metabolism 2004; 30:203–207.

85 Pelaez-Luna M, Takahashi N, Fletcher JG, et al. Resectability of presymptomatic pancreatic cancer and its relationship to onset of diabetes: a retrospective review of CT scans and fasting glucose values prior to diagnosis. American Journal of Gastroenterology 2007; 102:2157–2163.

86 Chari ST, Leibson CL, Rabe KG, et al. Pancreatic cancer-associated diabetes mellitus: prevalence and temporal association with diagnosis of cancer. Gastroenterology 2005; 129:504–511.

87 Brentnall TA, Bronner MP, Byrd DR, et al. Early diagnosis and treatment of pancreatic dysplasia in patients with a family history of pancreatic cancer. Annals of Internal Medicine 1999; 131:247–255.

88 Jin SM, Choi SH, Choi DW, et al. Glucagon/insulin ratio in preoperative screening before pancreatic surgery: correlation with hemoglobin A_{1c} in subjects with and without pancreatic cancer. Endocrine 2014; 47:493–499.

89 Hart PA, Baichoo E, Bi Y, et al. Pancreatic polypeptide response to a mixed meal is blunted in pancreatic head cancer associated with diabetes mellitus. Pancreatology 2015; 15:162–166.

90 Pfeffer F, Koczan D, Adam U, et al. Expression of connexin-26 in islets of Langerhans is associated with impaired glucose tolerance in patients with pancreatic carcinoma. Pancreas 2004; 29:284–290.

91 Basso D, Greco E, Fogar P, et al. Pancreatic cancer-derived S100A8 N-terminal peptide: a diabetes cause? Clinica Chimica Acta 2006; 372:120–128.

92 Huang H, Dong X, Kang MX, et al. Novel blood biomarkers of pancreatic cancer-associated diabetes mellitus identified by peripheral blood-based gene expression profiles. American Journal of Gastroenterology 2010; 105:1661–1669.

93 He XY, Yuan YZ. Advances in pancreatic cancer research: moving towards early detection. World Journal of Gastroenterology 2014; 20:11241–11248.

94 Sah RP, Nagpal SJS, Mukhopadhyay D, Chari ST. New insights into pancreatic cancer-induced paraneoplastic diabetes. Nature Reviews Gastroenterology & Hepatology 2013; 10:423–433.

95 Hinson JP, Kapas S, Smith DM. Adrenomedullin, a multi-functional regulatory peptide. Endocrine Reviews 2000; 21(2):138–167.

96 Afghani E, Sinha A, Singh V. An overview of the diagnosis and management of nutrition in chronic pancreatitis. Nutrition in Clinical Practice 2014; 29:295–311.

97 Nathan DM, Holman RR, Buse JB, et al. Medical management of hyperglycemia in type 2 diabetes: a consensus algorithm for the initiation and adjustment of therapy: a consensus statement of the American Diabetes Association and the European Association for the Study of Diabetes. Diabetes Care 2009; 32:193–203.

98 Riccardi G, Giacco R, Parillo M, et al. Efficacy and safety of acerbose in the treatment of type 1 diabetes mellitus: a placebo-controlled, double-blind, multicenter study. Diabetic Medicine 1999; 16:228–232.

99 Nair S, Wilding JP. Sodium glucose co-transporter 2 inhibitors as a new treatment for diabetes mellitus. Journal of Clinical Endocrinology and Metabolism 2010; 95:35–42.

100 Bao B, Wang Z, Ali S, et al. Metformin inhibits cell proliferation, migration and invasion by attenuating CSC function mediated by deregulating miRNAs in pancreatic cancer cells. Cancer Prevention Research 2012; 5:355–364.

101 Couet C, Genton P, Pointel JP. et al. The prevalence of retinopathy is similar in diabetes mellitus secondary to chronic pancreatitis with or without pancreatectomy and in idiopathic diabetes mellitus. Diabetes Care 1985; 8:323–328.

Nutrition without a pancreas: how does the gut do it?

William Lancaster[1], Matthew Kappus[2] & Robert Martindale[3]

[1] *Department of Surgery, Medical University of South Carolina, Charleston, SC, USA*
[2] *Division of Gastroenterology, Department of Medicine, Duke University, Durham, NC, USA*
[3] *Department of Surgery, Oregon Health and Sciences University, Portland, OR, USA*

Introduction

Chronic pancreatitis (CP) is a disease of chronic inflammation of the pancreas leading to progressive fibrosis and loss of functional parenchyma. Pancreatic insufficiency results when there is insufficient exocrine pancreatic function. Most patients only become symptomatic when 90% of the exocrine pancreas is nonfunctional [1]. Despite surgical resections of the pancreas usually only removing 30–70%, the majority of major pancreatic resections, estimated 56–98% of patients undergoing pancreaticoduodenectomy (PD), will experience pancreatic exocrine insufficiency postoperatively with an estimated 12–80% of patients with distal or central resections will experience exocrine insufficiency [2]. The clinical manifestations are most commonly chronic abdominal pain and exocrine and endocrine insufficiency related to loss of pancreatic acinar cells and islet cells, respectively. The estimated incidence in the United States is approximately 5 new cases per 100,000 persons per year. The cost burden is primary related to repeat hospitalization with an estimated 19,000 hospitalizations per year at a yearly cost of $172 million [3]. There are multiple etiologies for exocrine pancreatic insufficiency (EPI), the most common etiologies being cystic fibrosis, CP, and loss of functional pancreatic tissue following necrotizing pancreatitis. Others include surgical resection for benign or malignant disease, obstruction of the main

pancreatic duct from stones, neoplasm or stricture, acid-mediated inactivation of pancreatic enzymes in hypersecretory states such as in Zollinger–Ellison syndrome, and secondary causes of exocrine dysfunction from loss of stimulatory capacity such as in the settings of autoimmune enteropathy, short-gut syndrome with enteropathy, inflammatory bowel disease [4], or maldigestion or inadequate mixing of food and exocrine pancreatic enzymes following foregut surgery [5]. Essentially, 100% patients who undergo total pancreatectomy for islet cell transplantation or malignancy suffer from pancreatic insufficiency symptoms and require meticulous attention to enzyme replacement therapy and dietary restriction [6].

Pancreatic function in normal digestion

The pancreas secretes a bicarbonate-rich fluid that contains multiple enzymes that aid in the digestion of carbohydrates, protein, and fat into component molecules that are then absorbed by the gut using a variety of transport mechanisms. The majority of pancreatic enzymes, except amylase, are secreted as inactive precursor molecules called zymogens that are ultimately activated by enzymatic cleavage in the gut lumen. The activity of pancreatic enzymes and thus the function of the pancreas in digestion are highly dependent on intestinal pH. The bicarbonate in pancreatic fluid is essential in creating a postprandial environment suitable for enzymatic activity.

Exocrine pancreatic insufficiency

EPI can be broadly defined as inadequate pancreatic exocrine function to meet the nutritional and metabolic needs of the patient. The etiology of EPI can be classified as either primary or secondary. Primary EPI results from either loss of functional pancreatic parenchyma, for example, surgical resection, CP with parenchymal fibrosis, or from absence of delivery of pancreatic secretions to the intestinal lumen such as an ampullary tumor or stricture causing obstruction of the main pancreatic duct. Secondary EPI implies that pancreatic function is preserved but there are other processes that create a clinical syndrome consistent with exocrine insufficiency. An example would be Zollinger–Ellison syndrome with high gastric acid output leading to acidic inactivation of pancreatic enzymes. Another less common scenario is an enteropathy causing loss of intestinal brush border function with associated malabsorption in conditions such as autoimmune enteropathy, short-gut syndrome with enteropathy, or inflammatory bowel disease. The distinction of primary versus secondary EPI highlights the important fact that EPI is not always attributable to loss of pancreatic enzymes in the intestinal lumen and that pancreatic function in digestion is highly dependent on other associated factors including luminal pH, relative intestinal blood flow, as well as intestinal motility and brush border integrity [2, 4].

Carbohydrate digestion

Carbohydrate digestion begins in the mouth with salivary amylase, which breaks down complex carbohydrates into component polysaccharides. This process continues in the stomach and duodenum, where pancreatic amylase functions similarly to salivary amylase. The final step in carbohydrate digestion lies with intestinal brush border enzymes that further break down polysaccharides into monosaccharides. The end product monosaccharides are then absorbed [7].

Amylorrhea is defined as inadequate digestion of carbohydrates such that they are lost in stool. The clinical symptoms associated with amylorrhea are abdominal distention, flatulence, and loose stools [8, 9]. While amylorrhea can occur with pancreatic insufficiency, it is not a common initial finding because digestion of carbohydrates is not solely dependent on pancreatic secretions. Because of the redundancy of enzymes that participate in carbohydrate digestion, loss of pancreatic amylase can be compensated for and amylorrhea is seldom seen clinically. This specifically occurs by salivary amylase and brush border enzymes such as α-glucosidase, sucrase, maltase, and lactase. In addition, amylase is much less susceptible to acidic and proteolytic mechanisms in the intestinal lumen and has been shown to have approximately 35% activity in the ileum [10]. Carbohydrate digestion can occur rather effectively in the setting of EPI and complete pancreatectomy as long as dietary recommendations are followed.

Protein digestion

Protein digestion begins in the stomach where gastric pepsin cleaves dietary proteins, primarily the intramolecular protein bonds, thereby essentially unraveling the complex structure of the protein and revealing enzymatic targets for the proteases in the small bowel lumen. Gastric pepsin is secreted as an inactive zymogen and is activated by the acidic environment in the stomach lumen. The next phase occurs in the duodenum where pancreatic secretions include numerous enzymes including trypsin, chymotrypsin, and an assortment of carboxypeptidases. These enzymes continue the process of breaking down polypeptides into smaller oligopeptides and amino acids. Finally, intestinal brush border peptidases cleave oligopeptides into dipeptides and tripeptides, which are then absorbed into the enterocyte and further broken down by cytosolic peptidases to amino acids to be absorbed at the basolateral membrane by facilitated diffusion, entering the portal system. The process of absorption of di- and tripeptides from the intestinal lumen into the enterocyte is largely governed by a broad-specificity transport protein, peptide transporter-1 (PEPT-1). PEPT-1 is a sodium-specific cotransporter, utilizing a sodium–hydrogen ATPase to create an electrochemical gradient. The PEPT-1 transporter is a very nonspecific transporter and can transport an estimated 8000 combinations of di- and tripeptides. Ultimately, approximately

70% of consumed protein mass is absorbed as small peptides via PEPT-1 [11, 12].

Azotorrhea is defined as greater than 2.5 g fecal protein loss and associated with ascites and peripheral edema. While pancreatic insufficiency can lead to malabsorption of proteins, the loss of significant protein calories is relatively uncommon, provided there is a functioning intestinal brush border. Intestinal brush border peptidases, including aminopeptidases, dipeptidyl-aminopeptidase, and dipeptidases, can compensate for much of the loss of pancreatic peptidases in many cases [12].

Lipid digestion

Dietary lipids are essential for myriad physiologic processes that make them essential for normal metabolism. Independent of the human requirement for the essential fatty acids, linolenic and linoleic acids, lipids are energy dense and aid in the absorption of fat-soluble vitamins. They are also crucial for cell membrane function and fluidity, gene expression, cell signaling pathways, eicosanoid metabolism, and cytokine production [13]. Lipid digestion begins first with the formation of micelles in which the ingested lipids are enveloped by amphipathic molecules and stabilized for enzymatic degradation. This stabilizes the lipid in an aqueous environment. The lipids within micelles are then cleaved into monoacylglycerol and fatty acids by pancreatic lipase. Absorption of fatty acids occurs in the proximal one-third of the small intestine and transported to the portal bloodstream or lymphatics. The majority of fatty acids with carbon chains greater than 14 carbons are required to pass via the lymphatics as chylomicrons. The medium-chain fatty acid and short-chain fatty acid (SCFA) can pass into the portal vein or the lymphatics, and the majority pathway will depend on conditions in the gastrointestinal tract [14]. Unlike carbohydrate and protein digestion, the pancreas plays a crucial role in lipid absorption. Pancreatic lipase is responsible for 90% of fat digestion [15], and there is little redundancy in lipid metabolism that compensates for absent pancreatic function. The normal pancreas produces over 700,000 units of lipase per day, and 90% of pancreatic function must be lost before symptoms of fat malabsorption are present. In addition, pancreatic insufficiency is associated with decreased bicarbonate secretion, which

decreases duodenal pH where pancreatic lipase is much more susceptible to luminal degradation. Thus, the effects of decreased lipase production are typically seen before those of carbohydrate or protein malabsorption. Steatorrhea is defined as greater than 7 g fecal fat per day, and because 90% of pancreatic function must be lost before steatorrhea is present, it can be seen as a clinical marker of severe EPI [16].

Vitamin malabsorption

Specific receptors have now been described for the absorption of all the water-soluble vitamins. These include SVCT-1 (ascorbic acid), SMVT (biotin), PCFT and RFC (folate), and THTR and THTR-1 (thiamine). Our knowledge of the mechanisms and regulation of intestinal absorption of water-soluble vitamins under normal physiological conditions has greatly expanded. The water-soluble vitamins share the feature of being essential for normal cellular functions, growth, and development, and their deficiency leads to a variety of clinical abnormalities including anemia, growth retardation, and neurologic disorders. Since these water-soluble vitamins cannot be synthesized by the human body, interference with intestinal absorption, can lead to significant deficiency [17, 18].

The fat-soluble vitamins A, D, E, and K may also be affected in EPI, but less so. Vitamins E and A are relatively easy to replace, but are generally low in most studies of EPI. Vitamin K malabsorption is usually not as much of a problem as more than 50% of vitamin K is produced by colonic bacteria. Vitamin D supplementation can be a problem, and patients generally begin having clinical evidence of deficiency when 25-OH vitamin D levels are less than 20 ng/dL [17, 18].

Nutritional issues

The nutritional disturbances observed in EPI can be related to the destruction of functional gland, pancreatic duct obstruction, or altered anatomy secondary to surgical resection, and the most immediate consequence is weight loss. Regardless of etiology, exocrine insufficiency is associated with clinical manifestations of diarrhea, bloating, and steatorrhea. Importantly, these symptoms are consistently linked to the poor quality of life associated with EPI [19, 20].

Nutritional assessment

Though malnutrition in patients with pancreatic insufficiency is accepted as an important sequelae of the disease process, it is not entirely clear how often and how severely patients are affected. Using indirect indicators of malnutrition such as low body mass index (BMI) and decreased lean body mass, conservative estimates range from 20% to 30% of patients being malnourished, though these estimates are probably quite low, especially with CP [21]. Thorough assessment of the patient with suspected EPI begins with the assessment of malnutrition. A multidisciplinary approach is preferred [22]. While it is important to assess for clinical indicators of maldigestion such as bloating, flatulence, and steatorrhea, significant malabsorption and malnutrition may be present before these symptoms appear [22]. Thus, in assessing for malnutrition, specific inquiry must be made regarding recent weight loss and current dietary intake and limitations as well as measurement of BMI [23]. Assessment should provide insights into the cause of malnutrition in the event it is suspected. In patients with pancreatic insufficiency, the cause is either due to lack of nutrients, that is, underconsumption secondary to pain, nausea and vomiting, or anorexia, or secondary to malabsorption due to EPI. A useful adjunct to assessing the patient's nutritional status is anthropometric measurement, which involves measurements of arm circumference and triceps skinfold. Whereas BMI and body weight can be misleading in certain cases such as shifts in patient volume status, anthropometrics offers measurements that can be compared with normative standards. However, it is important to note that both arm circumference and triceps skinfold thickness may be affected by tissue edema. Indeed, it has been shown that patients may be obese according to BMI and malnourished according to other clinical indicators [24]. Historically, serum markers, namely albumin and prealbumin, have been used as objective measures of nutritional status but recent guidelines have discouraged this practice because they are felt to be markers of inflammation and do not reliably correlate with weight loss or calorie restriction [25]. Visceral protein biomarkers may be considered in stable patients where

acute inflammation is playing less of a role. However, it should be noted that there is currently little consensus with respect to screening for malnutrition nor is there consensus as to what defines malnutrition [26]. There may be additional tools for assessment in the future including cross-sectional assessment of muscle wasting and body composition. This may be done using axial computed tomography, magnetic resonance imaging, or ultrasonography [27].

Pancreatic function testing is also necessary. The most invasive test is the secretin/CCK test, which involves IV administration of secretin and CCK with measurement of gastric and duodenal luminal secretions. This test carries the highest potential sensitivity with moderate specificity (86–94% sensitive and 67–70% specific) [18]. Although this test provides the most direct assessment of pancreatic function, it is invasive and considered impractical in certain settings [28]. Indirect testing is commonly done using quantitative fecal fat testing is used as a surrogate for exocrine insufficiency. While protocols vary, the patient typically consumes 100 g of dietary fat followed by stool collection for 72 hours with 15 g per day of fecal fat considered severe steatorrhea [29]. A newer test that is becoming increasingly available is fecal elastase-1 measurement. The test is easily performed from a stool specimen and is a good approximation of pancreatic enzyme production. However, because of limited sensitivity it does not detect mild and moderate insufficiency [30]. The ^{13}C-triglyceride breath test requires a 6-hour exam but is a very accurate test and can be used for compliance testing and efficacy of treatment [18].

Dietary recommendations

The essential paradigm of recommended diet is provision of adequate calories in order to meet energy demands, macro and micronutrient requirements, and ultimately maintain weight and lean body mass. Other important considerations include improved quality of life with reduction in symptoms and increased functional capacity. Abstinence from alcohol is essential. Most agree that dietary habits should consist of several (4–8) small meals per day with limitation on the amount of carbohydrates consumed. Special emphasis is placed on the importance of not skipping meals. Protein consumption should be approximately 1.5–2 g/kg/day.

As stated earlier, in contrast to fat digestion, the enzymatic redundancy within the mucosal border allows for compensation for EPI in carbohydrate and protein digestion, provided that dietary recommendations are followed. Carbohydrates should be complex if possible, but also note that too much fiber will decrease the activity of pancreatic enzyme replacement therapy (PERT). Patients are advised to minimize high-sugar foods or fluids as these may lead to osmotic diarrhea. The main source of macronutrient loss is malabsorption of dietary long-chain fat (LCT). Since fat is energy dense yielding 9 calories per gram, malabsorption of fat plays a major role in weight loss and malnutrition. It is recommended that 30–40% of calories consist of dietary fat. In the event of persistent weight loss or severe steatorrhea, a diet containing additional medium-chain triglycerides (MCTs) and less LCTs can be attempted. MCTs are absorbed without the participation of pancreatic lipase and, therefore, can provide a valuable source of lipid calories in EPI. The limitations of this approach are side effects including bloating, cramping, and diarrhea; therefore, small amounts with gradual increase should be started. In addition, consumption of MCTs is limited to 50 g/day. Patients should be provided a standard multivitamin supplementation with periodic testing for deficiencies. To ensure adequate nutritional intake, it is advised that patients be seen regularly for assessment by a dietician familiar with EPI, and consider the use of a detailed food diary for ensure adequate intake.

Options for nutritional support in the setting of inability to maintain weight and persistent malnutrition include enteral nutrition (EN) and parenteral nutrition (PN). EN can be considered in cases where the primary source of malnutrition is inadequate delivery of calories either due to altered anatomy, decreased absorptive surface area, or patient symptoms preventing adequate intake. In CP, tube feeding is indicated in only about 5% of patients with parenteral feeding being required on <1% of patients [18]. In EPI resulting from resectional therapy or even total pancreatectomy, enteral and parenteral requirements are higher but still should be less than 10–15%. EN can be pursued either as a short-term intervention via a nasoenteral tube or through more permanent enteral access. The goal is to provide adequate calories and micronutrients and this can be accomplished in either a supplementary fashion or, if needed, a patient's entire dietary needs can be met. Specialized EN is needed in less than 5% of

cases, and elemental or semi-elemental formulas can be considered, but no large trials have been done and most of the data on selection of the type of enteral formula is considered expert opinion based on theory and not data. Notably, there is no consistent data for the use of immune or metabolic formulas. PN should be limited to only severe cases in which there is complete inability to tolerate EN or if there is insufficient intestinal length to absorb adequate nutrients [31]. PN is associated with the loss of intestinal mucosal architecture and immune barrier. It is also associated with serious complications including central line infections and bacteremia as well as parenteral nutrition–associated liver disease (PNALD) noted clinically first as cholestatic jaundice [32]. If needed, PN is typically used only for short intervals. Its long-term use has not been studied in patients with EPI. More recent dietary considerations include probiotic supplementation. *Lactobacillus plantarum* has been found to have a high lipase activity, remaining active at a maximum pH of 7.5, and still having 40% activity at a lower pH of 5.

Final consideration includes the use of colon to scavenge carbohydrates via the process of fermentation. When carbohydrates and soluble fiber enter the colon, bacteria can ferment these nonabsorbed carbohydrates into SCFAs. Known substrates include resistant starch, nonstarch polysaccharides, nondigestible oligosaccharides, and some nonabsorbed mono- and disaccharides. Acetate, propionate, and butyrate comprise 83% of SCFAs. They enhance the structure and function of the colonic mucosa by causing mucosal proliferation in the colon, ileum, and jejunum, and improve transport activity, in addition to being a source of calories absorbed by the colon. The colon can be a source of up to 300–500 calories per day in patients with severe malabsorption in the proximal gut, in short-bowel syndrome, and in some cases EPI [33].

If the aforementioned are not controlling symptoms, or patients continue to experience symptoms of abdominal pain, bloating, or steatorrhea/diarrhea, consider small-bowel bacterial overgrowth (SBO). SBO is reported in up to 40% of patients with CP and occurs due to the degradation of carbohydrate by enteric bacteria with the production of SCFAs, carbon dioxide, hydrogen, and methane. Patients experience acidic stools, abdominal distension, pain, and flatulence. Hydroxylated fatty acids stimulate the secretion of water and electrolytes along with bile acids, leading to watery diarrhea [2]. Signs include macrocytic anemia due to vitamin B_{12} deficiency, large joint arthritis due to toxin production by bacteria, and it is important to recognize that altered gut motility is a complex issue secondary to opiates and previous surgery.

Pancreatic enzyme replacement therapy

PERT is essential in EPI. The goals of enzyme replacement are twofold. The first is to improve the digestion of carbohydrates, protein, and fat, thereby improving nutritional status, and the second is to alleviate the symptoms associated with the loss of pancreatic enzymes, for example, steatorrhea. The instrumental role PERT plays in nutritional management is attributable to replacing pancreatic lipase. It has been shown that the greatest benefit received is among patients with greater than 15 g/day fecal fat excretion [34, 35]. Several randomized, blinded studies have demonstrated improved fat absorption with PERT, with improvements ranging from 10% to 20% from baseline absorption [36]. It has also been shown that enzyme supplementation significantly improves BMI and reduces stool frequency. However, these effects were not seen until 6 months to 1 year of therapy.

Though there are several commercial preparations available, all enzyme replacement products contain pancrelipase, which is a mixture of amylase, protease, and lipase [37]. Dosing is based on the lipase component. It is estimated that 1000 units of lipase are needed to digest 1 g of fat. A common starting regimen is 40,000 units with meals and 20,000 units with snacks. The dose can be increased based on patient symptoms and nutritional improvement [38]. The preparations are available in both enteric-coated and non-enteric-coated formulations. The enteric-coated formulations are intended to resist gastric degradation and become active in the relatively alkaline environment in the duodenum. It is recommended that the non-enteric formulations be administered with concurrent proton pump inhibitor (PPI) therapy. Though this is in theory not required with enteric-coated formulations, consideration must be given when desired effects are not seen with appropriate dosing, especially in cases of altered anatomy or gastrointestinal function, for example, gastroparesis. Administration with or after meals has been shown to be more effective than dosing prior to meals [38]. Efficacy of enzyme supplementation is primarily determined by clinical response in terms of weight gain, reduction in steatorrhea, and improvement in symptoms. Pancreatic function tests such as fecal fat excretion or fecal elastase can also be used to monitor treatment response [39].

Summary

EPI can result in malnutrition and maldigestion, but the good news is that most patients can be managed if a thoughtful and practical nutrition plan is devised and the patient is compliant. By combining dietary support with compliance, use of PERT, as well as cessation of both tobacco and alcohol use, the vast majority of patients can be managed successfully [18]. Requirements for nutritional intervention will depend on the remaining functional pancreatic parenchyma and mucosal enzymatic integrity. The extreme of total pancreatectomy with or without islet transplantation will need intensive nutritional training to maintain lean body mass and a multidisciplinary team should being involved with routine follow-up. Future treatment possibilities include use of lipid nanoparticles, more targeted probiotic therapy to secrete lipase, and the use of resistance exercise with high protein intake to improve lean body tissue synthesis and prevent loss. Exercise in combination with adequate amino acid/protein consumption has been shown to be anabolic in multiple models, including ICU, burn, and cancer patients [40]. Better understanding of existing therapies may have an added role to already effective treatment of these patients.

References

1 Berry AJ. Pancreatic enzyme replacement therapy during pancreatic insufficiency. Nutrition in Clinical Practice 2014; 29:312–321.

2 Phillips ME. Pancreatic exocrine insufficiency following pancreatic resection. Pancreatology 2015; 15:449–455.

3 Yadav D, Timmons L, Benson JT, et al. Incidence, prevalence, and survival of chronic pancreatitis: a population-based study. American Journal of Gastroenterology 2011; 106:2192–2199.

4 Lindkvist B Diagnosis and treatment of pancreatic exocrine insufficiency. World Journal of Gastroenterology 2014; 19:7258–7266.

5 Pongprasobchai S Maldigestion from pancreatic exocrine insufficiency. Journal of Gastroenterology and Hepatology 2013;28 Suppl 4:99–102.

6 Bellin MD, Freeman ML, Gelrud A, et al. Total pancreatectomy and islet autotransplantation in chronic pancreatitis: recommendations from PancreasFest. Pancreatology 2014; 14:27–35.

7 Wright E et al. Sugar absorption. In: Johnson L (ed), Physiology of the Gastrointestinal Tract 4th edn. San Diego, Academic Press. 2006: 1653–1666.

8 Sjölund K, Häggmark A, Ihse I, et al. Selective deficiency of pancreatic amylase. Gut 1991; 32:546–548.

9 Frederiksen HJ, Mogensen NB, Magid E. The clinical significance of salivary amylase in duodenal aspirates in evaluation of exocrine pancreas function. Scandinavian Journal of Gastroenterology 1985;20:1046–1048.

10 Hammer HF. Pancreatic exocrine insufficiency: diagnostic evaluation and replacement therapy with pancreatic enzymes. Digestive Diseases 2010; 28:339–343.

11 Pieri M, Gan C, Bailey P, Meredith D. The transmembrane tyrosines Y56, Y91 and Y167 play important roles in determining the affinity and transport rate of the rabbit proton-coupled peptide transporter PepT1. International Journal of Biochemistry and Cell Biology 2009;41:2204–2213.

12 Ganapathy V, Martindale R. Protein digestion and absorption. In: Johnson L (ed), Physiology of the Gastrointestinal Tract 4th edn. San Diego, Academic Press. 2006: 1667–1692.

13 Calder PC. Functional roles of fatty acids and their effects on human health. Journal of Parenteral and Enteral Nutrition 2015; 39:18S–32S.

14 Abumrad N, Storch J. Role of membrane and cytosolic fatty acid binding proteins in lipid processing by the small intestine. In: Johnson L (ed), Physiology of the Gastrointestinal Tract 4th edn. San Diego, Academic Press. 2006: 1693–1710.

15 DiMagno EP, Go VL. Exocrine pancreatic insufficiency. Current concepts of pathophysiology. Postgraduate Medicine. 1972;52:135–140.

16 Gupte AR, Forsmark CE. Chronic pancreatitis. Current Opinion in Gastroenterology 2014; 30:500–505.

17 Rasmussen HH, Irtun O, Olesen SS, et al. Nutrition in chronic pancreatitis. World Journal of Gastroenterology 2013; 19:7267–7275.

18 Afghani E, Sinha A, Singh VK. An overview of the diagnosis and management of nutrition in chronic pancreatitis. Nutrition in Clinical Practice 2014; 29:295–311.

19 Epelboym I, Winner M, DiNorcia J, et al. Quality of life in patients after total pancreatectomy is comparable with quality of life in patients who undergo a partial pancreatic resection. Journal of Surgical Research 2014; 187:189–196.

20 Barbier L, Jamal W, Dokmak S, et al. Impact of total pancreatectomy: short- and long-term assessment. Hepato Pancreato Biliary (Oxford). 2013; 15:882–892.

21 Armbrecht U Chronic pancreatitis: weight loss and poor physical performance - experience from a specialized rehabilitation centre. Rehabilitation (Stuttg) 2001; 40:332–336.

22 Duggan S, O'Sullivan M, Feehan S, et al. Nutrition treatment of deficiency and malnutrition in chronic pancreatitis: a review. Nutrition in Clinical Practice 2010; 25:362–370.

23 Sorensen J, Kondrup J, Prokopowicz J, et al. EuroOOPS: an international, multicentre study to implement nutritional risk screening and evaluate clinical outcome. Clinical Nutrition 2008; 27:340–349.

24 Duggan SN, Smyth ND, O'Sullivan M, et al. The prevalence of malnutrition and fat-soluble vitamin deficiencies in chronic pancreatitis. Nutrition in Clinical Practice 2014;29:348–354.

25 White JV, Guenter P, Jensen G, et al. Consensus statement of the Academy of Nutrition and Dietetics/American Society for Parenteral and Enteral Nutrition: characteristics recommended for the identification and documentation of adult malnutrition (undernutrition). Journal of the Academy of Nutrition and Dietetics 2012; 112:730–738.

26 Soeters PB, Reijven PL, van Bokhorst-de van der Schueren MA, et al. A rational approach to nutritional assessment. Clinical Nutrition 2008; 27:706–716.

27 Prado CM, Heymsfield SB, Lean tissue imaging: a new era for nutritional assessment and intervention. Journal of Parenteral and Enteral Nutrition 2014; 38:940–953.

28 Tran TC, van Lanschot JJ, Bruno MJ, van Eijck CH. Functional changes after pancreatoduodenectomy: diagnosis and treatment. Pancreatology 2009; 9:729–737.

29 Nakajima K, Oshida H, Muneyuki T, Kakei M. Pancrelipase: an evidence-based review of its use for treating pancreatic exocrine insufficiency. Core Evidence 2012; 7:77–91.

30 Benini L, Amodio A, Campagnola P, et al. Fecal elastase-1 is useful in the detection of steatorrhea in patients with pancreatic diseases but not after pancreatic resection. Pancreatology 2013; 13:38–42.

31 Seres DS, Valcarcel M, Guillaume A. Advantages of enteral nutrition over parenteral nutrition. Therapeutic Advances in Gastroenterology 2013;6: 157–167.

32 Beath SV, Kelly DA. Total parenteral nutrition-induced cholestasis: prevention and management. Clinics in Liver Disease 2016; 20:159–176.

33 Pezzilli R Chronic pancreatitis: maldigestion, intestinal ecology and intestinal inflammation. World Journal of Gastroenterology 2009; 15:1673–1676.

34 Domínguez-Muñoz JE, Iglesias-García J, Vilariño-Insua M, Iglesias-Rey M. 13C-mixed triglyceride breath test to assess oral enzyme substitution therapy in patients with chronic pancreatitis. Clinical Gastroenterology and Hepatology 2007; 5:484–488.

35 Domínguez-Muñoz JE. Chronic pancreatitis and persistent steatorrhea: what is the correct dose of enzymes? Clinical Gastroenterology and Hepatology 2011; 9:541–546.

36 Thorat V, Reddy N, Bhatia S, et al. Randomised clinical trial: the efficacy and safety of pancreatin enteric-coated minimicrospheres (Creon 40000 MMS) in patients with pancreatic exocrine insufficiency due to chronic pancreatitis--a double-blind, placebo-controlled study. Alimentary Pharmacology and Therapeutics 2012; 36: 426–436.

37 Whitcomb DC, Lehman GA, Vasileva G, et al. Pancrelipase delayed-release capsules (CREON) for exocrine pancreatic insufficiency due to chronic pancreatitis or pancreatic surgery: a double-blind randomized trial. American Journal of Gastroenterology 2010; 105:2276–2286.

38 Domínguez-Muñoz JE, Iglesias-García J, Iglesias-Rey M, et al. Effect of the administration schedule on the therapeutic efficacy of oral pancreatic enzyme supplements in patients with exocrine pancreatic insufficiency: a randomized, three-way crossover study. Alimentary Pharmacology and Therapeutics 2005; 21:993–1000.

39 Dumasy V, Delhaye M, Cotton F, Deviere J. Fat malabsorption screening in chronic pancreatitis. American Journal of Gastroenterology 2004; 99:1350–1354.

40 Morton RW, McGlory C, Phillips SM. Nutritional interventions to augment resistance training-induced skeletal muscle hypertrophy. Frontiers in Physiology 2015; 6:245.

CHAPTER 15

PART A: Endoscopic management of chronic pancreatitis

Wiriyaporn Ridtitid[1,2] & Stuart Sherman[1]

[1] *Division of Gastroenterology and Hepatology, Indiana University School of Medicine, Indianapolis, IN, USA*

[2] *Division of Gastroenterology and Hepatology, Chulalongkorn University, King Chulalongkorn Memorial Hospital, Thai Red Cross Society, Bangkok, Thailand*

Introduction

Chronic abdominal pain is the main symptom in patients with chronic pancreatitis (CP). The mechanisms of pain in CP are multifactorial, involving pancreatic duct (PD) obstruction with increased PD pressure, ischemia, and neural inflammatory processes. Complications of CP such as PD/common bile duct (CBD) strictures, pseudocysts, and PD fistulas can contribute to abdominal pain. Treatment focused on treating only one mechanism of pain may fail to alleviate the patient's pain. Medical management in CP includes dietary alterations, discontinuing alcohol, analgesics/octreotide administration, pancreatic enzyme supplements, reducing oxidant stress, and neuromodulators. Interventional treatment with endotherapy is based on the theory that PD hypertension is the cause for pain in patients with CP. Certain pathologic alterations of PD, CBD, and/or sphincter lend themselves to endoscopic treatment. Endoscopic modalities, including endoscopic retrograde cholangiopancreatography (ERCP) and endoscopic ultrasound (EUS), can provide duct decompression and pseudocyst drainage. Furthermore, celiac plexus block performed during EUS can be helpful for CP pain. In this chapter, we present the role of endoscopy in the management of CP, with a particular emphasis on PD/CBD strictures and pancreatic pseudocysts.

Endotherapy in chronic pancreatitis

Both endoscopic and surgical interventions play an important role in the treatment for patients with painful obstructive CP. To date, there are two randomized controlled trials (RCTs) comparing endoscopic and surgical management in patients with painful CP with ductal obstruction [1, 2]. In Dite and colleagues' study (64 for endotherapy vs. 76 for surgery), pain relief (92% vs. 92%) as well as weight gain (66% vs. 60%) were similar between both groups at the 1 year follow up period [1]. Nevertheless, at 5 years, patients undergoing surgery reported better pain control (86% vs. 65%; $P = 0.009$) and gained more weight (52% vs. 27%; $P = 0.002$) compared to those having endoscopic intervention. Similarly, Cahen and colleagues demonstrated significantly better pain relief in patients treated with surgery compared to endotherapy after 2 years (75% vs. 32%; $P = 0.007$) [2]. Patients having surgery were more likely to have better pain control than those undergoing endoscopic intervention for those followed for 5 years (80% vs. 38%; $P = 0.042$) [3]. Patients having surgical treatment required significantly fewer procedures than those treated endoscopically [3]. There was no significant difference in Izbicki pain score, quality of life scores, health utility scores, exocrine/endocrine insufficiency, length of hospital stay, and overall cost

---

between groups at 5 years [3]. Although these RCTs suggested that surgery provides better pain control compared with endotherapy, the strength of these data are limited by small sample size and the various endoscopic and surgical techniques performed. Due to its less invasive approach, endoscopic treatment is recommended as the first-line approach for properly selected patients with painful obstructive CP who do not respond to medical therapy or who are poor surgical candidates [4–7]. According to a European Society of Gastrointestinal Endoscopy (ESGE) guideline, factors independently associated with long-term (≥2 years) pain relief following endotherapy include obstructing stones in the pancreatic head, short disease duration, low frequency of pain attacks, complete main PD stone clearance, absence of main PD stricture at initial treatment, and discontinuation of alcohol and tobacco during follow-up [4].

Pancreatic duct strictures

Role of endotherapy in PD strictures

Benign PD strictures, which occur as a consequence of periductal fibrosis or acute inflammatory changes around the main PD, are common complications of CP [8, 9]. It is critical that malignancy be ruled out once a PD stricture is found. A contrast-enhanced CT scan and/or EUS ± fine-needle aspiration (FNA) can be helpful for cancer diagnosis. In addition, tissue sampling can be performed at the stricture site during ERCP if no mass is identified. The endoscopic

management of benign PD strictures includes pancreatic sphincterotomy and stent placement (Figures 15A.1a–c and 15A.2a–d). Dilatation of PD stricture can be performed using a balloon-dilatation catheter or graduated dilating catheter. However, simple balloon dilatation is not adequate for long-term patency due to the dense fibrosis of PD strictures [10]. Therefore, one or more pancreatic stents are required to expand the lumen chronically. In general, the stent caliber should not exceed the diameter of the downstream duct. In order to prevent stent migration, we prefer to use a pancreatic stent with an external pigtail and an internal flange. Single or multiple 5–10 Fr stents are usually placed. The best candidates for endoscopic PD stricture management are patients with symptomatic CP having a focal head stricture with upstream duct dilation [9–12]. Patients with complex multifocal strictures, small diameter ducts, and diffuse duct disease are at risk of a poor outcome after pancreatic stent placement.

Results of endotherapy in PD strictures

In patients with CP, the response rate of pancreatic stent placement depends on PD morphology. Patients with no PD dilation/stricture, either PD stricture or dilation, and PD stricture with upstream dilation improved in 47%, 64%, 67%, and 100%, respectively ($P = 0.003$). Based on the results of selected studies (12 series during 1988–2013; $n = 556$) [9, 13–23], technical success of pancreatic stent placement was reported in 91% for patients with CP with a dominant stricture. During a mean follow-up period of 34 months,

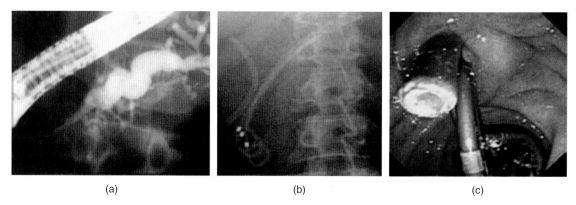

| (a) | (b) | (c) |

Figure 15A.1 (a) Main pancreatic duct stricture in the head of pancreas. (b) and (c) Multiple pancreatic stents placed. Note that a biliary stent was placed for a bile duct stricture.

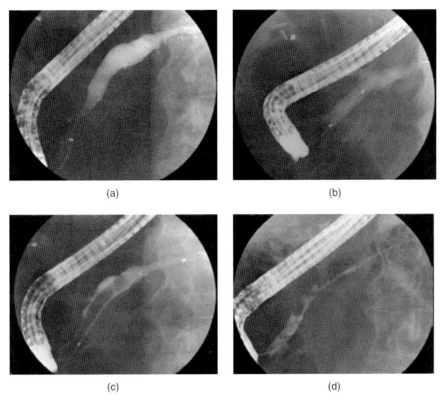

(a)   (b)

(c)   (d)

Figure 15A.2 (a) Main pancreatic duct stricture in the head of pancreas. (b) Balloon dilation of pancreatic duct stricture in the head of pancreas. (c) Fully covered self-expandable metallic stent placement. (d) Pancreatic duct stricture resolution after temporary fully covered self-expandable metallic stent was removed.

symptom improvement was identified in 62%. Major complications were seen in 18% with a 0.6% mortality rate. Although placement of a single plastic stent (PS) provided good short-term pain relief (70–94%) in patients with CP with PD stricture, repeated stent change/surgery was required due to persistent and recurrent PD strictures. Given the excellent outcomes associated with treating postoperative biliary strictures with multiple PS, the efficacy of multiple PS was evaluated in a study of 19 patients with refractory PD strictures [22]. The feasibility and safety of placement of multiple 8.5–11.5 Fr PS were demonstrated with 95% stricture resolution rate and 11% recurrent strictures. The median number of stents was 3 placed for 6–12 months. During a median follow-up period of 38 months, 84% of patients were symptom free after stent removal. Although placement of multiple simultaneous PS may have a better outcome in the long term compared with single PS insertion, RCTs comparing

single versus multiple PS are required to confirm this benefit.

Based on earlier studies with PS placement [9, 13–23], refractory/recurrent PD strictures were reported in 10–38%. Due to its larger diameter (8 or 10 mm), the insertion of a self-expandable metal stent (SEMS) has been reported in an effort to maintain PD patency long-term for benign PD stricture treatment [24–27]. In the Brussels study of SEMS placement for benign PD obstruction, 20 patients treated with uncovered SEMS (USEMS) had immediate pain relief [24]. Nevertheless, 55% of patients developed stent occlusion because of epithelial hyperplasia and tissue ingrowth. Moreover, USEMS are not removable. Thus, this modality is not an option for the long-term treatment of dominant PD strictures. Fully covered SEMS (FCSEMS) provide potential advantages, including superior patency, maximal dilation during the first ERCP, requiring less number of procedures, and removability. Recently, in three series, all 47 patients had stricture resolution after 4 months of temporary FCSEMS placement [25–27]. At 5–20 months follow-up, symptom improvement was reported in 85%; 13% had recurrent strictures. The disadvantages of FCSEMS include stent oversizing, stent migration, high cost, and obstruction of side branches leading to pancreatitis. Furthermore, long-term follow-up data are lacking. A recent systemic review ($n = 80$) compared FCSEMS versus multiple PS for refractory PD strictures in CP [28]. There was no significant difference in technical success rate (100% vs. 100%), pain improvement (85.2% vs. 84.2%), stent migration (8.2% vs. 10.5%), and re-intervention rate (9.8% vs. 15.8%) between the groups.

Although the ESGE guideline recommends treating dominant main PD strictures with a single 10-Fr PS, with stent exchange performed at regular intervals (e.g., 3 months) for 1 year duration [4], refractory/recurrent strictures are common with a single PS placement. The role of multiple PS and FCSEMS warrants further study. Based on earlier RCTs comparing endotherapy versus surgery in patients with painful obstructive CP, surgery appears to be more durable. Endotherapy may predict response to surgical drainage and may also be applied as a bridge to surgery [29]; however, this does not preclude subsequent surgery.

Chronic pancreatitis-induced common bile duct strictures

Role of endotherapy in CP-induced CBD strictures

Biliary strictures occur in 3–23%% of patients with CP [30]. The patients may present with pain, jaundice, cholangitis, and secondary biliary cirrhosis [31, 32]. Malignancy should be ruled out with CT scan and EUS ± FNA once CBD strictures are identified in the setting of CP [11]. Benign CBD strictures may be secondary to acute inflammation, chronic scar formation leading to a periductal fibrotic stenosis or the development of a pancreatic pseudocyst causing extrinsic compression on the BD [32]. The indications for biliary drainage include jaundice, cholangitis, biliary cirrhosis, complicating CBD stones, progression of bile duct stricture, and persistent alkaline phosphatase elevation for more than 1 month (2–3 times above the upper normal limit) [4, 33–35]. Traditionally, surgical drainage has been recommended

as the definitive treatment for symptomatic patients with a CP-induced CBD stricture. However, there are some disadvantages for surgical intervention such as high morbidity, long recovery time, anastomotic stenosis leading to ascending cholangitis, and high cost [36]. An endoscopic approach is an alternative to surgery in the management of symptomatic biliary strictures in the setting of CP [35, 37]. Endoscopic treatment for CP-induced CBD stricture include PS or SEMS placement (Figures 15A.3a–c and 15A.4a–d). Currently, USEMS are not recommended due to its lack of removability [38, 39]. Moreover, long-term failure because of tissue ingrowth limits their use [40]. Although covered SEMSs have recently been increasingly utilized as a treatment of benign CBD strictures, previous studies showed a lower resolution rate of CP-induced CBD strictures in comparison with other causes (46–77% vs. 80–100%) [41, 42]. In a prospective follow-up study, calcifications of the pancreatic head were identified as a risk factor for failure of endoscopic stenting of CBD strictures in CP (17-fold increased risk of failure of a 12-month course of stent placement) [43].

Results of endotherapy in CP-induced CBD strictures

Previous studies (9 series from 1990 to 2005; $n = 350$) showed excellent short-term relief with use of a single stent for CBD strictures in CP [36, 37, 43–49]. However, stricture resolution rarely occurs during long-term follow-up; treatment success was reported in 31% during a mean follow-up period of 42 months after stent removal. Clogging and migration have been reported as major complications (0–36% and 1–23%). Three small series ($n = 50$) demonstrated long-term success of 66% with multiple PS during a mean follow-up period of 45 months after stent removal in patients with CP-induced CBD strictures [36, 50, 51]. Compared with single stent placement, multiple simultaneous stents provided better clinical success rate (reduction in liver function tests, episodes of cholangitis, and the diameter of the CBD stenosis before and after treatment) (24% vs. 92%, $P < 0.01$) [36]. During long-term follow-up (4 years), 92% of patient with multiple PS remained symptom free after stent therapy, whereas 38% of patients with single PS had persistently elevated liver function tests that required intermittent stent exchange [36]. Although multiple PS may provide long-term benefit in patients with CP with CBD strictures, several ERCP sessions are

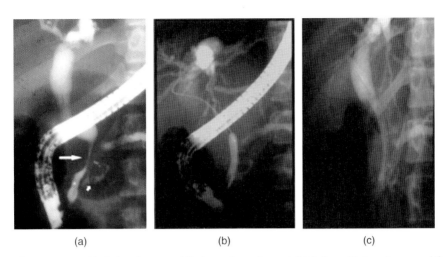

(a)   (b)   (c)

Figure 15A.3 (a) Chronic pancreatitis–induced common bile duct stricture (arrow). (b) Balloon dilation of common bile duct stricture. (c) Multiple plastic stents placed.

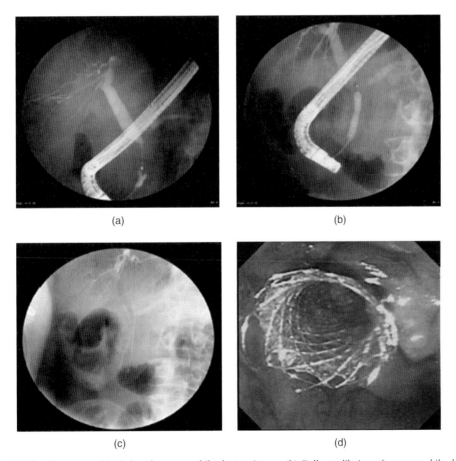

(a)   (b)

(c)   (d)

Figure 15A.4 (a) Chronic pancreatitis–induced common bile duct stricture. (b) Balloon dilation of common bile duct stricture. (c) and (d) Fully covered self-expandable metallic stent placement.

required for stent exchange to prevent cholangitis and to resolve the stricture. Due to its larger diameter, SEMS has become an established therapy for malignant biliary obstruction, but its role is unclear for benign biliary strictures [38, 42, 52–54]. Six published series between 2008 and 2014 ($n = 153$) showed the efficacy of FCSEMS for CP-induced CBD strictures [54–59]. Stricture resolution was reported in 69% after a mean stenting duration of 7 months. Stricture recurrence occurred in 13% during a mean follow-up time of 23 months. However, a major adverse event of FCSEMS is stent migration. RCTs comparing multiple PS versus FCSEMS are required to clarify the best option of endoscopic stenting in properly selected patients with CP-induced CBD stricture.

Pancreatic pseudocysts

Role of endotherapy in pancreatic pseudocysts

Pancreatic pseudocysts are defined as localized collection of pancreatic juice enclosed by a nonepithelialized wall. These can arise as a consequence of acute pancreatitis, CP, or pancreatic trauma and typically require 4 weeks or more to form [60]. Pancreatic pseudocysts occur in 20–40% of patients during the course of CP [61–63]. Based on the American Society for Gastrointestinal Endoscopy (ASGE) guideline, pseudocyst drainage is required in symptomatic patients, rapidly enlarging collections, and/or complications (such as gastric outlet/duodenal/biliary obstruction or infection) [64]. Pseudocyst drainage can be performed by surgical, endoscopic, or percutaneous approaches. A recent RCT of 40 patients with pseudocyst demonstrated equal success rate of endoscopic ($n = 20$) and open surgical cystogastrostomy ($n = 20$) (95% vs. 100%; $P = 0.50$) [65]. After a follow-up period of 24 months, there was no pseudocyst recurrence in patients undergoing endoscopic drainage and 1 in the surgically treated group ($P = 0.50$). Complications were lower in patients undergoing endoscopic approach compared with those having surgical drainage (0% vs. 10%; $P = 0.24$). In addition, endoscopic treatment was associated with a shorter hospital stay (2 days vs. 6 days; $P < 0.001$) and lower costs ($7011 vs. $15,052; $P = 0.003$). Recently, a retrospective study demonstrated similar clinical success rates for symptomatic pseudocysts treated by endoscopic and percutaneous methods (71% vs. 72%; $P = 0.36$) [66]. Nevertheless, the percutaneous approach was associated with significant higher rates of re-intervention (42% vs. 10%; $P = 0.001$), longer length of hospital stay (15 days vs. 6 days; $P = 0.001$), and increased number of follow-up abdominal imaging studies (6 vs. 4; $P = 0.02$).

Endoscopic drainage of a pseudocyst can be performed by conventional techniques using a duodenoscope (or end viewing scope) or under EUS guidance (Figures 15A.5a–f and 15A.6a–e). The route of endoscopic therapy for pseudocysts involves transpapillary, transmural (cystogastrostomy or cystoduodenostomy), or combined techniques. The transpapillary approach is preferred if a relatively small pseudocyst (less than 5 cm) communicates with the main PD. Endoscopic cystoenterostomy may be considered without EUS guidance if there is a visible luminal bulge, absence of collateral vessels, and the cyst-to-lumen distance is less than 1 cm [11]. The aim of cystoenterostomy is to create a communication between the cyst cavity and gastric or duodenal lumen. Currently, EUS techniques have expanded the patient population eligible for endoscopic treatment. EUS-guided drainage compared with blind puncture provides potential advantages including avoidance of intervening vascular structures, assessment of degree of necrosis, determination of cyst wall maturity, and the ability to perform cyst sampling for exclusion of a mucinous neoplasm. Moreover, the number of patients eligible for endoscopic drainage has been expanded, as a visible bulge is not necessary for drainage [4]. The first step of the transmural technique is to puncture the gastric/duodenal wall at the visible bulge using a needle-knife via a duodenoscope, or a 19-guage FNA needle via a linear echoendoscope. Under fluoroscopy, a guidewire is subsequently advanced through the needle knife or FNA needle into the cyst cavity and looped at least twice to maintain secure access. Then, a balloon dilator (8–10 mm) is utilized for expanding the cystoenterostomy tract. Due to aggressive flow of pseudocyst fluid from the cyst cavity to the gut lumen, head elevation of the fluoroscopy table and suction should be performed to prevent aspiration. In general, at least two double-pigtail stents are placed transmurally into the cyst cavity and can be removed when the pseudocyst resolves. However, several attempts to access the cyst cavity are needed for multiple PS insertion. Moreover, a 10-Fr PS may be hard to deploy through the relative

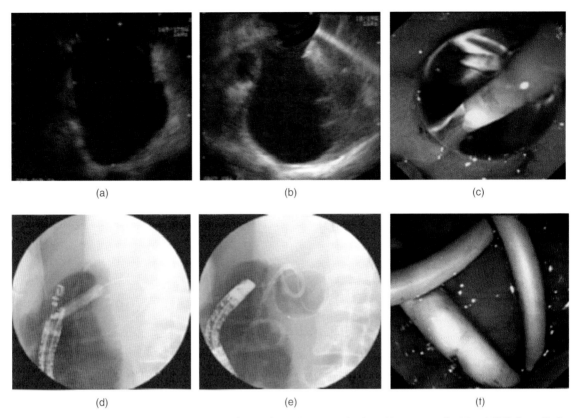

Figure 15A.5 (a) Pancreatic pseudocyst seen on EUS. (b) Pseudocyst is punctured using a 19-guage needle. (c) and (d) Balloon dilation to enlarge the cystogastrostomy tract. (e) and (f) Two double-pigtail plastic stents placed transmurally.

small 3.7-mm channel of the therapeutic linear echoendoscope. Recent studies have demonstrated the feasibility of temporary FCSEMS placement for transmural pseudocyst drainage [67–71]. The potential advantage of placing FCSEMS for this indication is the use of a single stent that has a larger diameter than the PS. However, FCSEMS may have higher rate of stent migration. Placement of a double pigtail PS through the FCSEMS has been shown to be an effective way to reduce migration [67]. In the setting of CP, it is very important that associated ductal disease be treated to obtain the best outcome.

Results of endotherapy in pancreatic pseudocysts

Previous studies showed the technical success rate of endoscopic pseudocyst drainage, ranging from 73% to 100% [14, 72–80]. Initial resolution of pancreatic pseudocysts was reported in approximately 90%.

Recurrence and complications were estimated in 13% and 14%, respectively. Recently, a meta-analysis of four studies (two RCTs and two prospective nonrandomized trials) compared EUS guided drainage and conventional techniques [81]. Due to the failure of conventional techniques when a visible bulge is not present, EUS guidance provided a significantly higher technical success rate than conventional drainage. A total of 18 patients who failed conventional drainage were successfully treated by EUS guidance on crossover. Nevertheless, EUS-guided drainage was not superior to conventional drainage regarding short- or long-term resolution. Several studies of PS placement for transmural pseudocyst drainage demonstrated successful treatment in 84–94% [82–85]. In a recent retrospective study of patients having single or multiple, 7 or 10 Fr double-pigtail PS placement for transmural drainage of uncomplicated pancreatic pseudocysts, the stent size (OR 1.54) and number (OR 1.15) were not associated

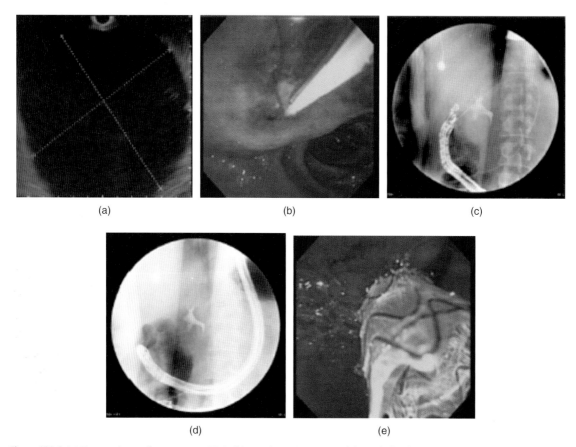

(a)
(b)
(c)

(d)
(e)

Figure 15A.6 (a) Pancreatic pseudocyst seen on EUS. (b) Pseudocyst is punctured through the duodenal wall using a 19-guage needle. (c) A guidewire is looped twice to maintain secure access. (d) and (e) Fully covered self-expandable metallic stent placed transmurally.

with the number of interventions required for treatment success when adjusted for pseudocyst size, location, drainage modality, the presence or absence of PD stent, and luminal compression [84]. Although, the evidence showed a high treatment success rate (78–100%) of temporary FCSEMS placement for transmural drainage [67–71], there are no RCTs comparing FCSEMS and PS for pseudocyst drainage regarding treatment efficacy, complication, and recurrence.

Conclusion

Management of symptomatic CP requires a multidisciplinary team approach to achieve the best treatment outcome. Although the evidence appears to favor surgery in patients with obstructive CP, endotherapy

may still be the first-line treatment option in a properly selected group due to its less invasive approach. In patients with dominant PD head strictures, PS placement provides an acceptable short-term treatment of pain/pancreatitis. However, refractory and recurrent strictures commonly occur with a single PS insertion. The role of multiple PS and FCSEMS in the management of PD strictures warrants further study. PS placement is a good alternative to surgery for short-term treatment of CP-induced CBD strictures complicated by cholestasis, jaundice, or cholangitis. The long-term efficacy of single PS insertion is much less satisfactory as stricture resolution rarely occurs. More data on long-term outcome with multiple PS and FCSEMS for treating CP-induced CBD strictures are needed. Endoscopic pseudocyst drainage has similar efficacy as open surgery at lower cost and shorter hospital stay. For the bulging pseudocyst, conventional transmural techniques can be performed. EUS guidance is preferred when there is a nonbulging lesion or collateral vessels are present. Further RCTs comparing the efficacy of FCSEMS and PS are required to determine the best option of endoscopic stent placement for transmural pseudocyst drainage.

References

1 Dite P, Ruzicka M, Zboril V, et al. A prospective, randomized trial comparing endoscopic and surgical therapy for chronic pancreatitis. Endoscopy 2003; 35: 553–558.

2 Cahen DL, Gouma DJ, Nio Y, et al. Endoscopic versus surgical drainage of the pancreatic duct in chronic pancreatitis. New England Journal of Medicine 2007; 356: 676–684.

3 Cahen DL, Gouma DJ, Laramee P, et al. Long-term outcomes of endoscopic vs surgical drainage of the pancreatic duct in patients with chronic pancreatitis. Gastroenterology 2011; 141: 1690–1695.

4 Dumonceau JM, Delhaye M, Tringali A, et al. Endoscopic treatment of chronic pancreatitis: European Society of Gastrointestinal Endoscopy (ESGE) Clinical Guideline. Endoscopy 2012; 44: 784–800.

5 Reddy DN, Ramchandani MJ, Talukdar R. Individualizing therapy for chronic pancreatitis. Clinical Gastroenterology and Hepatology 2012; 10: 803–804.

6 Clarke B, Slivka A, Tomizawa Y, et al. : Endoscopic therapy is effective for patients with chronic pancreatitis. Clinical Gastroenterology and Hepatology 2012; 10: 795–802.

7 Forsmark CE. Management of chronic pancreatitis. Gastroenterology 2013; 144: 1282–1291.

8 Kalady MF, Peterson B, Baillie J, et al. Pancreatic duct strictures: identifying risk of malignancy. Annals of Surgical Oncology 2004; 11: 581–588.

9 Cremer M, Deviere J, Delhaye M, et al. Stenting in severe chronic pancreatitis: results of medium-term follow-up in seventy-six patients. Endoscopy 1991; 23: 171–176.

10 Attasaranya S, Abdel Aziz AM, Lehman GA. Endoscopic management of acute and chronic pancreatitis. The Surgical Clinics of North America 2007; 87: 1379–1402.

11 Avula H, Sherman S. What is the role of endotherapy in chronic pancreatitis? Therapeutic Advances in Gastroenterology 2010; 3: 367–382.

12 Oza VM, Kahaleh M. Endoscopic management of chronic pancreatitis. World Journal of Gastrointestinal Endoscopy 2013; 5: 19–28.

13 McCarthy J, Geenen JE, Hogan WJ. Preliminary experience with endoscopic stent placement in benign pancreatic diseases. Gastrointestinal Endoscopy 1988; 34: 16–18.

14 Grimm H, Meyer WH, Nam VC, et al. New modalities for treating chronic pancreatitis. Endoscopy 1989; 21: 70–74.

15 Kozarek RA, Patterson DJ, Ball TJ, et al. Endoscopic placement of pancreatic stents and drains in the management of pancreatitis. Annals of Surgery 1989; 209: 261–266.

16 Binmoeller KF, Jue P, Seifert H, et al. Endoscopic pancreatic stent drainage in chronic pancreatitis and a dominant stricture: long-term results. Endoscopy 1995; 27: 638–644.

17 Ponchon T, Bory RM, Hedelius F, et al. Endoscopic stenting for pain relief in chronic pancreatitis: results of a standardized protocol. Gastrointestinal Endoscopy 1995; 42: 452–456.

18 Smits ME, Badiga SM, Rauws EA, et al. Long-term results of pancreatic stents in chronic pancreatitis. Gastrointestinal Endoscopy 1995; 42: 461–467.

19 Vitale GC, Cothron K, Vitale EA, et al. Role of pancreatic duct stenting in the treatment of chronic pancreatitis. Surgical Endoscopy 2004; 18: 1431–1434.

20 Eleftherladis N, Dinu F, Delhaye M, et al. Long-term outcome after pancreatic stenting in severe chronic pancreatitis. Endoscopy 2005; 37: 223–230.

21 Weber A, Schneider J, Neu B, et al. Endoscopic stent therapy for patients with chronic pancreatitis: results from a prospective follow-up study. Pancreas 2007; 34: 287–294.

22 Costamagna G, Bulajic M, Tringali A, et al. Multiple stenting of refractory pancreatic duct strictures in severe chronic pancreatitis: long-term results. Endoscopy 2006; 38: 254–259.

23 Weber A, Schneider J, Neu B, et al. Endoscopic stent therapy in patients with chronic pancreatitis: a 5-year follow-up study. World Journal of Gastroenterology 2013; 19: 715–720.

24 Eisendrath P, Deviere J. Expandable metal stents for benign pancreatic duct obstruction. Gastrointestinal Endoscopy Clinics of North America 1999; 9: 547–554.

25 Sauer B, Talreja J, Ellen K, et al. Temporary placement of a fully covered self-expandable metal stent in the pancreatic duct for management of symptomatic refractory chronic pancreatitis: preliminary data (with videos). Gastrointestinal Endoscopy 2008; 68: 1173–1178.

26 Moon SH, Kim MH, Park DH, et al. Modified fully covered self-expandable metal stents with antimigration features for benign pancreatic-duct strictures in advanced chronic pancreatitis, with a focus on the safety profile and reducing migration. Gastrointestinal Endoscopy 2010; 72: 86–91.

27 Giacino C, Grandval P, Laugier R. Fully covered self-expanding metal stents for refractory pancreatic duct strictures in chronic pancreatitis. Endoscopy 2012; 44: 874–877.

28 Shen Y, Liu M, Chen M, et al. Covered metal stent or multiple plastic stents for refractory pancreatic ductal strictures in chronic pancreatitis: a systematic review. Pancreatology 2014; 14: 87–90.

29 DuVall GA, Scheider DM, Kortan P, et al. Is the outcome of endoscopic therapy of chronic pancreatitis predictive of surgical success? Gastrointestinal Endoscopy 1996; 43: 405.

30 Kaffes AJ, Liu K. Fully covered self-expandable metal stents for treatment of benign biliary strictures. Gastrointestinal Endoscopy 2013; 78: 13–21.

31 van Berkel AM, Cahen DL, van Westerloo DJ, et al. Self-expanding metal stents in benign biliary strictures due to chronic pancreatitis. Endoscopy 2004; 36: 381–384.

32 Abdallah AA, Krige JE, Bornman PC. Biliary tract obstruction in chronic pancreatitis. Hepato Pancreato Biliary (Oxford) 2007; 9: 421–428.

33 Frey CF, Suzuki M, Isaji S. Treatment of chronic pancreatitis complicated by obstruction of the common bile duct or duodenum. World Journal of Surgery 1990; 14: 59–69.

34 Arslanlar S, Jain R. Benign biliary strictures related to chronic pancreatitis: balloons, stents, or surgery. Current Treatment Options in Gastroenterology 2007; 10: 369–375.

35 Nguyen-Tang T, Dumonceau JM. Endoscopic treatment in chronic pancreatitis, timing, duration and type of intervention. Best Practice & Research Clinical Gastroenterology 2010; 24: 281–298.

36 Catalano MF, Linder JD, George S, et al. Treatment of symptomatic distal common bile duct stenosis secondary to chronic pancreatitis: comparison of single vs. multiple simultaneous stents. Gastrointestinal Endoscopy 2004; 60: 945–952.

37 Smits ME, Rauws EA, van Gulik TM, et al. Long-term results of endoscopic stenting and surgical drainage for biliary stricture due to chronic pancreatitis. British Journal of Surgery 1996, 83: 764–768.

38 Siriwardana HP, Siriwardena AK. Systematic appraisal of the role of metallic endobiliary stents in the treatment of benign bile duct stricture. Annals of Surgery 2005; 242: 10–19.

39 van Boeckel PG, Vleggaar FP, Siersema PD. Plastic or metal stents for benign extrahepatic biliary strictures: a systematic review. BMC Gastroenterology 2009; 9: 96.

40 Deviere J, Cremer M, Baize M, et al. Management of common bile duct stricture caused by chronic pancreatitis with metal mesh self expandable stents. Gut 1994; 35: 122–126.

41 Poley JW, Cahen DL, Metselaar HJ, et al. A prospective group sequential study evaluating a new type of fully covered self-expandable metal stent for the treatment of benign biliary strictures (with video). Gastrointestinal Endoscopy 2012; 75: 783–789.

42 Kahaleh M, Behm B, Clarke BW, et al. Temporary placement of covered self-expandable metal stents in benign biliary strictures: a new paradigm? (with video). Gastrointestinal Endoscopy 2008; 67: 446–454.

43 Kahl S, Zimmermann S, Genz I, et al. Risk factors for failure of endoscopic stenting of biliary strictures in chronic pancreatitis: a prospective follow-up study. American Journal of Gastroenterology 2003; 98: 2448–2453.

44 Deviere J, Devaere S, Baize M, et al. Endoscopic biliary drainage in chronic pancreatitis. Gastrointestinal Endoscopy 1990; 36: 96–100.

45 Barthet M, Bernard JP, Duval JL, et al. Biliary stenting in benign biliary stenosis complicating chronic calcifying pancreatitis. Endoscopy 1994; 26: 569–572.

46 Vitale GC, Reed DN, Jr., Nguyen CT, et al. Endoscopic treatment of distal bile duct stricture from chronic pancreatitis. Surgical Endoscopy 2000; 14: 227–231.

47 Farnbacher MJ, Rabenstein T, Ell C, et al. Is endoscopic drainage of common bile duct stenoses in chronic pancreatitis up-to-date? American Journal of Gastroenterology 2000; 95: 1466–1471.

48 Eickhoff A, Jakobs R, Leonhardt A, et al. Endoscopic stenting for common bile duct stenoses in chronic pancreatitis: results and impact on long-term outcome. European Journal of Gastroenterology and Hepatology 2001; 13: 1161–1167.

49 Cahen DL, van Berkel AM, Oskam D, et al. Long-term results of endoscopic drainage of common bile duct strictures in chronic pancreatitis. European Journal of Gastroenterology and Hepatology 2005; 17: 103–108.

50 Draganov P, Hoffman B, Marsh W, et al. Long-term outcome in patients with benign biliary strictures treated endoscopically with multiple stents. Gastrointestinal Endoscopy 2002; 55: 680–686.

51 Pozsar J, Sahin P, Laszlo F, et al. Medium-term results of endoscopic treatment of common bile duct strictures in chronic calcifying pancreatitis with increasing numbers of stents. Journal of Clinical Gastroenterology 2004; 38: 118–123.

52 Davids PH, Groen AK, Rauws EA, et al. Randomised trial of self-expanding metal stents versus polyethylene stents for distal malignant biliary obstruction. Lancet 1992; 340:1488–1492.

53 Knyrim K, Wagner HJ, Pausch J, et al. A prospective, randomized, controlled trial of metal stents for malignant obstruction of the common bile duct. Endoscopy 1993; 25: 207–212.

54 Mahajan A, Ho H, Sauer B, et al. Temporary placement of fully covered self-expandable metal stents in benign biliary strictures: midterm evaluation (with video). Gastrointestinal Endoscopy 2009; 70: 303–309.

55 Cahen DL, Rauws EA, Gouma DJ, et al. Removable fully covered self-expandable metal stents in the treatment of common bile duct strictures due to chronic pancreatitis: a case series. Endoscopy 2008; 40: 697–700.

56 Behm B, Brock A, Clarke BW, et al. Partially covered self-expandable metallic stents for benign biliary strictures due to chronic pancreatitis. Endoscopy 2009; 41: 547–551.

57 Irani S, Baron TH, Akbar A, et al. Endoscopic treatment of benign biliary strictures using covered self-expandable

metal stents (CSEMS). Digestive Diseases and Sciences 2014; 59: 152–160.

58 Wagh MS, Chavalitdhamrong D, Moezardalan K, et al. Effectiveness and safety of endoscopic treatment of benign biliary strictures using a new fully covered self expandable metal stent. Diagnostic and Therapeutic Endoscopy 2013; 2013: 183513.

59 Kahaleh M, Brijbassie A, Sethi A, et al. Multicenter trial evaluating the use of covered self-expanding metal stents in benign biliary strictures: time to revisit our therapeutic options? Journal of Clinical Gastroenterology 2013; 47: 695–699.

60 Bradley EL 3rd., A clinically based classification system for acute pancreatitis. Summary of the International Symposium on Acute Pancreatitis, Atlanta, Ga, September 11 through 13, 1992. Archives of Surgery 1993; 128: 586–590.

61 Grace PA, Williamson RC. Modern management of pancreatic pseudocysts. British Journal of Surgery 1993; 80: 573–581.

62 Adler DG, Lichtenstein D, Baron TH, et al. The role of endoscopy in patients with chronic pancreatitis. Gastrointestinal Endoscopy 2006; 63: 933–937.

63 Andren-Sandberg A, Dervenis C. Pancreatic pseudocysts in the 21st century. Part I: classification, pathophysiology, anatomic considerations and treatment. Journal of the Pancreas 2004; 5: 8–24.

64 Jacobson BC, Baron TH, Adler DG, et al. ASGE guideline: the role of endoscopy in the diagnosis and the management of cystic lesions and inflammatory fluid collections of the pancreas. Gastrointestinal Endoscopy 2005; 61: 363–370.

65 Varadarajulu S, Bang JY, Sutton BS, et al. Equal efficacy of endoscopic and surgical cystogastrostomy for pancreatic pseudocyst drainage in a randomized trial. Gastroenterology 2013; 145: 583–590.

66 Akshintala VS, Saxena P, Zaheer A, et al. A comparative evaluation of outcomes of endoscopic versus percutaneous drainage for symptomatic pancreatic pseudocysts. Gastrointestinal Endoscopy 2014; 79: 921–928.

67 Penn DE, Draganov PV, Wagh MS, et al. Prospective evaluation of the use of fully covered self-expanding metal stents for EUS-guided transmural drainage of pancreatic pseudocysts. Gastrointestinal Endoscopy 2012; 76: 679–684.

68 Itoi T, Binmoeller KF, Shah J, et al. Clinical evaluation of a novel lumen-apposing metal stent for endosonography-guided pancreatic pseudocyst and gallbladder drainage (with videos). Gastrointestinal Endoscopy 2012; 75: 870–876.

69 Berzosa M, Maheshwari S, Patel KK, et al. Single-step endoscopic ultrasonography-guided drainage of peripancreatic fluid collections with a single self-expandable metal stent and standard linear echoendoscope. Endoscopy 2012; 44: 543–547.

70 Fabbri C, Luigiano C, Cennamo V, et al. Endoscopic ultrasound-guided transmural drainage of infected pancreatic fluid collections with placement of covered self-expanding metal stents: a case series. Endoscopy 2012; 44: 429–433.

71 Weilert F, Binmoeller KF, Shah JN, et al. Endoscopic ultrasound guided drainage of pancreatic fluid collections with indeterminate adherence using temporary covered metal stents. Endoscopy 2012; 44: 780–783.

72 Kozarek RA, Ball TJ, Patterson DJ, et al. Endoscopic transpapillary therapy for disrupted pancreatic duct and peripancreatic fluid collections. Gastroenterology 1991; 100: 1362–1370.

73 Catalano MF, Geenen JE, Schmalz MJ, et al. Treatment of pancreatic pseudocysts with ductal communication by transpapillary pancreatic duct endoprosthesis. Gastrointestinal Endoscopy 1995; 42: 214–218.

74 Smits ME, Rauws EA, Tytgat GN, et al. The efficacy of endoscopic treatment of pancreatic pseudocysts. Gastrointestinal Endoscopy 1995; 42: 202–207.

75 Binmoeller KF, Seifert H, Walter A, et al. Transpapillary and transmural drainage of pancreatic pseudocysts. Gastrointestinal Endoscopy 1995; 42: 219–224.

76 Baron TH, Harewood GC, Morgan DE, et al. Outcome differences after endoscopic drainage of pancreatic necrosis, acute pancreatic pseudocysts, and chronic pancreatic pseudocysts. Gastrointestinal Endoscopy 2002; 56: 7–17.

77 Kahaleh M, Shami VM, Conaway MR, et al. Endoscopic ultrasound drainage of pancreatic pseudocyst: a prospective comparison with conventional endoscopic drainage. Endoscopy 2006; 38: 355–359.

78 Park DH, Lee SS, Moon SH, et al. Endoscopic ultrasound-guided versus conventional transmural drainage for pancreatic pseudocysts: a prospective randomized trial. Endoscopy 2009; 41: 842–848.

79 Varadarajulu S, Christein JD, Tamhane A, et al. Prospective randomized trial comparing EUS and EGD for transmural drainage of pancreatic pseudocysts (with videos). Gastrointestinal Endoscopy 2008; 68: 1102–1111.

80 Hookey LC, Debroux S, Delhaye M, et al. Endoscopic drainage of pancreatic-fluid collections in 116 patients: a comparison of etiologies, drainage techniques, and outcomes. Gastrointestinal Endoscopy 2006; 63: 635–643.

81 Panamonta N, Ngamruengphong S, Kijsirichareanchai K, et al. Endoscopic ultrasound-guided versus conventional transmural techniques have comparable treatment outcomes in draining pancreatic pseudocysts. European Journal of Gastroenterology and Hepatology 2012; 24: 1355–1362.

82 Varadarajulu S, Bang JY, Phadnis MA, et al. Endoscopic transmural drainage of peripancreatic fluid collections: outcomes and predictors of treatment success in 211 consecutive patients. Journal of Gastrointestinal Surgery 2011; 15: 2080–2088.

83 Sadik R, Kalaitzakis E, Thune A, et al. EUS-guided drainage is more successful in pancreatic pseudocysts compared with abscesses. World Journal of Gastroenterology 2011; 17: 499–505.

84 Bang JY, Mel Wilcox C, Trevino JM, et al. Relationship between stent characteristics and treatment outcomes in endoscopic transmural drainage of uncomplicated pancreatic pseudocysts. Surgical Endoscopy 2014; 28: 2877–2883.

85 Seewald S, Ang TL, Richter H, et al. Long-term results after endoscopic drainage and necrosectomy of symptomatic pancreatic fluid collections. Digestive Endoscopy 2012, 24: 36–41.

Shocking and fragmenting pancreatic ductal stones

Rupjyoti Talukdar[1,2] & Duvvur Nageshwar Reddy[1]

[1] Department of Gastroenterology, Asian Institute of Gastroenterology, Hyderabad, India
[2] Wellcome DBT India Alliance Laboratory, Asian Healthcare Foundation, Hyderabad, India

Introduction

Pain is the dominant and most compelling symptom of chronic pancreatitis (CP) that mandates intense medical attention. Pain in CP is multifactorial. From a broad mechanistic perspective, pain results from a composite of persistent inflammation and neurobiologic interactions that involves the pancreatic nerves, dorsal root ganglia, and the pain-modulating architecture within the brain [1]. It has long been held that ductal hypertension that results from obstructing pancreatic duct calculi and strictures is a major driver of pancreatic pain [2]. Experimental studies have recently shown that ductal hypertension can cause activation of pancreatic stellate cells, which generates oxidative stress and inflammation [3]. These observations justify ductal decompression as a major approach to ameliorate pain. Several surgical and endoscopic modalities have evolved over the years.

We discuss the current status of endotherapy for pancreatic ductal stones, with emphasis on shockwave lithotripsy.

Modalities for stone fragmentation

The primary goal of endotherapy is to break the calculi into small fragments. This can be achieved directly during endoscopic retrograde cholangiopancreatography (ERCP) (with mechanical, electrohydraulic, or laser-guided lithotripsy) or with extracorporeal shockwave lithotripsy (ESWL).

ERCP methods

Endotherapy usually involves a pancreatic sphincterotomy [4] and standard accessories (balloons, baskets, and biopsy forceps) are used to extract stones and fragments [5]. Stents may be placed to facilitate extraction of fragments after ESWL, especially in patients with concomitant ductal strictures.

ERCP-directed lithotripsy techniques are far less successful (and more risky) than when applied in the bile duct because stones are often very hard and because of the natural tortuosity of the duct.

Intraductal mechanical lithotripsy is now rarely used because of a low success rate and significant complications [6, 7]. A particular problem for through-the-scope mechanical lithotripsy is the potential for the baskets to get trapped or broken, sometimes requiring surgical removal [8].

Electrohydraulic and laser lithotripsy techniques are performed under direct visualization using pancreatoscopes, which is important since the duct wall is easily damaged if the energy is misdirected. This risk can be reduced by using a dual-laser system that recognizes its target before firing. Experience with these methods is limited, results are suboptimal, and long-term follow-up data are nonexistent [9–11]. Currently, EHL and laser lithotripsy may be considered only as a second option for stones refractory to a technically sound ESWL.

Pancreatitis: Medical and Surgical Management, First Edition.
David B. Adams, Peter B. Cotton, Nicholas J. Zyromski and John Windsor.
© 2017 John Wiley & Sons, Ltd. Published 2017 by John Wiley & Sons, Ltd.

Extracorporeal shockwave lithotripsy (ESWL)

ESWL has emerged as the preferred method for managing large stones and has been recommended as the first-line treatment by the ESGE [12]. This is particularly true for large (>5 mm) obstructive calculi located in the head and body regions. The goal is to reduce the stones to fragments smaller than 3 mm.

Techniques: ESWL machines have four different components: a shockwave generator, a focusing system, a coupling mechanism, and a localizing unit [13]. Currently available third-generation lithotripters are equipped with bi-dimensional fluoroscopic and ultrasonic targeting systems, which have shown better results (as opposed to the older generation lithotripters) in patients of any age and stage of the disease. In the presence of multiple ductal stones, the ones nearest to the duct orifice should be targeted first. Isolated intraductal stones located in the tail need not be treated with ESWL. A maximum of 5000 shocks per session with an intensity of 15,000–16,000 Kv and 90 shocks per minute are usually delivered [14]. The mean number of sessions required in our cases is 3, with a range of 1–8. ERCP with pancreatic sphincterotomy is usually performed after ESWL to remove the stone fragments. Stenting may be performed in select situations, for example, in the presence of a pancreatic ductal stricture. ESWL has been described as effective in some patients without any use of ERCP/sphincterotomy, before or afterward [15]. In patients with radiolucent stones, pancreatic sphincterotomy and nasopancreatic tube placement are performed before ESWL to facilitate targeting [16]. However, radiolucent stones tend to be soft and can often be managed with ERCP extraction techniques alone.

The addition of secretin stimulation for pancreatic ESWL was recommended recently. It produces a fluid–stone interface, akin to that in ureteral stones that is supposed to result in more efficient fragmentation. Choi et al. reported in a cohort of 233 patients that intravenous administration of 16 mcg secretin prior to ESWL resulted in a 63% stone clearance compared with 46% when secretin was not used [17]. Analysis showed that secretin and pre-ESWL pancreatic stenting were independent predictors of complete or near-complete stone clearance.

Anesthesia: ESWL has traditionally been performed under general anesthesia. In our experience, thoracic epidural anesthesia (TEA) with bupivacaine 0.25% (with or without clonidine) to cause D6–D12 segmental block had yielded favorable results. TEA also offers the advantage of a reduced procedural time when compared with the use of standard anesthesia [18].

Precautions: ESWL should be avoided in patients with stones only in the pancreatic tail, stones all along the main pancreatic duct, multiple ductal strictures, and presence of moderate to massive ascites, large pancreatic pseudocysts, and pancreatic head masses [19].

Efficacy: Several studies have reported rates of complete stone fragmentation, stone clearance, and pain relief with or without ERCP (Table 15B.1). Recently, we have demonstrated complete pain relief in 69% and 60% patients on intermediate (2–5 years) and long-term (>5 years) follow-up, respectively, after ESWL in a cohort of 636 patients [25]. ESWL resulted in complete clearance of stones in 77% and 76% in the intermediate and long-term follow-up groups, respectively. Fourteen percent of patients in the intermediate follow-up group and 22.8% in the long-term group had stone recurrence. However, repeat ESWL was required in only 4% of patients on intermediate follow-up while none in the long-term follow-up patients. This study suggested that pain relief is likely to persist for a longer duration if ESWL is initiated early on.

In a previous retrospective study of 120 patients by Seven et al. [24], complete pain relief was observed in 50%, along with a significant improvement in quality-of-life scores (VAS) [7.3 (2.7) vs. 3.7 (2.4); $P < 0.001$]. Pain relief was observed in 85% patients after a mean follow-up of 4.3 years. Longest follow-up period in this study was over 7 years. Proportion of pain-free patients followed-up for over 4 years was significantly higher than those who underwent surgery [61% vs. 21%; $P = 0.009$]. This was in contrast to the study by Tandan et al., in which most patients were below the age of 40 years and nearly all of them were idiopathic [25].

ESWL is effective in stone clearance and amelioration of pain across different age groups and all etiologies. We have recently demonstrated that ESWL can be performed for large stones safely and effectively in children [26]. In this study, 34.9% children who had pancreatic ductal calculi greater than 5 mm size were treated with a total of 57 ESWL sessions (range 1–3 session per patient). There were no intraprocedural

Table **15B.1** Studies evaluating the efficacy of ESWL with or without ERCP for the treatment of pancreatic ductal calculi.

Author	Year	Treatment	Follow-up in months	N	Complete duct clearance (%)	Overall (complete) pain relief (%)
Kozarek et al. [20]	2002	ESWL + ERCP	30	40	NA	80
Farnbacher et al. [7]	2002	ESWL + ERCP	29	125	64	(48)
Delahaye et al. [21]	2004	ESWL + ERCP	173	56	48	66
Inui et al. [22]	2005	ESWL + ERCP	44	237	73	91
		ESWL		318	70	
Dumonceau et al. [23]	2007	ESWL + ERCP	52	29	NA	55
		ESWL		26	NA	58
Tandan et al. [18]	2010	ESWL + ERCP	6	1006	76	84
Seven et al. [24]	2012	ESWL + ERCP	51	120	NA	50
Tandan et al. [25]	2013	ESWL + ERCP	96	636	76	60.6

adverse events, and only eight (4.8%) patients overall (which also included children undergoing only ERCP) developed postprocedure adverse events in the form of mild AP in two and abdominal pain in six patients.

Adverse events: ESWL has a much better safety profile compared with that of mechanical and electrohydraulic lithotripsy. Usual complications include acute pancreatitis, splenic injury, skin petechiae, bleeding, steinstrasse, and perforation, with acute pancreatitis being the most important. A recent study on 1470 pancreatic ESWL procedures on 634 patients reported an overall complication rate of 6.7%. Presence of pancreas divisum and the interval between diagnosis of CP and ESWL were risk factors for developing post-ESWL complications with odds ratios of 1.28 each. On the other hand, male gender, diabetes, and steatorrhea were associated with odds ratios for complications of 0.50, 0.45, and 0.19, respectively, indicating that these are protective factors. Out of these three, male gender emerged as the single independent protective factor against moderate-to-severe complications (odds ratio 0.19) [27].

Conclusion

The published literature and our own large experience show that ESWL, with or without ERCP, is a major advance in the management of pancreatic stones. The technology and specific methods deserve to be more widely applied, akin to the universal popularity of ESWL for kidney stones.

References

1 Talukdar R, Reddy DN. Pain in chronic pancreatitis: managing beyond the pancreatic duct. World Journal of Gastroenterology, 2013; 19: 6319–6328.

2 Talukdar R. Pathogenesis of acute and chronic pancreatitis. In: Reddy DN (Ed). Recent Advances in Pancreas. Elsevier. New Delhi. 2012: 27–53.

3 Asaumi H, Watanabe S, Taguchi M, Tashiro M, Otsuki M. Externally applied pressure activates pancreatic stellate cells through the generation of intracellular reactive oxygen species. American Journal of Physiology: Gastrointestinal and Liver Physiology 2007; 293: G972–G978.

4 Choi EK, Lehman GA. Update on endoscopic management of main pancreatic duct stones in chronic calcific pancreatitis. Korean Journal of Internal Medicine 2012; 27: 20–29.

5 Tandan M, Nageshwar Reddy D. Endotherapy in chronic pancreatitis. World Journal of Gastroenterology 2013; 19: 6156–6164.

6 Freeman ML. Mechanical lithotripsy for pancreatic duct stones. Gastrointestinal Endoscopy 1996; 44: 333–336.

7 Farnbacher MJ, Schoen C, Rabenstein T, et al. Pancreatic duct stones in chronic pancreatitis: criteria for treatment intensity and success. Gastrointestinal Endoscopy 2002; 56: 501–506.

8 Thomas M, Howell DA, Carr-Locke D, et al. Mechanical lithotripsy of pancreatic and biliary stones: complications and available treatment options collected from expert centers. American Journal of Gastroenterology 2007; 102: 1896–1902.

9 Howell DA, Dy RM, Hanson BL, et al. Endoscopic treatment of pancreatic duct stones using a 10F pancreatoscope and electrohydraulic lithotripsy. Gastrointestinal Endoscopy 1999; 50: 829–833.

10 Chen YK, Taransky PR, Raijman I, et al. Peroral pancreatic stone therapy and investigation of suspected pancreatic

lesions- first human experience using the spyglass direct visualization system (SDVS). Gastrointestinal Endoscopy 2008; 67: AB108.

11 Maydeo A, Kwek BE, Bhandari S, et al. Single-operator cholangioscopy-guided laser lithotripsy in patients with difficult biliary and pancreatic ductal stones (with videos). Gastrointestinal Endoscopy. 2011;74(6):1308–1314.

12 Dumonceau JM, Delhaye M, Tringali A, Dominguez-Munoz JE, Poley JW, et al. Endoscopic treatment of chronic pancreatitis: European Society of Gastrointestinal Endoscopy (ESGE) Clinical Guideline. Endoscopy 2012 ; 44: 784–800.

13 Nguyen-Tang T, Dumonceau J-M. Endoscopic treatment in chronic pancreatitis, timing, duration and type of intervention. Best Practice & Research Clinical Gastroenterology 2010; 24: 281–298.

14 Ong WC, Tandan M, Reddy V, Rao GV, Reddy DN. Multiple pancreatic duct stones in tropical chronic pancreatitis: safe clearance with extracorporeal shock wave lithotripsy. Journal of Gastroenterology and Hepatology 2006; 21: 1514–1518.

15 Ohara H, Hoshino M, Hayakwa T, et al. Single application extracorporeal shock wave lithotripsy is the first choice for patients with pancreatic duct stones. American Journal of Gastroenterology 1996; 91: 1388–1394.

16 Tandan M, Reddy DN, Santosh D, et al. Extracorporeal shock wave lithotripsy and endotherapy for pancreatic calculi- a large single center experience. Indian Journal of Gastroenterology 2010; 29: 143–148.

17 Choi EK, McHenry L, Watkins JL, et al. Use of intravenous secretin during extracorporeal shock wave lithotripsy to facilitate endoscopic clearance of pancreatic duct stones. Pancreatology 2012; 12: 272–275.

18 Darisetty S, Tandan M, Reddy DN, et al. Epidural anesthesia is effective for extracorporeal shock wave lithotripsy of pancreatic and biliary calculi. World Journal of Gastrointestinal Surgery 2010; 2: 165–168.

19 Tringali A, Boskoski I, Costamagna G, et al. The role of endoscopy in the therapy of chronic pancreatitis. Best Practice & Research Clinical Gastroenterology 2008; 22: 145–165.

20 Kozarek RA, Brandabur JJ, Ball TJ, et al. Clinical outcomes in patients who undergo extracorporeal shock wave lithotripsy for chronic calcific pancreatitis. Gastrointestinal Endoscopy 2002; 56: 496–500.

21 Delahaye M, Aravantakis M, Verset G, et al. Long-term clinical outcome after endoscopic pancreatic ductal drainage of patients with painful chronic pancreatitis. Clinical Gastroenterology and Hepatology 2004; 2: 1096–1106.

22 Inui K, Tazuma S, Yamaguchi T, et al. Treatment of pancreatic stones with extracorporeal lithotripsy: results of a multicenter survey. Pancreas 2005; 30: 26–30.

23 Dumonceau JM, Costamagna G, Tringali A, et al. Treatment of painful chronic calcific pancreatitis: extracorporeal shock wave lithotripsy versus endoscopic treatment: a randomized controlled trial. Gut 2007; 56: 545–552.

24 Seven G, Schreiner MA, Ross AS, et al. Long-term outcomes associated with pancreatic extracorporeal shock wave lithotripsy for chronic calcific pancreatitis. Gastrointestinal Endoscopy 2012; 75: 997–1004.

25 Tandan M, Reddy DN, Talukdar R, et al. Long-term clinical outcomes of extracorporeal shockwave lithotripsy in painful chronic calcific pancreatitis. Gastrointestinal Endoscopy 2013; 78: 726–733.

26 Agarwal J, Nageshwar Reddy D, Talukdar R, et al. ERCP in the management of pancreatic diseases in children. Gastrointestinal Endoscopy 2014; 79: 271–278.

27 Li BR, Liao Z, Du TT, et al. Risk factors for complications of pancreatic extracorporeal shock wave lithotripsy. Endoscopy 2014: 46: 1092–1100.

PART C: Endoscopic management: celiac plexus blockade

Vikesh K. Singh

Division of Gastroenterology, Johns Hopkins University School of Medicine, Baltimore, MD, USA

Introduction

Pain is the dominant symptom for many patients with chronic pancreatitis (CP), and its management is difficult. Opioid analgesics are often prescribed, but they carry the risk of tolerance, addiction, and a myriad of gastrointestinal side effects with prolonged use.

Blocking the relevant afferent nerves in the celiac plexus is a logical approach to treatment. This has been achieved during surgery, and by percutaneous injection, which was first described in 1914 [1]. Localization of the site of injection by fluoroscopy was superseded by CT guidance; more recently, endoscopic ultrasound (EUS) has become the preferred method.

Technique

The patient is placed in the left lateral decubitus position and sedation is administered. A linear array echoendoscope is advanced to the takeoff of the celiac artery from the aorta, which is seen just after traversing the gastroesophageal junction. The celiac plexus is located anterolateral to the celiac artery and is composed of paired ganglia. Under Doppler guidance, a fine-needle aspiration (FNA) needle, without a stylet and preflushed with saline to remove air, is advanced into the soft tissue anterocephalad to the celiac artery (central injection; see Figures 15C.1–15C.3), into the soft tissue on either side of and caudal to the celiac artery (bilateral injection) or directly into the celiac ganglia (oblong hypoechoic structures with hyperechoic

foci; see Figures 15C.1 and 15C.4). The 19-gauge needle is more difficult to insert, particularly when there is a short distance between the gastric wall and the intended site or structure for injection, but generally allows for easier injection due to its larger diameter. Conversely, the 22-gauge needle is easier to insert but more difficult to inject through given its smaller diameter. Care must be taken to evaluate the anatomic structures near the celiac artery takeoff, particularly the left adrenal gland, which can be easily mistaken for a celiac ganglion; to aspirate prior to each injection to ensure no return of blood; and to administer prophylactic antibiotics. The injectate for a celiac plexus block typically consists of a local anesthetic (usually 20 cc of 0.25% bupivacaine) and a corticosteroid (usually 80 mg of triamcinolone). This is in contrast to a celiac plexus neurolysis where alcohol is used instead of a corticosteroid in order to ablate the plexus. The total quantity of injectate can be administered centrally or into the ganglia or divided in half for bilateral injections.

Complications

Minor but more frequently occurring complications of celiac plexus blockade are due to sympathetic blockade and include transient hypotension, diarrhea, and an increase in pain. This suggests that they should be considered to be side effects as opposed to true complications of the procedure. Major but infrequent complications that have been previously reported include retroperitoneal abscess and bleeding, ischemia, and empyema. It is possible that retroperitoneal abscesses are more likely to occur in patients

Pancreatitis: Medical and Surgical Management, First Edition.
David B. Adams, Peter B. Cotton, Nicholas J. Zyromski and John Windsor.
© 2017 John Wiley & Sons, Ltd. Published 2017 by John Wiley & Sons, Ltd.

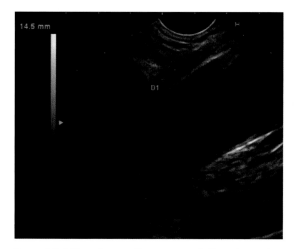

Figure 15C.1 The celiac ganglia, measuring 1.45 cm, is seen just anterior to the takeoff of the celiac artery from the aorta.

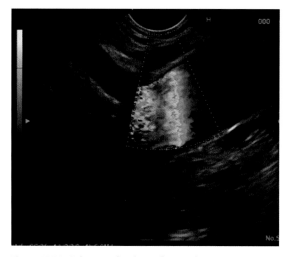

Figure 15C.2 Color Doppler shows flow in the aorta.

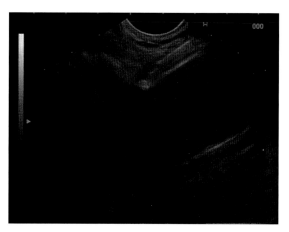

Figure 15C.3 A 19-gauge needle is inserted into the celiac ganglia.

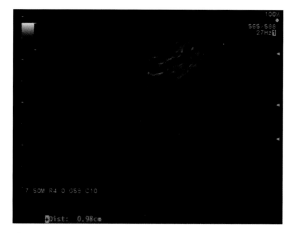

Figure 15C.4 A 1-cm celiac ganglia is seen as a hypoechoic oblong structure with hyperechoic foci.

who either do not receive prophylactic antibiotics or use acid suppressive therapies. A recent large case series evaluated 128 patients who underwent a total of 189 procedures and reported a total complication rate of 1.6%, with 0.5% and 1.1% categorized as major and minor, respectively, and 0.5% considered minor and lasting for greater than 48 hours [2]. When the authors pooled their results with those of prior studies, they reported a total complication rate of 4.7% with 0.6% and 4%, categorized as major and minor, respectively, and 1.9% considered minor and lasting for greater than 48 hours [2]. There have been two reports of fatality after EUS-guided celiac plexus neurolysis, one occurring after inadvertent injection into the celiac artery [3] and the other after 13 procedures over 4 years resulted in gastric and aortic necrosis and perforation [4]. While there have been six reports of permanent paraplegia [5–10] as well as three reports of reversible paraplegia [11–13] occurring after percutaneous celiac plexus blockade, permanent paraplegia due to the endoscopic approach has been only reported once [14].

Outcomes

Despite the heterogeneity of prior studies of endoscopic celiac plexus blockade with regard to patient selection, technique, and assessment of outcome, two reviews reported pooled rates of pain relief of 51.5% [15] and 59.5% [16]. These reviews incorporated unpublished abstracts and studies that utilized the same patients in two separate publications. However, even after excluding these abstracts and duplicated patients, the pooled pain relief rates for endoscopic celiac plexus blockade is 50% (see Table 15C.1). Unfortunately, the mean duration of pain relief has been reported to be approximately 1 month [16].

Two randomized trials have compared endoscopic versus percutaneous celiac plexus blockade. The first by Gress et al. randomized a total of 18 patients: 10 to endoscopic and 8 to percutaneous bilateral celiac plexus blockade with short-term pain relief rates of 50% and 25%, respectively. The median pain score decreased from 8 to 1 versus 10 to 9 at weeks in the endoscopic versus percutaneous arms, respectively [23]. Overall, 30% of patients had relief at 24 weeks in the endoscopic arm but only 12% did at 12 weeks in the percutaneous arm. The second study randomized a total of 56 patients: 27 to endoscopic and 29 to percutaneous bilateral celiac plexus blockade with pain response in 70% versus 30% ($P = 0.04$), respectively [20]. Both studies were small and had methodologic limitations. However, the endoscopic approach may better localize the site of injection as there is considerable topographic variation of the celiac artery and, therefore, location of the celiac plexus [24]. This is also one potential reason why there have been no differences between central versus bilateral celiac plexus blockade. A cohort study evaluating central versus bilateral injection for blockade and neurolysis in patients with CP ($n = 79$) and pancreatic cancer ($n = 72$), respectively, found that bilateral injection is an independent predictor of pain relief (OR 3.55, 95% CI: 1.72–7.34, $P = 0.001$) [24] but this was not supported by a recent trial utilizing this technique for celiac plexus neurolysis in patients with pancreatic cancer [25]. There have also been no differences in rates of pain relief between 1 or 2 injections in patients undergoing celiac plexus blockade for CP [19] or celiac plexus neurolysis for pancreatic cancer [26].

Levy et al. demonstrated that direct visualization and injection of the celiac ganglia in patients with CP resulted in pain relief in 80% (4/5 undergoing neurolysis) and 38% (5/13 undergoing blockade) [17]. Subsequent studies have established the superiority of celiac ganglia over celiac plexus neurolysis for pain relief in patients with pancreatic cancer [27, 28]; however, there have been no trials evaluating celiac ganglia blockade in patients with CP. It is possible that the celiac ganglia are more commonly visualized in patients with pancreatic cancer, particularly in advanced stages, due to metastases to the celiac axis. There have been other techniques used for pain relief in patients with pancreatic cancer, including EUS-guided insertion of radioactive seeds into the celiac plexus [29] and broad plexus neurolysis over the superior mesenteric artery [30]. However, neither is in widespread use and neither have been evaluated for CP.

Table 15C.1 Studies evaluating celiac plexus block for chronic pancreatitis.

Author [Refs]	Year	Number of patients	Response	Number of EUS criteria	Calcifications?	ERCP
Levy [17]	2008	18	5/13 steroid 4/5 alcohol	≥4	Not stated	No
Gress [18]	2001	90	50/90	Not stated	Not stated	Cambridge classification
Leblanc [19]	2009	50	31/50 10% in those who had repeat block	≥3	Yes	Cambridge classification, 49% with mild CP
Santosh [20]	2009	27	19/27	≥6	Yes	No
Sahai [21]	2009	79	Not reported for CP	≥5	Yes	No
Stevens [22]	2012	40	6/40	Rosemont Indeterminate or higher	Not stated	No

While alcohol was used to perform neurolysis in five patients with CP in the study by Levy et al. [17], alcohol is typically avoided in benign conditions such as CP for two reasons. The first is the theoretical concern that permanent ablation of the celiac plexus will lead to unopposed parasympathetic activity. However, a small study of six patients undergoing percutaneous celiac plexus neurolysis found that permanent denervation does not occur as cardiovascular parameters (blood pressure, pulse) returned to normal after 1 day, pancreatic hormone levels remained constant, and pain returned 1 week after neurolysis [31] possibly because the celiac plexus is only partially destroyed on histologic examination [32]. The second is the concern that the use of alcohol in CP could lead to a desmoplastic reaction that could make subsequent pancreatic surgery more difficult and unsafe but there is no data to support or refute this claim.

A recent well-designed randomized trial of bilateral celiac plexus blockade in patients with CP compared bupivacaine ($n = 19$) versus the combination of bupivacaine and triamcinolone ($n = 21$) and found 1 month response rates of 15.8% versus 14.3% ($P = 0.64$), respectively [22]. The study concluded that the addition of triamcinolone did not augment the effect of bupivacaine alone.

Editorials on endoscopic celiac plexus blockade have been advocating for a sham-controlled trial for many years [33, 34], and this led to a multicenter effort to conduct a randomized, double-blinded, and sham-controlled trial of patients with painful CP. The interim analysis of this trial, presented at DDW 2014, showed a significant reduction in pain scores at 1 month, assessed by the visual analog scale, of $-29 \pm 46\%$ versus $+1 \pm 26\%$ for bilateral endoscopic celiac plexus block ($n = 18$) and sham ($n = 18$) ($P = 0.011$), respectively. However, there was no difference in the use of morphine between the two groups. The planned enrollment is 40 patients per arm [35].

Limitations of celiac plexus blockade

There are two primary limitations of all studies evaluating celiac plexus blockade for pain relief in CP. The first is the method by which CP was defined as there is no "gold-standard" for the diagnosis of noncalcific CP.

While histopathology has commonly been used as the "gold standard," there is no consensus among pathologists on the quantity and extent of fibrosis and chronic inflammation necessary to diagnose noncalcific CP. Since tissue acquisition can cause acute pancreatitis and histologic evaluation often demonstrates focal and patchy disease in noncalcific CP, routine biopsy is not performed. It is also known that histologic fibrosis is commonly found in asymptomatic individuals who are older [36], consume alcohol [37] and/or smoke [38], and are obese [39]. Upper abdominal pain alone is neither sensitive nor specific for noncalcific CP as a number of other conditions present with similar symptoms. Even in patients with established findings of CP on CT imaging, there is a poor correlation between those findings and pain [40]. Histology is often obtained at the time of surgical intervention in most patients with CP, which biases the performance characteristics of any preoperative diagnostic test to those with more severe disease.

EUS was the primary diagnostic test used to diagnose CP in prior studies evaluating celiac plexus blockade (see Table 15C.1). Based on studies utilizing histology as the reference standard, EUS was reported to have sensitivities of 75–91% and specificities of 80–100% for CP [41–43]. However, these studies had many limitations, including surgical resection for cancer in 95% [41], high pretest probability of CP based on smoking (72%) and history of acute pancreatitis (94%) [43], and variable thresholds of fibrosis utilized to define CP [41–43]. Only one study to date, published in abstract form, evaluated the ability of EUS to diagnose noncalcific CP in 50 patients undergoing total pancreatectomy over a 2.5-year period [44]. EUS demonstrated poor discrimination with an AUC of 0.59. The positive predictive value for an abnormal EUS was 72% when six or more criteria were present. There was a clear selection bias for patients with severe or suspected severe disease, and it is not known whether this cohort represented consecutive patients or only patients in whom histology was obtained. Overall, the lower threshold for EUS criteria increases sensitivity, whereas the higher threshold increases specificity for a diagnosis of CP. Given the high interobserver variability for the standard EUS criteria [45, 46], the Rosemont criteria were developed in 2009 as a four-level probability classification system that assigns weights and numerical thresholds to the different EUS criteria [47]. However, the Rosemont criteria are more cumbersome, based on expert opinion as opposed to a histological standard, and have not improved interobserver variability [48, 49].

The second and more important limitation of endoscopic celiac plexus blockade is the lack of recognition that the mechanisms of pain in CP are complex. It is clear that ongoing peripheral nociceptive input from a chronically inflamed pancreas results in altered central pain processing [50]. For this reason, endoscopic and surgical interventions have variable efficacy and most patients ultimately will require opioid analgesics for the management of their pain, which only increase central sensitization, lead to tolerance, and a myriad of gastrointestinal side effects, including narcotic bowel syndrome. Opioid dependence has been shown to be a factor associated with a reduced pain response in patients with CP undergoing celiac plexus blockade [51] as well as another denervation procedure, thoracic splanchnicectomy [52]. Peripheral nerves also display a remarkable ability to regenerate [53], and this might also explain the limited efficacy of celiac plexus blockade.

Indications

The technique and risks of endoscopic celiac plexus blockade are now well established, and it has an unequivocal palliative role in patients with pancreatic cancer. However, the rather short duration of any benefit (weeks or months) reduces its value in patients with CP. It should also be noted that the role of celiac plexus blockade for the treatment of chronic upper abdominal pain of unclear etiology has not been established. There are limits to the number of times the procedure should be repeated. The respite from pain may be valuable as a temporizing measure and as a bridge to more definitive surgical therapy or chronic pain management. Some practitioners advocate the use of celiac plexus blockade as a patient selection tool for total pancreatectomy but this requires further study.

Conclusion

Endoscopic celiac plexus blockade is a useful tool in managing painful CP, but with limited indications.

References

1 Jain P, Dutta A, Sood J. Celiac plexus blockade and neurolysis: an overview. Indian Journal of Anaesthesia. 2006: 50 (3); 169–177.

2 O'Toole TM, Schmulewitz N. Complication rates of EUS-guided celiac plexus blockade and neurolysis: results of a large case series. Endoscopy 2009; 41: 593–597.

3 Gimeno-Garcia AZ, Elwassief A, Paquin SC et al. Fatal complication after endoscopic ultrasound-guided celiac plexus neurolysis. Endoscopy 2012; 44 Suppl 2: E267.

4 Loeve US, Mortensen MB. Lethal necrosis and perforation of the stomach and the aorta after multiple EUS-guided celiac plexus neurolysis procedures in a patient with chronic pancreatitis. Gastrointestinal Endoscopy 2013; 77: 151–152.

5 Woodham MJ, Hanna MH. Paraplegia after celiac plexus block. Anaesthesia 1989; 44: 487–489.

6 Kinoshita H, Denda S, Shimoji K et al. Paraplegia following celiac plexus block by anterior approach under direct vision. Masui 1996; 45: 1244–1246.

7 Hayakawa J, Kobayashi O, Murayama H. Paraplegia after intraoperative celiac plexus block. Anesthesia and Analgesia 1997; 84: 447–448.

8 Galizia EJ, Lahiri SK. Paraplegia following celiac plexus block with phenol. Case Report. British Journal of Anaesthesia 1974; 46: 539–540.

9 De Conno F, Caraceni A, Aldrighetti L et al. Paraplegia following coeliac plexus block. Pain 1993; 55: 383–385.

10 van Dongen RT, Crul BJ. Paraplegia following celiac plexus block. Anaesthesia 1991; 46: 862–863.

11 .Kumar A, Tripathi SS, Dhar D et al. A case of reversible paraparesis following celiac plexus block. Regional Anesthesia and Pain Medicine 2011; 26: 75–78.

12 Wong GY, Brown DL. Transient paraplegia following alcohol celiac plexus block. Regional Anesthesia 1995; 20: 352–355.

13 Jabbal SS, Hunton J. Reversible paraplegia following celiac plexus block. Anaesthesia 1992; 47: 857–858.

14 Fujii L, Clain JE, Morris JM et al. Anterior spinal cord infarction with permanent paralysis following endoscopic ultrasound celiac plexus neurolysis. Endoscopy 2012; 44 Suppl 2: E265–E266.

15 Kaufman M, Singh G, Das S et al. Efficacy of endoscopic ultrasound-guided celiac plexus block and celiac plexus neurolysis for managing abdominal pain associated with chronic pancreatitis and pancreatic cancer. Journal of Clinical Gastroenterology 2010; 44: 127–134.

16 Puli SR, Reddy JB, Bechtold ML et al. EUS-guided celiac plexus neurolysis for pain due to chronic pancreatitis or pancreatic cancer pain: a meta-analysis and systematic review. Digestive Diseases and Sciences 2009; 54: 2330–2337.

17 Levy MJ, Topazian MD, Wiersema MJ et al. Initial evaluation of the efficacy and safety of endoscopic ultrasound-guided direct ganglia neurolysis and block. American Journal of Gastroenterology 2008; 103: 98–103.

18 Gress F, Schmidt C, Sherman S et al. Endoscopic ultrasound-guided celiac plexus block for managing abdominal pain associated with chronic pancreatitis: a

prospective single center experience. American Journal of Gastroenterology 2001; 96: 409–416.

19 Leblanc JK, DeWitt J, Johnson C et al. A prospective randomized trial of 1 versus 2 injections during EUS-guided celiac plexus block for chronic pancreatitis pain. Gastrointestinal Endoscopy 2009; 69: 835–842.

20 Santosh D, Lakhtakia S, Gupta R et al. Clinical trial: a randomized trial comparing fluoroscopy guided percutaneous technique vs. endoscopic ultrasound guided technique of coeliac plexus block for treatment of pain in chronic pancreatitis. Alimentary Pharmacology and Therapeutics 2009; 29: 979–984.

21 Sahai AV, Lemelin V, Lam E et al. Central vs. bilateral endoscopic ultrasound-guided celiac plexus block or neurolysis: a comparative study of short term effectiveness. American Journal of Gastroenterology 2009; 104: 326–329.

22 Stevens T, Costanzo A, Lopez R et al. Adding triamcinolone to endoscopic ultrasound-guided celiac plexus blockade does not reduce pain in patients with chronic pancreatitis. Clinical Gastroenterology and Hepatology 2012; 10: 186–191.

23 Gress F, Schmitt C, Sherman S et al. A prospective randomized comparison of endoscopic ultrasound- and computer tomography-guided celiac plexus block for managing chronic pancreatitis pain. American Journal of Gastroenterology 1999; 94: 900–905.

24 Yang IY, Oraee S, Viejo C et al. Computed tomography celiac trunk topography relating to celiac plexus block. Regional Anesthesia and Pain Medicine 2011; 36: 21–25.

25 Tellez-Avila FI, Romano-Munive AF, Herrera-Esquivel Jde J et al. Central is as effective as bilateral endoscopic ultrasound-guided celiac plexus neurolysis in patients with unresectable pancreatic cancer. Endoscopic Ultrasound 2013; 2: 153–156.

26 LeBlanc JK, Al-Haddad M, McHenry L et al. A prospective, randomized study of EUS-guided celiac plexus neurolysis for pancreatic cancer: one injection or two? Gastrointestinal Endoscopy 2011; 74: 1300–1307.

27 Doi S, Yasuda I, Kawakami H et al. Endoscopic ultrasound-guided celiac ganglia neurolysis vs. celiac plexus neurolysis: a randomized multicenter trial. Endoscopy 2013; 45: 362–369.

28 Ascunce G, Ribeiro A, Reis I et al. EUS visualization and direct celiac ganglia neurolysis predicts better pain relief in patients with pancreatic malignancy (with video). Gastrointestinal Endoscopy 2011; 73: 267–274.

29 Wang KX, Jin ZD, Du YQ et al. EUS-guided celiac ganglion irradiation with iodine-125 seeds for pain control in pancreatic carcinoma: a prospective pilot study. Gastrointestinal Endoscopy 2012; 76: 945–952.

30 Sakamoto H, Kitano M, Kamata K et al. EUS-guided broad plexus neurolysis over the superior mesenteric artery using a 25-gauge needle. American Journal of Gastroenterology 2010; 105: 2599–2606.

31 Myhre J, Hilsted J, Tronier B et al. Monitoring of celiac plexus block in chronic pancreatitis. Pain 1989; 38: 269–274.

32 Vranken JH, Zuurmond WW, Van Kemenade FJ et al. Neurohistopathologic findings after a neurolytic celiac plexus block with alcohol in patients with pancreatic cancer pain. Acta Anaesthesiologica Scandinavica 2002; 46: 827–830.

33 Sahai AV, Wyse J. EUS guided celiac plexus block for chronic pancreatitis: a placebo-controlled trial should be the first priority. Gastrointestinal Endoscopy 2010; 71: 430–431.

34 Wilcox CM. Tinkering with a tarnished technique: isn't it time to abandon celiac plexus blockade for the treatment of abdominal pain in chronic pancreatitis? Clinical Gastroenterology and Hepatology 2012; 10: 106–108.

35 https://clinicaltrials.gov/ct2/show/NCT01318590. Accessed May 12, 2015.

36 Bhutani MS, Arantes VN, Verma D, et al. Histopathologic correlation of endoscopic ultrasound findings of chronic pancreatitis in human autopsies. Pancreas 2009; 38: 820–824.

37 Yusoff IF, Sahai AV. A prospective, quantitative assessment of the effect of ethanol and other variables on the endosonographic appearance of the pancreas. Clinical Gastroenterology and Hepatology 2004; 2: 405–409.

38 van Geenen EJ, Smits MM, Schreuder TC, et al. Smoking is related to pancreatic fibrosis in humans. American Journal of Gastroenterology 2011; 106: 1161–1166.

39 Al-Haddad M, Khashab M, Zyromski N, et al. Risk factors for hyperechogenic pancreas on endoscopic ultrasound. Pancreas 2009; 38: 672–675.

40 Wilcox MC, Yadav D, Ye T et al. Chronic pancreatitis pain pattern and severity are independent of abdominal imaging findings. Clinical Gastroenterology and Hepatology 2015; 13: 552–560.

41 Varadarajulu S, Eltoum I, Tamhane A, et al. Histolopathologic correlates of noncalcific chronic pancreatitis by EUS: a prospective tissue characterization study. Gastrointestinal Endoscopy 2007; 66: 501–509.

42 Chong AK, Romagnuolo J, Hoffman BJ, et al. Diagnosis of chronic pancreatitis with endoscopic ultrasound: a comparison with histopathology. Gastrointestinal Endoscopy 2007; 65: 808–814.

43 Albashir S, Bronner M, Parsi M, et al. Endoscopic ultrasound, secretin endoscopic pancreatic function test, and histology: correlation in chronic pancreatitis. American Journal of Gastroenterology 2010; 105: 2498–2503.

44 Vega-Peralta J, Manivel C, Attam R, et al. Accuracy of EUS for diagnosis of minimal change chronic pancreatitis (MCCP): correlation with histopathology in 50 patients undergoing total pancreatectomy (TP) with islet autotransplantation (IAT). Pancreas 2011; 40: 1361.

45 Wallace MB, Hawes RH, Durkalski V, et al. The reliability of EUS for the diagnosis of chronic pancreatitis: interobserver

agreement among experienced endosonographers. Gastrointestinal Endoscopy 2001; 53: 294–299.

46 Gardner TB, Gordon SR. Interobserver agreement for pancreatic endoscopic ultrasonography determined by same day back-to-back examinations. Journal of Clinical Gastroenterology 2011; 45: 542–545.

47 Catalano MF, Sahai A, Levy M, et al. EUS-based criteria for the diagnosis of chronic pancreatitis: the Rosemont classification. Gastrointestinal Endoscopy 2009; 69: 1251–1261.

48 Stevens T, Adler DG, Al-Haddad MA, et al. Multicenter study of interobserver agreement of standard endoscopic ultrasound scoring and Rosemont classification for diagnosis of chronic pancreatitis. Gastrointestinal Endoscopy 2010; 71: 519–526.

49 Del Pozo D, Poves E, Tabernero S, et al. Conventional versus Rosemont endoscopic ultrasound criteria for chronic pancreatitis: interobserver agreement in same day back to back procedures. Pancreatology 2012; 12: 284–287.

50 Bouwense SA, de Vries M, Schreuder LT et al. Systematic mechanism-oriented approach to chronic pancreatitis pain. World Journal of Gastroenterology 2015; 21: 47–59.

51 Busch EH, Atchison SR. Steroid celiac plexus block for chronic pancreatitis: results in 16 cases. Journal of Clinical Anesthesia 1989; 1: 431–433.

52 Stefaniak T, Vingerhoets A, Makarewicz W et al. Opioid use determines success of videothoracoscopic splanchnicectomy in chronic pancreatic pain patients. Langenbeck's Archives of Surgery 2008; 393: 213–218.

53 Navarro X, Vivo M, Valero-Cabre A. Neural plasticity after peripheral nerve injury and regeneration. Progress in Neurobiology 2007; 82: 163–201.

CHAPTER 16

PART A: A brief history of modern surgery for chronic pancreatitis

Michael G. Sarr[1], Charles F. Frey[2] & Thomas Schnelldorfer[3]

[1] *Department of Surgery, Mayo Clinic, Rochester, MN, USA*

[2] *Department of General Surgery, University of California Sacramento, Sacramento, CA, USA*

[3] *Department of Surgery, Lahey Clinic, Burlington, MA, USA*

Although the history of pancreatic surgery extends functionally back into the late 1800s, what we call the start of our understanding of modern pancreatic surgery for chronic pancreatitis really began in the 1940s. Indeed, pancreatic surgery lagged behind the surgery of other visceral organs, probably because of several aspects well voiced by von Mikulicz-Radecki in 1903 [1]: "The cause of the tardy development of the surgery of the pancreas … three reasons … 1) the topographical relations to other organs; 2) the difficulty in diagnosis; and 3) the operation … is more dangerous than an operation upon any other abdominal organ." When one considers these points pre-1940, experience with pancreatectomy (for cancer) was just beginning, because of several reasons: an objective, radiographic diagnosis was not possible, and the concepts of critical care medicine were only starting to develop. Specifically, for chronic pancreatitis, no imagining procedure could differentiate dilated from nondilated pancreatic ducts preoperatively (no CT, MRI, ERCP, etc.) or reliably recognize the extent of the inflammation (or lack thereof), and many (if not most) of the patients were alcoholics and malnourished. Thus, our starting point of modern pancreatic surgery begins at about 1940. This review focuses primarily on the seminal publications/thoughts that laid the foundation for our current understanding of the surgical approaches to chronic pancreatitis.

The approaches to treating chronic pancreatitis that have persisted to date are as follows:

a. denervation of the pancreas – visceral, autonomic splanchnicectomy
b. pancreatic resection – distal based versus proximal based
c. ductal drainage (± an element of resection)
d. islet (auto)transplantation after resection.

These are the principles from which our current operative strategies to the treatment of chronic pancreatitis derive. This review represents our interpretation and is not exhaustive, but it is rather a recounting of what we consider to be the important surgeons and operative procedures introduced.

Pancreatic denervation

The primary symptom of chronic pancreatitis is PAIN – and the visceral, autonomic nerves rather than the somatic nerves mediate this form of deep-seated, boring epigastric and back pain. The approach to the pain of chronic pancreatitis differed radically from the approach to the management of pancreatic neoplasms. Moreover, in the 1940s, pancreatic resection was fraught with multiple problems related to the reconstruction of the upper gut after a major resection, pancreatic fistulas, and nutritional support in often malnourished patients, many of whom were alcoholics. Indeed, experience was limited, and a neurectomy from a translumbar approach was a much less morbid operation. From 1942 onward, Mallet-Guy and colleagues [2–4] from Lyons, France,

Pancreatitis: Medical and Surgical Management, First Edition.
David B. Adams, Peter B. Cotton, Nicholas J. Zyromski and John Windsor.
© 2017 John Wiley & Sons, Ltd. Published 2017 by John Wiley & Sons, Ltd.

and DeTakats and Walter did much to popularize (and study) the procedure of operative splanchnicectomy and celiac ganglionectomy for "chronic relapsing pancreatitis" having diverse etiologies. According to Mallet-Guy, those patients with dilated pancreatic ducts, pancreatic duct calculi, and patients with pancreatic cysts were not suitable candidates for splanchnicectomy or celiac ganglionectomy. Consequently, his procedure excluded more than half the patient population with chronic pancreatitis. Interestingly, Mallet-Guy maintained that the operation was not directed at so much the pain but rather at the process of recurrent, relapsing pancreatitis. Thomas White in 1965 spent a year in Lyon, France, while on a Guggenheim fellowship reviewing the records of all patients undergoing splanchnicectomy and celiac ganglionectomy performed by Mallet-Guy up to 1965 [5]. White felt many of the patients' records he reviewed had acute gallstone pancreatitis from which they recovered after cholecystectomy and remained pain free. Indeed, many of this group of patients would have been expected to remain pain free with or without splanchnicectomy, as well as incurring further damage to the pancreatic parenchyma. Others who tried to duplicate Mallet-Guy's procedure at the time found that a large percentage of their patients failed to obtain or sustain pain relief.

The early 1990s saw a transient resurgence of interest in splanchnicectomy for chronic pain with the ability to perform a splanchnic nerve transection thoracoscopically; results have been mixed and did not yield a long duration of pain relief [6, 7].

Pancreatic resection

Prior to the 1950s, pancreatectomy was not performed commonly, and especially so for chronic pancreatitis. Experience with resection for pancreatic cancer was growing via work by Whipple, Brunschwig, and many others [1] – remember, there was no cross-sectional imaging available, so most resections were explorations for "painless jaundice" for presumed pancreatic cancer. Distal pancreatectomy avoided the need for pancreato or bilioenteric anastomosis, and (probably) the assumption that the amount of pain was proportional to the amount of diseased parenchyma or to preserve the duodenum led to the left-to-right-sided approach to resection; that is, a 60% distal pancreatectomy to 80% subtotal

pancreatectomy to 95% near total pancreatectomy to 100% pancreatectomy – total pancreatectomy. Many centers adopted this approach of "creeping" proximal resections suggested early on by Child, Frey, Braasch, Warren, Clagett, Longmire, White, Cattell, Jordan, and others [8–12].

Parenchymal resections of ≥80% produced pain relief in 80% of patients, which was no better than operations such as pancreatoduodenectomy that preserved a greater amount of pancreatic parenchyma. Extensive pancreatic resections (80% or more) were abandoned by their proponents including Child and Frey after they presented their results with 77 patients at the American Surgical Association due to the devastating consequences of the procedure, which led to brittle diabetes and pancreatic insufficiency in a majority of patients. As stated by Dr Child who originated the 95% distal pancreatectomy, "it was an experiment which failed" even surprisingly after total pancreatectomy and eventuated in pancreatic insufficiency in an already difficult patient population (largely alcoholics).

The success of the 95% distal pancreatectomy and pancreatoduodenectomy focused attention to the head of the pancreas as the principal anatomic target in pain relief. Longmire referred to the head of the pancreas as "the pacemaker of pain" (Traverso, personal communication). This concept led Longmire in the United States to suggest a proximal resection (pancreatoduodenectomy) [13] and Beger in Germany [14] to concentrate on resecting the head of the pancreas as the source of the majority of the pain in chronic pancreatitis. Their approach designed to preserve the parenchyma of the body and tail of the pancreas had surprisingly good results (prolonged pain relief in up to 85% of patients). The concomitant growing experience with pancreatectomy for pancreatic cancer further supported this practice and offered operative experience with the technical aspects and postoperative care of the post-pancreatic patient. Currently, this approach of proximal resection persists for small-duct chronic pancreatitis.

Ductal drainage (± partial, nonanatomic resection)

Two types of chronic pancreatitis were noted both intra-operatively and preoperatively with the development of cross-sectional imaging: small-duct disease and large-duct disease. The latter was presumed to be related to ductal obstruction with related increases in *intraductal pressure leading to* the presumed associated pain of chronic pancreatitis – thus the concept of "ductal drainage" by some form of pancreaticoenterostomy. One of the earliest "successful" ductal drainage procedures was a true tube pancreatostomy by Link in 1909 [15]; this surgeon mobilized the body/tail of the pancreas, filleted open the dilated pancreatic duct, placed a tube within the duct, closed the duct/parenchymal pancreatic incision (pancreatotomy), brought the gland through the mesocolon, and exteriorated the tube (wow!). Thereafter, a number of anecdotal attempts at enteric ductal drainage were made but were unsuccessful. Similarly, an era of interest in sphincterotomy of the ampullary sphincter ensued under the impression that proximal "relief" of the ductal obstruction by sphincterotomy would prevail [16, 17], but results were inconsistent.

The first real breakthrough came from the work of DuVal in 1954 [18] in which he performed a limited resection of the tail of the pancreas (with splenectomy) to which a Roux limb was sewn for retrograde drainage of the pancreatic duct in two patients with good results. Over the next 6 years, modifications of the pancreatojejunostomy were evaluated. The procedure was improved on by Puestow and Gillesby in 1958 [19], when they reported their experience with 22 patients in whom they not only performed the short distal pancreatectomy (with splenectomy) to help locate the pancreatic duct, but they also filleted open the duct proximally and sewed a Roux limb onto this filleted-open pancreatic ductotomy. Their work was based on their five basic principles (the following four of which are still largely believed to be true today): (i) the pain of chronic pancreatitis is secondary to increased intraductal pressure; (ii) calcification/stone formation is from calcium-soap formation within the duct (stasis); (iii) the pancreatic duct often has multiple sites of obstruction, all of which require drainage; and (iv) inflammation of the ductal system occurs when strictures are present that prevent free communication of ductal fluid throughout the duct. This concept of multiple sites of ductal obstruction proved to be a major advance in our understanding of the success of ductal drainage procedures and appears to be why proximal-based sphincterotomy and distal-based drainage alone (per DuVal) did not always work.

Besides, it is often overlooked that they also described a pancreaticogastrostomy as well. Partington and Rochelle [20] further improved the technique by accomplishing a similar, total ductal drainage via a side-to-side pancreaticojejunostomy but without the added morbidity of a distal (albeit limited) pancreatectomy and without the need for a concomitant splenectomy and its morbidity.

These forms of ductal drainage persisted as the procedure of choice for large duct disease until the 1980s, when the work of Frey and Smith [21] extended this concept by adding a concomitant, nonanatomic, subtotal pancreatic head resection to the ductal drainage. This procedure was based on their observations that drainage of the main duct alone often left multiple side branches undrained usually in the head of the gland (where the duct dives posteriorly) due to inflammatory obstruction of segmented ducts and on occasion an enlarged head of the gland. This concept was influenced by the success of the 95% pancreatectomy in achieving pain relief with the removal of the head of the pancreas and also possibly influenced by the work of Beger [14] as well as Longmire's contention that the pacemaker of the pain was in the head of the pancreas. Frey and Smith "cored out" the head of the pancreas without the need for full mobilization of the posterior surface of the gland, often the trickiest part of the mobilization for either a Beger procedure or a pancreatoduodenectomy, and especially so in some patients with severe, chronic inflammatory changes involving the retropancreatic superior mesenteric vein.

Islet cell autotransplantation

With the growing success of organ transplantation, the transplant surgeons approached this disorder in a different and complimentary fashion in the mid- to late-1960s. From a metabolic standpoint, one of the major drawbacks of any pancreatic resective procedure is the potential for the development of pancreatic insufficiency and especially the brittle diabetes that can ensue in an already compromised (often alcoholic) patient. Why not resect the offending organ (the pancreas), but then (auto)transplant the islets to prevent (or at the least ameliorate) the resultant diabetes. While some groups were developing whole organ pancreatic transplants for diabetes [22], others were concentrating on selective forms of islet cell (auto)transplantation.

A major advance was the use of collagenase digestion by Moskalewski [23] to help disperse the islet cells from the pancreatic tissue. Lindal et al. [24] improved the islet cell purification via the use of Ficoll gradient separation, although yields were low. Nevertheless, Ballinger and Lacy [25] first reported the success of these islets in reversing the diabetes in rats as a proof of principle. Mirkovitch and Campiche [26] approached the concept of auto islet cell transplantation by using digested pancreatic tissue rather than isolated islets. Their concept was adopted clinically by others [27, 28] with some success, but the process of infusion of "digested" pancreatic tissue into the portal system had too many potential side effects. Since then, the work of many groups (Sutherland, Lacy, Najarian, Sharp, and others) have further perfected the isolation and culture of pancreatic islets and sparked our current programs in total or near-total pancreatectomy with auto islet transplantation in selected patients with chronic pancreatitis.

Summary

Our current approach to the operative treatment of chronic pancreatitis is founded on this prior work of many different innovative investigators around the world and still remains founded on the concepts of neural mediation of pancreatic pain, resection of the inflamed pancreatic parenchyma, ductal drainage, and auto islet transplantation. But admittedly, we treat the symptoms. Maybe the next advance will be its prevention through genetic screening for identifying the population at risk for developing pancreatitis (not all alcoholics develop acute or chronic pancreatitis), environmental "epigenomic" factors, nutritional or anti-inflammatory supplements, and of course, a more effective educational program of intervention BEFORE the process becomes established.

References

1 Schnelldorfer T, Adams DB, Warshaw AL, Lillemoe KD, Sarr MG: Forgotten pioneers of pancreatic surgery: beyond the favorite few. Annals of Surgery 2008; 247:191–202.

2 Mallet-Guy PA, Jeanjean R, Servettaz P. Results eloignes de la splanchniecetomie unilaterale dans le traitement des pancreatite chroniques. Lyon Chirurgical 1945; 40:293–314.

3 Mallet-Guy PA: Late and very late results of resections of the nervous system in the treatment of chronic relapsing pancreatitis. American Journal of Surgery 1983; 145:234–238.

4 DeTakats G and Walter LE. The treatment of pancreatic pain by splanchnic nerve transection. Surgery, Gynecology & Obstetrics 1947; 95:742–746.

5 White TT, Lawinski M, Stacher G, Pang T, Tea J, Michoulier J, Murat J, Mallet-Guy P. Treatment of pancreatitis by left splanchnicectomy and celiac ganglionectomy. Analysis of 146 cases. American Journal of Surgery 1966; 112:195–199.

6 Cuschieri A, Shimi SM, Crosthwaite G, Joypaul V. Bilateral endoscopic splanchnicectomy through a posterior thoracoscopic approach. Journal of the Royal College of Surgeons of Edinburgh 1994; 39:44–48.

7 Baghdadi S, Abbas MH, Albouz F, Ammori BJ. Systematic review of the role of thoracoscopic splanchnicectomy in palliating the pain of patients with chronic pancreatitis. Surgical Endoscopy 2008; 22:580–588.

8 Frey CF, Child GG, III, Fry W. Pancreatectomy for chronic pancreatitis. Annals of Surgery 1976; 184:403–408.

9 Longmire WP, Jordan PH, Briggs JD. Experience with resection of the pancreas in the treatment of chronic relapsing pancreatitis. Annals of Surgery 1956; 144:681–690.

10 Cattell RB and Warren KW. Pancreatic surgery. New England Journal of Medicine 1951; 244:941–945.

11 Braasch JW, Vito L, Nugent FW. Total pancreatectomy for end-stage chronic pancreatitis. Annals of Surgery 1978; 188:317 322.

12 Clagett OT. Total pancreatectomy for chronic pancreatitis with calcification. Proceedings of the Staff Meetings of the Mayo Clinic 1946; 21:32–36.

13 Traverso LW, Tompkins RK, Urrea PT, Longmire WP. Surgical treatment of chronic pancreatitis. Annals of Surgery 1979; 190:312–317.

14 Beger HG, Krautzberger W, Bittner R, Buchler M, Limmer J. Duodenum-preserving resection of the head of the pancreas in patients with severe chronic pancreatitis. Surgery 1983; 97:467–473.

15 Link G. The treatment of chronic pancreatitis by pancreatostomy. Annals of Surgery 1911; 53:768–782.

16 Doubilet HJ and Mulholland JH. Recurrent acute pancreatitis: observations on etiology and surgical treatment. Annals of Surgery 1948; 128:609.

17 Doubilet H and Mulholland JH. Eight year study of pancreatitis and sphincterotomy. JAMA 1956; 160:521.

18 DuVal MK. Caudal pancreaticojejunostomy for chronic relapsing pancreatitis. Annals of Surgery 1954; 140:775–785.

19 Puestow CB and Gillesby WJ. Retrograde surgical drainage of pancreas for chronic relapsing pancreatitis. AMA Archives of Surgery 1958; 76:898–907.

20 Partington PF and Rochelle RE. Modified Puestow procedure for retrograde drainage of the pancreatic duct. Annals of Surgery 1960; 152:1037–1043.

21 Frey CF and Smith GJ. Description and rationale of a new operation for chronic pancreatitis. Pancreas 1987; 2:701–707.

22 Kelly WD, Lillehei RC, Merkel FK, et al. Autotransplantation of the pancreas and duodenum along with the kidney in diabetic nephropathy. Surgery 61:827, 1967.

23 Moskalewski S. Isolation and culture of the islets of Langerhans of the guinea pig. General and Comparative Endocrinology 1965; 5:342–348.

24 Lindal AW, Steffes M, Sorensen R. Immunoassayable content of subcellular fractions of rat islets. Endocrinology 1969; 85:218–230.

25 Ballinger WF and Lacy P E. Transplantation of intact islets in rats. Surgery 1972; 72:175–181.

26 Mirkovitch V, Campiche M. Successful intrasplenic autotransplantation of pancreatic tissue in totally pancreatectomized dogs. Transplantation 1976; 21:265–273.

27 Najarian JS, Sutherland DER, Matas AJ, Goetz FC. Human islet autotransplantation following pancreatectomy. Transplantation Proceedings 1979; 11:336–340.

28 Cameron JL, Mehigan DG, Broe PJ, Zuidema GD. Distal pancreatectomy and islet autotransplantation for chronic pancreatitis. Annals of Surgery 1981; 193:312–317.

PART B: Surgery for chronic pancreatitis: indications and timing of surgery

Philippus C. Bornman[1,2], Dirk J. Gouma[3] & Jake E. J. Krige[1,2]

[1] Department of Surgery, University of Cape Town, Cape Town, South Africa
[2] Groote Schuur Hospital, Cape Town, South Africa
[3] Academic Medical Center, Amsterdam, the Netherlands

Introduction

With the development of subspecialization in the field of pancreatic diseases over the last two decades, there has been a gradual paradigm shift away from the nihilistic view that other than for complicated disease, surgery has a limited role in the management of pain in patients with chronic pancreatitis (CP), in particular in the alcohol-induced group. In the past, surgery has not enjoyed a good track record because of the morbidity and mortality of major resection operations, the development of exocrine and endocrine insufficiency, and shortened life expectancy. In the 1980s, the conservative school enjoyed further support when the Zurich group introduced the concept of the "pancreatic burn out syndrome." Their long-term studies on the natural history of CP showed that pain relief developed *pari passu* with the deterioration of pancreatic function and that this followed a predictable pattern [1]. They and others [2] championed the view that by waiting long enough, less patients would require surgery for pain. However, subsequent studies have challenged this concept [3–6]. These showed that at best relief of pain occurred mostly in the subgroup of patients with mild recurrent relapsing pancreatitis and not in the group with severe and persistent pain who required opiates for pain control. In the words of Warshaw [7], *It seems unreasonable to tell a patient to wait an indeterminate number of years in the hope of spontaneous subsidence of pain when surgery can offer a 75% success rate.* Yet, it took some time for the "burn out" concept to be debunked in the context of delaying surgery in suitable cases. In recent times, the advent of endoscopic stenting and extracorporeal shockwave lithotripsy (ESWL) [8] has,

to a certain extent, changed the pattern of referral of patients for surgery.

Subspecialization in pancreatic surgery has significantly improved the results after surgery in CP by virtue of increasingly sophisticated imaging and, refinement of surgical procedures with the emphasis on maximum organ preservation. In addition, improved quality of anesthesia and ICU care and minimally invasive procedures has further reduced post operative morbidity [9]. As a consequence, tailoring of the procedure according to morphological changes of the pancreas has improved and made these much safer operations in the hands of expert pancreatic surgeons. Satisfactory pain relief can now be achieved with acceptable preservation of pancreatic function [10]. Whether these improved results have resulted in an increase in the number of referrals for surgery remains unclear but at least surgery has now assumed an important role in the treatment of patients with persistent and intractable pain who have failed to improve despite receiving adequate conservative treatment.

Indications for surgery

Failure of conservative treatment measures to control intractable pain in uncomplicated disease

Patients should only be considered for invasive interventional procedures once all forms of conservative treatment have been exhausted in order to achieve satisfactory relief of intractable pain over a reasonable period of time. Such a period may vary from patient to patient but it is advisable to err on the conservative side

Pancreatitis: Medical and Surgical Management, First Edition.
David B. Adams, Peter B. Cotton, Nicholas J. Zyromski and John Windsor.
© 2017 John Wiley & Sons, Ltd. Published 2017 by John Wiley & Sons, Ltd.

unless there is concern about opiate dependency (see Section "Timing of surgery").

Details of conservative treatment are discussed in Chapters 11 and 14. The reader is also referred to recent published guidelines on CP [11–13].

In summary, the following principles should be adhered to.

i. Multidisciplinary care

It is imperative that these patients should be managed by a multidisciplinary subspecialist group experienced in the management of patients with CP. At the very least, the team should consist of a medical gastroenterologist, hepatopancreaticobiliary (HPB) surgeon, an experienced endoscopic interventionist, and an HPB radiologist. It is prudent to have further support from a psychiatrist/psychologist, a social worker, a dietician, and a pain management team. Close cooperation between gastroenterologists and surgeons are of paramount importance to avoid unnecessary and prolonged conservative treatment on the one hand and premature intervention on the other (discussed later).

ii. Behaviour modification

Abstinence from both alcohol [14, 15] and smoking [16] remains the cornerstone of conservative treatment. This can best be achieved with the assistance of an alcohol dependency counselor or psychologist. In many countries, patients with alcohol-induced pancreatitis live in a poor socioeconomic environment. Under these circumstances, the assistance of a social worker is invaluable to provide a holistic approach to patient management.

There are now well-documented pain control regimes based on a sequential step-up approach [11–13, 17]. The mechanisms of pain in CP are poorly understood and may differ among patients and change in the individual patient over a period of time. Two categories mostly seen are those who present with frequent acute attacks of pain requiring hospitalization with pain-free periods in between and those who suffer from severe intractable pain [4–6]. It is important to exclude other causes of pain that may mimic pancreatic pain (i.e., NSAID-induced ulcer disease) and to be aware of the development of possible complications such as pancreatic fluid collections (PFCs), when there is a change in the severity or pattern of the pain.

For all the aforementioned reasons, it is important to monitor the patient's progress over a reasonable period of time before a decision is taken to intervene.

Complications

The most common complications seen in CP are biliary obstruction and PFCs. Duodenal obstruction and bleeding from segmental portal hypertension or false aneurysms are much less common. Apart from bleeding or secondary infections of PFCs, there is seldom a need for urgent intervention in the other complications and in many instances these can be managed conservatively (see Chapter 16c).

Another important indication for surgery is a strong suspicion of an associated malignancy, which cannot be excluded on preoperative imaging.

Timing of surgery

The decision and timing of both surgery and other interventional procedures remain controversial. It is important to stress that while the indications for less invasive nonoperative procedures are currently the same as for surgery [18], this may change in future with the refinement and further development of minimally invasive techniques.

The main purpose of any interventional procedure is to relieve pain so that patients no longer require opioids, to preserve maximal pancreatic function, and to restore the quality of life (QOL) [19]. There is a fine line between the risks associated with surgery and the problem of addiction to opioids when conservative treatment is unnecessarily prolonged [18]. There is now good evidence that prolonged usage of opioids is one of the important predictors of failure after surgery, both in terms of pain relief and QOL [20–24]. In addition to the problem of opioid dependency, there is evidence to suggest that poor pain outcome after surgery is associated with greater central sensitization and more pronociceptive descending modulation, which results after periods of prolonged pain [25]. It is questionable whether earlier surgery will prevent this phenomenon. Trials on this important issue of timing of intervention are currently being performed. At present, there are no clear guidelines on how long it is safe to keep patients on maintenance opioid therapy before it compromises the results of surgery and other interventional procedures.

On balance, it would seem reasonable to consider some form of intervention when opioids are required for adequate pain control for periods longer than 6 months. However, the decision to intervene early may be delayed by other factors such as the severity of comorbid disease and those with small-duct disease, which often limits the choice of organ-preserving operations.

Prolonged and repeated pancreatic stenting has been identified as a risk factor for failure after subsequent rescue surgery [22]. Apart from the delay in referral for definitive surgery, it is conceivable that stent-induced pancreatitis and a "foreign body" effect may be additional contributing factors. There is now ample evidence that surgical drainage operations afford patients significantly better long-term pain relief and improved QOL when compared with endoscopic drainage of the pancreatic duct [23, 25, 26]. Endoscopic drainage with or without ESWL will continue to play an important role in the management of these patients but it is important to identify those who will benefit most from this less invasive interventional approach. In this regard, guidelines such as those provided by the European Society of Gastrointestinal Endoscopy (ESGED) [27] have been invaluable although further refinement based on level 1 studies are eagerly awaited.

Similarly, guidelines are required for the timing of referral for surgery when endoscopic drainage has failed. The proposed randomized trial by the Dutch Pancreatic Study Group on Early Surgery versus Optimal Step-up Practice for Chronic Pancreatitis (which will include endoscopic drainage) may provide answers to these questions [28]. It is also anticipated that the study will shed more light on the supposition that early drainage surgery preserves or improves pancreatic function [29–31]. This will probably be the most difficult question to answer because progressive deterioration in pancreatic function is usually inevitable in the majority of patients despite successful surgical drainage procedures [10].

Summary and conclusion

Much of the success in the treatment of patients with CP who have intractable pain depends on a detailed and holistic approach by a multidisciplinary team of experts. It is important to ensure, however, that these patients,

who require considerable support, are not stranded between the various disciplines within the team framework. Ideally, they should primarily be evaluated by and cared for by a medical gastroenterologist in order to establish a rapport with the emphasis on monitoring response to pain control and to adjust medication requirements accordingly. The recent development of guidelines with treatment algorithms are encouraging as are the proposed studies to improve the timing and selection of interventional procedures.

References

1 Ammann RW, Akovbiantz A, Largiadér F, et al Course and outcome of chronic pancreatitis. Longitudinal study of a mixed medical-surgical series of 245 patients. Gastroenterology 1984; 82:820–828.

2 Van Esch AA, Ahmed AU, Van Goor H, et al. A wide variation in the diagnosis and therapeutic strategies in chronic pancreatitis: a Dutch national survey. Journal of the Pancreas 2012; 13: 394–401.

3 Lankisch PG, Löhr-Happe A, Otto J, et al. Natural course in chronic pancreatitis. Pain, exocrine and endocrine pancreatic insufficiency and prognosis of the disease. Digestion 1993; 54:148–155.

4 Layer P, Yamamoto H, Kalthoff L, et al. The different courses of early-and late-onset idiopathic and alcoholic chronic pancreatitis. Gastroenterology 1994; 107:1481–1487.

5 Ammann RW, Muellhaupt B, Group ZPS. The natural history of pain in alcohol chronic pancreatitis. Gastroenterology 1999; 116: 1132–1140.

6 Bornman PC, Marks IN, Girdwood AH, et al. Pathogenesis of pain in chronic pancreatitis - An ongoing enigma. World Journal of Surgery 2003; 27. 1175–1182.

7 Warshaw AL. Pain in chronic pancreatitis. Patients, patience and the impatient surgeon. Gastroenterology 1984; 86: 987–989.

8 Rosch T, Daniel S, Scholz M, et al. Endoscopic treatment of chronic pancreatitis: a multicentre study of 1000 patients with long-term follow-up. Endoscopy 2002; 34: 765–771.

9 Anderson DK, Frey CF. The evolution of surgical treatment of chronic pancreatitis. Annals of Surgery 2010; 251: 18–32.

10 Diener MK, Rahbari NN, Fisher L, et al. Duodenum-preserving pancreatic head resection versus pancreaticoduodenectomy for surgical treatment of chronic pancreatitis. A systematic review and meta-analysis. Annals of Surgery 2008; 247: 950–961.

11 Forsmark CE. Management of chronic pancreatitis. Gastroenterology 2013; 144: 1282–1291.

12 Bornman PC, Botha JF, Ramos JM, et al. Guidelines for the diagnosis and treatment of chronic pancreatitis. South African Medical Journal 2010; 100: 845–860.

13 Conwell DL, Lee LS, Yadav D, et al. American Pancreatic Association practice guidelines in chronic pancreatitis: evidence-based report on diagnostic guidelines. Pancreas 2014; 43: 1143–1162.

14 Strum WB. Abstinence in alcoholic chronic pancreatitis. Effect on pain and outcome. Journal of Clinical Gastroenterology 1995; 20: 4–5.

15 Nordback I, Pelli H, Lappalainen-Lehto R, et al. The recurrence of alcohol-associated pancreatitis can be reduced: a randomized controlled study. Gastroenterology 2008; 136: 848–855.

16 Maisonneuve P, Lowenfels AB, Mullhaupt B, et al. Cigarette smoking accelerates progression of alcoholic pancreatitis. Gut 2005; 54:510–514.

17 Chauhan S, Forsmark CE. Pain management in chronic pancreatitis: a treatment algorithm. Best Practice & Research Clinical Gastroenterology 2010; 24: 323–335.

18 Bornman PC. Chronic pancreatitis. In: Garden OJ (Ed). A Companion to Specialist Surgical Practice-Hepatobiliary and Pancreatic Surgery. 4th ed. New York. WB Saunders Co. 2009: 259–283.

19 Bachmann K, Kutup A, Mann O, et al. Surgical treatment in chronic pancreatitis timing and type of procedure. Best Practice & Research Clinical Gastroenterology 2010; 24: 299–310.

20 Negi S, Singh A, Chaudhary A. Pain relief after Frey's procedure for chronic pancreatitis. British Journal of Surgery 2010; 97: 1087–1095.

21 Van der Gaag NA, van Gulik TM, Busch OR, et al. Functional and medical outcomes after tailored surgery for pain due to chronic pancreatitis. Annals of Surgery 2012; 255:763–770.

22 Ahmed AU, Nieuwenhuijs VB, van Eijck CH, et al. Clinical outcome in relation to timing of surgery in chronic pancreatitis. A nomogram to predict pain relief. Archives of Surgery 2012; 147: 925–932.

23 Issa Y, van Santvoort HC, van Goor H, et al. Surgical and endoscopic treatment of pain in chronic pancreatitis: a multidisciplinary update. Digestive Surgery 2013; 30: 35–50.

24 Cahen DL, Gouma DJ, Nio Y, et al. Endoscopic versus surgical drainage of the pancreatic duct in chronic pancreatitis. New England Journal of Medicine 2007; 356: 676–684.

25 Bouwense SA, Ahmed AU, ten Broek RP, et al. Altered central pain processing after pancreatic surgery for chronic pancreatitis. British Journal of Surgery 2013; 100: 1797–1804.

26 Cahen DL, Gouma DJ, Laramée P, et al. Long-term outcomes of endoscopic vs surgical drainage of the pancreatic duct in patients with chronic pancreatitis. Gastroenterology 2011; 141: 1690–1695.

27 Dumonceau JM, Delhey M, Tringgali A, et al. Endoscopic treatment of chronic pancreatitis: European Society of Gastrointestinal Endoscopy(ESGED) clinical guidelines. Endoscopy 2012; 44:784–800.

28 Ahmed AU, Issa Y, Bruno MJ, et al. Early surgery versus optimal current step-up practice for chronic pancreatitis (ESCAPE): design and rationale of a randomised trial. BMC Gastroenterology 2013; 13:49.

29 Nealon WH, Thompson JC. Progressive loss of pancreatic function impairment is delayed by main pancreatic duct decompression. A longitudinal prospective analyses of the modified Puestow procedure. Annals of Surgery 1993;217: 485–486.

30 Maartense S, Ledeboer M, Bemelman WA, et al. Effect of surgery for chronic pancreatitis on pancreatic function: pancreatico-jejunostomy and duodenum-preserving resection of the head of the pancreas. Surgery 2004; 135: 125–130.

31 Lamme B, Boermeester MA, Straatsburg IH, et al. Early versus late surgical drainage for obstructive pancreatitis in an experimental model. British Journal of Surgery 2007; 94: 849–854.

PART C: Chronic pancreatitis: surgical strategy in complicated diseases

Philippus C. Bornman[1,2], Jake E. J. Krige[1,2] & Sandie R. Thomson[2,3]

[1] Department of Surgery, University of Cape Town, Cape Town, South Africa
[2] Groote Schuur Hospital, Cape Town, South Africa
[3] Division of Gastroenterology, Department of Medicine, University of Cape Town, Cape Town, South Africa

Introduction

Complications occur in about a third of patients with chronic pancreatitis (CP) during the course of the disease and may lead to considerable morbidity if not managed appropriately. Modern imaging has become invaluable in the assessment of the nature and extent of these complications, while radiological and endoscopic interventional procedures have broadened the treatment armamentarium. This section provides basic guidelines on management strategies in CP with an emphasis on a multidisciplinary approach to the most common complications.

Pancreatic fluid collections

Pathogenesis and pathology

Pancreatic fluid collection (PFC) is now the accepted nomenclature for the commonly used term pseudocyst. It is important to stress that PFCs in CP differ from those seen as a consequence of acute necrotizing pancreatitis. The fluid content seldom contains overt necrotic material; PFCs have a higher incidence of persistent communication with the pancreatic duct, are often rich in amylase, and are less likely to resolve spontaneously. The pathogenesis is thought to be due to one of two mechanisms: either "retention cysts" secondary to ductal obstruction or duct disruption with leakage of pancreatic juice due to focal pancreatic necrosis after an episode of acute CP [1]. The former tend to present as "intrapancreatic cysts" and occur most commonly in the head of the pancreas [2] (Figure 16C.1a), while the latter are "extrapancreatic" and are confined to the lesser sac (Figure 16C.1b,c) or, occasionally, to the tail region with or without extension into the subcapsular plane of the spleen (Figure 16C.1d). These extrapancreatic fluid collections may leak into the peritoneal cavity resulting in pancreatic ascites or may extend along the retroperitoneal space into the pleural cavity and present as an isolated left-sided pleural effusion (Figure 16C.2a). The leak may also extend into the mediastinum or rarely into the pericardial sac causing cardiac tamponade. Other complications include secondary infection (pancreatic abscess) or compression of the bile duct and duodenum causing obstructive jaundice and gastric outlet obstruction. These amylase-rich fluid collections may erode into a contiguous visceral artery causing a false aneurysm, which may bleed into the PFC or the pancreatic duct, resulting in hemosuccus pancreaticus.

Management

The treatment of PFCs is determined by several factors. These include the severity of the patient's symptoms, whether their symptoms are attributable solely to the PFC, the development of secondary complications, the nature of the PFCs (i.e., intra- or extrapancreatic), and, importantly, the morphological changes of the remainder of the pancreas. Careful evaluation of the patient's general state of health, severity of symptoms, and detailed imaging of the pancreas and biliary system are required to individualize treatment. CT and MRI/MRCP are the key investigations used to select the appropriate treatment. Endoscopic ultrasound (EUS) has become an important adjunct, both diagnostically to exclude an

Pancreatitis: Medical and Surgical Management, First Edition.
David B. Adams, Peter B. Cotton, Nicholas J. Zyromski and John Windsor.
© 2017 John Wiley & Sons, Ltd. Published 2017 by John Wiley & Sons, Ltd.

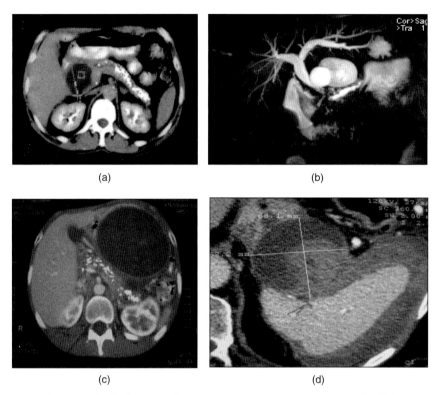

(a)

(b)

(c)

(d)

Figure 16C.1 Spectrum of pancreatic fluid collection in chronic pancreatitis. (a) CT: Intra-pancreatic head. (b) MRCP: pancreatic duct obstruction and lesser sac collection. (c) CT: extra-pancreatic lesser sac collection. (d) CT: extra-pancreatic tail of pancreas collection.

underlying malignancy and therapeutically for trans-mural endoscopic drainage (ED) [3–5]. ERCP is now reserved for transampullary endoscopic intervention.

Asymptomatic PFCs

Asymptomatic or minimally symptomatic PFCs are often discovered incidentally while investigating a patient with CP. Asymptomatic cysts can usually be observed but there is a notion that cysts >5–6 cm and those which persist for longer than 6 weeks should be drained because these do not resolve spontaneously and there is a higher risk of complications [6]. However, the data from which this recommendation was formulated were retrospective studies that included postnecrotic PFCs. In general, asymptomatic PFCs can be safely observed [7, 8].

Symptomatic PFCs

Most patients with symptomatic PFCs will require drainage, but under certain circumstances conservative treatment can be tried first if, for example, there is concern about the "maturity" of the PFC or when major surgery will be required to address associated pancreatic pathology.

There is a paucity of level I evidence to support any particular method of drainage, but there is now accumulated evidence that when feasible, either trans-duodenal or transgastric ED should be the first line of treatment [9] preferably with EUS guidance [3–5]. ED is less invasive than surgical drainage, is safe in skilled hands, and has a high success rate [8, 10]. Transpapillary stent drainage is mostly reserved for smaller cysts that are not amenable to transmural drainage and when there is communication with the pancreatic duct or an associated stricture [11]. Intuitively, surgery with a lateral pancreaticojejunostomy would be the first choice if there is associated pancreatic duct obstruction with pancreatic dilatation. However, there is scant data to support this approach other than that surgical drainage of the pancreatic duct in this setting is all that is required [12]. On the other hand, it could be

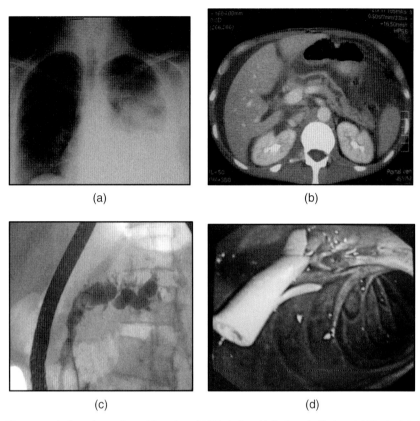

(a)   (b)

(c)   (d)

Figure 16C.2 (a) CT: pancreatic duct obstruction with ascites. (b) XR: Isolated left pleural effusion. (c) ERCP: showing an obstructed pancreatic duct with stones. (d) Endoscopy: Pancreatic duct stent.

argued that when considering the safety record and high success rate of ED of PFCs, patients should have ED first and that surgery should be reserved for failures of ED [13].

Surgery has now taken a secondary role in the management of PFCs unless concomitant complications such as biliary obstruction need to be addressed. A Frey procedure would be the operation of choice when intrapancreatic cysts in the head of the pancreas coincides with upstream pancreatic duct dilatation.

Pancreatic ascites and pleural effusions

Pancreatic ascites and pleural effusions occur when there is disruption or a leak from an extrapancreatic fluid collection and may be associated with a PFC/pseudocyst (Figure 16C.2a,b). The typical presentation is the insidious onset of ascites, which is often mistaken for ascites secondary to decompensated liver disease. The

natural history of pancreatic ascites varies but given time will resolve spontaneously in a substantial number of cases. This has made it difficult to determine the efficacy of conventional treatment aimed at "resting the pancreas" by nutritional support (parenteral/or nasojejunal feeding), paracentesis, and suppression of pancreatic secretion by somatostatin analogs [14]. Prolonged conservative treatment increases the risk of sepsis in these patients who are usually poorly nourished.

Endoscopic intervention (papillotomy/stenting) with the aim of sealing the leak (Figure 16C.2c,d) is an attractive alternative [15–17] and should now be considered earlier when rapid response to conventional treatment is not apparent. In more advanced disease, placement of a stent beyond the leak or obstruction may be more difficult to achieve in which case a pancreatic duct drainage operation remains a viable alternative.

Bile duct obstruction

Pathogenesis and pathology

Bile duct obstruction (BDO) is commonly seen during the advanced stages of CP when there is an associated inflammatory mass and calcification in the head of the pancreas. The obstruction can be caused by edema during an acute on chronic attack, compression of a contiguous intrapancreatic fluid collection, or fibrosis. The presentation and natural history vary according to the predominant underlying pathology. The clinical spectrum ranges from an incidental finding on imaging with a disproportionately raised alkaline phosphatase level to overt obstructive jaundice with associated severe pain. The natural history is often unpredictable but it should be noted that jaundice may resolve in half of patients after resolution of an acute on chronic attack [18]. There are conflicting reports on the risk of developing secondary biliary cirrhosis. In 11 publications, the overall incidence was 7.3% and in 4 of these no case with cirrhosis was reported [19].

Management

There are several clinical and morphological factors that need to be considered in order to achieve optimal treatment of a BDO in CP.

In addition to the patient's physical fitness, the four elective clinical scenarios to consider are as follows:

1 an incidental finding in a nonjaundiced patient with minimal symptoms;
2 clinical jaundice with or without minimal pain;
3 a combination of jaundice and pain;
4 low-grade BDO (dilated biliary system with biochemical cholestasis) in patients who require surgery for pain.

With regard to pancreatic morphology, consideration should be given to the following factors:

a. the presence of an inflammatory mass in the head of the pancreas;
b. bile duct compression by an intrapancreatic fluid collection;
c. size of the pancreatic duct;
d. presence of segmental portal hypertension;
e. concern about an underlying malignancy.

As with PFCs, the morphological changes of the pancreas and biliary system need to be carefully mapped by CT and MRI/MRCP (Figure 16C.3). EUS and biopsy are indicated when there is a concern about an underlying malignancy.

Based on the aforementioned information, the management can be individualized with the size of the pancreatic duct having a pivotal role in the decision making (Figure 16C.4).

1 Asymptomatic or minimally symptomatic low-grade strictures should be treated conservatively and monitored every 6 month with repeated liver function tests. Stenting should be avoided as this will result in bacterial colonization of the biliary system and an unnecessary long-term commitment to stenting. The need for a biliary drainage when the alkaline phosphatase remains >2–3 times higher than the upper range of normal [9] remains unclear as are the proposed rationale and timing for surveillance liver biopsies [20].
2 Cholecystectomy and hepatico-jejunostomy are the treatments of choice for patients with persistent jaundice and minimal pain. A Frey procedure should be considered when there is an associated inflammatory mass and a dilated pancreatic duct because an appreciable number of these patients will eventually return with significant pain.
3 In those patients who have significant pain associated with jaundice, a hepatico-jejunostomy in combination with a Frey procedure is the ideal operation in the presence of an inflammatory mass in the head of the pancreas and a dilated pancreatic duct.
4 Whether a bile duct drainage procedure (hepatico-jejunostomy) should be added to a Frey procedure in patients with a low-grade BD stricture (without jaundice) is unclear but it would seem reasonable to proceed if the bile duct is significantly dilated. It is often difficult to determine at the time of the operation whether the bile duct is adequately decompressed after "coring out" the inflammatory mass in the head. The addition of a bile duct drainage procedure to the Frey procedure does not seem to increase the morbidity [21].
5 A pylorus-preserving pancreatico-duodenectomy (PPPD) should be performed if there is doubt about the presence of an underlying cancer.
6 The surgical options when encountering scenarios 3 and 4 in the presence of a nondilated duct are a PPPD, Berger procedure, or one of the other hybrid duodenal preserving operations. Personal preference and experience will dictate the choice of operation.

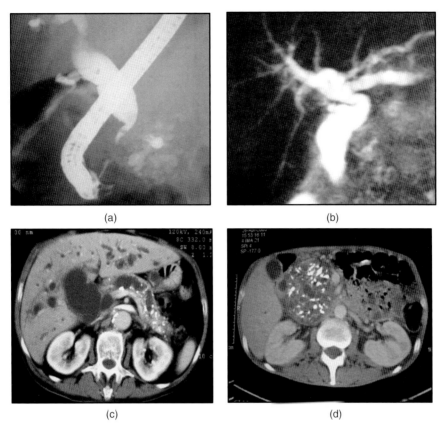

(a) (b)

(c) (d)

Figure 16C.3 (a and b) ERCP and MRCP: high grade distal bile duct obstruction. (c). CT: grossly dilated bile duct and pancreatic duct. (d) CT: demonstrating large calcified mass in head of pancreas without dilated pancreatic duct.

Endoscopic treatment

Stenting is the preferred treatment option in patients who are unfit for surgery and those with associated portal hypertension. In addition, stenting has an important role in patients who present with cholangitis. In some cases with an intrapancreatic fluid collection, drainage may suffice but underlying fibrosis and calcifications may prevent complete resolution.

Long-term stenting (plastic or expandable) has a variable track record which is marred by recurrent blockage and biliary septic complications [8, 9, 22], although a recent RCT reports, with a 6 month stenting period, minimal septic complications and a 90% stricture resolution after five years, in those randomized to removable covered metal stents [23]. While stents are frequently employed for BDO, surgical bypass remains the most definitive long-term treatment and should be considered in all patients who are fit for surgery or

can be made fit when their infective and nutritional complications have resolved.

Summary

The management algorithm of BDO in CP may at times become convoluted both in terms of timing and selection of treatment options. Careful evaluation of symptoms and morphological changes of the pancreas are required to tailor the appropriate surgical procedures. Since jaundice frequently resolves spontaneously there is no need for urgent intervention unless there is associated cholangitis. The overzealous use of stenting should be avoided when there is asymptomatic low-grade BDO [13, 22].

Duodenal obstruction

Overt duodenal obstruction is less frequently seen in CP but many patients with advanced disease will

Treatment strategy based on clinical features and pancreatic morphology

Clinical presentation	Morphological changes
1. Jaundice and minimal pain	A. Inflammatory mass
2. Pain and jaundice	B. Pancreatic duct > 5 mm.
3. Pain and low-grade obstruction	C. Cancer concern

Treatment algorithm for bile duct obstruction in the presence of a dilated pancreatic duct

1 + A & B	2 + A & B	3 + A & B	C
H-J +? Frey	H-J + Frey	Frey + H-J	PPPD

Treatment algorithm for bile duct obstruction in absence of a dilated pancreatic duct

1 + A & B	2 + A & B	3 + A & B	C
H-J +? B or H	H-J + B or H	B or H + H-J	PPPD

H-J, hepatico-jejunostomy; Frey, Frey procedure; B or H, Beger
PPPD, pylorus preserving pancreatico-duodenectomy;

Figure 16C.4 Management algorithm for bile duct obstruction according to the size of the main pancreatic duct.

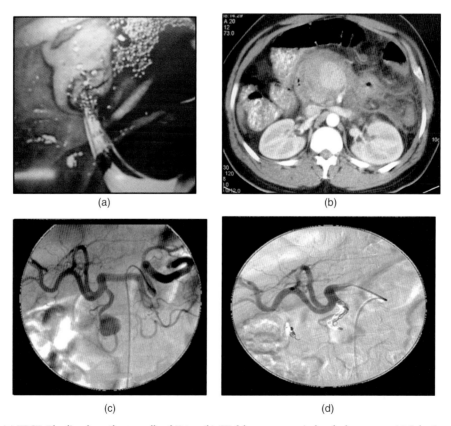

(a)

(b)

(c)

(d)

Figure 16C.5 (a) ERCP: Bleeding from the ampulla of Vater. (b) CT: false aneurysm in head of pancreas. (c) Selective angiography: false aneurysm arising from gastro-duodenal artery. (d) Selective angiography: successful embolization.

have subclinical evidence of delayed gastric emptying. As with biliary obstruction, an inflammatory mass is frequently present in the head of the pancreas and occasionally a contiguous PFC may be an important contributing factor.

There is no clear consensus on the best surgical bypass procedure for persistent duodenal obstruction. The options are kocherization of the duodenum if the cause is a dominant fibrotic band or a bypass operation (i.e., duodenoduodenostomy or gastroenterostomy). A PPPD should be considered when duodenal obstruction is associated with a BDO and an inflammatory mass in the head of the pancreas.

Temporary duodenal stenting may be an option in poorly nourished patients and those who are unfit for surgery.

Hemorrhage

Hemorrhage associated with CP may be due to analgesic-induced peptic ulcer disease, false aneurysms (Figure 16C.5a,b) related to PFCs or gastric varices secondary to segmental portal hypertension. Surprisingly, the risk of bleeding from gastric varices is low and there is no need for prophylactic intervention. Most cases with bleeding from false aneurysms can be successfully managed by selective angiographic embolization) [24] (Figure 16C.5c,d). Surgery should be the last resort and is aimed at vascular control rather than performing a major resection unless the aneurysm is situated in the body or tail of the pancreas.

Overall summary

Complications in CP may occur in isolation or in combination in about a third of patients during the course of their disease and are often associated with pain. Before embarking on therapy, a multidisciplinary approach is essential and should be based on a full morphological and clinical assessment. There is robust evidence for the use of minimally invasive solutions for PFC, hemorrhage, and pancreatic ascites as first-line and often definitive therapy. Surgery remains the most definitive treatment for the drainage of symptomatic BDO. Additional procedures on the pancreas are often required when severe pain is associated with BDO.

References

1 D'Egidio A and Schein M. Pancreatic pseudocysts: a proposed classification and its management implications. British Journal of Surgery 1991;78:981–984.

2 Apostolou C, Krige JEJ, Bornman PC, et al. Pancreatic pseudocysts. South African Journal of Surgery 2006;44:148–154.

3 Varadarajulu S Christein JD, Tamhani A, et al. Prospective randomized trial comparing EUS and EGD for transmural drainage of pancreatic pseudocysts. Gastrointestinal Endoscopy 2008;68: 1102–1111.

4 Park DH, Lee S, Moon S-H, et al. Endoscopic ultrasound-guided versus conventional transmural drainage for pancreatic pseudocysts: a prospective randomized trial. Endoscopy 2009;41:842–848.

5 Larsen M, Kozarek R. Management of pancreatic duct leaks and fistula. Journal of Gastroenterology and Hepatology 2014;29: 1361–1370.

6 Bachmann K, Kutup A, Mann O, et al. Surgical treatment in chronic pancreatitis timing and type of procedure. Best Practice & Research Clinical Gastroenterology 2010; 24: 299–310.

7 Jacobson BC, Baron TH, Alder DG. ASGE guidelines: the role of endoscopy in the diagnosis and the management of cystic lesions and inflammatory collections of the pancreas. Gastrointestinal Endoscopy 2005; 61: 363–370.

8 Nguyen-Tang T, Dumonceau J-M. Endoscopic treatment in chronic pancreatitis, timing, duration and type of intervention. Best Practice & Research Clinical Gastroenterology 2010; 24: 281–298.

9 Dumonceau JM, Delhey M, Tringgali A, et al. Endoscopic treatment of chronic pancreatitis: European Society of Gastrointestinal Endoscopy (ASGED) clinical guidelines. Endoscopy 2012;44:784–800.

10 Varadarajulu S, Bang JI, Sutton BS, et al. Equal efficacy of endoscopic and surgical cystgastrostomy for pancreatic pseudocyst drainage in a randomized trial. Gastroenterology 2013;145:583–590.

11 Barthet M, Lamblin G, Gasini M, et al. Clinical usefulness of a treatment algorithm for pancreatic pseudocysts. Gastrointestinal Endoscopy 2008; 67: 245–252.

12 Nealon WH, Walser E. Duct drainage alone is sufficient in the operative management of pancreatic pseudocyst in patients with chronic pancreatitis. Annals of Surgery 2003; 237: 614–622.

13 Bornman PC, Botha JF, Ramos JM, et al. Guidelines for the diagnosis and treatment of chronic pancreatitis. South African Medical Journal 2010; 100: 845–860.

14 Gomes-Cerezo J, Barbado-Cano A, Suarez I, et al. Pancreatic ascites: study of therapeutic options by analyses of case reports and case series between 1975–2000. American Journal of Gastroenterology 2003;93: 568–577.

15 Kozarek RA, Ball TJ, Patterson DJ, et al. Endoscopic treatment of pancreatic ascites. American Journal of Surgery 1994; 168: 223–226.

16 Bracher GA, Manocha AP, De Banto JR, et al. Endoscopic pancreatic duct stenting to treat pancreatic ascites. Gastrointestinal Endoscopy 1999; 49:710–715.

17 Pai GC, Suvarna D, Bhat G. Endoscopic treatment as first line therapy for pancreatic ascites and pleural effusions. Journal of Gastroenterology and Hepatology 2009;24:1196–1202.

18 Kalvaria I, Bornman PC, Marks IN, et al. The spectrum and natural history of common bile duct stenosis in chronic alcohol induced pancreatitis. Annals of Surgery 1989; 210: 608–613.

19 Abdullah A, Krige JEJ, Bornman PC. Bile duct obstruction in chronic pancreatitis. Hepato Pancreato Biliary 2007;9:421–428.

20 Vijungco J, Prinz R. Management of biliary and duodenal complications of chronic pancreatitis. World Journal of Surgery 2003;27: 1258–1270.

21 Cauchy F, Regimbeau JM, Fuks D, et al. Influence of bile duct obstruction on the results of Frey's procedure for chronic pancreatitis. Pancreatology 2014; 14: 21–26.

22 Waldthaler A, SchÜtte K, Weigt J, et al. Long-term outcome of self-expandable metal stents for biliary obstruction in chronic pancreatitis. Journal of the Pancreas 2013;14:57–62.

23 Carola H, Leena K, Marianne U, et al. Randomized multicenter study of multiple plastic stents vs. covered self-expandable metallic stent in the treatment of biliary stricture in chronic pancreatitis. Endoscopy 2015; 47: 605–610.

24 Chiang K-C, Chen T-H, Hsu J-t. Management of chronic pancreatitis complicated with a bleeding pseudoaneurysm. World Journal of Gastroenterology 2014; 20: 16132–16137.

PART D: Surgery for chronic pancreatitis: pancreatic duct drainage procedures

Dirk J. Gouma[1] & Philippus C. Bornman[2,3]

[1] Academic Medical Center, Amsterdam, the Netherlands
[2] Department of Surgery, University of Cape Town, Cape Town, South Africa
[3] Groote Schuur Hospital, Cape Town, South Africa

Introduction

The first pancreatic duct drainage procedure was described by DuVal in 1954, which entailed a distal pancreatectomy and caudal pancreaticojejunostomy [1]. The operation was then modified by Puestow who introduced the longitudinal pancreaticojejunostomy of the body and tail, and shortly thereafter it was modified to a side-to-side anastomosis. This longitudinal side-to-side Roux-en-Y pancreaticojejunostomy (LPJ) was later described in detail by Partington–Rochelle [2] to whom this operation is now commonly referred to. This operation is less commonly referred to as a "modified Puestow procedure."

This section covers pancreatic duct drainage procedures for pain in uncomplicated chronic pancreatitis (CP). The surgical strategies for complications such as bile duct obstruction, pancreatic cysts, and duodenal obstruction are reviewed in Chapter 16C. Other new concepts of combining the drainage of the duct and (organ sparing) resection, the so-called hybrid procedures such as the Frey procedure [3, 4], and the Beger procedure and Bern procedure are described in detail in Chapter 16E.

Patient selection

Persistent uncontrolled pain after adequate medical treatment is the most common indication for surgical drainage procedures [5–8]. As with other interventional procedures, patients should first undergo an adequate trial of intensive medical therapy before a pancreatic drainage operation is considered. This should include eliminating etiologic factors such as alcoholic consumption, optimal pain medication in a step-up fashion, and when appropriate administration of pancreatic enzymes for exocrine insufficiency and control of diabetes mellitus [5–8]. Autoimmune pancreatitis is a separate entity with the opportunity to start with specific treatment options such as corticosteroids, which might even be effective in management of ductal stenosis [5–7].

The selection for either a minimally invasive endoscopic drainage procedure or one of the different surgical procedures will depend mainly on morphological features as determined by contrast-enhanced computed tomography (CT) or magnetic resonance imaging (MRI) [5–8]. The most common morphological changes are an inflammatory mass and local fibrosis, pancreatic duct dilatation and stenosis, and ductal stones. Associated complications such as pseudocysts, bile duct stenosis, and duodenal stenosis are also frequently encountered. Considering surgical series from major centers around the world, there seems to be a remarkable difference in the morphological changes between series from the United States and some countries in Europe [9]. When comparing the median sizes of the pancreatic heads in patients who underwent surgery, Keck et al. showed a significantly larger pancreatic head mass in the German group (4.5 cm) when compared with an American group (2.6 cm) [9]. This resulted in a different surgical approach. They suggested that the population might be different in Europe [9]. The results of a recent analysis from the Netherlands mirrored the American experience showing that 65% of the patients underwent a drainage procedure because of a small

Pancreatitis: Medical and Surgical Management, First Edition.
David B. Adams, Peter B. Cotton, Nicholas J. Zyromski and John Windsor.
© 2017 John Wiley & Sons, Ltd. Published 2017 by John Wiley & Sons, Ltd.

pancreatic head mass while only 18% had a pancreatic head resection [10]. It remains difficult to explain these differences of treatment in the same area in Europe. This might be due to a different treatment philosophy; delay in referral may also result in more advanced disease by the time patients come to surgery. A survey from the Netherlands indeed highlighted a conservative approach among internists and gastroenterologists who consider (local) inflammation in the pancreas as a self-limiting disease, which should "burn out" over the years, while patients with dilated ducts and stones are treated primarily with interventional endoscopic procedures [11]. An inflammatory mass in the head of the pancreas is a relative contraindication for a drainage procedure; these are best treated by a resection or a hybrid procedure (resection and drainage). Patients best suited for a pancreatic drainage procedure are those without an inflammatory mass and dilated main pancreatic duct greater than 5 mm in diameter.

Pancreaticojejunostomy (Partington–Rochelle procedure)

A bilateral subcostal incision provides the best exposure of the pancreas. This is achieved by full Kocherization of the duodenum, mobilization of the hepatic flexure of the colon, and division of the gastrocolic ligament toward the splenic flexure of the colon. The neck of the pancreas is usually the best site to enter the pancreatic duct. The pancreatic duct is identified using palpation and a syringe or, if these fail, by intraoperative

ultrasonography. The longitudinal incision into the main pancreatic duct is extended as far as possible toward the tail and the head. The extension into the head, as in the Frey procedure, is a new addition to the original description of the operation and helpful to remove stones. When the pancreatic duct is exposed, a biopsy is taken for frozen section if there is any doubt about a malignancy and stones are removed. The side-to-side anastomosis with the jejunal limb is carried out with a one layer continuous or inter-rupted monofilament 4/0 sutures. The longitudinal pancreaticojejunostomy is shown in Figure 16D.1. The Roux-en-Y loop is then completed with a one layer continuous 3/0 monofilament sutures.

Results of lateral pancreaticojejunostomy (LPJ)

LPJ is associated with a low morbidity (20%) and mortality (1%) rate. The early and long-term pain relief is reported to vary between 42% and 100% [3–7, 12, 13]. The outcome of LPJ in studies that included >20 patients is summarized in Table 16D.1 [13]. In these studies, long-term pain relief was better in patients with a dilated duct >7 mm, while pain relief is relatively low in patients with nondilated ducts with some studies achieving only 50% pain relief after 5 years. These poor results have been attributed to undrained side duct in an inflammatory mass in the pancreas head and those with small-duct disease. The alternative drainage operation for small-duct disease is the V-shaped excision

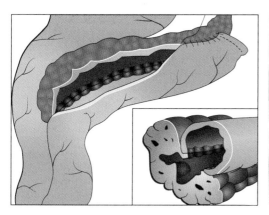 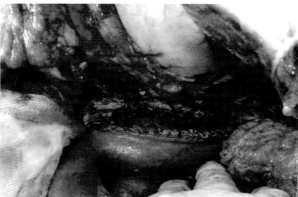

Figure 16D.1 The longitudinal side-to-side pancreaticojejunostomy. The opened pancreatic duct with ductal mucosa. The posterior layer is sutured and a start is made for the anterior layer at the schematic drawing.

Table 16D.1 Results of drainage procedure by pancreaticojejunostomy in series of >20 patients.

Reference	No. of patients	Complete or partial pain relief (%)	Mortality (%)	Mean follow-up (months)
Sarles et al. [14]	69	85	4	60
Warshaw [12]	33	83	3	43
Morrow et al. [15]	46	80	0	72
Sato et al. [16]	43	100	0	110
Bradley [17]	48	66	0	69
Nealon et al. [18, 19]	41	93	0	15
Drake and Fry [20]	23	90	0	60
Greenlee and Prinz [21][a]	86	80	3	95
Adloff et al. [22]	105	93	2	65
Wilson et al. [23]	20	76	5	60
Delcore et al. [24][b]	28	86	0	42
Adams et al. [25]	85	55	0	76
Buhler et al. [26][c]	35	42	0	48
Sielezneff et al. [27]	57	84	0	65
Sakorafas et al. [28]	120	81	0	96
Boerma et al. [29, 30]	50	88	0	27
Mean results (±SD)	889	80.1 ± 14.8	1.1 ± 1.7	62.7 ± 24.9

[a]Study consisted of 91 patients, 5 omitted who underwent a caudal PJ.
[b]Eighty nine percent of the patients without dilated pancreatic ducts.
[c]Either ductal or cyst drainage.
Adapted from van der Gaag et al. [13], Aliment Pharmacol Ther 2007; 26 Suppl 2:221–232.

operation described by Izbicki and the Hamburg group [31]. By excision of the ventral pancreas and removing a small segment of parenchyma, the duct is opened and partly a new artificial channel for drainage is created. It is also a combination of drainage and decompression of the pancreas [31]. A low morbidity (20%) and mortality (0%) have been reported, with long-term complete pain relief in 73% of patients after a median follow-up of 83 months. These results appear to be superior to the standard LPJ for small-duct disease, but the downside of this operation is a relatively high rate of new onset exocrine and endocrine insufficiency. The V-shaped excision procedure is not widely practiced and as such there is a paucity of data to support the Hamburg experience.

Surgical versus endoscopic drainage procedures

Endoscopic stenting techniques with and without extra-corporeal shockwave lithotripsy (ESWL) have been introduced in the 1990s as alternative minimally inva-sive therapy to surgical drainage operations. Apart from less morbidity and mortality, these minimally invasive options may also be associated with fewer new-onset endocrine and exocrine pancreatic insufficiencies. As a consequence, endoscopic interventional procedures have enjoyed increasing support as first-line treatment for pain due to CP. A review of the short-term results of endoscopic pancreatic duct drainage for painful CP showed complete or partial pain relief in 74% of cases [13]. However, the initial enthusiasm for endoscopic intervention has been dampened by subsequent studies showing disappointing long-term results of pain relief [32, 33]. The first randomized controlled trial (RCT) by Dite et al. compared endoscopic drainage and different types of surgical treatment and showed significantly better pain control in the surgical arm [32]. In the second RCT, the Dutch group restricted the surgical procedure to an LPJ, which eliminated the bias in favor of surgery when there is an inflammatory mass in the head of the pancreas [33]. After 24-month follow-up, patients who underwent surgery had lower Izbicki pain

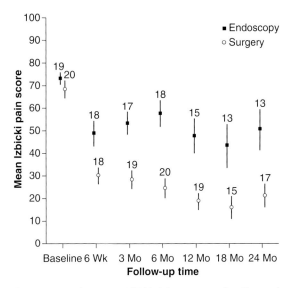

Figure 16D.2   The mean Izbicki Pain scores at baseline and 6 weeks up to 24 months after endoscopic and surgical drainage. Adapted from the Cahen et al. [33], NEJM 2007; 356:676–684.

scores (25 vs. 51) and better physical health scores compared with those who were treated endoscopically (Figure 16D.2). Complete or partial pain relief was obtained in 75% after surgery compared with 32% after endoscopic therapy [33]. A recent analysis with a longer follow-up period of 79 months showed that 68% of patients treated by endoscopy needed repeated endoscopic drainage. About half of these patients needed surgery as opposed to 5% in the surgical group [34]. Pain relief in the surgery and endoscopy groups was 80% and 38%, respectively. Costs of surgery were also lower compared with endoscopy treatment. A recent meta-analysis confirmed that surgery is superior to endoscopy in patients with a dilated pancreatic duct [35].

While it should be conceded that the current studies comparing surgery with endoscopic treatment for CP are small and have methodological shortcomings, there is mounting evidence that surgery provides superior long-term pain relief when compared with current endoscopic interventional procedures. Therefore, the current recommendation from the recent guideline of the ESGE that endoscopic intervention should be considered as first-line interventional therapy for pain in CP should be revisited [36].

Timing for surgical drainage in relation to other procedures

Considering the relatively high percentage of patients who need additional surgery after long-term stenting and on the other hand the good relatively early results, the choice first stenting, and timing of surgery in this ongoing disease process needs to be evaluated further. Older studies did not show a negative effect of previous stenting [29], but a recent series from the Academic Medical Center demonstrated that poor response to surgical treatment for CP in terms of pain relief and good quality of life was related to increasing numbers of stenting procedures prior to surgery [37]. Surgery after more than 3 years of symptomatic disease was another important risk factor [38]. An experimental study in pigs also suggested that early surgery resulted in less histological damage and better exocrine function [30]. The fact that surgical intervention is generally performed at a later stage of disease a trial comparing early surgery versus optimal current step-up practice for CP is currently performed [39]. In the previous RCT, it was not allowed to perform a Frey procedure because only surgical and endoscopic drainage of the pancreatic duct should be compared [34]. In patients with intraductal stones in the pancreatic head area, it is sometimes difficult to remove these stones without removing a wedge of the pancreatic tissue ventrally to the duct. Therefore, pancreatic parenchyma in this area toward the duodenum/papilla is now more frequently removed to have better access to the duct and this concept is also accepted in the new ESCAPE trial [39]. Many surgeons believe nowadays that, therefore, resection should be part of a surgical procedure. This might be an explanation for the increasing popularity of the Frey procedure and other organ-sparing resection procedures such as the Beger and Bern procedure (Chapter 16E).

Summary and conclusion

The longitudinal pancreaticojejunostomy (LPJ) has been used for decades as the only therapeutic drainage procedure in CP and is nowadays a relatively safe procedure, but with certain limitations for long-term pain relief. The introduction of duodenal preserving resection operations with or without drainage of the pancreatic duct has to a large extent superseded LPJ, especially in those cases with an inflammatory mass in the head of the pancreas. Yet, this operation still deserves its rightful place when there is a dilated main pancreatic duct without an inflammatory mass in the head of the pancreas. There is good reason to believe that LPJ should yield results that are similar to the duodenum-preserving resection operations if the operation is restricted to these selection criteria. The proposed RCT comparing Frey and LPJ operations to endoscopic stenting should throw more light on the overall role of LPJ in the management of patients with CP with intractable pain. Timing of surgical drainage procedures (combined with partial resection) in relation to long-term outcome, pain relief, and function is an important subject for new studies.

References

1 DuVal MK Jr., Caudal pancreatico-jejunostomy for chronic relapsing pancreatitis Annals of Surgery 1954;140:775–785.

2 Partington PF, Rochelle RE. Modified Puestow procedure for retrograde drainage of the pancreatic duct. Annals of Surgery 1960; 152:1037–1043

3 Frey CF, Smith GJ. Description and rationale of a new operation for chronic pancreatitis. Pancreas. 1987;2(6):701–707.

4 Andersen DK, Frey CF. The evolution of the surgical treatment of chronic pancreatitis. Annals of Surgery 2010; 251: 18–32.

5 Forsmark CE. Management of chronic pancreatitis. Gastroenterology. 2013;144(6):1282–1291; e3. doi: 10.1053/j.gastro.2013.02.008. Review

6 Conwell DL, Lee LS, Yadav D, Longnecker DS, Miller FH, Mortele KJ, Levy MJ, Kwon R, Lieb JG, Stevens T, Toskes PP, Gardner TB, Gelrud A, Wu BU, Forsmark CE, Vege SS. American Pancreatic Association practice guidelines in chronic pancreatitis: evidence-based report on diagnostic guidelines. Pancreas. 2014;43(8):1143–1162.

7 Issa Y, Bruno MJ, Bakker OJ, Besselink MG, Schepers NJ, van Santvoort HC, Gooszen HG, Boermeester MA. Treatment options for chronic pancreatitis. Nature Reviews Gastroenterology & Hepatology. 2014;11(9):556–564. DOI: 10.1038/nrgastro.2014.74. Epub 2014 Jun 10. Review

8 Bornman PC, Botha JF, Ramos JM, Smith MD, Van der Merwe S, Watermeyer GA, Ziady CC. Guideline for the diagnosis and treatment of chronic pancreatitis. South African Medical Journal. 2010;100(12 Pt 2):845–860.

9 Keck T, Marjanovic G, Fernandez-del CC, et al. The inflammatory pancreatic head mass: significant differences in the anatomic pathology of German and American patients with chronic pancreatitis determine very different surgical strategies. Annals of Surgery 2009; 249:105–110.

10 van der Gaag NA, Boermeester MA, Gouma DJ. The inflammatory pancreatic head mass. Annals of Surgery 2009; 250:352–353.

11 van Esch AA, Ahmed Ali U, van Goor H, Bruno MJ, Drenth JP. A wide variation in diagnostic and therapeutic strategies in chronic pancreatitis: a Dutch national survey. Journal of the Pancreas. 2012;13(4):394–401.

12 Warshaw AL, Popp JW, Jr., Schapiro RH. Long-term patency, pancreatic function, and pain relief after lateral pancreaticojejunostomy for chronic pancreatitis. Gastroenterology 1980; 79(2):289–293.

13 van der Gaag NA, Gouma DJ, van Gulik TM, Busch OR, Boermeester MA. Review article: surgical management of chronic pancreatitis. Alimentary Pharmacology and Therapeutics 2007; 26 Suppl 2:221–232.

14 Sarles JC, Nacchiero M, Garani F, Salasc B. Surgical treatment of chronic pancreatitis. Report of 134 cases treated by resection or drainage. American Journal of Surgery 1982; 144: 317–321.

15 Morrow CE, Cohen JI, Sutherland DE, Najarian JS. Chronic pancreatitis: long term surgical results of pancreatic duct drainage, pancreatic resection, and near-total pancreatectomy and islet autotransplantation. Surgery 1984; 96: 608–616.

16 Sato T, Miyashita E, Yamauchi H, Matsuno S. The role of surgical treatment for chronic pancreatitis. Annals of Surgery 1986; 203: 266–271.

17 Bradley EL III,. Long-term results of pancreatojejunostomy in patients with chronic pancreatitis. American Journal of Surgery 1987; 153: 207–213.

18 Nealon WH, Walser E. Duct drainage alone is sufficient in the operative management of pancreatic pseudocyst in patients with chronic pancreatitis. Annals of Surgery 2003; 237: 614–620.

19 Nealon WH, Townsend CM Jr, Thompson JC. Operative drainage of the pancreatic duct delays functional impairment in patients with chronic pancreatitis. A prospective analysis. Annals of Surgery 1988; 208: 321–329.

20 Drake DH, Fry WJ. Ductal drainage for chronic pancreatitis. Surgery 1989; 105: 131–140.

21 Greenlee HB, Prinz RA, Aranha GV. Long-term results of side-to-side pancreaticojejunostomy. World Journal of Surgery 1990; 14: 70–76.

22 Adloff M, Schloegel M, Arnaud JP, Ollier JC. Role of pancreaticojejunostomy in the treatment of chronic pancreatitis. A study of 105 operated patients. Chirurgie 1991; 117: 251–256.

23 Wilson TG, Hollands MJ, Little JM. Pancreaticojejunostomy for chronic pancreatitis. Australian and New Zealand Journal of Surgery 1992; 62: 111–115.

24 Delcore R, Rodriguez FJ, Thomas JH, Forster J, Hermreck AS. The role of pancreatojejunostomy in patients without

dilated pancreatic ducts. American Journal of Surgery 1994; 168: 598–601.

25 Adams DB, Ford MC, Anderson MC. Outcome after lateral pancreaticojejunostomy for chronic pancreatitis. Annals of Surgery 1994; 219: 481–487.

26 Buhler L, Schmidlin F, de Perrot M, Borst F, Mentha G, Morel P. Long-term results after surgical management of chronic pancreatitis. Hepatogastroenterology 1999; 46: 1986–1989.

27 Sielezneff I, Malouf A, Salle E, Brunet C, Thirion X, Sastre B. Long term results of lateral pancreaticojejunostomy for chronic alcoholic pancreatitis. European Journal of Surgery 2000; 166: 58–64.

28 Sakorafas GH, Farnell MB, Farley DR, Rowland CM, Sarr MG. Long-term results after surgery for chronic pancreatitis. International Journal of Pancreatology 2000; 27: 131–142.

29 Boerma D, van Gulik TM, Rauws EA, Obertop H, Gouma DJ. Outcome of pancreaticojejunostomy after previous endoscopic stenting in patients with chronic pancreatitis. European Journal of Surgery. 2002;168(4):223–228.

30 Lamme B, Boermeester MA, Straatsburg IH, van Buijtenen JM, Boerma D, Offerhaus GJ, et al. Early versus late surgical drainage for obstructive pancreatitis in an experimental model. British Journal of Surgery 2007; 94(7): 849–854.

31 Yekebas EF, Bogoevski D, Honarpisheh H, Cataldegirmen G, Habermann CR, Seewald S, Link BC, Kaifi JT, Wolfram L, Mann O, Bubenheim M, Izbicki JR. Long-term follow-up in small duct chronic pancreatitis: a plea for extended drainage by "V-shaped excision" of the anterior aspect of the pancreas. Annals of Surgery. 2006;244(6):940–946; discussion 946–948.

32 Dite P, Ruzicka M, Zboril V, Novotny I. A prospective, randomized trial comparing endoscopic and surgical therapy for chronic pancreatitis. Endoscopy 2003; 35(7):553–558.

33 Cahen DL, Gouma DJ, Nio Y, Rauws EA, Boermeester MA, Busch OR, et al. Endoscopic versus surgical drainage of the pancreatic duct in chronic pancreatitis. New England Journal of Medicine 2007; 356(7):676–684.

34 Cahen DL, Gouma DJ, Laramee P, Nio Y, Rauws EA, Boermeester MA, et al. Long-term outcomes of endoscopic vs surgical drainage of the pancreatic duct in patients with chronic pancreatitis. Gastroenterology 2011; 141(5):1690–1695.

35 Ahmed Ali U, Pahlplatz JM, Nealon WH, van Goor H, Gooszen HG, Boermeester MA. Endoscopic or surgical intervention for painful obstructive chronic pancreatitis. Cochrane Database of Systematic Reviews 2012;1:CD007884.

36 Dumonceau JM, Delhaye M, Tringali A, Dominguez-Munoz JE, Poley JW, Arvanitaki M, Costamagna G, Costea F, Devière J, Eisendrath P, Lakhtakia S, Reddy N, Fockens P, Ponchon T, Bruno M. Endoscopic treatment of chronic pancreatitis: European Society of Gastrointestinal Endoscopy (ESGE) Clinical Guideline. Endoscopy. 2012;44(8):784–800.

37 van der Gaag NA, van Gulik TM, Busch OR, Sprangers MA, Bruno MJ, Zevenbergen C, Gouma DJ, Boermeester MA. Functional and medical outcomes after tailored surgery for pain due to chronic pancreatitis. Annals of Surgery. 2012;255(4):763–770.

38 Usama Almed Ali, Nieuwenhuijs VB, van Ejck CH, Gooszen HG, van Dam RM, Busch OR, et al. Clinical outcome in relation to Timing of surgery in chronic pancreatitis. A nomogram to predict pain relief. Archives of Surgery 2012, 147:925–932.

39 Ahmed Ali U, Issa Y, Bruno MJ, van Goor H, van Santvoort H, Busch OR, et al.Dutch Pancreatitis Study Group. Early surgery versus optimal current step-up practice for chronic pancreatitis (ESCAPE): design and rationale of a randomized trial. BMC Gastroenterology. 2013;13:49.

PART E: Surgical management: resection and drainage procedures

Chronic pancreatitis – hybrid procedures

Tobias Keck[1], Ulrich Wellner[1] & Ulrich Adam[2]

[1] *Department of Surgery, University Medical Center Schleswig Holstein, Lübeck, Germany*
[2] *Department of Surgery, Vivantes Hospital Humboldt, Berlin, Germany*

Introduction

All hybrid procedures share the concept of resection of the so-called pacemaker of progression of chronic pancreatitis (CP), the inflammatory pancreatic head, while on the other hand the duodenum is preserved. Duodenum-preserving pancreatic head resection in the last 20 years has augmented the armamentarium of the pancreatic surgeon to efficiently address pain and complications in CP. All procedures – the Berne, Frey, and Beger procedures – have been proven to be highly efficient in pain reduction, improvement of life quality, and avoidance of progression to organ complications of CP such as duodenal obstruction, bile duct stenosis, or portal vein thrombosis. In addition, it has been demonstrated that these procedures can be performed with a low perioperative morbidity and mortality, preservation of endocrine and exocrine function of the organ, and low recurrence rates. The procedures vary in their extent of resection of the pancreatic head, the extent of portal vein decompression, and the inclusion of a biliary anastomosis. Accordingly, the procedures in part vary in the technical approach and technical level of difficulty performing these operations.

Indications for surgery

Pain is the leading symptom of recurrent CP. After failure of initial limited conservative treatment, operative treatment for CP is indicated. It is of essential importance to know that conservative treatment is limited in its efficacy for pain control and has been shown to be inferior in the efficacy of pain control in comparison to operative drainage of the pancreatic duct [1, 2]. Pathophysiologically, pain has been attributed to multifactorial genesis inxcluding ductal and intra-parenchymatous hypertension as well as peripancreatic neuromodular nociception [3, 4]. Procedures addressing the inflammatory pancreatic head mass (IPHM), the so-called pacemaker of the inflammation [5], have been shown in several studies to be even more efficient than drainage procedures addressing the pancreatic duct alone [6, 7] (Figures 16E.1 and 16E.2).

Apart from pain, long-lasting pancreatitis might lead to further mechanical complications in direct proximity of the pancreatic head such as duodenal stenosis, cholestasis due to biliary duct stenosis within the pancreatic head, and partial or complete obstruction of the mesentericoportal axis leading to portal hypertension. Local, relatively seldom complications might also include pseudocyst formation, pancreaticopleural fistula formation, or pseudoaneurysms at the gastroduodenal or splenic artery. In the choice of the most effective hybrid procedure, these mechanical complications have to be considered when choosing the most effective operation among the hybrid procedures for CP.

Duodenum preservation or no duodenum preservation – is that the question?

Alternatively, procedures that resect the duodenum together with the pancreatic head usually used for

Pancreatitis: Medical and Surgical Management, First Edition.
David B. Adams, Peter B. Cotton, Nicholas J. Zyromski and John Windsor.
© 2017 John Wiley & Sons, Ltd. Published 2017 by John Wiley & Sons, Ltd.

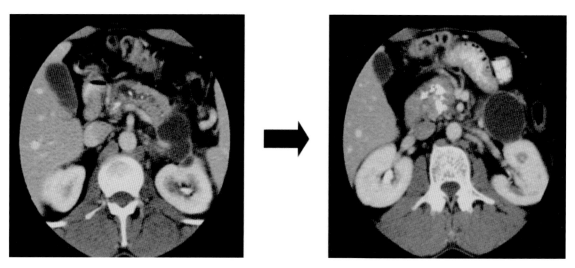

Figure 16E.1 Progression of the pancreatic head tumor 2 years after a drainage operation. Limiting the operation to the pancreatic duct in the pancreatic body and tail of the pancreas might lead to persistent symptoms due to the pacemaker function of the pancreatic head.

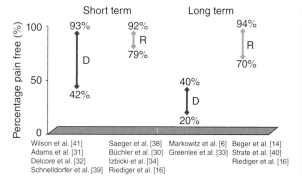

Figure 16E.2 Comparison of long- and short-term results comparing drainage procedures (D) to resection procedures (R). On the long-term procedures resecting the pancreatic head are more effective than simple drainage procedures. Cumulated data from 13 studies, adapted from [19].

	Büchler (1995)	Izbicki et al. [23]	Keck et al. [24]
	n = 40	*n* = 61	*n* = 85
P.o. mortality	O	O	O
P.o. morbidity	+	O	O
Endocrine function	+	O	O
Exocrine function	+	O	O
Pain	+	O	O
QOL	+	+	O

Figure 16E.3 Randomized controlled trials comparing duodenum-preserving operations (Frey and Beger) to oncological operations (PPPD and Whipple operation). o, no difference; +, superiority of duodenum-preserving operation; p.o., postoperative; QOL, quality of life.

oncologic patients also have been promoted for CP. The pylorus-preserving pancreatoduodenectomy (PPPD) [20] and the classic Whipple operation [21, 22] have been compared with duodenum-preserving operations in several randomized controlled trials (RCTs; Figure 16E.3). Whereas the long-term results of these trials show no difference in the endocrine and exocrine functions of the remaining pancreas, the efficacy of pain reduction, and the patients' quality of life (QOL), two trials have shown a potential benefit of the duodenum-preserving operation in a short-term perioperative evaluation.

Today, we know from bariatric surgery that preservation of the duodenum additionally has several beneficial effects on the hormonal axis in the gastrointestinal tract that have not been in the focus of the RCTs conducted earlier for duodenum preservation in CP. It has been shown, however, that duodenum preservation leads to a faster recovery of weight and a better glucose homeostasis [25].

Beger operation – duodenum-preserving pancreatic head resection

Comparative studies have shown that there are differences between the determination of size of the inflammatory head mass between Germany and the United States [26]. In 1972, Beger et al. [27] developed an operation to specifically address the IPHM in CP and at the same time preserve the function of the duodenum. This hybrid operation combined elements of resection and drainage. During this procedure, the pancreas is transected over the mesentericoportal axis and a subtotal resection of the pancreatic head is performed leaving a small rim of pancreatic tissue on the duodenal aspect of the pancreas. Leaving this rim not too small is important for the arterial perfusion of the duodenum (Figure 16E.4). The reconstruction is performed using a retrocolic-guided Roux-en-Y loop. One anastomosis is performed as terminolateral pancreaticojejunostomy to the pancreatic tail; to this same loop, the second anastomosis is performed as a laterolateral pancreatojejunostomy to the remaining pancreatic rim on the duodenum, and a third anastomosis is performed as an anastomosis between the common bile duct in its intrapancreatic course and the jejunal loop, usually as a laterolateral anastomosis. The addition of the biliary anastomosis is necessary in around 25% of the cases when a Beger procedure is performed [27, 17]. Throughout the development of this procedure, several modifications have been published by the group. One modification is the extension of the resection to the pancreatic tail and the combination of the original Beger operation with a drainage procedure leading to a laterolateral pancreatojejunostomy instead of a terminolateral anastomosis in the aforementioned first anastomosis [28]. In any case, a revision of the pancreatic duct for potential pancreatic stones in the remaining pancreatic tail has to be performed during this operation. Fresh frozen sections of pancreatic tissue have to be examined for the detection of potential occult small pancreatic cancer within the CP.

Given the complexity of the operation, this operation has the most benefits in cases where due to partial obstruction of the portal vein this needs to be liberated. Biliary obstruction in the context of CP is another good indication; however, there is a biliary restenosis rate of approximately 4% requiring secondary reoperation or intervention in the long run after the Beger operation

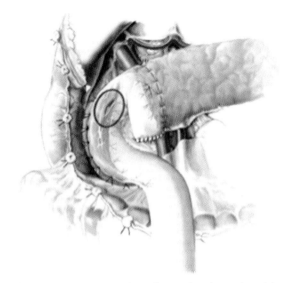

Figure 16E.4 Beger operation. After a subtotal resection of the pancreatic head two anastomoses are performed to the remaining pancreatic tail and a rim of pancreas on the duodenum. The operation can be combined with a biliary anastomosis to the intrapancreatic part of the biliary duct.

[15]. A comparison of the different hybrid operations for CP is presented in Figure 16E.5.

Frey operation – duodenum-preserving pancreatic head resection

Following the aforementioned Beger operation, several other hybrid operations have been developed. In 1987, Charles Frey presented an operation that combined a duodenum-preserving wide excavation of the pancreatic head with a side-to-side pancreaticojejunostomy (Figure 16E.6) [29]. This operation does not need a dissection of the pancreas at the mesentericoportal axis, which makes it much easier to perform especially in the context of severe portal hypertension when dissection in the plain of the mesentericoportal axis in some cases might not be possible anymore. Longitudinal resection of the tissue covering the pancreatic duct is obligatory in this operation leading to a long laterolateral pancreaticojejunostomy. The wide excavation including the uncinate process is an important step of the operation, and some authors suggest weighing the resected volume of the pancreatic tissue in the pancreatic head to guarantee an adequate resection of the pancreatic head tumor.

Procedure	Beger	Frey	Berne
Duodenum preservation	+	+	+
Pancreatic head resection	+	±	±
Portal vein liberation	+	−	−
Bile duct anastomosis	±	−	±
Pancreatic duct longitudinal decompression	−	+	−
Required technical skills	Difficult	Easy	Easy
Described long-term secondary complications	Secondary biliary stenosis	Recurrence of pancreatic head tumor	Secondary biliary stenosis

Figure 16E.5 Comparison of the various commonly used hybrid techniques. +, always performed; ±, sometimes performed; −, rarely performed.

The Frey operation by some authors is considered a limited resection of the pancreatic head [30] in comparison to the subtotal resection achieved with the Beger procedure. Comparative studies between the Frey and the Beger operations, however, do not show significant differences between those two procedures concerning pain, QOL, as well as postoperative endocrine and exocrine functions (Figure 16E.7). Given the fact that both procedures are equally effective, the Frey operation is much easier to perform and, therefore, is the first procedure of choice in many centers for the surgical treatment of CP without further organ complications.

Berne operation – duodenum-preserving pancreatic head resection

In 2001, Büchler and his group in Berne, Switzerland [31], published a modified hybrid technique that was later named the Berne procedure. This operation is a true hybrid as it combines parts of the Beger operation and the Frey operation. In detail, the more extended pancreatic head excavation of the Frey operation is combined with an anastomosis to the intrapancreatic common bile duct within the cavity of the pancreatic head. The Berne operation does not include a long laterolateral pancreaticojejunostomy. By this procedure, a common cavity of bile and pancreatic juice is generated in the pancreatic head excavation. Similar to the Frey operation, there is no dissection of the pancreas on the mesentericoportal axis. This fact and the limitation of necessary reconstructive work have shown, in an RCT with 32/33 patients in each group and a follow-up of 2 years, that the time of the operation and the length of stay in the hospital were significantly reduced in comparison to the Beger operation with similar functional results [32, 33].

Comparison of hybrid procedures and PPPD/Whipple operation

There is a very good basis for the evaluation of duodenum-preserving operations versus non-duodenum-preserving pancreatic head resection from a variety of randomized clinical trials. Currently, five RCTs address this question [23, 24, 34–36]. A recent meta-analysis by Diener et al. [37], which included the first four RCTs, did not show differences in perioperative morbidity. All RCTs have in common that surgery for CP is associated with excellent perioperative results, and low morbidity and mortality rates. In addition, there was no difference between the duodenum-preserving and non-preserving operations [23, 24, 34–36]. The

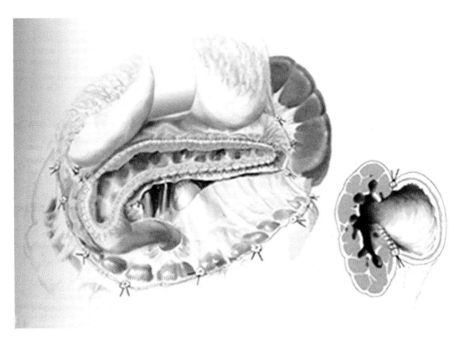

Figure 16E.6 Frey operation. A wide excision of the pancreatic head is combined with a longitudinal drainage procedure. A latero-lateral pancreaticojejunostomy is performed in a Roux-en-Y fashion.

Author/year	Beger vs. Frey	Differences	Follow-up
Izbicki et al. [36]	20 vs. 22	NS	≈ 1.5 yrs
Izbicki et al. [35] f/u	38 vs. 36	NS	≈ 2.5 yrs
Strate et al. [40] f/u	34 vs. 33	NS	≈ 9 yrs
Keck et al. [24, 37]	42 vs. 50	NS	≈ 5 yrs

Figure 16E.7 Comparison between the Frey and the Beger operations as short- and long-term observations. f/u, follow-up of the previous study; NS, no differences in pain, QOL, and endocrine and exocrine functions.

meta-analysis of the first four RCTs [37] and the latest study, not included in this meta-analysis [24], all showed that the time for the operation was shorter in the duodenum-preserving group. In the last study where the Beger and Frey operations were included, this was attributable to the Frey operation [24]. Long-term observation of functional results did not show a significant difference as to endocrine and exocrine functions in those RCTs. Postoperative weight gain, however, was significantly improved in the duodenum-preserving groups when evaluated [34, 36]. The current prospective multicenter RCT ChroPac demonstrates whether these results can be transferred to a wider group of surgeons [41].

References

1 Cahen DL, Gouma DJ, Nio Y, et al. Endoscopic versus surgical drainage of the pancreatic duct in chronic pancreatitis. New England Journal of Medicine 2007;356:676–684. DOI: 10.1056/NEJMoa060610

2 Dite P, Ruzicka M, Zboril V, Novotný I. A prospective, randomized trial comparing endoscopic and surgical therapy for chronic pancreatitis. Endoscopy 2003;35:553–558. DOI: 10.1055/s-2003-40237

3 Ceyhan GO, Bergmann F, Kadihasanoglu M, et al. Pancreatic neuropathy and neuropathic pain--a comprehensive pathomorphological study of 546 cases. Gastroenterology 2009;136:177–186; e1.

4 Demir IE, Tieftrunk E, Maak M, et al. Pain mechanisms in chronic pancreatitis: of a master and his fire. Langenbeck's Archives of Surgery 2011;396:151–160.

5 Beger HG, Buchler M. Duodenum-preserving resection of the head of the pancreas in chronic pancreatitis with inflammatory mass in the head. World Journal of Surgery 1990;14:83–87.

6 Markowitz JS, Rattner DW, Warshaw AL. Failure of symptomatic relief after pancreaticojejunal decompression for chronic pancreatitis. Strategies for salvage. Archives of Surgery 1994;129:374–379; discussion 379–380.

7 Niederau C, Schönberg M. New developments in the pathophysiology of inflammatory pancreatic disease. Hepato-Gastroenterology 1999;46:2722.

8 Wilson TG, Hollands MJ, Little JM. Pancreaticojejunostomy for chronic pancreatitis. Australian and New Zealand Journal of Surgery 1992;62:111–115.

9 Adams DB, Ford MC, Anderson MC. Outcome after lateral pancreaticojejunostomy for chronic pancreatitis. Annals of Surgery 1994;219:481–489.

10 Delcore R, Rodriguez FJ, Thomas JH, et al. The role of pancreatojejunostomy in patients without dilated pancreatic ducts. American Journal of Surgery 1994;168:598–601; discussion 601–602.

11 Schnelldorfer T, Lewin DN, Adams DB. Operative management of chronic pancreatitis: longterm results in 372 patients. Journal of the American College of Surgeons 2007;204:1039–1045; discussion 1045–1047. DOI: 10.1016/j.jamcollsurg.2006.12.045

12 Saeger HD, Schwall G, Trede M. The Whipple partial duodenopancreatectomy: its value in the treatment of chronic pancreatitis. Zentralblatt Für Chirurgie 1995;120:287–291.

13 Büchler MW, Friess H, Müller MW, et al. Randomized trial of duodenum-preserving pancreatic head resection versus pylorus-preserving Whipple in chronic pancreatitis. American Journal of Surgery 1995;169(1):65–69; discussion 69–70.

14 Izbicki JR, Bloechle C, Knoefel WT, et al. Complications of adjacent organs in chronic pancreatitis managed by duodenum-preserving resection of the head of the pancreas. British Journal of Surgery 1994;81:1351–1355.

15 Riediger H, Adam U, Fischer E, et al. Long-term outcome after resection for chronic pancreatitis in 224 patients. Journal of Gastrointestinal Surgery 2007;11:949–959; discussion 959–960.

16 Greenlee HB, Prinz RA, Aranha GV. Long-term results of side-to-side pancreaticojejunostomy. World Journal of Surgery 1990;14:70–76.

17 Beger HG, Schlosser W, Friess HM, Buchler MW. Duodenum-preserving head resection in chronic pancreatitis changes the natural course of the disease: a single-center 26-year experience. Annals of Surgery 1999;230:512–519; discussion 519–523.

18 Strate T, Taherpour Z, Bloechle C, et al. Long-term follow-up of a randomized trial comparing the Beger and Frey procedures for patients suffering from chronic pancreatitis. Annals of Surgery 2005;241:591–598.

19 Keck T, Hopt UT, Erkrankungen des Pankreas. In: Beger et al. (Ed). Operative Gangdrainage bei Chronischer Pankreatitis. Springer, Berlin, Heidelberg 2013: 123.

20 Traverso LW, Longmire WP. Preservation of the pylorus in pancreaticoduodenectomy a follow-up evaluation. Annals of Surgery 1980;192:306–310.

21 Kausch W. Das Carcinom der Papilla Duodeni und seine radikale Entfernung. Beitrage zur Klinische Chirurgie 1912;78:439–486.

22 Whipple AO, Parsons WB, Mullins CR. Treatment of carcinoma of the ampulla of vUater. Annals of Surgery 1935;102:763–779.

23 Izbicki JR, Bloechle C, Broering DC, et al. Extended drainage versus resection in surgery for chronic pancreatitis: a prospective randomized trial comparing the longitudinal pancreaticojejunostomy combined with local pancreatic head excision with the pylorus-preserving pancreatoduodenectomy. Annals of Surgery 1998;228:771–779.

24 Keck T, Adam U, Makowiec F, et al. Short- and long-term results of duodenum preservation versus resection for the management of chronic pancreatitis: a prospective, randomized study. Surgery 2012;152:S95–S102. DOI: 10.1016/j.surg.2012.05.016

25 Waleczek H, Kozuschek W. Pylorus preservation--"a never-ending story". Deutsche Medizinische Wochenschrift (1946) 1994;119:1372–1373.

26 Keck T, Marjanovic G, Fernandez-del Castillo C, et al. The inflammatory pancreatic head mass: significant differences in the anatomic pathology of German and American patients with chronic pancreatitis determine very different surgical strategies. Annals of Surgery 2009;249:105–110.

27 Beger HG, Witte C, Krautzberger W, Bittner R. Experiences with duodenum-sparing pancreas head resection in chronic pancreatitis. Chirurg 1980;51:303–307.

28 Beger HG, Bittner R. Duodenum-preserving pancreas head resection. Chir Z Für Alle Geb Oper Medizen 1987;58:7–13.

29 Frey CF, Smith GJ. Description and rationale of a new operation for chronic pancreatitis. Pancreas 1987;2:701–707.

30 Frey CF, Amikura K. Local resection of the head of the pancreas combined with longitudinal pancreaticojejunostomy in the management of patients with chronic pancreatitis. Annals of Surgery 1994;220:492–507.

31 Gloor B, Friess H, Uhl W, Büchler MW. A modified technique of the Beger and Frey procedure in patients with chronic pancreatitis. Digestive Surgery 2001;18:21–25. DOI: 50092

32 Köninger J, Seiler CM, Sauerland S, et al. Duodenum-preserving pancreatic head resection--a randomized controlled trial comparing the original Beger procedure with the Berne modification (ISRCTN No. 50638764). Surgery 2008;143:490–498. DOI: 10.1016/j.surg.2007.12.002

33 Müller MW, Dahmen RP, Köninger J, et al. The techniques of duodenum preserving head resection of the pancreas in the treatment of chronic pancreatitis. Chirurgia Italiana 2006;58:273–283.

34 Farkas G, Leindler L, Daroczi M, Farkas G. Prospective randomised comparison of organ-preserving pancreatic head resection with pylorus-preserving pancreaticoduodenectomy. Langenbeck's Archives of Surgery 2006;391:338–342.

35 Klempa I, Spatny M, Menzel J, et al. Pancreatic function and quality of life after resection of the head of the pancreas in chronic pancreatitis. A prospective, randomized comparative study after duodenum preserving resection of the head of the pancreas versus Whipple's operation. Chirurg 1995;66:350–359.

36 Müller MW, Friess H, Martin DJ, et al. Long-term follow-up of a randomized clinical trial comparing Beger with pylorus-preserving Whipple procedure for chronic pancreatitis. British Journal of Surgery 2008;95:350–356. DOI: 10.1002/bjs.5960

37 Diener MK, Rahbari NN, Fischer L, et al. Duodenum-preserving pancreatic head resection versus pancreatoduodenectomy for surgical treatment of chronic pancreatitis: a systematic review and meta-analysis. Annals of Surgery 2008;247:950–961.

38 Izbicki JR, Bloechle C, Knoefel WT, et al. Duodenum-preserving resection of the head of the pancreas in chronic pancreatitis. A prospective, randomized trial. Annals of Surgery 1995;221:350–358.

39 Izbicki JR, Bloechle C, Knoefel WT, et al. Drainage versus resection in surgical therapy of chronic pancreatitis of the head of the pancreas: a randomized study. Chirurg 1997;68:369–377.

40 Keck T, Wellner UF, Riediger H, et al. Long-term outcome after 92 duodenum-preserving pancreatic head resections for chronic pancreatitis: comparison of Beger and Frey procedures. Journal of Gastrointestinal Surgery 2010;14:549–556. DOI: 10.1007/s11605-009-1119-9

41 Diener MK, Bruckner T, Contin P, et al. ChroPac-trial: duodenum-preserving pancreatic head resection versus pancreatoduodenectomy for chronic pancreatitis. Trial protocol of a randomised controlled multicentre trial. Trails 2010;11:47.

PART F: The role of pancreatoduodenectomy in the management of chronic pancreatitis

Kristopher P. Croome[1] & Michael B. Farnell[2]

[1] Division of Transplant Surgery, Mayo Clinic Florida, Jacksonville, FL, USA
[2] Department of Surgery, Mayo Clinic Rochester, Rochester, MN, USA

Introduction

Chronic pancreatitis (CP) is a debilitating disease characterized by pain, local mechanical complications such as biliary or duodenal obstruction, and endocrine and exocrine insufficiency that may lead to a poor quality of life (QOL) in many patients. Over the last 30 years, significant developments in the philosophy of management of CP have occurred. This has been driven by improvements in imaging, endoscopic techniques, and the advent of innovative surgical approaches such as the Frey and the Beger procedures, as well as total pancreatectomy and islet autotransplantation. The history of the evolution of surgical approaches to management of CP is covered in detail in Chapter 16A. There now exist a variety of surgical options for managing CP, which begs the question of the precise role of pancreatoduodenectomy (PD) among the surgical alternatives currently available. In this chapter, we endeavor to define both the indications and the selection of candidates for PD in patients with CP.

Although the surgical options available have expanded, the indications for intervention in patients with CP have remained the same; namely, chronic pain, either intermittent or constant, is by far the most common indication. Mechanical complications such as pseudocysts, pancreatic duct leak or obstruction, obstructive jaundice, duodenal or colonic obstruction, hemorrhage, and portal venous obstruction are well recognized and may need surgical or in some cases endoscopic intervention. Lastly, at times, distinguishing an inflammatory mass from a neoplastic head mass may be difficult and head resection may be necessary to exclude malignancy.

Conservative management with analgesic medications is typically the initial treatment. Nonoperative approaches have generally been employed and exhausted by the time surgical consultation is obtained. In patients whose QOL has been significantly compromised by pain or mechanical complications, delaying operative intervention may be counterproductive. Once the patient has developed neuropathic pain and narcotic dependence, even complete removal of the pancreas may not result in pain relief [1]. Moreover, in randomized controlled trials (RCTs), surgical intervention has been shown to be superior to endoscopic treatment [2–4].

Surgical options for management of chronic pancreatitis

The choice of operation for patients with CP should be tailored to both the indication for operation as well as the morphology of the pancreas itself. With regard to morphology, patients can be categorized as having large-duct (7 mm or greater) or small-duct disease. Drainage procedures such as the lateral pancreaticojejunostomy have been shown to be effective in large-duct disease and are particularly suitable when there is not an inflammatory mass in the head of the gland. Drainage procedures are covered in Chapter 16E. Conversely, small-duct disease (6 mm or less) has been best managed with some form of pancreatic resection. Ideally, the operation chosen should match the morphology of the gland and address the indications for operation. If a patient has small-duct disease and a resective procedure is chosen, it should address

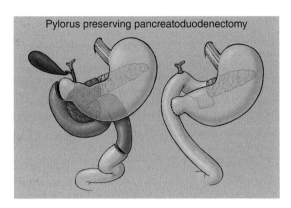

Figure 16F.1 Pylorus-preserving pancreatoduodenectomy. Note the end-to-side mucosa-to-mucosa pancreaticojejunostomy. If the pancreatic duct in the distal pancreatic remnant is very dilated (greater than 7 mm) lateral pancreatoduodenectomy is an alternative.

pain, any mechanical complications, if present, and both exclude and surgically treat malignancy if this is an issue preoperatively. Although improvements in cross-sectional imaging have decreased the frequency with which this question needs to be addressed, the distinction between benign and malignant disease remains a dilemma in 6–8% of patients [5].

The resective procedures include the standard PD (with distal gastrectomy), the pylorus-preserving pancreatoduodenectomy (PPPD) (Figure 16F.1), the duodenum-preserving pancreatic head resection (DPPHR) (Beger procedure) (Figure 16F.2), and the local resection of the pancreatic head with longitudinal pancreaticojejunostomy (LR-LPJ) (Frey procedure) (Figure 16F.3). The latter two procedures are theoretically attractive because they appear to interfere less with postprandial digestive physiologic function (gastric emptying) and the postprandial milieu (preservation of duodenal enteroendocrine cells).

Duodenum-preserving pancreatic head resection (Beger procedure) and local head resection of the pancreatic head and longitudinal pancreaticojejunostomy (Frey procedure)

Extensive literature has focused on the comparison of PD to duodenum-preserving operations such as the

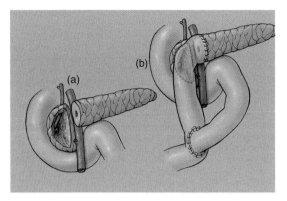

Figure 16F.2 (a) Beger procedure with near complete resection of pancreatic head. Note the preservation of posterior capsule of pancreas and bile duct. If obstructed, the intrapancreatic portion of the common bile duct can be opened in the proximal pancreatic head remnant and included in the proximal side to-side pancreaticojejunostomy. (b) Note two pancreatic anastomoses for reconstruction: end-to-end pancreaticojejunostomy to the distal pancreatic remnant and a-side to-side pancreaticojejunostomy to the proximal pancreatic remnant.

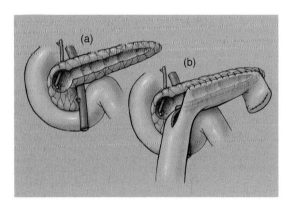

Figure 16F.3 (a) Frey procedure with filleting of the pancreas longitudinally from splenic hilum to medial wall of duodenum. The head of the gland is unroofed or "cored out." Care needs to be taken to protect the common bile duct as it courses posteriorly. (b) Longitudinal pancreaticojejunostomy includes the filleted portion of the pancreatic duct in the neck, body, and tail as well as the excavation cavity in the head of the gland.

Beger [6] and Frey [7] procedures. Multiple RCTs comparing the short-term outcomes of PD with the Beger and Frey procedures have been performed, demonstrating lower morbidity with both when compared with PD. Klempa et al. [8] compared Whipple ($n = 22$) with Beger ($n = 21$) and demonstrated that patients who underwent the Beger procedure experienced a more rapid convalescence of 16.5 versus 21.7 days. Buchler et al. [9] compared PPPD ($n = 20$) with the Beger procedure ($n = 20$) and demonstrated that after duodenum- and pylorus-preserving resections, morbidity was 15% and 20%, respectively. After 6 months, patients who underwent the duodenum-preserving resection had less pain, greater weight gain, better glucose tolerance, and a higher insulin secretion capacity [9]. Izbicki et al. [10] compared PPPD ($n = 32$) with the Frey procedure ($n = 32$) and found that in-hospital complications were 53.3% and 19.4% ($P < 0.05$), respectively. They noted delayed gastric emptying in 9 of 32 patients in the PPPD group. Mechanical complications of adjacent organs were definitively resolved in 100% in the PPPD group and 93.5% in the Frey group. The pain score decreased by 95% after PPPD and 94% after the Frey procedure. Global QOL improved by 43% in the PPPD group and 71% in the Frey group ($P < 0.01$). Farkas et al. [11] compared PPPD ($n = 20$) with an "organ-sparing pancreatic head resection" ($n = 20$) and demonstrated that the mortality rate was zero for each, and the morbidity rates observed were 40% in the former and 0% in the latter ($P < 0.05$). After 1 year, the pain relief was equally effective in both groups.

A meta-analysis including the aforementioned RCTs was performed by Diener et al. [12] comparing PPPD to both the Beger and Frey procedures. No significant difference relative to postoperative pain relief was detected, but concerning the QOL, the Beger and Frey procedures were found to be superior to PPPD. In addition, operating time, duration of hospital stay, and the need for blood replacement were reduced after both Beger and Frey procedures. With regard to weight gain and occupational rehabilitation, the organ-preserving resections were superior as well.

Although short-term follow-up has favored the organ-sparing pancreatic head resections after the techniques of Beger and Frey, long-term outcomes in comparison to PD have been recently reported and are most interesting.

Long-term follow-up of PPPD versus Beger operation for chronic pancreatitis

Muller et al. [13] performed an updated analysis of the 40 patients in the aforementioned RCT by Buchler et al. [5] at a median follow-up of 14 years. When comparing PPPD with Beger, no differences were noted in pain status and exocrine pancreatic function. Loss of appetite was significantly worse in the PPPD group at 14-year follow-up, but there were no other differences in QOL parameters examined. After 14 years, diabetes mellitus was present in 7 of 15 patients who had the Beger procedure and 11 of 14 patients after PPPD resection ($P = 0.128$). Long-term survival was similar, however, two patients in the Beger cohort required reoperation for bile duct stenosis and stricture of the pancreaticojejunostomy.

Long-term follow-up of PPPD versus Frey procedure for chronic pancreatitis

Strate et al. [14] performed an intermediate analysis (median follow-up 7 years) of the previously mentioned study by Izbicki [10] comparing PPPD ($n = 32$) to Frey ($n = 32$) and found that both procedures were equally effective in pain control with no differences in long-term functional or symptom-related QOL scores or endocrine or exocrine parameters of pancreatic function. This study also showed that several patients in the Frey group required reoperations for mechanical complications not relieved by the initial procedure. This suggested that PPPD may be superior in managing biliary and duodenal stenosis. Long-term follow-up of this same cohort was reported with a median follow-up of 15 years by Bachmann et al. [15]. No difference in pain scores were observed between the two groups. QOL was better with regard to physical status after the Frey procedure. A higher long-term mortality was noted after PPPD (53%) than that found after the Frey procedure (30%), resulting in a longer mean survival (14.5 vs. 11.3 years; $P = 0.037$). The authors concluded that both provide good pain relief, but the Frey procedure is superior due to better short-term results, better QOL with long-term follow-up, and survival.

Differences in patient populations

Although a number of randomized trials support superiority of the Beger and Frey procedures relative to PPPD for the surgical management of CP, these data should be placed in perspective. It is noteworthy that all such trials

Table 16F.1 Results of Pancreatoduodenectomy for Chronic Pancreatitis.

Source	No. of patients	Operative mortality (%)	Operative morbidity (%)	Pain relief (%)	Follow-up (years)
Stapleton and Williamson [18]	52	0	46	80	4.5
Martin et al. [19]	54	1.8	30	92	5.2
Rumstadt et al. [20]	134	0.7	18	88	8.3
Traverso and Kozarek [21]	47	0	NA	100	3.5
Sakorafas et al. [17]	105	3.0	32	89	6.6
Jimenez et al. [22]	72	1.4	45	70	3.6
Schnelldorfer et al. [23]	97	1.0	51	34	4.9
Croome et al. [24]	166	1.8	30	7.9 ± 3.5 preoperative[a]	15
				1.6 ± 2.6 postoperative	

NA, not available.

[a]Mean preoperative and postoperative (±SD) pain scores (on scale 1–10) in 54 of 81 surviving patients responding to survey median of 15 years following pancreatoduodenectomy for chronic pancreatitis ($P < 0.001$).

Adapted from Sakorafas et al. [17]. Pancreatoduodenectomy for Chronic Pancreatitis. Long-term Results in 105 Patients. Arch Surg. 2000 May;135:517–524. Used with permission. (Copyright (2000) AMA. All rights reserved.)

have been conducted in Germany. There is reasonable evidence to suggest that the morphology and mechanical complications encountered in the US and German populations are different. In an intercontinental comparison, patients in Germany were found to have a significantly larger head mass when compared with a US cohort (4.5 vs. 2.6 cm, $P < 0.001$) [16]. The different morphology, anatomic complications, and indications for surgery may explain why German surgeons select duodenum pancreatic head resection more frequently than in the United States. Moreover, when the inflammatory mass causes portal hypertension, anatomic pancreatic head resection may be unsafe. In such circumstances, a "coring out" of the pancreatic head such as a Frey procedure or the Berne modification of the Beger procedure may be a safer option. The latter procedure consists of excavation of the pancreatic head without attempting to develop a plane between the neck of the pancreas anteriorly and the pancreas posteriorly.

Mayo Clinic experience with pancreatoduodenectomy for chronic pancreatitis

The Mayo Clinic experience with the Whipple procedure for CP in 105 patients was previously published [17]. In that study, the operation was found to be safe with a morbidity of 32% and a mortality of 3%. Of patients with pain prior to operation, relief was substantial or complete in 89% with a median follow-up of 6.6 years. See Table 16F.1 for selected series of patients undergoing PD for CP.

In preparation for the International Symposium on the Medical and Surgical Treatment of Chronic Pancreatitis held in Kiawah Island, South Carolina, in February 2014, the authors conducted a review of the Mayo Clinic experience with 166 consecutive patients undergoing PD for CP between 1976 and 2013. This study comprised both the 105 patients previously reported and included 61 additional consecutively treated patients. Our goals were to update our experience and to assess our patients with an extended follow-up period. The study was approved by the institutional review board. The data were presented at the International Symposium in February 2014 and have been published [25]. Alcohol was the most common underlying etiology (51%), while the most common clinical manifestation was abdominal pain in 146 patients (88%). Uncertainty or suspicion of malignancy prior to surgery was identified in 48% of patients. A low operative mortality (1.8%) and low rate of pancreatic leak were observed (8%). It should be noted that an operative mortality has not been experienced since 1997.

A survey including the SF-12 questionnaire was administered to all eligible patients. On the SF-12, mean physical component score (PCS) was 43.8 ± 11.8 and mental component score (MCS) was 54.3 ± 7.9. Patients were significantly lower on the PCS ($P < 0.001$) and significantly better on the MCS ($P = 0.001$) than the general US population. Mean pain score out of 10 was significantly lower after surgery (1.6 ± 2.6) than before surgery (7.9 ± 3.5; $P < 0.001$). In our long-term follow-up, we demonstrated a relatively high prevalence of insulin-dependent diabetes mellitus (34%) with new onset of diabetes since the time of surgery in 28% of patients. As previous studies have shown, we found the patients to experience a good QOL regardless of pancreatic insufficiency, underscoring the impact of chronic pain on the patient's QOL [14]. Survey results are shown in Table 16F.2. Of the 81 patients alive and eligible for the survey, 54 subjects (67%) participated. Three patients refused, and 24 patients were unable to be contacted despite multiple attempts. Median follow-up for those that completed the survey was 15 years.

Long-term survival was examined in all patients. We found an inferior survival compared with the age-matched US population in patients undergoing PD for CP (Figure 16F.4). This finding is consistent with previous studies examining the natural history of CP [26]. We speculate that the inferior survival observed is due to both the underlying CP as well as comorbidities inherent in this population. This is underscored by the large proportion of alcoholic pancreatitis observed in our study (51%) and the deaths secondary to causes such as alcoholic cirrhosis seen in the follow-up period. Previous epidemiologic studies in patients with CP have demonstrated frequent alcohol abuse and cigarette smoking with high rates of related deaths due to causes such as cirrhosis of the liver, cardiovascular disease, and malignancies of the mouth, esophagus, and lungs [27]. It should be noted, however, that our Kaplan–Meier survival curves become parallel for the study patients and the matched general US population beyond 10 years of follow-up. Survival beyond 10 years in this cohort suggests survival similar to age-matched controls thereafter (Figure 16F.4).

Preoperative considerations

Cross-sectional imaging is critical in the surgical planning process in patients with CP. Our preference is

Table 16F.2 Long-term results from survey of 54 Mayo Clinic patients undergoing pancreatoduodenectomy for chronic pancreatitis (median follow-up 15 years).

	$N = 54$	P value
SF-12 Score[a]		
Physical (PCS)[b]	43.8 ± 11.8	<0.001[c]
Mental (MCS)[d]	54.3 ± 7.9	<0.001[c]
Pain (scale 1–10)[e]		
Before	7.9 ± 3.5	<0.001[f]
After	1.6 ± 2.6	
Pain medication		
None	35 (65%)	
Non-narcotic	9 (17%)	
Occasional narcotic	3 (6%)	
Regular narcotic use	7 (13%)	
Endocrine insufficiency		
Insulin	17 (31%)	
Oral drugs	2 (4%)	
Diet controlled	2 (4%)	
New diabetes since surgery	15 (28%)	
Pancreatic enzymes	23 (43%)	
Frequent diarrhea	8 (15%)	
Weight		
Increased	21 (39%)	
Decreased	13 (24%)	
Same	20 (37%)	
Resumed drinking		
Never	34 (63%)	
Occasionally	16 (30%)	
Frequently	4 (7%)	
Return to work after surgery		
No	10 (19%)	
Yes	31 (57%)	
Not applicable	13 (24%)	
Working now		
No	34 (63%)	
Retired	22 (41%)	
Too ill	12 (22%)	
Yes	20 (37%)	
Reoperation related to pancreatoduodenectomy[g]	3 (6%)	
Readmission	16 (24%)	

[a]SF-12 – 12-item short-form health survey.
[b]PCS – mean physical component score on SF-12.
[c]Significantly different compared with general population.
[d]MCS – mean mental component score on SF-12.
[e]Pain – mean pain score $\pm$ standard deviation on scale 1–10.
[f]Significantly different preoperatively compared with postoperatively.
[g]One completion pancreatectomy, one bowel obstruction, one incisional hernia.

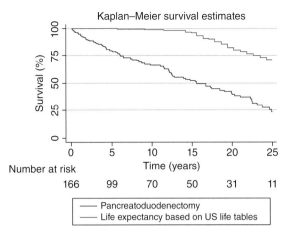

Kaplan–Meier survival estimates

Number at risk

| 166 | 99 | 70 | 50 | 31 | 11 |

—— Pancreatoduodenectomy
—— Life expectancy based on US life tables

Figure 16F.4 Kaplan–Meier survival curves for 166 patients undergoing pancreatoduodenectomy at Mayo Clinic from 1976 to 2013 (blue) and for age-matched control patients with life expectancy based on US life tables (red). Survival was significantly less for patients with chronic pancreatitis.

triple phase, thin-slice helical abdominal computed tomography (CT). This is used to evaluate the morphology of the pancreas, the presence of stones, ductal dilation if present, and importantly to ascertain if the inflammatory process extends beyond the pancreatic parenchyma to involve the surrounding vasculature (see Figure 16F.5). Precise pancreatic and biliary ductal anatomy is also very important. Endoscopic retrograde cholangiopancreatography (ERCP) is the gold standard and our preference (see Figure 16F.6). We acknowledge that well-performed magnetic resonance imaging with magnetic resonance cholangiopancreatography (MRCP) is a useful noninvasive alternative for mapping ductal anatomy. Endoscopic ultrasound (EUS) is used selectively. While EUS allows for fine-needle aspiration or, if possible, core-needle biopsy of the pancreas, if there is suspicion of malignancy, a negative biopsy does not exclude cancer and therefore resection may be indicated. Also, biopsy may be useful when autoimmune pancreatitis is suspected.

Evaluation preoperatively of the peripancreatic vascular anatomy is crucial for the following reasons. First, celiac stenosis, either due to atherosclerotic disease or median arcuate ligament compression, may result in hepatic ischemia if not recognized prior to pancreatic head resection. While celiac stenosis can be seen on sagittal views of the celiac and superior mesenteric arteries, suspicion of celiac artery stenosis should be raised by seeing a plethora of arterial collaterals coursing through the head of the pancreas on arterial phase of the abdominal CT on axial and coronal images. In such patients, if resection is to be undertaken, a plan for dealing with the celiac artery stenosis should be developed prior to operation. Options include preoperative catheter-based angioplasty, intraoperative median arcuate ligament release, celiac artery angioplasty, or bypass. Second, extrahepatic portal hypertension due to either entrapment of the portomesenteric vein by the inflammatory process or portomesenteric thrombosis is a contraindication to Whipple resection in our hands. Pancreatic head resection in this setting may be fraught with massive intraoperative hemorrhage, postoperative hepatic portal venous ischemia, or mesenteric venous congestion.

The extent of the peripancreatic inflammatory process should be evaluated on preoperative imaging as well. If tissue planes around the peripancreatic vasculature are obliterated by inflammation, safe development of dissection planes between the pancreas and surrounding arterial and venous structures may be extremely hazardous and result in hemorrhage or vascular injury. If pancreatic head resection is contemplated in such circumstances, a "coring out" of the head of the pancreas without dissecting out vessels would be advised. Either the Frey procedure or the "Berne modification" of the Beger procedure would be a viable option (see Chapter 16D, Hybrid Procedures).

In addition to alcohol abuse, most patients with painful CP have long-standing narcotic dependence. We do insist that patients be abstinent from alcohol before considering surgery. Because of the severity of the pain experienced by such patients, it is neither practical nor humane to insist on abstinence from narcotics preoperatively. Accordingly, management of pain in the postoperative period is a substantial challenge, and we engage a dedicated pain management service to help not only with pain control but also with a weaning protocol for controlled substance withdrawal.

Pancreatoduodenectomy for chronic pancreatitis in perspective

While this chapter addresses the role of Whipple procedure in patients with CP, a few comments regarding our overall surgical approach to the disease is in order. For

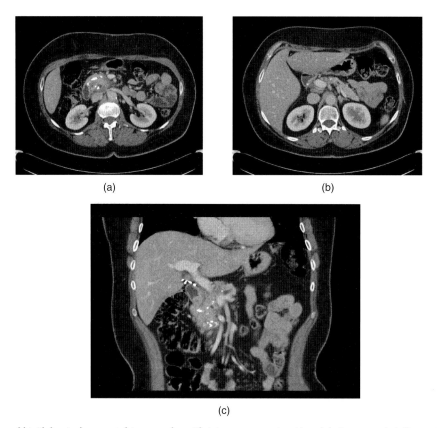

(a)   (b)

(c)

Figure 16F.5 (a and b) Abdominal computed tomography with intravenous contrast in axial views reveals inflammatory pancreatic head mass and macrocalcification. Note the patency of portal vein and preservation of tissue planes between the pancreas and the peripancreatic vessels. (c) Coronal image in same subject with inflammatory head mass, macrocalcification, and moderate pancreatic duct dilation noted in proximal body of the pancreas. The patient underwent pylorus-preserving pancreatoduodenectomy with satisfactory outcome.

patients with large-duct disease (greater than 7 mm), our preference is to perform a Frey procedure. If the patient has large-duct disease and a head mass or too large a stone burden in the head to "core out," our preference is to perform a PPPD with a lateral pancreaticojejunostomy. For head dominant, small-duct disease, our preference is the PPPD. In those patients with chronic obstructive pancreatitis resulting in a disconnected segment of pancreas, we typically perform a distal pancreatectomy. Lastly, total pancreatectomy with islet autotransplantation is recommended for those patients with hereditary pancreatitis and intractable pain. We do not recommend total pancreatectomy in patients with hereditary pancreatitis prophylactically in the absence of intractable pain.

To provide context and to place the role of PD in perspective, in a recent 2-year period (2009–2010), 49 patients underwent operation for CP. A drainage procedure was performed in 13 (27%) and resection in 36 (73%). Of the 36 patients who underwent resection, standard or pylorus-preserving Whipple procedure was performed in 14, which is 39% of the patients undergoing resection for CP and 29% of patients undergoing any type of operation for CP. The remaining 22 patients undergoing resective procedures included 15 distal pancreatectomy, 5 total pancreatectomies, 1 Beger procedure, and 1 central pancreatectomy. The senior author considers the Frey procedure, a drainage procedure, and during the same 2-year period, five such procedures were performed [28].

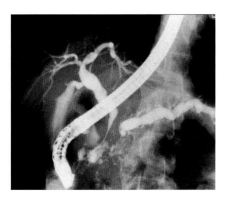

Figure 16F.6 Endoscopic retrograde cholangiopancreatography in a different patient with intractable abdominal pain, weight loss, and impending obstructive jaundice. Double duct sign suspicious for malignancy. Head mass and duodenal stenosis was present. Pylorus-preserving pancreatoduodenectomy was chosen to rule out malignancy and to treat both intractable pain and mechanical complications.

Summary

Pancreatoduodenectomy is a viable option for selected patients in need of a resective procedure for CP. DPPHRs such as the Beger and Frey procedures have been shown to have advantages in the short term, but these advantages are less evident with very long-term (15 year) follow-up. All of the prospective, randomized trials comparing Beger and Frey procedures with PD were conducted in Germany. There is evidence that both the morphology and mechanical complications differ between US and German populations. Candidates for PD include patients with CP with intractable pain, small-duct, head-dominant disease in whom perivascular tissue planes are preserved and portal hypertension is absent. In such patients, biliary or duodenal obstruction, and particularly suspicion of malignancy, should prompt the surgeon to consider PD as the procedure of choice. In experienced hands, the operation can be performed safely and provides good QOL and durable pain relief in more than 80% of patients. Operation does not alter the inexorable development of endocrine and exocrine insufficiency. Long-term survival of patients with CP is less than that of the general population.

References

1 Ceyhan GO, Bergmann F, Kadihasanoglu M, Altintas B, Demir IE, Hinz U, Muller MW, Giese T, Buchler MW, Giese NA, Friess H. Pancreatic neuropathy and neuropathic pain – a comprehensive pathomorphological study of 546 cases. Gastroenterology 2009;136:177–186.

2 Cahen DL, Gouma DL, Nio Y, Rauws EAJ, Boermeester MA, Busch OR, Stoker J, Lameris JS, Dijkgraaf MGW, Huibregtse K, Bruno MJ. Endoscopic versus surgical drainage of the pancreatic duct in chronic pancreatitis. New England Journal of Medicine 2007;356:676–684.

3 Cahen DL, Gouma DJ, Laramee P, Nio Y, Rauws EAJ, Boermeester MA, Busch OR, Fockens P, Kuipers EJ, Pereira SP, Wonderling D, Dijkgraaf MGW, Bruno MJ. Long-term outcomes of endoscopic vs surgical drainage of the pancreatic duct in patients with chronic pancreatitis. Gastroenterology 2011;141:1690–1695.

4 Dite P, Ruzicka M, Zboril V, Novotny I. A prospective, randomized trial comparing endoscopic and surgical therapy for chronic pancreatitis. Endoscopy 2003;35:553–558.

5 Buchler MW, Warshaw AL. Resection versus drainage in treatment of chronic pancreatitis. Gastroenterology 2008;134(5):1605–1607.

6 Beger HG, Witte C, Krautzberger W, Bittner R. Experiences with duodenal-sparing pancreas head resection in chronic pancreatitis. Chirurgie 1980; 51(5):303–307.

7 Frey CF, Smith GJ. Description and rationale of a new operation for chronic pancreatitis. Pancreas 1987;2(6):701–707.

8 Klempa I, Spatny M, Menzel J, Baca I, Nustede R, Stockmann F, Arnold W. Pancreatic function and quality of life after resection of the head of the pancreas in chronic pancreatitis. A prospective, randomized comparative study after duodenum preserving resection of the head of the pancreas versus Whipple's operation. Chirurgie 1995;66(4):350–359.

9 Buchler MW, Friess H, Muller MW, Wheatley AM, Beger HG. Randomized trial of duodenum-preserving pancreatic head resection versus pylorus-preserving Whipple in chronic pancreatitis. American Journal of Surgery 1995;169(1):65–69; discussion 69–70.

10 Izbicki JR, Bloechle C, Broering DC, Knoefel WT, Kuechler T, Broelsch CE. Extended drainage versus resection in surgery for chronic pancreatitis: a prospective randomized trial comparing the longitudinal pancreaticojejunostomy combined with local pancreatic head excision with the pylorus-preserving pancreatoduodenectomy. Annals of Surgery 1998;228(6):771–779.

11 Farkas G, Leindler L, Daroczi M, Farkas G Jr., Prospective randomized comparison of organ-preserving pancreatic head resection with pylorus-preserving pancreaticoduodenectomy. Langenbecks Archives of Surgery 2006;391:338–342.

12 Diener MK, Rahbari NN, Fischer L, Antes G, Buchler MW, Seiler CM. Duodenum-preserving pancreatic head resection versus pancreatoduodenectomy for surgical treatment of chronic pancreatitis: a systematic review and meta-analysis. Annals of Surgery 2008;247:950–961.

13 Muller MW, Friess H, Martin DJ, Hinz U, Dahmen R, Buchler MW. Long-term follow-up of a randomized clinical trial comparing Beger with pylorus-preserving Whipple procedure for chronic pancreatitis. British Journal of Surgery 2008;95(3):350–356.

14 Strate T, Bachmann K, Busch P, Mann O, Schneider C, Bruhn JP, Yekebas E, Kuechler T, Bloechle C, Izbicki JR. Resection vs drainage in treatment of chronic pancreatitis: long-term results of a randomized trial. Gastroenterology 2008;134(5):1406–1411.

15 Bachmann K, Tomkoetter L, Kutup A, Erbes J, Vashist Y, Mann O, Bockhorn M, Izbicki JR. Is the Whipple procedure harmful for long-term outcome in treatment of chronic pancreatitis? 15-years follow-up comparing the outcome after pylorus-preserving pancreatoduodenectomy and Frey procedure in chronic pancreatitis. Annals of Surgery 2013;258(5):815–821.

16 Keck T, Marjanovic G, Fernandez-del Castillo C, Makowiec F, Schafer AO, Rodriguez JR, Razo O, Hopt UT, Warshaw AL. Significant differences in the anatomic pathology of German and American Patients with chronic pancreatitis determine very different surgical strategies. Annals of Surgery 2009;249(1):105–110.

17 Sakorafas GH, Farnell MB, Nagorney DM, Sarr MG, Rowland CM. Pancreatoduodenectomy for chronic pancreatitis. Archives of Surgery 2000;135:517–524.

18 Stapleton GN, Williamson RCN. Proximal pancreatoduodenectomy for chronic pancreatitis. British Journal of Surgery 1996;83:1433–1440.

19 Martin RF, Rossi RL, Leslie KA. Long-term results of pylorus-preserving pancreatoduodenectomy for chronic pancreatitis. Archives of Surgery 1996;131:247–252.

20 Rumstadt B, Forssmann K, Singer MV, Trede M. The Whipple partial duodenopancreatectomy for the treatment of chronic pancreatitis. Hepatogastroenterology 1997;44:1554–1559.

21 Traverso LW, Kozarek RA. Pancreatoduodenectomy for chronic pancreatitis: anatomic selection criteria and subsequent long-term outcome analysis. Annals of Surgery 1997;226:429–438.

22 Jimenez RE, Fernandez-del Castillo C, Rattner DW, Chang Y, Warsaw AL. Outcome of pancreaticoduodenectomy with pylorus preservation or with antrectomy in the treatment of chronic pancreatitis. Annals of Surgery 2000;231:293–300.

23 Schnelldorfer T, Lewin DN, Adams DB. Operative management of chronic pancreatitis: long-term results in 372 patients. Journal of the American College of Surgeons 2007;204(5):1039–1047.

24 Croome KP, Farnell MB. Who needs a Whipple procedure for chronic pancreatitis? Presented at: The International Symposium on the Medical and Surgical Treatment of Chronic Pancreatitis. 2014 February 6–8; Kiawah Island, South Carolina.

25 Croome KP, et al. Pancreatoduodenectomy for chronic pancreatitis: results of a pain relief and quality of life survey 15 years following operation. Journal of Gastrointestinal Surgery 2015;19:2146–2153.

26 Sakorafas GH, Farnell MB, Nagorney DM, Sarr MG. Surgical management of chronic pancreatitis at the Mayo Clinic. Surgical Clinics of North America 2001;81(2):457–465. Review.

27 Cavallini G, Frulloni L, Pederzoli P, Talamini G, Bovo P, Bassi C, De Francesco V, Vaona B, Falconi M, Sartori N, Angelini G, Brunori MP, Filippini M. Long-term follow-up of patients with chronic pancreatitis in Italy. Scand Journal Gastroenterology 1998;33(8):880–889.

28 Farnell MB, Levendale A. Chronic pancreatitis surgery. Commentary. In: Mantke R, Lippert H, Buchler MW, Sarr MG (Eds). International Practices in Pancreatic Surgery. Springer-Verlag. Heidelberg. 2013. 105–115.

CHAPTER 17

PART A: Total pancreatectomy and islet cell autotransplantation: patient selection

Sydne Muratore, Martin Freeman & Greg Beilman

Department of Surgery & Medicine, University of Minnesota, Minneapolis, MN, USA

Introduction

Worldwide, over 1000 total pancreatectomy islet auto-transplants (TPIATs) have been reported in the literature to date since its inception in 1977 at the University of Minnesota [1]. Selecting total pancreatic extirpation as the treatment for chronic pancreatitis (CP) or relapsing acute pancreatitis (RAP) is complicated given the potential lifelong risks of insulin and pancreatic enzyme dependence. This must be carefully weighed against the potential therapeutic benefits of pain relief and mitigation of diabetic side effects by islet autotransplant.

Correct diagnosis

Despite the presence of abdominal pain in the majority of CP/RAP patients, there is no pathognomonic pattern or rate of progression to guide the clinician's approach to diagnosis and management [2]. Commonly associated symptoms include nausea, vomiting, food intolerance, and diarrhea. Due to this, thorough evaluation to rule out other causes of abdominal pain must be undertaken. This can include an exhaustive list of imaging and testing, depending on the patient and clinical scenario. Cessation of alcohol and tobacco use, evaluation for constipation or gastroparesis, treatment of peptic ulcers, evaluation for biliary obstruction or dyskinesia, and evaluation for pancreatic lesions (benign or malignant) are common considerations.

In order to guide clinicians in making the correct diagnosis, the only published criteria for TPIAT come from the University of Minnesota [3, 4] and was recently adapted and included in the summary of the National Institute of Diabetes and Digestive and Kidney Diseases 2014 Workshop [5] (see Table 17A.1). This includes radiographic evaluation to detect morphologic changes within the pancreas using computed tomography (CT), magnetic resonance imaging (MRI), ultrasound, magnetic resonance cholangiopancreatography (MRCP), endoscopic retrograde cholangiopancreatography (ERCP), and/or endoscopic ultrasound using Rosemount classification: hyperechoic parenchymal foci, hypoechoic lobules, cysts, main duct contour irregularity, ductal dilation, strands, hyperechoic duct walls, side branch dilation, stones, and calcifications [6]. Utilization of pancreatic function testing with secretin stimulation may also help identify exocrine insufficiency. Particularly in young patients, or those with a family history of pancreatitis, genetic counseling and testing should also be considered early, as those patients may be appropriate to intervene with TPIAT at an earlier stage given some evidence of improved pain response in patients with genetic mutations and the increased risk of malignancy with advancing years [7]. PRSS1 is the most common genetic mutation followed by SPINK1 and CFTR. Additional gene variations continue to be identified as conferring increased risk of developing CP [7].

Pancreatitis: Medical and Surgical Management, First Edition.
David B. Adams, Peter B. Cotton, Nicholas J. Zyromski and John Windsor.
© 2017 John Wiley & Sons, Ltd. Published 2017 by John Wiley & Sons, Ltd.

Table 17A.1 TPIAT University of Minnesota criteria [4].

DEFINITIONS

(must have one of the following: A, B, or C)

A) Chronic Pancreatitis: *(must have one of 1, 2, or 3)* Patients with chronic abdominal pain, lasting >6 months, features consistent with that of pancreatitis, and evidence of CP as evidenced by at least one of the following:

1) Morphologic/functional evidence of CP [CT of abdomen with evidence of CP (calcifications), or ERCP evidence of pancreatitis]

2) EUS of ≥6/9 criteria positive of CP

3) At least two of the following three findings:
   – Secretin MRCP or ERCP, with findings suggestive of CP (abnormal duct/side branch) or MRI T2 evidence of fibrosis
   – EUS with ≥4/9 criteria positive for pancreatitis
   – Abnormal exocrine pancreatic function tests (peak bicarbonate <80)

B) Relapsing Acute Pancreatitis: *(must have both)*
   • Three or more episodes of documented AP with ongoing episodes over >6 months.
   • No evidence of current gallstone disease or other correctable etiology such as autoimmune pancreatitis

C) Documented hereditary pancreatitis with compatible clinical history.

INDICATIONS

(must have each of the following: 1–5)

Documented CP or relapsing AP with chronic or severe abdominal pain, directly resulting in at least one of the following:

1) Chronic narcotic dependence (patient requires narcotics on a daily or nearly daily basis for >3 months)

2) Impaired quality of life, defined by at least one of the following:
   • Loss of job
   • Inability or significantly reduced ability to work or attend school
   • Frequent absences from school
   • Frequent hospitalizations
   • Loss of ability to participate in usual age-appropriate activities

3) Complete evaluation, with no reversible cause of CP or relapsing AP present or untreated

4) Unresponsive to maximal medical therapy and endoscopic therapy, with ongoing abdominal pain requiring routine narcotics for CP or relapsing AP

5) Adequate islet cell function (nondiabetic or noninsulin-requiring diabetes with C-peptide positive)

AP, acute pancreatitis; CP, chronic pancreatitis; CT, computed tomography; ERCP, endoscopic retrograde cholangiopancreatography; MRCP, magnetic resonance cholangiopancreatography; MRI, magnetic resonance imaging; EUS, endoscopic ultrasonography.
To be considered for TPIAT, patients must meet criteria mentioned in sections I and II and have no contraindications.

Failure of medical and surgical therapy

To ensure that the patient does not have a reversible cause of CP or RAP, exhaustion of medical and endoscopic therapies should be completed. That being said, careful consideration must be taken for balancing the risk of islet mass burnout with protracted exposure to the inflammation, fibrosis, and atrophy of CP. In addition, the clinician should take into account the potential years of lost time at work or school, and increasing risk of narcotic bowel syndrome and opioid-induced hyperalgesia associated with chronic narcotics and pain [8]. In order to optimize the balance

of these challenges, evaluation for TPIAT should be done within a multidisciplinary team who will direct pre-, peri-, and postoperative care to ensure comprehensive assessment and close adherence to follow-up care.

Attenuation of pancreatitis pain should first be approached with non-narcotic analgesics if possible. Though with refractory pain, many progress to requiring narcotics and adjuncts such as tricyclic antidepressants, selective and nonselective serotonin reuptake inhibitors, and alpha 2-delta inhibitors. Pancreatic enzymes can be used to help with symptoms associated with pancreatic insufficiency as well as an attempt at pain mitigation. Radiographic or endoscopically guided celiac ganglion blocks or neurolysis with alcohol injections offer pain relief for a small number of patients, though often only transiently [2]. ERCP with sphincterotomy, gallstone removal, stent placement, or balloon dilatation may be undertaken as appropriate. Patients should be evaluated for potential cholecystectomy. Some patients are candidates for partial resection such as a distal pancreatectomy in the setting of a disrupted duct or tail-only disease. Surgical drainage procedures (Puestow, Beger, Frey, etc.) can sometimes be utilized for main pancreatic duct dilation. This should be considered with caution, however, given the growing evidence that prior pancreatic procedures significantly decrease islet yield, which can in turn affect long-term metabolic outcomes if a patient has progressive disease or is unresponsive to this treatment and later requires TPIAT [9–12].

Disability

In a paper examining published quality-of-life evaluations for CP, the authors found that, of possible factors related to this condition, pain was the only factor able to impair all eight domains evaluated by the questionnaires [13]. Patients with impairment in ability to function in normal life activities should have increasing consideration for more definitive treatment, such as TPIAT, as appropriate. Longer duration of pain is generally associated with higher patient disability, with exceptions. These disabilities include inability to work, go to school, or perform normal daily activities. This is often coupled with repeated hospitalization and countless emergency department and office visits. Presence of pain greater than 6 months with a constant narcotic requirement has been suggested as a requirement for consideration in institutional criteria for TPIAT [3, 4].

Preoperative evaluation

Preoperative assessment to determine appropriateness to undergo major abdominal surgery and postoperative treatment regimens should occur early. Malnutrition may be amenable to improvement prior to surgery with enteral or parenteral nutrition. The patient should be assessed for the presence of diabetes with a fasting glucose and hemoglobin A_{1c}, using diabetes diagnosis criteria set forth by the American Diabetes Association

(fasting glucose ≥ 126 mg/dL or $HbA_{1c} \geq 6.5\%$) [9, 14]. Although C-peptide-positive diabetes is not a contraindication to surgery, patients have a higher chance of postoperative insulin independence if not already diabetic [15]. Islet function is assessed with stimulatory testing. Evaluation can be done with orally administered glucose or mixed meal test, or intravenously dosed glucose or arginine; the latter being the most informative study, particularly in patients with impaired fasting glucose [5]. Assessment of liver health and patency of portal vein is also necessary. Portal hypertension or thrombosis, cirrhosis, or advanced liver disease is a relative contraindication to major pancreatic surgery, and consideration must be given to the increased risk of portal vein thrombosis associated with embolization of islets to the liver. Finally, the clinician should ensure appropriate immunization status prior to surgery if concurrent splenectomy is planned or likely.

Contraindications

Patients who are determined to be medically unsuitable for a major abdominal operation should not undergo TPIAT. This includes conditions such as end-stage pulmonary disease, cirrhosis, or severe atherosclerotic heart disease. Given the complexity of postoperative management, patients with poorly controlled psychiatric conditions or those unable to comply with postoperative treatment regimens are poor candidates for this treatment, and alternate therapies should be sought or resources provided to mitigate these factors prior to consideration for surgery. TPIAT is contraindicated in patients who are unable to comply with pain medication tapers, adherence to diabetes care, close follow-up, and pancreatic enzyme treatment. Other contraindications within the United States include active alcoholism, current illegal drug use, pancreatic cancer, and intraductal papillary mucinous neoplasm. TPIAT has been performed in the setting of the latter two conditions outside of the United States, however, that remains a contraindication here due to the risk of dissemination of malignancy with islet autotransfusion. Finally, patients with C-peptide-negative diabetes or type 1 diabetes are currently not thought to benefit from islet autotransfusion given the lack of functioning islets; therefore, TPIAT is not recommended for this subset of patients at this time [9].

References

1 Muratore S, Freeman M, Beilman G. Total pancreatectomy and islet auto transplantation for chronic pancreatitis. In: Pancreapedia. http://www.pancreapedia.org/reviews/total-pancreatectomy-and-islet-auto-transplantation-for-chronic-pancreatitis. Accessed February 20, 2015.

2 Chauhan S, Forsmark CE. Pain management in chronic pancreatitis: a treatment algorithm. Best Practice & Research Clinical Gastroenterology. 2010; 24(3):323–335.

3 Bellin MD, Freeman ML, Schwarzenberg SJ, et al. Quality of life improves for pediatric patients after total pancreatectomy and islet autotransplant for chronic pancreatitis. Clinical Gastroenterology and Hepatology. 2011;9(9):793–799.

4 Dudeja V, Beilman GJ, Vickers SM. Total pancreatectomy with islet autotransplantation in patients with malignancy: are we there yet? Annals of Surgery. 2013;258(2):219–220.

5 Bellin MD, Gelrud A, Arreaza-Rubin G, et al. Total pancreatectomy with islet autotransplantation: summary of an NIDDK workshop. Annals of Surgery. 2015; 261(1):21–29.

6 Catalano MF, Sahai A, Levy M, et al. EUS-based criteria for the diagnosis of chronic pancreatitis: the rosemont classification. Gastrointestinal Endoscopy 2009;69(7):1251–1261.

7 Chinnakotla S, Radosevich DM, Dunn TB, et al. Long-term outcomes of total pancreatectomy and islet auto transplantation for hereditary/genetic pancreatitis. Journal of the American College of Surgeons 2014; 218: 530–543

8 Muratore S, Beilman G. Total pancreatectomy should be offered early in the course of chronic pancreatitis. *AGA Perspectives Online.* http://www.gastro.org/journals-publications/aga-perspectives/octobernovember2014/total-pancreatectomy-should-be-offered-early-in-the-course-of-chronic-pancreatitis. Nov 14, 2014. Accessed March 2, 2015.

9 Bellin MD, Freeman ML, Gelrud A, et al. Total pancreatectomy and islet autotransplantation in chronic pancreatitis: recommendations from PancreasFest. Pancreatology. 2014; 14(1):27–35.

10 Lundberg R, Beilman GJ, Dunn TB, et al. Metabolic assessment prior to total pancreatectomy and islet autotransplant: utility, limitations and potential. American Journal of Transplantation. 2013; 13(10):2664–2671.

11 Sutherland DE, Radosevich DM, Bellin MD, et al. Total pancreatectomy and islet autotransplantation for chronic pancreatitis. Journal of the American College of Surgeons. 2012;214(4):409–424

12 Wang H, Desai KD, Dong H, et al. Prior surgery determines islet yield and insulin requirement in patients with chronic pancreatitis. Clin Gastroenterol Hepatol. 2011 Sep;9(9):793–9. Transplantation. 2013;95(8):1051–1057.

13 Pezzilli R, Bini L, Fantini L, et al. Quality of life in chronic pancreatitis. World Journal of Gastroenterology. 2006; 12(39):6249–6251.

14 American Diabetes Association. Diagnosis and classification of diabetes mellitus. Diabetes Care 2015;38(Suppl 1):S8–S16.

15 Bellin MD, Beilman GJ, Dunn T, et al. Islet autotransplantation to preserve beta cell mass in selected patients with chronic pancreatitis and diabetes mellitus undergoing total pancreatectomy. Pancreas. 2013;42(2):317–321.

PART B: Total pancreatectomy and islet cell autotransplantation: the science of islet cell preservation, from pancreas to liver

Appakalai N. Balamurugan[1,2] & Melena D. Bellin[3]

[1] Clinical Islet Cell Laboratory, Cardiovascular Innovation Institute, Department of Surgery, University of Louisville, Louisville, KY, USA
[2] Islet Transplantation Program, University of Louisville, Louisville, KY, USA
[3] Schulze Diabetes Institute, University of Minnesota, Minneapolis, MN, USA

Introduction

Carefully selected candidates with chronic pancreatitis (CP) may undergo total pancreatectomy and islet autotransplantation (TPIAT) for definitive disease management at a center experienced with the surgical procedure and with an onsite or a collaborative remote islet-processing facility. The pancreatic resection procedure involves complete resection of the pancreas, partial duodenectomy, restoration of gastrointestinal luminal, and biliary system continuity (usually with Roux-en-Y or duodenoduodenostomy, and choledochojejunostomy or choledochoduodenostomy), with or without splenectomy [1]. Islets, which make up only 2% of the pancreatic mass, are separated from the exocrine portions of the pancreas using enzymatic and mechanical digestion performed in a good manufacturing practices cell-manufacturing facility, and are subsequently returned back to the patient, most commonly by infusion into a tributary of the portal vein [2] (Figure 17B.1); intrahepatic islet engraftment is gradual over the following months. The first successful islet autotransplantation (IAT) procedure was reported in 1977, in a recipient who achieved insulin independence [3].

The technical procedure of intraportal IAT is similar to that performed for patients with labile type 1 diabetes who receive allogenic islet transplants from cadaveric donors. However, unlike a conventional transplant, patients receiving autologous islet infusions after total pancreatectomy are not at risk for rejection of their islet graft, and thus do not need require immunosuppressive therapy; probably for this reason, autologous islet grafts have better function relative to the number of islets transplanted [4, 5]. However, similar to allogenic islet transplants, autologous islet grafts are susceptible to damage from innate inflammation triggered by intraportal infusion, activation of beta-cell apoptotic pathways, and hyperglycemic stress during islet engraftment in the liver [6–11]. Thus, the technical challenge of IAT lies in facilitating as successful as possible the recovery of healthy islets from the native pancreas and transfer into the new "home" of the liver. The first step is to successfully isolate islets from the pancreas; the second step is to optimize conditions for engraftment and function after transplantation into the liver. We discuss both of these critical steps in the subsequent sections.

Islet isolation techniques for maximizing islet yield

Despite many advances in the technical aspects of human islet isolation, it still remains a challenging procedure. The single most critical factor predicting insulin independence after transplantation is the islet cell mass acquired from the isolation procedure [12]. We have successfully optimized the islet isolation process, especially the pancreas digestion phase, to yield a higher islet mass in those pancreases affected by CP [13]. In contrast to islet allografts, autografts are routinely conducted in the absence of factors affecting cadaveric donors. The islet isolation process involves specialized techniques for obtaining a maximum number of islets,

Pancreatitis: Medical and Surgical Management, First Edition.
David B. Adams, Peter B. Cotton, Nicholas J. Zyromski and John Windsor.
© 2017 John Wiley & Sons, Ltd. Published 2017 by John Wiley & Sons, Ltd.

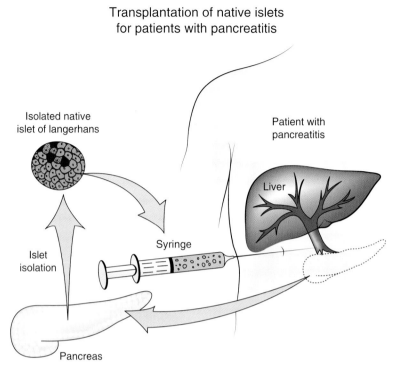

Transplantation of native islets for patients with pancreatitis

Figure 17B.1 Illustration of the procedure of total pancreatectomy and intraportal islet infusion. Following the complete resection of the pancreas, the islets are isolated and gently infused back into the portal vein of the patient. Blondet 2007 [1]. Reproduced with permission of Elsevier.

in particular taking into account some of the specific features in the CP pancreas, such as fibrosis.

The islet isolation procedure is divided into the following essential steps: ductal cannulation, enzyme distention, tissue digestion, tissue recombination, islet purification, islet viability assessment, and final transplant preparation [14]. There are points in each step designed to be adaptable to the different situations that may arise with the wide variety of CP pancreases. Adequate laboratory preparation prior to the isolation procedure is important so that the team is ready to begin as soon as the pancreas arrives to the clean-room facility.

Pancreas transport and pancreas trimming

After pancreatectomy, the pancreas is immersed immediately in a cold organ preservation solution. The pancreas is then packed in cold conditions according to the hospital's protocol and transported to the islet isolation facility. The pancreas is transported for a short distance so that the two-layer pancreas preservation method, hypothermic machine perfusion, hypothermic persufflation, and/or gaseous oxygen perfusion methods are not required [15]. It is critical that the pancreas be kept cold from the time of organ removal to the initiation of enzymatic digestion [16]. Once the pancreas arrives at the facility, the organ is unpacked inside a biosafety cabinet using sterile techniques. Before touching the pancreas, a sample of the transport solution is taken and sent to the microbiology lab to determine the presence of any contamination prior to the isolation process.

After visual inspection, the pancreas is then placed into a sterile pan and the dissection step begins. Excess fat and connective tissue are removed aseptically. The pancreatic capsule should be intact to reduce the likelihood of enzyme leakage during ductal perfusion. The pancreas is submerged in antibiotic solution or povidone iodine that has been checked against potential patient allergies before treating the pancreas. The gross morphology of every pancreas is different and we assess each as mild, moderate, or severe to determine enzyme dose and digestion conditions [14].

Pancreas cannulation

The pancreas typically arrives as a whole, intact organ. However, in some cases, due to surgical complications an organ may arrive as a partial organ or a whole organ in multiple pieces. When the organ is intact, there has been more success in distention when the head and the body–tail portions are cannulated individually. Severely fibrotic organs may require a metal or Christmas catheter, while less fibrotic organs typically require catheters in the range of 14–24 G [14] (Figure 17B.2).

Pancreas distention with collagenase enzymes

Enzymatic tissue dissociation has been used to separate the exocrine and endocrine components of the pancreas and the best tissue dissociation resulting after the ductal perfusion of a blend of collagenase (Col) and neutral protease (NP) enzymes into the main pancreatic duct. This can be done by either hand syringe injection or using a semi-automated system with a peristaltic pump connected to the main pancreatic duct of a whole or segmented (head and body/tail sections) pancreas. The infused enzyme blends digest the extracelluar matrix of pancreas and release islets and exocrine cells.

The pancreas distention with enzyme is the critical step in islet isolation. Any problems that arise during the distention phase must be addressed immediately and resolved effectively to ensure proper enzyme distribution throughout the pancreas. Leaks may be solved using hemostats and ductal occlusions may be bypassed with catheters of a higher gauge.

In some pancreases, the tissue is so fibrotic that ductal enzyme perfusion is insufficient at distributing the enzyme solution throughout the whole organ. When this is the case, interstitial perfusion can be employed to inject enzyme into the rest of the pancreas. Interstitial perfusion is performed by continuously injecting the

enzyme solution manually with a needle and syringe throughout the pancreas. In addition, if the pancreas is distended as a whole organ, partial distention may occur. This is due to ductal inflammation or calcification deposits that obstruct the flow of the enzyme to the rest of the pancreas. In these cases, it is acceptable to make a complete transverse cut before the distal section after the proximal end has finished distending, and recannulate the distal end to attempt further distention in this area.

We have continuously improved the islet yield using new enzymes and combinations in different quantities [13, 17]. The enzyme dose delivered to the pancreas should be based on the degree of fibrosis of the pancreas. The standard dose of 18–26 W U of Col (Collagenase HA, VitaCyte LLC, Indianapolis, IN), and 0.75–1.75 DMC U of NP (SERVA Electrophoresis GmbH, Heidelberg, Germany) per gram pancreas is delivered to minimally diseased pancreases by diluting the enzyme in 350 mL of Hanks Balanced Salt Solution with 10 U/mL heparin. This standard dose can be, and is often, modified by increasing the amount of enzyme for more fibrotic, and younger donor pancreases.

During enzyme distention, infusion pressure (60–180 mmHg), enzyme flow rate (>30 mL/min), enzyme temperature (6–16 °C), and time (~12 minutes) are carefully monitored. Initially, the enzyme solution is perfused at a minimal flow rate. The flow rate is gradually increased throughout the distention period. Enzyme flow is important than distention pressure for CP pancreas.

Because distention is the most important step, all efforts should be employed to distribute enzyme throughout the entire pancreas so as to maximize digestion efficiency. Once the pancreas has been distended, a quick, final trimming is performed to remove any excess surface fat and connective tissue that may interfere with the digestion phase. The pancreas is then cut into small pieces of 2–5 cm in diameter and placed in the Ricordi chamber along with any enzyme solution remaining after the distention phase [14].

Pancreas digestion using semi-automated method

The digestion phase begins immediately after the post-distention trimming and utilizes a semi-automated

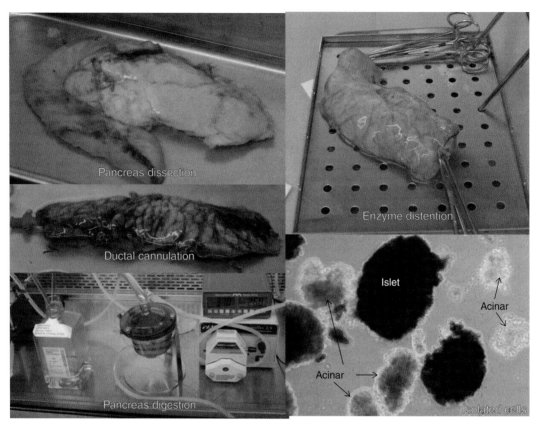

Figure 17B.2 Islet isolation process: pancreas dissection, ductal cannulation, collagenase enzyme distention, digestion setup, and isolated islets.

method of tissue dissociation. The digestion system consists of a specialized Ricordi chamber [18] with a wire mesh screen and marbles to add a mechanical aspect of digestion, a closed circuit consisting of silicon tubing and clamps, a sample port for monitoring the digestion progress, and a peristaltic pump for circulating the solution throughout the system. A heating coil is attached to the tubing and placed in a water bath to maintain the desired temperature range.

After the pancreas is transferred to the Ricordi chamber, a known volume of solution is added to the circuit and the pump begins circulating the fluid through the heating coil. The heating coil is suspended in a water bath that has been heated to 40–42 °C prior to receipt of the pancreas. The initial flow rate of the solution is 200 mL/min as the solution is heated to 34–35 °C over the first several minutes. Once the solution reaches the desired temperature, the flow is reduced to 100 mL/min

and the chamber is shaken vigorously. After about 8 minutes, samples of 1–2 mL are taken and stained with dithizone then observed under a microscope to monitor the extent of dissociation. Phase-1 of digestion is considered complete when successive samples contain large quantities of free islets.

As phase-2 begins, the flow rate is increased to 200 mL/min and the temperature inside the chamber is reduced. The circuit is opened at one end by manipulating clamps on the tubing, and tissue is collected into collection (Erlenmeyer) flasks that have been prefilled with cold collection media (RPMI 1640 + 2.5% HSA). RPMI 1640 is added as a dilution media to replace dispensed volume. As the tissue is collected in the flasks, any remaining enzyme is deactivated by the drop in temperature and the presence of serum albumin to protect against any further damage to the islets.

Samples should continue to be collected at 5, 10, and 20 minutes postswitch to assess the efficiency of the dissociation. Once samples beyond 20 minutes do not contain islets, the end of phase-2 begins, and air is introduced to the system. The remaining digest slurry is emptied, and the amount of undigested tissue is assessed.

The extent of chemical and mechanical agitation can be controlled by islet technicians by manipulating temperature and the level of mechanical agitation. By increasing the temperature in the system, the activity of the enzyme is increased and a more chemical dissociation is achieved. A more chemical dissociation is favorable when samples reveal large chunks of acinar tissue containing islets embedded within. If dissociation is slow to begin during phase-1, additional enzyme may be added directly to the digest circuit. It is imperative to minimize the amount of undigested tissue left in the chamber. Therefore, it is essential that islet isolation technicians understand how manipulating digestion parameters may affect the quality and rate of tissue dissociation [14].

Tissue recombination

The recombination phase begins as soon as the first collection flask is filled with tissue and serves to collect and combine the digested product into a single tissue pellet. The slurry in each collection flask is divided into four 250 mL conicals and centrifuged at $140 \times g$ to obtain small pellets. The supernatant is poured off and the tissue pellets are transferred to a single recombination flask filled with Cold Storage/Purification Stock solution (Mediatech, Inc.) with 2% Penta Starch and 10 U/mL of heparin.

After all digested slurry has been transferred into the single recombination flask, it is once again divided into four 250 mL conicals and centrifuged once more. The four conicals are then combined into a single conical for final tissue characterization. Two samples are taken from the final conical and stained with dithizone for a postdigest count. Both quality and quantity are noted, along with apparent purity and proportion of embedded islets. As the samples are being evaluated, the final tissue suspension should be washed with media and centrifuged to remove any dead cells. Heavily diseased CP pancreases may have calcification present in the pellet after several

centrifugations. These calcifications should be removed by aspiration. After the final wash, the tissue volume is estimated [14].

Tissue purification

Whether purification should be performed or not depends on several factors. If a small tissue volume (<15 mL) is obtained from the digestion phase, purification is generally not necessary as smaller volumes can be safely infused into the portal infusion site. A tissue volume of 20 mL or greater is generally always purified to reduce tissue volume and prevent potential portal hypertension following infusion [19]. As the total IEQ/kg recipient weight infused is currently the most well-known predictor of a successful clinical outcome [20, 21], the decision to purify should be carefully weighed in each unique case.

The current purification method utilizes a continuous density gradient with iodixanol gradient solutions in combination with a COBE 2991 cell processor. A volume of 125 mL of gradient stock solution (density = 1.110 g/cm^3) is loaded into the COBE bag with a peristaltic pump. A gradient maker is then used to gradually mix heavy (1.100 g/cm^3) and light (1.060 g/cm^3) solutions as they are loaded into the COBE machine that is spinning at 1800 rpm. Acinar tissue has a heavier density and will gravitate toward the heavier gradient at the bottom of the bag. Pure islets, with a lighter density, will remain on the top of the bag. After 3 minutes of centrifugation, the tissue is pushed out of the machine via a diaphragm into twelve 25-mL fractions diluted by 225 mL of cold CMRL media. A sample is taken from each fraction and stained with dithizone to assess the purity and quantity of islets. As a post-COBE islet count is taken, the fractions are centrifuged to determine the final pellet volume [14].

Transplant product preparation

A final sterility sample is taken from the supernatant of the tissue before the bags are filled. In addition, 100 μL of suspended islets are taken to determine viability. While not currently standard routine, newer techniques to assess islet quality have been reported, including beta-cell counts and islet viability by oxygen consumption ratios (OCR) in the islet product [22, 23].

Following the assessment of the post-COBE fractions, the isolation staff will choose which combination of fractions will produce the most efficient product (most IEQ per mL of packed tissue), while keeping in mind that the tissue limit for each transplant infusion bag is 10 mL of tissue. Infusion bags are prepared by adding up to 10 mL of packed tissue suspended in 100 mL of transplant media, along with ciprofloxacin (1% = 10,000 µg/mL). If the program director decides to increase the total IEQ brought to the OR, additional infusion bags may be used and the transplant surgeon should be notified. If this happens, the infusion bag with the highest IEQ/volume should be infused first. In this way, in the event that the surgeon must stop intraportal infusion of the islets due to patient safety concerns, an alternate site may be chosen for the less pure transplant bags. The ultimate goal is to transplant as many IEQ as possible into the portal venous system, the most effective islet engraftment site [1], in order to increase the probability of transplant success.

Islet infusion, from pancreas to liver

Within the native pancreas, islets are highly vascularized and innervated. Although islets comprise only 2% of the pancreatic mass, they receive up to 15% of the arterial blood flow [24]. There is a low rate of beta-cell turnover within the native pancreas, although the sources of new beta cells in adult humans are not entirely clear; beta-cell replication or neogenesis from ductal precursors are proposed [25], the latter directly observed in some younger patients with severe CP [26]. This native environment is invariably disrupted when islets are isolated from the pancreas and infused into the intrahepatic environment.

During isolation, islets are unavoidably devascularized, deinnervated, and removed from the potentially supportive structure of the surrounding pancreas. Histological and functional evidence of reinnervation have been reported in rodent models of islet transplant [27, 28] although it is not clear if functional islet reinnervation occurs in clinical IAT recipients. Revascularlization occurs over a period of 14 days to 3 months posttransplant [29–32], triggered by vascular endothelial growth factor secretion from the transplanted islets [33]. In a murine model of syngeneic intraportal islet transplant, hypoxia was frequent in 1-day- and 1-month-old islet grafts but significantly lower by 3 months after transplant, corresponding to a time during which vascular density was increasing within the islet grafts [31]. Thus, transplanted islets are exposed to conditions of relative hypoxia for the first 1–3 months after intraportal islet infusion. Large islets may be more vulnerable than small islets to central necrosis and beta-cell loss during this period of hypoxia [34, 35]. In IAT recipients with a marginal islet mass transplanted, grafts with a greater predominance of small islets were superior in restoring insulin independence posttransplant [36].

Isolation and subsequent postinfusion events trigger beta-cell apoptosis at a rate significantly higher than in the healthy pancreas [9, 10]. In animal models, beta-cell apoptosis remains even at 30 days after islet transplantation and is upregulated by both inflammatory cytokine exposure and hyperglycemia [11, 37]. To best protect islet mass, insulin should be administered in the peri- and postoperative periods. In murine models, as many as twice as many islets are required to reverse diabetes when hyperglycemia is not controlled with insulin treatment [11]. Thus, in clinical IAT recipients, maintenance of euglycemia is targeted after islet infusion, with intravenous insulin infusion and subcutaneous insulin analogs.

When islets are infused into the portal blood stream, tissue factor expressed on the surface of the islets an instant blood-mediated inflammatory reaction (IBMIR), in which complement and coagulation cascades are activated and innate inflammation is triggered. This nonspecific inflammatory response is proposed to contribute to substantial islet loss in some recipients [6, 7, 38, 39]. Multiple proinflammatory cytokine/chemokine pathways are upregulated in the 1-week period following surgery in clinical IAT recipients [6, 40]. Anti-inflammatory approaches are currently under study to target this potential source of islet loss [8].

Islet physiology and function following TPIAT

Ultimately, the goal of the IAT is to preserve endogenous insulin secretion in those patients who require total pancreatectomy for relief of severe, unrelenting pancreatic pain. Total pancreatectomy alone often results in labile diabetes mellitus (DM), due to complex medical disease, malabsorption from exocrine insufficiency, lack of any basal or counter-regulatory glucagon production, and, importantly, the complete reliance on subcutaneous insulin injections [41]. Simply restoring some ability to endogenously regulate insulin secretion, even in the absence of insulin independence, significantly reduces the risk for this labile form of DM. TPIAT confers a long-term survival advantage over total pancreatectomy alone for CP [42].

Glucose-dependent insulin secretion is preserved in the transplanted islets. Thus, as ambient blood glucose rises, glucose travels freely into the beta cell through an insulin-independent glucose transporter and stimulates the secretion and synthesis of insulin. The pulsatile pattern of insulin secretion, which is present in the native pancreas, is restored in intrahepatic islet transplant recipients [43]. Islet function and insulin dependence are highly dependent upon the islet mass transplanted [21, 44]. Overall, islet function is present in about 90% and insulin independence is achieved in about 30% of IAT recipients in the first year after surgery (Figure 17B.3), although attrition of insulin independence occurs over time [4, 21, 45, 46]. While surgery is approached cautiously in younger children, the youngest IAT recipients are frequently insulin independent, and this insulin independence is sustained long term [20, 47]. Because prior surgical resection or surgical drainage procedures (Puestow, or similar) reduce the islet mass available for transplant, a history of prior pancreatic surgery reduces the likelihood of islet

autotransplant success [21, 48]; thus, such procedures are often avoided as a temporizing measure in those likely to require IAT such as young patients with genetic disease [49, 50].

When islets are transplanted intrahepatically, the alpha cells produce normally basal and arginine (protein)-stimulated glucagon. However, in contrast, the expected elevation of glucagon in response to hypoglycemia is absent in IAT recipients with intrahepatic islet grafts, even when a large number of islets are transplanted. This appears to be a transplant site–specific defect; when a portion of the islets are placed in the peritoneal cavity, a normal counter-regulatory rise of glucagon during hypoglycemia is restored [51]. At this time, intraportal infusion remains the preferred approach to IAT, based on the vast experience with this site, clear potential for beta-cell longevity, and superior performance of this site historically in animal models. However, alternative sites remain under study, with the potential advantage of restoring glucagon counter-regulation, as well as other benefits including avoidance of IBMIR and exposure to toxins in the liver [29].

Conclusions

Recent advances in islet autotransplantation have expanded our ability to successfully isolate islets from patients with CP. Once transplanted into the intrahepatic environment, islets require several weeks to months to engraft and reestablish a vascular supply. However, remarkably once transplanted and engrafted, islets can function nearly normally and sustain function for years. Control of detrimental factors such as posttransplant beta-cell apoptosis and control of the IBMIR will be critical to continue to advance our success with this procedure.

References

1 Blondet JJ, Carlson AM, Kobayashi T, Jie T, Bellin M, et al. The role of total pancreatectomy and islet autotransplantation for chronic pancreatitis. The Surgical Clinics of North America 2007;87:1477–1501.

2 Bellin MD, Balamurugan AN, Pruett TL, Sutherland DE. No islets left behind: islet autotransplantation for surgery-induced diabetes. Current Diabetes Reports 2012;12:580–586.

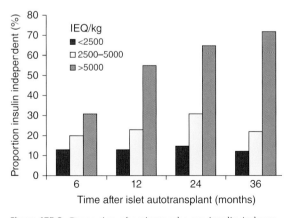

Figure 17B.3 Proportion of patients who are insulin independent at various time points after TPIAT, by the number of islets (IEQ/kg) transplanted. Bellin 2012 [2]. Reproduced with permission from Springer.

3 Najarian JS, Sutherland DE, Matas AJ, Steffes MW, Simmons RL, et al. Human islet transplantation: a preliminary report. Transplantation Proceedings 1977;9:233–236.

4 Sutherland DE, Gruessner AC, Carlson AM, Blondet JJ, Balamurugan AN, et al. Islet autotransplant outcomes after total pancreatectomy: a contrast to islet allograft outcomes. Transplantation 2008;86:1799–1802.

5 Bellin MD, Sutherland DE, Beilman GJ, Hong-McAtee I, Balamurugan AN, et al. Similar islet function in islet allotransplant and autotransplant recipients, despite lower islet mass in autotransplants. Transplantation 2011;91:367–372.

6 Naziruddin B, Iwahashi S, Kanak MA, Takita M, Itoh T, et al. Evidence for instant blood-mediated inflammatory reaction in clinical autologous islet transplantation. American Journal of Transplantation 2014;14:428–437.

7 Moberg L. The role of the innate immunity in islet transplantation. Upsala Journal of Medical Sciences 2005;110:17–55.

8 Citro A, Cantarelli E, Piemonti L. Anti-inflammatory strategies to enhance islet engraftment and survival. Current Diabetes Reports 2013;13:733–744.

9 Negi S, Park SH, Jetha A, Aikin R, Tremblay M, et al. Evidence of endoplasmic reticulum stress mediating cell death in transplanted human islets. Cell Transplantation 2012;21:889–900.

10 Paraskevas S, Maysinger D, Wang R, Duguid TP, Rosenberg L. Cell loss in isolated human islets occurs by apoptosis. Pancreas 2000;20:270–276.

11 Biarnes M, Montolio M, Nacher V, Raurell M, Soler J, et al. Beta-cell death and mass in syngeneically transplanted islets exposed to short- and long-term hyperglycemia. Diabetes 2002;51:66–72.

12 Morrison CP, Wemyss-Holden SA, Dennison AR, Maddern GJ. Islet yield remains a problem in islet autotransplantation. Archives of Surgery (Chicago, Ill: 1960) 2002;137:80–83.

13 Balamurugan AN, Loganathan G, Bellin MD, Wilhelm JJ, Harmon J, et al. A new enzyme mixture to increase the yield and transplant rate of autologous and allogeneic human islet products. Transplantation 2012;93:693–702.

14 Balamurugan AN, Gopalakrishnan L, Lockridge A, Soltani SM, Wilhelm JJ, Beilman GJ, Hering BJ, Sutherland DER. Islet isolation from pancreatitis pancreas for autologous islet isolation. In: Islam M (Ed). Islet of Langerhans. Second edition, Springer, 2014.

15 Pepper AR, Gala-Lopez B, Kin T. Advances in clinical islet isolation. In: Islam M (Ed). Islet of Langerhans, Springer, 2014.

16 Lakey JR, Kneteman NM, Rajotte RV, Wu DC, Bigam D, et al. Effect of core pancreas temperature during cadaveric procurement on human islet isolation and functional viability. Transplantation 2002;73:1106–1110.

17 Anazawa T, Balamurugan AN, Bellin M, Zhang HJ, Matsumoto S, et al. Human islet isolation for autologous transplantation: comparison of yield and function using SERVA/Nordmark versus Roche enzymes. American Journal of Transplantation: Official Journal of the American Society of Transplantation and the American Society of Transplant Surgeons 2009;9:2383–2391.

18 Ricordi C, Lacy PE, Finke EH, Olack BJ, Scharp DW. Automated method for isolation of human pancreatic islets. Diabetes 1988;37:413–420.

19 Wilhelm JJ, Bellin MD, Balamurugan AN, Beilman GJ, Dunn TB, et al. A proposed threshold for dispersed-pancreatic tissue volume infused during intraportal islet autotransplantation after total pancreatectomy to treat chronic pancreatitis. Pancreas 2011;40:1363.

20 Bellin MD, Freeman ML, Schwarzenberg SJ, Dunn TB, Beilman GJ, et al. Quality of life improves for pediatric patients after total pancreatectomy and islet autotransplant for chronic pancreatitis. Clinical Gastroenterology and Hepatology 2011;9:793–799.

21 Sutherland DE, Radosevich DM, Bellin MD, Hering BJ, Beilman GJ, et al. Total pancreatectomy and islet autotransplantation for chronic pancreatitis. Journal of the American College of Surgeons 2012;214:409–424.

22 Keymeulen B, Gillard P, Mathieu C, Movahedi B, Maleux G, et al. Correlation between beta cell mass and glycemic control in type 1 diabetic recipients of islet cell graft. Proceedings of the National Academy of Sciences of the United States of America 2006;103:17444–17449.

23 Kitzmann JP, O'Gorman D, Kin T, Gruessner AC, Senior P, et al. Islet oxygen consumption rate dose predicts insulin independence for first clinical islet allotransplants. Transplantation Proceedings 2014;46:1985–1988.

24 Ballian N, Brunicardi FC. Islet vasculature as a regulator of endocrine pancreas function. World Journal of Surgery 2007;31:705–714.

25 Weir GC, Bonner-Weir S. Islet beta cell mass in diabetes and how it relates to function, birth, and death. Annals of the New York Academy of Sciences 2013;1281:92–105.

26 Soltani SM, O'Brien TD, Loganathan G, Bellin MD, Anazawa T, et al. Severely fibrotic pancreases from young patients with chronic pancreatitis: evidence for a ductal origin of islet neogenesis. Acta Diabetologica. 2013;50:807–814.

27 Gardemann A, Jungermann K, Grosse V, Cossel L, Wohlrab F, et al. Intraportal transplantation of pancreatic islets into livers of diabetic rats. Reinnervation of islets and regulation of insulin secretion by the hepatic sympathetic nerves. Diabetes. 1994;43:1345–1352.

28 Juang JH, Peng SJ, Kuo CH, Tang SC. Three-dimensional islet graft histology: panoramic imaging of neural plasticity in sympathetic reinnervation of transplanted islets under the kidney capsule. American Journal of Physiology Endocrinology and Metabolism 2014;306:E559–E570.

29 Pepper AR, Gala-Lopez B, Ziff O, Shapiro AM. Revascularization of transplanted pancreatic islets and role of the transplantation site. Clinical & Developmental Immunology 2013;2013:352315.

30 Menger MD, Yamauchi J, Vollmar B. Revascularization and microcirculation of freely grafted islets of Langerhans. World Journal of Surgery 2001;25:509–515.

31 Olsson R, Olerud J, Pettersson U, Carlsson PO. Increased numbers of low-oxygenated pancreatic islets after intraportal islet transplantation. Diabetes 2011;60:2350–2353.

32 Jansson L, Carlsson PO. Graft vascular function after transplantation of pancreatic islets. Diabetologia 2002;45:749–763.

33 Brissova M, Shostak A, Shiota M, Wiebe PO, Poffenberger G, et al. Pancreatic islet production of vascular endothelial growth factor--a is essential for islet vascularization, revascularization, and function. Diabetes 2006;55:2974–2985.

34 Giuliani M, Moritz W, Bodmer E, Dindo D, Kugelmeier P, et al. Central necrosis in isolated hypoxic human pancreatic islets: evidence for postisolation ischemia. Cell Transplantation 2005;14:67–76.

35 Li W, Zhao R, Liu J, Tian M, Lu Y, et al. Small islets transplantation superiority to large ones: implications from islet microcirculation and revascularization. Journal of Diabetes Research 2014;2014:192093.

36 Suszynski TM, Wilhelm JJ, Radosevich DM, Balamurugan AN, Sutherland DE, et al. Islet size index as a predictor of outcomes in clinical islet autotransplantation. Transplantation 2014;97:1286–1291.

37 Rabinovitch A, Sumoski W, Rajotte RV, Warnock GL. Cytotoxic effects of cytokines on human pancreatic islet cells in monolayer culture. Journal of Clinical Endocrinology and Metabolism 1990;71:152–156.

38 Gibly RF, Graham JG, Luo X, Lowe WL, Jr.,, Hering BJ, et al. Advancing islet transplantation: from engraftment to the immune response. Diabetologia 2011;54:2494–2505.

39 Bennet W, Groth CG, Larsson R, Nilsson B, Korsgren O. Isolated human islets trigger an instant blood mediated inflammatory reaction: implications for intraportal islet transplantation as a treatment for patients with type 1 diabetes. Upsala Journal of Medical Sciences 2000;105:125–133.

40 Itoh T, Iwahashi S, Kanak MA, Shimoda M, Takita M, et al. Elevation of high-mobility group box 1 after clinical autologous islet transplantation and its inverse correlation with outcomes. Cell Transplantation. 2014;23:153–165.

41 Slezak LA, Andersen DK. Pancreatic resection: effects on glucose metabolism. World Journal of Surgery 2001;25:452–460.

42 Garcea G, Pollard CA, Illouz S, Webb M, Metcalfe MS, et al. Patient satisfaction and cost-effectiveness following total pancreatectomy with islet cell transplantation for chronic pancreatitis. Pancreas 2013;42:322–328.

43 Meier JJ, Hong-McAtee I, Galasso R, Veldhuis JD, Moran A, et al. Intrahepatic transplanted islets in humans secrete insulin in a coordinate pulsatile manner directly into the liver. Diabetes 2006;55:2324–2332.

44 Ahmad SA, Lowy AM, Wray CJ, D'Alessio D, Choe KA, et al. Factors associated with insulin and narcotic independence after islet autotransplantation in patients with severe chronic pancreatitis. Journal of the American College of Surgeons 2005;201:680–687.

45 Webb MA, Illouz SC, Pollard CA, Gregory R, Mayberry JF, et al. Islet auto transplantation following total pancreatectomy: a long-term assessment of graft function. Pancreas 2008;37:282–287.

46 Wilson GC, Sutton JM, Abbott DE, Smith MT, Lowy AM, et al. Long-term outcomes after total pancreatectomy and islet cell autotransplantation: is it a durable operation? Annals of Surgery 2014;260:659–665; discussion 65–67.

47 Chinnakotla S, Bellin MD, Schwarzenberg SJ, Radosevich DM, Cook M, et al. Total pancreatectomy and islet autotransplantation in children for chronic pancreatitis: indication, surgical techniques, postoperative management, and long-term outcomes. Annals of Surgery 2014;260:56–64.

48 Morgan KA, Theruvath T, Owczarski S, Adams DB. Total pancreatectomy with islet autotransplantation for chronic pancreatitis: do patients with prior pancreatic surgery have different outcomes? American Surgeon 2012;78:893–896.

49 Chinnakotla S, Radosevich DM, Dunn TB, Bellin MD, Freeman ML, et al. Long-term outcomes of total pancreatectomy and islet auto transplantation for hereditary/genetic pancreatitis. Journal of the American College of Surgeons 2014;218:530–543.

50 Sutton JM, Schmulewitz N, Sussman JJ, Smith M, Kurland JE, et al. Total pancreatectomy and islet cell autotransplantation as a means of treating patients with genetically linked pancreatitis. Surgery 2010;148:676–685; discussion 85–86.

51 Bellin MD, Parazzoli S, Oseid E, Bogachus LD, Schuetz C, et al. Defective glucagon secretion during hypoglycemia after intrahepatic but not nonhepatic islet autotransplantation. American Journal of Transplantation 2014;14:1880–1886.

PART C: Total pancreatectomy and islet cell autotransplantation: long-term assessment of graft function

Giuseppe Garcea & Ashley Dennison

Department of Hepato-Pancreato-Biliary Surgery, Leicester General Hospital, University Hospitals of Leicester NHS Trust, Leicester, UK

Introduction

Diabetes and chronic pancreatitis

Any process that leads to the destruction/reduction of the pancreatic parenchyma and particularly the endocrine component (progressive fibrosis, surgery or trauma) will result in hormone deficiencies and altered responses of organs to these pancreatic hormones. This results in a type of impaired glucose metabolism known as pancreatogenic diabetes [1]. The American Diabetic Association classifies this type of diabetes mellitus as "other specific type of diabetes mellitus" [2] as opposed to the previous classification in 2003 as type lll.C.1 [3]. Pancreaticogenic diabetes following surgical resection differs from type 1 and type 2 diabetes in a number of respects. In particular, as type 1 diabetes mellitus is caused by cell-mediated autoimmune destruction of beta cells, it carries a significant risk of hyperglycemia and ketoacidosis both of which are uncommon with pancreaticogenic diabetes.

Pancreaticogenic diabetes is also unlike type 2 diabetes mellitus, which is characterized by insulin resistance and relative insulin deficiency, because patients with pancreatic diabetes are sensitive to insulin [1]. In addition, the increased peripheral sensitivity to insulin and reduced glucagon levels with pancreaticogenic diabetes means that exogenous insulin administration frequently causes hypoglycemic attacks, and this response is the reason for the use of the term "brittle diabetes." The consequence of this sensitivity is frequent iatrogenic hypoglycemia with exogenous insulin, which can be severe and cause hospitalization, irreversible central nervous system damage, and even fatalities [4–8]. As a consequence, glycemic control can be extremely challenging to manage with HbA_{1c} levels, which are generally high and not infrequently associated with chronic diabetic complications (nephropathy, neuropathy, and retinopathy) in the longer term [6, 9].

Diabetes following total pancreatectomy

Total pancreatectomy (TP) without an islet autotransplant has an inevitable consequence of diabetes, and (in addition to the brittle nature) it is believed that rapid intestinal transit due to pancreatic insufficiency results in unpredictable glucose absorption and exacerbates the recurrent episodes of iatrogenic hypoglycemia. Fear of this "brittle" diabetes is one of the main reasons that referral for surgery is often much delayed, which further contributes to the potential for complications in the long term [10, 11]. Islet autotransplantation following pancreatectomy offers the opportunity to ameliorate the complete loss of endocrine function normally associated with TP with resultant improvements in the quality of life (QoL) and diabetic control. Hence, long-term assessment of graft function must include QoL assessment, in addition to physiological parameters.

Quality of life

Quality of life in patients with chronic pancreatitis

Although QoL in patients suffering from CP is invariably poor and associated with significant domestic and social disruption, quantitative assessment is difficult. In the past, the Short Form-36 (SF-36) was used for measuring health in gastroenterology but was not validated for chronic pancreatitis. The European Organisation for Research and Treatment of Cancer

Pancreatitis: Medical and Surgical Management, First Edition.
David B. Adams, Peter B. Cotton, Nicholas J. Zyromski and John Windsor.
© 2017 John Wiley & Sons, Ltd. Published 2017 by John Wiley & Sons, Ltd.

Quality of Life Questionairre-30 (EORTC QLQ-C30) and the Quality of Life Questionnaire Pancreatic Cancer Module (QLQ-PAN28) have also been used to provide CP specific information [12–14]. Fitzsimmons and colleagues developed the EORTC QLC-C30 in a multicenter study of patients with chronic pancreatitis but did not validate it with appropriate controls. They also modified the QLQ-PAN26 (a pancreatic specific module) and produced a CP-specific module, which was renamed QLQ-PAN28 [15, 16]. They concluded that QLQ-C30 and QLQ-PAN26 showed strong associations between conceptually related scales and discriminated between patients on the basis of performance status and their requirements for opiate analgesics. More recently, The Short Form-12 Health Survey forms have been assessed and compared with the EORTC QLQ C30 in a number of different cohorts [17, 18] and are presently the accepted tools in CP.

The largest study ever conducted on the pain from CP was able to demonstrate that for all categories of CP pain including mild/moderate intermittent to patients with constant severe pain almost half used pain medication for their condition, almost a quarter were on disability allowance, and patients had been admitted a median of once in the preceding year. The same study also demonstrated that constant pain regardless of severity was significantly associated with higher levels of hospitalization [19]. Those with constant pain were more likely to have been hospitalized on more than 10 occasions in the last year and have a higher need for incapacity benefit compared with sufferers of intermittent pain of all severities (42.1% vs. 17.5%, OR 3.2 (95% CI 2.0–5.1). Based on these assessments, the authors made the suggestion that treatments that eradicate pain (radical surgery) rather than therapeutic options that reduce pain scores (celiac plexus block, Puestow (drainage) procedure, and pancreatic enzyme supplementation) are the most effective strategies.

It is also known that at least 50% of patients who suffer from CP will ultimately require some form of surgical intervention due to persistent refractory pain and/or complications of the disease [20–23]. With such a high proportion of patients ultimately requiring surgery TP (which has been shown to result in the eradication of CP-related pain in the majority of patients) [24] is indicated in those patients with small duct/minimal change disease and previously failed surgery where other forms of treatment are very unlikely to succeed.

Quality of life following total pancreatectomy with and without islet transplantation

The first TP was performed by Rockey in 1943 [25], but for several decades the procedure was only employed in an attempt to improve the clearance and R0 resection rates in patients with pancreatic malignancies. As the management of these patients improved, consideration was given to its use for other (nonadenocarcinoma) tumors and benign conditions such as chronic pancreatitis. Unfortunately, prior to the advent of islet autotransplantation, the inevitable consequence of the surgery was immediate and complete exocrine and endocrine deficiency, which produced malabsorption and "brittle" diabetes [26].

Improvements in surgical technique and postoperative care means that TP is now associated with a very low mortality and a dramatically reduced morbidity [24], but without a concomitant islet autotransplantation it is still associated with significant postoperative problems. The principle problem that affects the QoL in these patients is poor glycemic control despite the use of frequently very complex insulin regimens [27]. The impact of the diabetes following TP is demonstrated in a study by Billings and colleagues who demonstrated the safety of the procedure but found that QoL was significantly inferior to age- and gender-matched controls but was no different from comparable patients with diabetes [4].

Several groups have recently reexamined the QoL in these patients in the light of further advances in surgical technique and progress in the management of the diabetes. A study from Italy looked at the QoL and long-term complications in a tertiary referral center between 1994 and 2006 and used the EORTC QLQ-C30 questionnaire to evaluate surviving patients. Ninety one percent of patients complained of hypoglycemia (at least once a week in 72%), and steatorrhea and abdominal pain were found in 66%. These problems resulted in major impairments of leisure and work activities in 56% and 31%, respectively. There were similar findings in a study from the Mayo Clinic that examined patients having TP between 2002 and 2008 and found that patients lost about 8 kg in weight, which was also associated with elevated HbA_{1c} values and over 50% of patients requiring rehospitalization within 12 months [28].

The addition of an islet autotransplant is able to abrogate the majority of the symptoms and problems outlined here that are associated with TP alone [29–31]. In a study from Cincinnati examining the role of TP and islet cell autotransplantation for genetically linked pancreatitis, insulin requirements reduced to a mean of 15 U/days by 22 months and 25% of patients were insulin independent. Narcotic use fell dramatically following surgery with a 63% rate of narcotic independence (at last outpatient visit), which was also associated with a significantly improved QoL (analysis of the 36-item short-form health survey and the McGill pain questionnaire) [29]. There are similar findings in children having a TP and islet autotransplant by the Minneapolis group who used the Medical Outcome Study 36-item short form (SF-36) before and after surgery and demonstrated a below-average health-related QoL preoperatively (mean physical component summary (PCS) score of 30 and mental component summary (MCS) score of 34 (2 and 1.5 standard deviations, respectively, below the mean for the US population). By 1 year following surgery, the PCS and MCS scores had improved to 50 and 46, respectively (PCS $P < 0.001$, MCS $P = 0.06$) and mean scores had also improve for all eight-component subscales. In addition, more than 60% of patients were insulin independent or required minimal insulin [32].

A recent meta-analysis has also attempted to determine the reduction in morbidity and mortality conferred by the addition of an islet autotransplant to a TP [31]. The study found a very low 30-day mortality of between 1% and 2% (median of 0%) and insulin independence rates of 4.62 per 100-person years and 8.34% per 100-person years at last follow-up and transiently, respectively. Dong and colleagues did not examine the results for QoL related to insulin independence, reduced requirements, or glycemic control but this was examined in a study from the Cleveland Clinic this year [33]. The stated aim of the study was "to improve QoL by alleviating pain and discontinuing narcotics while preventing or minimizing surgical diabetes". Patients were examined pre- and postoperatively using the Depression Anxiety Stress Scale (DASS) and the Pain Disability Index (PDI). A visual analog pain scale was used to assess global pain and diabetes was examined by the use of HbA_{1c}. Depression and anxiety were classed as mild, moderate, severe, and extremely severe and the effect on family/home responsibilities, recreation, social activity, occupation, sexual behavior, self-care, and life-support activities studied. Results for the impact of

Table 17C.1 Improvements in quality of life following total pancreatectomy and islet autotransplantation for chronic pancreatitis.

	Pre-operative state	Post-operative state
Family/home responsibilities	12 (61%)	2 (10%)
Recreation	16 (80%)	4 (20%)
Social activities	13 (66%)	3 (15%)
Occupation	14 (70%)	3 (20%)
Sexual behavior	11 (55%)	2 (10%)
Self care	6 (39%)	0 (0%)
Life support activity	9 (45%)	1 (10%)
Depression	4 (19%)	0 (0%)
Anxiety	1 (4%)	1 (4%)
Pain scale	11 (55%)	2 (10%)

the surgery and islet autotransplant on those activities severely affected are shown in Table 17C.1. These results are extremely encouraging and demonstrate that there has been a steady improvement in the QoL of the patients over the last three decades, brought about by a standardization of surgical technique, the involvement of multidisciplinary teams in the postoperative period and refinements in islet isolation [34–38].

Assessment of graft function

Long-term follow-up protocols have been employed in Leicester since 1994. Patients are routinely assessed for the development of diabetes and attention paid to changes in blood glucose levels with adjustments in insulin doses as appropriate by a consultant diabetologist. In addition, there is protocol evaluation of diabetic status at 1, 3, 6 and 12 months and at yearly intervals thereafter. This includes the response to an oral glucose tolerance test as well as measurement of levels of C-peptide and HbA_{1c}. Formal evaluation of QoL is performed periodically using regular assessments by a medical psychologist. In this way, a full picture of the effects of surgery can be obtained, which includes the following:

1 Insulin requirements.
2 HbA_{1c} as an index of average glucose levels.
3 Responses to mixed meals and oral/intravenous glucose.

4 Formal assessment of QoL, including changes in pain and narcotic use performed by a consultant medical psychologist.

5 Assessment of development of diabetic complications including regular eye screening to monitor retinopathy, urine examination to look for microalbuminuria, and regular clinical examination to look for evidence of diabetic neuropathy.

6 Annual abdominal ultrasound examinations.

Annual ultrasound examination is part of the standard follow up of patients with bilioenteric anastomoses to prevent complications following an insidious bilioenteric stenosis. In addition, infusion of islets into the portal venous system may induce long-term structural changes in the liver. Several authors have described periportal hepatic steatosis in patients who have undergone islet transplantation [39, 40].The hepatic steatosis seen in islet transplant patients differs from that seen in the general population in that it produces a heterogeneous nodular or granular pattern of liver involvement. It can be seen as early as 6–12 months following an islet transplant (Figure 17C.1) but does not produce clinical

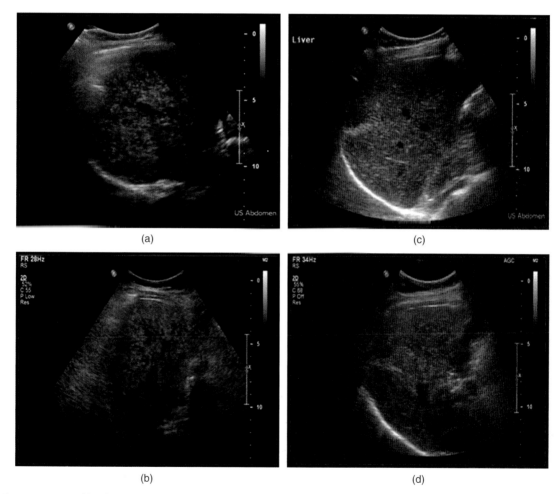

Figure 17C.1 (a and b) Abdominal ultrasound images of two patients following a pancreatectomy and islet cell autotransplant (more than 12 months earlier). The images demonstrate nodular echogenicity of the liver found in 25% of the patients. The changes occur from 6 to 12 months following the islet infusion and are not found in patients following a total pancreatectomy alone. (c and d) The liver appearances are not associated with clinical, biochemical, or radiological evidence of liver dysfunction or progression of the appearances once established. (c and d) show the same patient with stable ultrasound appearances over a 2-year period.

problems or abnormalities of liver function even in the long-term and does not progress on imaging. It is a benign condition thought to result from the paracrine action of high local concentrations of insulin and is believed to be a positive finding acting as a surrogate marker for persistent islet graft function. Magnetic resonance imaging (MRI) of these liver appearances suggests that the appearances are due to localized patch steatosis [41].

Although long-term prevention of diabetes remains the goal of the islet autotransplantation (IAT) procedure, significant insulin and C-peptide secretion is the main measure of the success of the procedure. Background C-peptide secretion will lessen the severity of diabetes even if some exogenous insulin is required, allowing easier control of blood glucose. The improved diabetic control will reduce or abrogate the onset of secondary chronic diabetic complications. Together with the improved control of blood glucose, cessation of narcotics will produce a significantly improved QoL.

Clinical outcomes following total pancreatectomy and islet autotransplantation

The Minneapolis program
Islet autotransplant programs throughout the world attempt to mimic the success of the Minneapolis transplant team (headed by Prof. David Sutherland), which was started in 1977 and now boasts the largest and most experienced team of islet autotransplant physicians and scientists in the world.

Insulin requirements
IAT has been shown to fully abrogate diabetes in approximately one-third of patients (32% were insulin independent at 1 year), while 65% of patients (also at 1 year) showed partial function and were classified as euglycemic recipients on once-daily long-acting insulin. The procedure has also been used to successfully treat 24 children to date with 56% showing insulin independence at 1 year posttransplant [42]. A more recent report following insulin requirements of patients with hereditary and nonhereditary chronic pancreatitis demonstrated that 16 of the 80 TP-IAT patients with hereditary/genetic chronic pancreatitis (HGP) attained complete insulin independence at some

time after islet infusion (20%). This compares with 133 of the 404 (32.9%) with a nonhereditary cause. Insulin requirements in general decreased for the first 2–3 years following TP/IAT with deterioration in the percentage of patients remaining insulin-free after this [43].

HGP was associated with a significantly reduced likelihood of insulin independence compared with nonhereditary causes (odds ratio [OR] = 0.33; 95% confidence limits [CL], 0.1 and 0.84; $P = 0.019$). Independent risk factors for insulin independence included recipient age, severity of pancreatic fibrosis, recipient body mass index, and transplant IEQ/kg body weight. The number of IEQs was the strongest independent predictor for insulin independence. C-Peptide levels were maintained in at least 80% of patients although the rate of decline was greater in patients with HGP [43]. Rates of long-term insulin independence were higher in a pediatric population of 75 patients undergoing TP/IAT at 41.3% [43]. By multivariate analysis, three factors were associated with insulin independence after TP-IAT: (i) male sex, (ii) lower body surface area, and (iii) higher total IEQ per kilogram body weight. Total IEQ (100,000) was the single factor most strongly associated with insulin independence (OR = 2.62; $P < 0.001$) [44].

Formal assessment of quality of life
QoL following TP/IAT was significantly improved in both pediatric and nonpediatric populations. Ninety percent of patients had statistically significant improvement in their pain and health-related QoL [43, 44]. As a global measure of physical health, PCS scale scores were unrelated to insulin status. However, in the aggregate, physical health declined more rapidly for those who were insulin dependent compared with those less dependent on insulin. Among those that were insulin dependent, the PCS scale scores dropped by a mean of 7.07 points. This is a marked decline considering that the MCS and PCS are standard normalized to have an SD of 10 points [43] emphasizing the impact of graft function on overall QoL.

Previous work by the Minneapolis group has shown that patients who had not had previous pancreatic surgery and those who had previously had procedures to the head of the pancreas were more likely to have a greater islet yield and achieve insulin independence. Patients who had previously had distal resections or hybrid techniques were more likely to require exogenous insulin administration and they consequently advocate TP and IAT at an early stage in the disease course [45].

The Leicester program

Within the Leicester group, 74% of patients who were treated presented with nonalcohol-induced CP with the onset of the disease reported as young as 6 years old. Sixty patients have undergone pancreatectomy and IAT to date, and a further 50 patients have had a pancreatectomy alone. The pancreatectomy-alone patients were on insulin at presentation, had severely abnormal GTTs, or were found (eight patients) to be unsuitable intraoperatively. Intraoperative problems related to a small number of patients where the calcification/fibrosis of the gland prevented the recovery of a significant or sufficient number of islets to justify autotransplantation. This represents the cohort where late diagnosis/referral was accompanied by the well-recognized reduction in islet mass and the onset of IDDM. In Leicester, IDDM or a severely abnormal GTT is considered to be a contraindication to attempting an IAT because the small increase in the risk of the procedure cannot be justified by the likely small islet yield (autotransplantation of very small numbers of islet does not produce significant endogenous insulin production in the long term, and these patients become C-peptide negative).

Insulin requirements

Thirty seven percent of patients have experienced insulin independence, and 32% were insulin free at 1 year posttransplant (Figure 17C.2). Unlike islet allotransplantation, optimal graft function was not achieved until 1 year following transplantation as evidenced by the highest serum C-peptide levels and lowest requirements of exogenous insulin. In those patients who are not insulin independent, the daily requirements are low with the majority requiring less than 20 units and C-peptide secretion preserved (Figure 17C.3) in response to glucose stimulation. Both C-peptide secretion and HbA_{1c} demonstrated some deterioration over time, but overall remained satisfactory throughout the follow-up period.

Formal assessment of quality of life

Following surgery, there was a significant reduction in the patients' visual analog pain score from 9.7 to 3.7 ($P < 0.001$) with a concomitant improvement in QoL (Figure 17C.4). Long-term follow-up showed that regular opiate use had reduced from 90.6% to 40.2% by the end of the first year following resection, to 15.9% at 5 years, and 7.9% at 10 years. This trend continued beyond 10 years, and at the maximum follow-up in the early patients in the series opiate use approaches zero. Finally, long-term follow-up of IAT

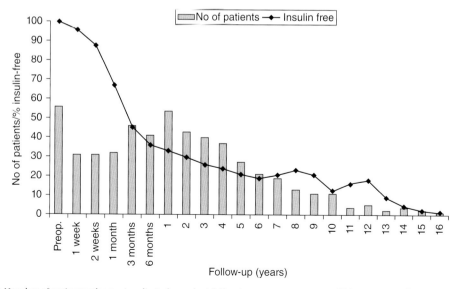

Figure 17C.2 Number of patients who are insulin independent following pancreatectomy and islet autotransplantation in the Leicester series.

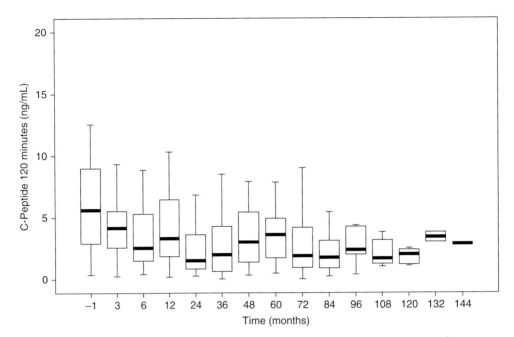

Figure 17C.3 C-Peptide levels at 120 minutes in patients who have had a pancreatectomy and islet autotransplant.

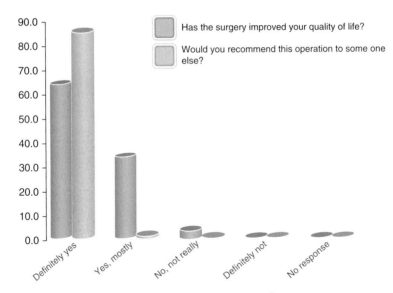

Figure 17C.4 Patient postoperative satisfaction survey. (Adapted from Garcea et al [46].)

patients demonstrated that survival was superior in patients with grafts than those undergoing TP alone (Figure 17C.5) suggesting (although not definitely proving) that functioning IAT could ameliorate long-term complications of diabetes [46].

Further developments in improving long-term graft function

As with all branches of transplant surgery, research and development allows progressive improvements in graft function and survival. The extensive global interest in

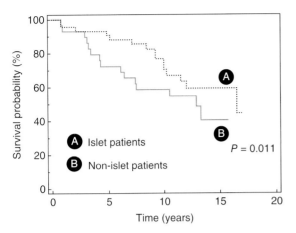

Figure 17C.5   Survival in islet and islet transplant patients following total pancreatectomy. (Adapted from Garcea et al [46].)

islet allotransplantation for the treatment of diabetes mellitus means that there are a plethora of research strategies to improve islet isolation and transplantation and to prolong graft survival. Although data on international budgets spent on islet-related research are not available, Diabetes UK spends an estimated £6 million per annum on islet research. A Pubmed search of islet-related research (search term: pancreatic islets) results in 41,298 peer-reviewed articles spanning 1907 to July 2011 and specifically 9039 related to islet transplantation. Research strategies developed for allotransplantation programs can be directly utilized to improve rates of insulin independence following auto-transplantation. Unpublished data (Leicester) suggests that the rates of insulin independence have improved with the last eight patients transplanted (five of eight patients have shown periods of insulin independence), and this coincides with the introduction of the newly formulated low endotoxin GMP-grade collagenase enzyme (Figure 17C.6).

Reproducible clinical success

Analysis of the three centers with the longest continuous islet autotransplant programs in the world shows remarkably similar patient outcomes, with low mortality (1–2% in the first year posttransplant) and insulin independence rates of between 32% and 40% at

1-year posttransplant. Although insulin independence rates appear relatively low compared with 85% at 1 year achieved following islet allotransplantation, it is difficult to directly compare these two groups. Pancreatectomy and IAT are performed as salvage procedures in patients whose pancreases are severely damaged (and has often been operated on previously) and when only one gland is available. Islet allografting is performed following harvesting of islets from (by definition) normal glands, and frequently multiple transplants from different donors are employed. Following transplantation, however, the situation is different and insulin requirements have been shown to remain relatively stable in islet autotransplant recipients. In Leicester, all patients transplanted since 1994 have retained insulin secretion based on continued C-peptide detection [47]. Based on the attributes of the three lead centers in the world and local experience, the key components needed for successful IAT program are as follows:

- Long-standing experience in complex pancreatic surgery in tertiary referral centers
- Experience in endocrine replacement therapy by transplantation
- Human tissue authority accredited clean room facilities
- Experienced islet isolation scientists with a keen interest in research and development
- A multidisciplinary team to fully assess patients' suitability for surgery and an islet autotransplant who will be involved in the long-term management of the recipients to follow-up the function of the islet graft.

What should be monitored postoperatively?

Following TP and IAT, patients should be carefully monitored for the development of diabetes. There should be protocolled evaluation of diabetic status at 1, 3, 6, and 12 months and at yearly intervals thereafter. These should include responses to an oral glucose tolerance tests as well as measurement of levels of C-peptide and HbA_{1c}. Continuous glucose monitoring sensors (CGMS) could be used to get detailed information about variation in glucose levels in normal life. Formal evaluation of QoL should also be assessed periodically by a medical psychologist. In this way, a full picture of the effects of surgery can be obtained and the results used

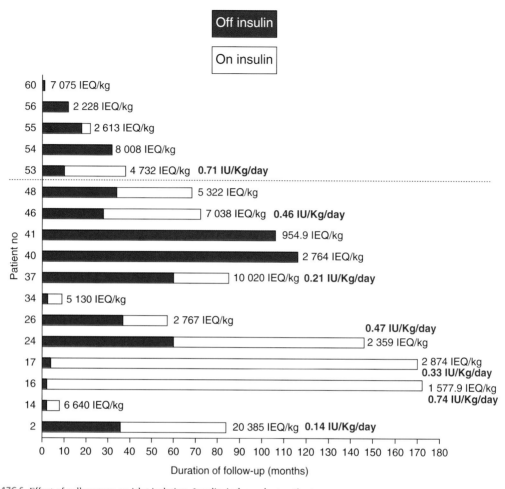

Figure 17C.6 Effect of collagenase on islet isolation: Insulin-independent patients.

to determine the success of TP/IAT and compare inter-group outcomes. Additional data need to be gathered by methods that assess whether patients have developed or are at risk of developing diabetic complications, including regular eye screening to monitor retinopathy, urine testing to look for microalbuminuria, and regular clinical examination to look for evidence of diabetic neuropathy.

Although long-term prevention of diabetes remains the goal of the IAT procedure, significant insulin and C-peptide secretion will remain the main measure of the success of the procedure. Background insulin secretion will lessen the severity of diabetes, allow easier control of blood glucose, improve QoL, and reduce or abolish the onset of secondary diabetic complications. Reductions in

pain and narcotic use are also important endpoints and together with the improved glycemic control will contribute to improvements in QoL and reduce or abolish hospital admissions.

The future of TPIAT

Increasingly centers are able to perform TPIAT and the availability of encouraging long-term results means that the number of procedures performed is likely to steadily increase. The surgical technique is largely established and advances in islet isolation continue; and this combined with the lack of an immune response in patients undergoing TPIAT provides valuable data for the islet allografting community. In addition, a number of units are considering approaches that may modify the immediate posttransplant environment to facilitate and improve early graft implantation. The ability to monitor the environment greatly facilities observations about the effect of a wide range of possible approaches, particularly improving portal oxygen levels and pharmacological manipulations. Access to the portal system for islet infusion can be performed using the recannulated umbilical vein and an indwelling catheter that can be left *in situ* for up to 6 days. This allows for hemodynamic measurements and potentially venous sampling to assess the effect of any pharmacological manipulation.

Nevertheless, the number of patients undergoing TPIAT is likely to remain modest and in the longer term more meaningful data are likely to accrue from a collaborative approach between units or ideally collaboration on a national level working to common protocols and maintaining a joint database. Presently, in the UK, consideration is being given by NHS England to designation of a National network for TPIAT. The proposed network is based upon four centers in Leicester, Oxford, Newcastle, and Kings College London and co-lead by a multidisciplinary group of pancreatic surgeons, transplant surgeons, physicians, diabetologists, and scientists who have examined and considered the available options and compared them with the latest data relating to TP and IAT. "State of the art" treatment of diabetes and its complications is available in the four centers and includes complex exogenous insulin regimens, segmental pancreatic autotransplantation, and pancreas allotransplantation. Of these options, none offers the potential to manage glycemic control as comprehensively or simply as TP/IAT, either due to problems with diabetic control or need for life-long immunosuppression. The consortium will work to common protocols and maintain a centralized database for collation. Audit and governance of the supraregional islet autotransplant program will be established and managed through the islet autotransplant consortium. Data collection will include details of the preoperative work-up and indications for surgery, operative procedure, and duration quality control of the islet isolation process in line with the current NHS England–funded islet allograft program, islet isolation number, and portal pressures during infusion. Postoperatively, surgical complications, insulin independence rates, analgesic usage, HbA$_{1c}$ levels, fasting and stimulated glucose tolerance, and C-peptide in addition to clinical outcomes including formal QoL assessment, pain scores, and hospital admission data will be collected. This collaborative approach will provide a complete long-term picture of the most appropriate work-up, perioperative care, postoperative management, and follow-up of patients following TPIAT.

References

1 Maeda H, Hanazaki K. Pancreatogenic diabetes after pancreatic resection. Pancreatology 2011; 11: 268–276.

2 American Diabetes Association. Diagnosis and classification of diabetes mellitus. Diabetes Care 2010; 33: S62–S69.

3 Expert Committee on the Diagnosis and Classification of Diabetes Mellitus. Report of the expert committee on the diagnosis and classification of diabetes mellitus. Diabetes Care 2003; 26: S5–S20.

4 Billings BJ, Christein JD, Harmsen WS, Harrington JR., Chari ST, Que FG, Farnell MB, Nagorney DM, Sarr MG. Quality-of-life after total pancreatectomy: is it really that bad on long-term follow-up? Journal of Gastrointestinal Surgery 2005; 9: 1059–1066; discussion 1066–1067.

5 Kahl S, Malfertheiner P. Exocrine and endocrine pancreatic insufficiency after pancreatic surgery. Best Practice & Research Clinical Gastroenterology 2004; 18: 947–955.

6 Jethwa P, Sodergren M, Lala A et al. Diabetic control after total pancreatectomy. Digestive and Liver Disease 2006; 38: 415–419.

7 Hutchins RR, Hart RS, Pacifico M, Bradley NJ, Williamson RC. Long-term results of distal pancreatectomy for chronic pancreatitis in 90 patients. Annals of Surgery 2002;236(5): 612–618.

8 Muller MW, Friess H, Kleeff J, Dahmen R, Wagner M, Hinz U, Breisch-Girbig D, Ceyhan GO, Buchler MW. Is there still a role for total pancreatectomy? Annals of Surgery 2007;246(6):966–974; discussion 974–975.

9 Deckert T. Late diabetic manifestations in pancreatogenic diabetes mellitus. Acta Medica Scandinavica 1960; 168: 439–446.

10 Dresler CM, Fortner JG, McDermott K, Bajorunas DR. Metabolic consequences of (regional) total pancreatectomy. Annals of Surgery 1991; 214: 131–140.

11 Duron F, Duron JJ. Pancreatectomy and diabetes. Annales de Chirurgie 1999; 53: 406–411.

12 Kalantar-Zadeh K, Kopple JD, Block G, Humphreys MH. Association among SF36 quality of life measures and nutrition, hospitalization, and mortality in hemodialysis. Journal of the American Society of Nephrology 2001 12: 2797–2806.

13 Forsmark CE. The early diagnosis of chronic pancreatitis. Clinical Gastroenterology and Hepatology 2008: 6; 1291–1293.

14 Aaronson NK, Ahmedzai S, Bergman B, et al. The European Organization for Research and Treatment of Cancer QLQ-C30: a quality-of-life instrument for use in international clinical trials in oncology. Journal of the National Cancer Institute 1993; 85: 365–376.

15 Fitzsimmons D, Johnson CD, George S et al. Development of a disease specific quality of life (QoL) questionnaire module to supplement the EORTC core cancer QoL questionnaire, the QLQ-C30 in patients with pancreatic cancer. EORTC Study Group on Quality of Life. European Journal of Cancer (Oxford, England: 1990) 1999;35(6): 939–941.

16 Fitzsimmons D, Kahl S, Butturini G, et al. Symptoms and quality of life in chronic pancreatitis assessed by structured interview and the EORTC QLQ-C30 and QLQ-PAN26. The American Journal of Gastroenterology 2005; 100: 918–926.

17 Pezzilli R, Morselli-Labate AM, Fantini L, et al. Quality of life and clinical indicators for chronic pancreatitis patients in a 2-year follow-up study. Pancreas 2007; 34: 191–196.

18 Pezzilli R, Morselli-Labate, AM, Fantini, L, et al. Assessment of the quality of life in chronic pancreatitis using Sf-12 and EORTC Qlq-C30 questionnaires. Digestive and Liver Disease 2007; 39: 1077–1086.

19 Mullady DK, Yadav D, Amann ST, et al. Type of pain, pain-associated complications, quality of life, disability and resource utilisation in chronic pancreatitis: a prospective cohort study. Gut 2011; 60: 77–84.

20 Mitchell RM, Byrne MF, Baillie J. Pancreatitis. Lancet 2003; 361: 1447–1455.

21 Buchler MW, Friess H, Bittner R, et al. Duodenum-preserving pancreatic head resection: long-term results. Journal of Gastrointestinal Surgery 1997; 1: 13–19.

22 Morrison CP, Wemyss-Holden SA, Partensky C, et al. Surgical management of intractable pain in chronic pancreatitis: past and present. Journal of Hepato-Biliary-Pancreatic Surgery 2002; 9: 675–682.

23 Frey CF, Suzuki M, Isaji S, et al. Pancreatic resection for chronic pancreatitis. The Surgical Clinics of North America 1989; 69: 499–528.

24 Garcea G, Weaver J, Phillips J, et al. Total pancreatectomy with and without islet cell transplantation for chronic pancreatitis: a series of 85 consecutive patients. Pancreas 2008; 38: 1–7.

25 Rockey EW. Total pancreatectomy for carcinoma : case report. Annals of Surgery 1943; 118: 603–611.

26 Cooper MJ, Williamson RC, Benjamin IS, et al. Total pancreatectomy for chronic pancreatitis. The British journal of Surgery 1987; 74: 912–915.

27 Parsaik AK, Murad MH, Sathananthan A, et al. Metabolic and target organ outcomes after total pancreatectomy: Mayo Clinic experience and meta-analysis of the literature. Clinical Endocrinology 2010; 73: 723–731.

28 Stauffer JA, Nguyen JH, Heckman MG, et al Patient outcomes after total pancreatectomy: a single centre contemporary experience. Hepato Pancreato Biliary 2009; 11: 483–492.

29 Sutton JM, Schmulewitz N, Sussman JJ, et al. Total pancreatectomy and islet cell autotransplantation as a means of treating patients with genetically linked pancreatitis. Surgery 2010; 148: 676–685.

30 Rodriguez Rilo HL, Ahmad SA, D'Alessio D, et al. Total pancreatectomy and autologous islet cell transplantation as a means to treat severe chronic pancreatitis. Journal of Gastrointestinal Surgery 2003; 7: 978–989.

31 Dong M, Parsaik AK, Erwin PJ, et al. Systematic review and meta-analysis: islet autotransplantation after pancreatectomy for minimizing diabetes. Clinical Endocrinology 2011; 75: 771–779.

32 Bellin MD, Freeman ML, Schwarzenberg SJ, et al. Quality of life improves for pediatric patients After total pancreatectomy and islet autotransplant for chronic pancreatitis. Clinical Gastroenterology and Hepatology 2011; 9: 793–799.

33 Aguilar-Saavedra JR, Lentz G, Scheman J, et al. Assessment of quality of life following total pancreatectomy and islet cells autotransplantation for chronic pancreatitis. Gastroenterology 2011;140(5;supplement 1): S-1010.

34 Hogle HH, Recemtsma K. Pancreatic autotransplantation following resection. Surgery 1978; 83: 359–360.

35 Rossi RL, Soeldner JS, Braasch JW, et al. Segmental pancreatic autotransplantation with pancreatic ductal occlusion after near total or total pancreatic resection for chronic pancreatitis. Results at 5- to 54-month follow-up evaluation. Annals of Surgery 1986; 203: 626–636.

36 Tamura K, Yano S, Kin S, et al. Heterotopic autotransplantation of a pancreas segment with enteric drainage after total or subtotal pancreatectomy for chronic pancreatitis. International Journal of Pancreatology 1993: 13: 119–127.

37 Gruessner RW, Sutherland DE, Dunn DL, et al Transplant options for patients undergoing total pancreatectomy for chronic pancreatitis. Journal of the American College of Surgeons 2004; 198: 559–567.

38 UK Transplant 2011/2010, September 2010-last update [2011, 8/1].

39 Ong L, Pollard C, Rees Y, et al. Ultrasound changes within the liver after total pancreatectomy and intrahepatic islet cell autotransplantation. Transplantation 2008; 85: 1773–1777.

40 Markmann JF, Rosen M, Siegelman ES, et al. Magnetic resonance-defined periportal steatosis following intraportal islet transplantation: a functional footprint of islet graft survival? Diabetes 2003; 52: 1591–1594.

41 Takita M, Naziruddin B, Matsumoto S, et al. Implication of pancreatic image findings in total pancreatectomy with islet autotransplantation for chronic pancreatitis. Pancreas 2011; 40:103–108.

42 Bellin MD, Sutherland DE. Pediatric islet autotransplantation: indication, technique, and outcome. Current Diabetes Reports 2010; 10: 326–331.

43 Chinnakotla S, Radosevich DM, Dunn TB, et al. Long-term outcomes of total pancreatectomy and islet auto transplantation for hereditary/genetic pancreatitis. Journal of the American College of Surgeons 2014; 218: 530–543.

44 Chinnakotla S, Bellin MD, Schwarzenberg SJ, et al. Total pancreatectomy and islet autotransplantation in children for chronic pancreatitis: indication, surgical techniques, postoperative management, and long-term outcomes. Annals of Surgery 2014; 260: 56–64.

45 Kobayashi T, Manivel JC, Bellin MD, et al. Correlation of pancreatic histopathologic findings and islet yield in children with chronic pancreatitis undergoing total pancreatectomy and islet autotransplantation. Pancreas 2010; 39: 57–63.

46 Garcea G, Pollard CA, Illouz S, et al Patient satisfaction and cost-effectiveness following total pancreatectomy with islet cell transplantation for chronic pancreatitis. Pancreas 2013;42: 322–328.

47 Webb MA, Illouz C, Pollard CA, et al. Islet auto transplantation following total pancreatectomy: a long-term assessment of graft function. Pancreas 2008; 37: 282–287.

Index

Pancreatitis: Medical and Surgical Management, First Edition.
David B. Adams, Peter B. Cotton, Nicholas J. Zyromski and John Windsor.
© 2017 John Wiley & Sons, Ltd. Published 2017 by John Wiley & Sons, Ltd.